Textbook of
Pharmacoepidemiology

Textbook of Pharmacoepidemiology

EDITED BY

Brian L. Strom, MD, MPH

Executive Vice Dean for Institutional Affairs
George S. Pepper Professor of Public Health and Preventive Medicine, Professor of Biostatistics and
Epidemiology, of Medicine, and of Pharmacology
Center for Clinical Epidemiology and Biostatistics
Center for Pharmacoepidemiology Research and Training
Perelman School of Medicine at the University of Pennsylvania
Philadelphia, PA
USA

Stephen E. Kimmel, MD, MSCE

Professor of Medicine and of Epidemiology
Center for Clinical Epidemiology and Biostatistics
Center for Pharmacoepidemiology Research and Training
Perelman School of Medicine at the University of Pennsylvania
Philadelphia, PA
USA

Sean Hennessy, PharmD, PhD

Associate Professor of Epidemiology and of Pharmacology
Center for Clinical Epidemiology and Biostatistics
Center for Pharmacoepidemiology Research and Training
Perelman School of Medicine at the University of Pennsylvania
Philadelphia, PA
USA

SECOND EDITION

WILEY Blackwell

This edition first published 2013 © 2013 by John Wiley & Sons Ltd

First Edition published 2006 by John Wiley & Sons Ltd.

Wiley-Blackwell is an imprint of John Wiley & Sons, formed by the merger of Wiley's global Scientific, Technical and Medical business with Blackwell Publishing.

Registered office: John Wiley & Sons, Ltd, The Atrium, Southern Gate, Chichester, West Sussex, PO19 8SQ, UK

Editorial offices: 9600 Garsington Road, Oxford, OX4 2DQ, UK

The Atrium, Southern Gate, Chichester, West Sussex, PO19 8SQ, UK

111 River Street, Hoboken, NJ 07030-5774, USA

For details of our global editorial offices, for customer services and for information about how to apply for permission to reuse the copyright material in this book please see our website at www.wiley.com/wiley-blackwell

Library of Congress Cataloging-in-Publication Data

Textbook of pharmacoepidemiology / edited by Brian L. Strom, Stephen E. Kimmel, Sean Hennessy. – 2nd ed.
    p. ; cm.
  Abridged version of: Pharmacoepidemiology. 5th ed. 2012.
  Includes bibliographical references and index.
  ISBN 978-1-118-34486-6 (pbk. : alk. paper)
  I. Strom, Brian L. II. Kimmel, Stephen E. III. Hennessy, Sean. IV. Pharmacoepidemiology.
  [DNLM: 1. Pharmacoepidemiology–methods. QZ 42]
  RM302.5
  615.7'042–dc23
                                                                                        2013002833

A catalogue record for this book is available from the British Library.

Wiley also publishes its books in a variety of electronic formats. Some content that appears in print may not be available in electronic books.

Cover image: iStock © FotografiaBasica, Karina Tischlinger
Cover design by Rob Sawkins for Opta Design

Set in 9/12pt Meridien by Thomson Digital, Noida, India.
Printed and bound in Malaysia by Vivar Printing Sdn Bhd

1   2013

Contents

Contributors

Trisha Acri
Formerly, Assistant Professor
of Family and Community Medicine
Temple University School
of Medicine
Philadelphia, PA
Currently, Director of Community
Research Health Services
AIDS Care Group
Sharon Hill, PA
USA

Susan E. Andrade
Senior Research Associate and
Research Associate Professor
Meyers Primary Care Institute
and
University of Massachusetts Medical
School
Worcester, MA
USA

Peter Arlett
Head
Pharmacovigilance and Risk
Management
European Medicines Agency
London, UK

Jerry Avorn
Professor of Medicine
Harvard Medical School
and
Chief
Division of
Pharmacoepidemiology and
Pharmacoeconomics
Brigham and Women's
Hospital
Boston, MA
USA

Jeffrey S. Barrett
Director
Laboratory for Applied
Pharmacokinetics and
Pharmacodynamics
Director
Pediatric Pharmacology Research Unit
The Children's Hospital of
Philadelphia
Research Professor of Pediatrics
Kinetic Modeling and Simulation
(KMAS) Core Director
Perelman School of Medicine at the
University of Pennsylvania
Colket Translational Research
Philadelphia, PA
USA

David W. Bates
Division of General Internal Medicine
and Primary Care
Brigham and Women's Hospital
and
Harvard Medical School
Boston, Massachusetts
USA

Jesse A. Berlin
Vice President
Epidemiology
Janssen Research & Development, LLC
Johnson & Johnson
Titusville, NJ
USA

Stella Blackburn
EMA Risk Management Development
and Scientific Lead
European Medicines Agency
London, UK

Denise M. Boudreau
Scientific Investigator
Group Health Research Institute
Seattle, WA
USA

M. Soledad Cepeda
Director
Epidemiology
Janssen Research & Development, LLC
Johnson & Johnson
Titusville, NJ
USA

Robert T. Chen
Medical Officer
Clinical Trials Team
Epidemiology Branch
Division of HIV/AIDS Prevention
Centers for Disease Control and
Prevention
Atlanta, GA
USA

Francesca Cunningham
Director
Center for Medication Safety
and
Program Manager
Outcomes Research PBM Services
Department of Veterans Affairs
Center for Medication Safety
Hines, IL
USA

Gerald J. Dal Pan
Director
Office of Surveillance and
Epidemiology
Center for Drug Evaluation and
Research
US Food and Drug Administration
Silver Spring, MD
USA

Hassy Dattani
Research Director (retired)
Cegedim Strategic Data Medical
Research Ltd
London, UK

Robert L. Davis
Director of Research
Center for Health Research
Southeast Kaiser Permanente
Atlanta, GA
USA

Antoine C. El Khoury
Director
Market Access and Health Economics
Johnson & Johnson Pharmaceutical
Horsham, PA
USA

Joel M. Gelfand
Associate Professor of Dermatology and
Epidemiology
Center for Clinical
Epidemiology and Biostatistics
Center for Pharmacoepidemiology
Research and Training
Perelman School of Medicine at the
University of Pennsylvania
Philadelphia, PA
USA

Kate Gelperin
Medical Officer
Division of Epidemiology
Office of Surveillance and
Epidemiology
Center for Drug Evaluation and
Research
US Food and Drug Administration
Silver Spring, MD
USA

Jason Glanz
Epidemiologist
Institute for Health Research
Kaiser Permanente Colorado
Department of Epidemiology Colorado
School of Public Health
Denver, CO
USA

Henry A. Glick
Professor of Medicine
Perelman School of Medicine at the
University of Pennsylvania
Philadelphia, PA
USA

Robert Gross
Associate Professor of Medicine and
Epidemiology
Center for Clinical Epidemiology and
Biostatistics
Center for Pharmacoepidemiology
Research and Training
Perelman School of Medicine at the
University of Pennsylvania
Philadelphia, PA
USA

Gordon H. Guyatt
Professor
Department of Clinical Epidemiology
and Biostatistics
McMaster University
Health Sciences Center
and
Department of Medicine
St Joseph's Hospital
Hamilton, Ontario
Canada

Katherine Haffenreffer
Project Administrator
Harvard Pilgrim Health Care Institute
and
Department of Population Medicine
Harvard Medical School
Boston, MA
USA

Sean Hennessy
Associate Professor of Epidemiology
and of Pharmacology
Center for Clinical Epidemiology and
Biostatistics
Director,
Center for Pharmacoepidemiology
Research and Training
Perelman School of Medicine at the
University of Pennsylvania
Philadelphia, PA
USA

Ron M.C. Herings
Director
PHARMO Institute
Utrecht, The Netherlands
and
Associate Professor of
Pharmaceutical Technology Assessment
Erasmus University Rotterdam
Rotterdam, The Netherlands

Roman Jaeschke
Professor of Clinical Epidemiology
and Biostatistics
McMaster University
Health Sciences Center
and
Professor of Medicine
St Joseph's Hospital
Hamilton, Ontario
Canada

Bradley C. Johnston
Assistant Professor of Clinical
Epidemiology and Biostatistics
McMaster University
Hamilton, Ontario
and
Assistant Professor
Institute of Health Policy
Management and Evaluation
and Department of Anesthesia & Pain
Medicine, University of Toronto
and
Scientist
The Hospital for Sick Children Research
Institute
Toronto , Ontario
Canada

Judith K. Jones
President and CEO
The Degge Group Ltd
Arlington, VA
and
Adjunct Professor
Georgetown University
Washington, DC
USA

Jason Karlawish
Professor of Medicine
Perelman School of Medicine at the
University of Pennsylvania
Philadelphia, PA
USA

David W. Kaufman
Associate Director
Slone Epidemiology Center at Boston
University
and
Professor of Epidemiology
Boston University School of
Public Health
Boston, MA
USA

Aaron S. Kesselheim
Assistant Professor of Medicine
Division of Pharmacoepidemiology
and Pharmacoeconomics
Brigham and Women's Hospital
Harvard Medical School
Boston, MA
USA

Stephen E. Kimmel
Professor of Medicine and
Epidemiology
Center for Clinical
Epidemiology and Biostatistics
Center for Pharmacoepidemiology
Research and Training
Perelman School of Medicine at the
University of Pennsylvania
Philadelphia, PA
USA

Karel Kostev
Senior Research Analyst
Centre of Excellence Patient Data
IMS Health GmbH & Co OHG
Frankfurt/Main, Germany

Sinéad M. Langan
NIHR Clinician Scientist
London School of Hygiene and
Tropical Medicine
and
Honorary Consultant Dermatologist
St John's Institute of Dermatology
London, UK

David Lee
Director
Technical Strategy and Quality
Center for Pharmaceutical
Management
Management Sciences for Health, Inc.
Arlington, VA
USA

Samuel M. Lesko
Medical Director
Northeast Regional Cancer Institute
Scranton, PA
and
Adjunct Professor of Basic Sciences
The Commonwealth Medical College
Scranton, PA
and
Adjunct Professor of Public Health
Sciences
Pennsylvania State University College
of Medicine
Hershey, PA
USA

Hubert G. Leufkens
Professor of Pharmacoepidemiology
and Clinical Pharmacotherapy
Utrecht Institute for Pharmaceutical
Sciences
Utrecht University
Utrecht, The Netherlands

Marie Lindquist
Director
Uppsala Monitoring Centre
WHO Collaborating Centre for
International Drug Monitoring
Uppsala, Sweden

Helene Levens Lipton
Professor of Pharmacy and Health
Policy
Schools of Medicine and Pharmacy
University of California at San
Francisco
San Francisco, CA
USA

Sumit R. Majumdar
Professor of Medicine
Faculty of Medicine and Dentistry
University of Alberta
Edmonton, Alberta
Canada

Claudia Manzo
Director
Division of Risk Management
Office of Surveillance and
Epidemiology
Center for Drug Evaluation and
Research
US Food and Drug Administration
Silver Spring, MD
USA

Danica Marinac-Dabic
Director
Division of Epidemiology
Office of Surveillance and Biometrics
Center for Devices and Radiological
Health
US Food and Drug Administration
Silver Spring, MD
USA

Allen A. Mitchell
Director
Slone Epidemiology Center at Boston
University
and
Professor of Epidemiology and
Pediatrics
Boston University Schools of Public
Health and Medicine
Boston, MA
USA

Jingping Mo
Senior Director
Epidemiology
Worldwide Research & Development
Pfizer Inc.
New York, NY
USA

Yola Moride
Full Professor
Faculty of Pharmacy
Université de Montréal
and
Researcher
CHUM Research Center (CRCHUM)
Montreal, Quebec
Canada

Sharon-Lise T. Normand
Professor of Health Care Policy
(Biostatistics)
Harvard Medical School
and
Professor of Biostatistics
Harvard School of Public Health
Boston, MA
USA

Alexis Ogdie
Instructor in Medicine
Division of Rheumatology
Center for Clinical Epidemiology and
Biostatistics
Center for Pharmacoepidemiology
Research and Training
Perelman School of Medicine at the
University of Pennsylvania
Philadelphia, PA
USA

Cristin Palumbo Freeman
Research Project Manager
Center for Clinical Epidemiology and
Biostatistics
Center for Pharmacoepidemiology
Research and Training
Perelman School of Medicine at the
University of Pennsylvania
Philadelphia, PA
USA

John Parkinson
Director
Clinical Practice Research Datalink
(CPRD)
Medicines and Healthcare Products
Regulatory Agency (MHRA)
London, UK

Pamala A. Pawloski
HealthPartners Institute for Education
and Research
Bloomington, MN
and
Adjunct Assistant Professor
University of Minnesota
College of Pharmacy
Minneapolis, MN
USA

Lars Pedersen
Professor of Clinical
Epidemiology
Department of Clinical Epidemiology
Aarhus University Hospital
Aarhus, Denmark

Richard Platt
Professor and Chair
Department of Population Medicine,
Harvard Medical School
and
Executive Director
Harvard Pilgrim Health Care Institute
Boston, MA
USA

Daniel Polsky
Executive Director, Leonard Davis
Institute for Health Economics
Professor of Medicine
Perelman School of Medicine at the
University of Pennsylvania
Philadelphia, PA
USA

Charles Poole
Associate Professor of Epidemiology
Gillings School of Global Public Health
University of North Carolina
Chapel Hill, NC
USA

Marsha A. Raebel
Investigator
Institute for Health Research
Kaiser Permanente Colorado
and
Clinical Professor
University of Colorado
Skaggs School of Pharmacy and
Pharmaceutical Sciences
Aurora, CO
USA

Timothy R. Rebbeck
Professor of Epidemiology
Center for Clinical
Epidemiology and Biostatistics
Perelman School of Medicine at the
University of Pennsylvania
Philadelphia, PA
USA

Shelby D. Reed
Associate Professor of Medicine
Duke University School of Medicine
Durham, NC
USA

Robert F. Reynolds
Vice President
Epidemiology
Worldwide Research & Development
Pfizer Inc.
New York, NY
USA

Mary Elizabeth Ritchey
Associate Division Director
Food and Drug Administration
Center for Devices and Radiological
Health
Silver Spring, MD
USA

Melissa A. Robb
Associate Director for Regulatory
Affairs
Office of Medical Policy Initiatives
Center for Drug Evaluation and
Research
US Food and Drug Administration
Silver Spring, MD
USA

Rita Schinnar
Senior Research Project Manager and
Analyst
Center for Clinical Epidemiology and
Biostatistics
Center for Pharmacoepidemiology
Research and Training
Perelman School of Medicine at the
University of Pennsylvania
Philadelphia, PA
USA

Sebastian Schneeweiss
Professor of Medicine and
Epidemiology
Harvard Medical School
and
Vice Chief
Division of Pharmacoepidemiology
Department of Medicine
Brigham & Women's Hospital
Boston, MA
USA

Kevin A. Schulman
Professor of Medicine and Gregory
Mario and Jeremy Mario Professor of
Business Administration
Duke University
Durham, NC
USA

Holger J. Schünemann
Professor and Chair
Department of Clinical Epidemiology
and Biostatistics
Health Sciences Center
and
Professor of Medicine
McMaster University
Hamilton, Ontario
Canada

Art Sedrakyan
Associate Professor of Public Health
New York Presbyterian Hospital
and
Weill Cornell Medical College
New York, NY
USA

Hanna M. Seidling
Head of Cooperation Unit Clinical
Pharmacy
Department of Clinical Pharmacology
and Pharmacoepidemiology
Cooperation Unit Clinical Pharmacy
University of Heidelberg
Heidelberg, Germany

Rachel E. Sherman
Associate Director for Medical Policy
Center for Drug Evaluation and
Research
US Food and Drug Administration
Silver Spring, MD
USA

Stephen B. Soumerai
Professor of Population Medicine
Director
Drug Policy Research Group
Harvard Medical School and Harvard
Pilgrim Health Care Institute
Boston, MA
USA

Brian L. Strom
Executive Vice Dean for Institutional
Affairs
George S. Pepper Professor of Public
Health and Preventive Medicine
Professor of Biostatistics and
Epidemiology, of Medicine, and of
Pharmacology
Center for Clinical
Epidemiology and Biostatistics
Center for Pharmacoepidemiology
Research and Training
Perelman School of Medicine at the
University of Pennsylvania
Philadelphia, PA
USA

Samy Suissa
James McGill Professor of
Epidemiology, Biostatistics and
Medicine
McGill University
and
Director
Centre for Clinical Epidemiology
Lady Davis Research Institute
Jewish General Hospital
Montreal, Quebec
Canada

Sengwee Toh
Assistant Professor of Population
Medicine
Harvard Medical School and Harvard
Pilgrim Health Care Institute
Boston, MA
USA

Claudia Vellozzi
Deputy Director
Immunization Safety Office
Division of Healthcare Quality
Promotion
Centers for Disease Control and
Prevention
Atlanta, GA
USA

Suzanne L. West
RTI Fellow and Senior Scientist
RTI International
Research Triangle Park, NC
and
Department of Epidemiology
Gillings School of Global Public
Health
University of North Carolina
Chapel Hill, NC
USA

Athena F. Zuppa
Associate Professor of Pediatrics,
Anesthesia and Critical Care Medicine
Laboratory for Applied
Pharmacokinetics and
Pharmacodynamics
Children's Hospital of Philadelphia
Perelman School of Medicine at the
University of Pennsylvania
Philadelphia, PA
USA

Preface

It was a remarkable 23 years ago that the first edition of Strom's *Pharmacoepidemiology* was published. The preface to that book stated that pharmacoepidemiology was a new field with a new generation of pharmacoepidemiologists arising to join the field's few pioneers. Over the ensuing 23 years, the field indeed has grown and no longer deserves to be called "new." Many of those "new generation" scientists (including two of the editors of this book) are now "middle-aged" pharmacoepidemiologists. Despite its relatively brief academic life, a short history of pharmacoepidemiology and review of its current state will set the stage for the purpose of this textbook.

Pharmacoepidemiology originally arose from the union of the fields of clinical pharmacology and epidemiology. Pharmacoepidemiology studies the use of and the effects of medical products in large numbers of people and applies the methods of epidemiology to the content area of clinical pharmacology. This field represents the science underlying postmarketing medical product surveillance, studies of the effects of medical products (i.e., drugs, biologicals, devices) performed after a product has been approved for use. In recent years, pharmacoepidemiology has expanded to include many other types of studies, as well.

The field of pharmacoepidemiology has grown enormously since the first publication of Strom. The International Society of Pharmacoepidemiology, an early idea when the first edition of this book was written, has grown into a major international scientific force, with over 1460 members from 54 countries, an extremely successful annual meeting attracting more than 1200 attendees, a large number of very active committees and scientific interest groups, and its own journal. In addition, a number of established journals have targeted pharmacoepidemiology manuscripts as desirable. As new scientific developments occur within mainstream epidemiology, they are rapidly adopted, applied, and advanced within our field as well. We have also become institutionalized as a subfield within the field of clinical pharmacology, with the Drug Safety Scientific Section of the American Society for Clinical Pharmacology and Therapeutics, and with pharmacoepidemiology a required part of the clinical pharmacology board examination.

Most of the major international pharmaceutical companies have founded dedicated units to organize and lead their efforts in pharmacoepidemiology, pharmacoeconomics, and quality-of-life studies. The continuing parade of drug safety crises emphasizes the need for the field, and some foresighted manufacturers have begun to perform "prophylactic" pharmacoepidemiology studies, to have data in hand and available when questions arise, rather than waiting to begin to collect data after a crisis has developed. Pharmacoepidemiologic data are now routinely used for regulatory decisions, and many governmental agencies have been developing and expanding their own pharmacoepidemiology programs. Risk evaluation and mitigation strategies are now required by regulatory bodies with the marketing of new drugs, as a means of improving drugs' benefit/risk balance, and manufacturers are identifying ways to respond. Requirements that a drug be proven to be cost-effective have been added to many national, local, and insurance health care systems, either to justify reimbursement or even to justify drug availability. A number of schools of medicine, pharmacy, and public health have established research programs in pharmacoepidemiology, and a few of them have also established pharmacoepidemiology training programs in response to a desperate need for more pharmacoepidemiology personnel. Pharmacoepidemiologic research funding is now more plentiful, and even limited support for training is available.

In the United States, drug utilization review programs are required, by law, of each of the 50 state

Medicaid programs, and have been implemented as well in many managed care organizations. Now, years later, the utility of drug utilization review programs is being questioned. In addition, the Joint Commission on Accreditation of Health Care Organizations now requires that every hospital in the country have an adverse drug reaction monitoring program and a drug use evaluation program, turning every hospital into a mini-pharmacoepidemiology laboratory. Stimulated in part by the interests of the World Health Organization and the Rockefeller Foundation, there is even substantial interest in pharmacoepidemiology in the developing world. Yet, throughout the world, the increased concern by the public about privacy has made pharmacoepidemiologic research much more difficult to conduct.

In recent years, major new changes have been made in drug regulation and organization, largely in response to a series of accusations about myocardial infarction caused by analgesics, which was detected in long-term prevention trials rather than in normal use of the drugs. For example, FDA has been given new regulatory authority after drug marketing, and has also begun developing the Sentinel Initiative, a program to conduct medical product safety surveillance in a population to exceed 100 million. Further, the development, since January 1, 2006, of Medicare Part D, a US federal program to subsidize prescription drugs for Medicare recipients, introduces to pharmacoepidemiology a new database with a stable population of about 25 million in what may be the largest healthcare system in the world. A new movement has arisen in the US of "comparative effectiveness research," which in many ways learns from much longer experience in Europe, as well as decades of experience in pharmacoepidemiology. These developments portend major changes for our field.

In summary, there has been tremendous growth in the field of pharmacoepidemiology and a fair amount of maturation. With the growth and maturation of the field, Strom's *Pharmacoepidemiology* has grown and matured right along. *Pharmacoepidemiology* thus represents a comprehensive source of information about the field. As a reflection of the growth of the field, the 4th Edition of Strom

was over twice as long as the first! We worked hard to avoid such growth in the 5th Edition, by aggressive pruning to go along with our additions.

So, why, one may ask, do we need a *Textbook of Pharmacoepidemiology*? The need arose precisely because of the growth of the field. With that, and the corresponding growth in the parent book, Strom's *Pharmacoepidemiology* has really become more of a reference book than a book usable as a textbook. Yet, there is increasing need for people to be trained in the field, and an increasing number of training programs. With the maturity of the field comes therefore the necessity for both comprehensive approaches (such as Strom's *Pharmacoepidemiology*) and more focused approaches. Therefore, *Textbook of Pharmacoepidemiology* was intended as a modified and shortened version of its parent, designed to meet the need of students. We believe that students can benefit from an approach that focuses on the core of the discipline, along with learning aids.

Textbook of Pharmacoepidemiology attempts to fill this need, providing a focused educational resource for students. It is our hope that this book will serve as a useful textbook for students at all levels: upper-level undergraduates, graduate students, post-doctoral fellows, and others who are learning the field. In order to achieve our goals, we have substantially shortened Strom's *Pharmacoepidemiology*, with a focus on what is needed by students, eliminating some chapters and shortening others. We also have provided case examples for most chapters and key points for all chapters. Each chapter is followed by a list of further reading.

So why update it? In looking at the 5th Edition of Strom, most chapters in the new edition were thoroughly revised. Ten new chapters were added, along with many new authors. The first edition of the textbook was simply getting out of date.

Specifically, we have tried to emphasize the methods of pharmacoepidemiology and the strengths and limitations of the field, while minimizing some of the technical specifications that are important for a reference book but not for students. Therefore, the first five chapters of Part I, "Introduction to Pharmacoepidemiology," lay out the cores of the discipline, and remain essentially unchanged from Strom's *Pharmacoepidemiology*, with the exception of the inclusion of key points and lists of further reading. We have also included a chapter on different perspectives of the field (from academia, industry, regulatory agencies, and the legal system), as a shortened form of several chapters from the reference book. Part II focuses on "Sources of Pharmacoepidemiology Data" and includes important chapters about spontaneous pharmacovigilance reporting systems, and other approaches to pharmacoepidemiology studies. A substantially shortened chapter on Examples of Automated Databases is included, focused on the strengths and limitations of these data sources rather than providing extensive details about the content of each database. Part III summarizes "Special Issues in Pharmacoepidemiology Methodology" that we feel are important to more advanced pharmacoepidemiology students. Although no student is likely to become an expert in all of these methods, they form a core set of knowledge that we believe all pharmacoepidemiologists should have. In addition, one never knows what one will do later in one's own career, nor when one may be called upon to help others with the use of these methods. Part IV concludes the textbook with a collection of "Special Applications" of the field, and speculation about its future, always an important consideration for new investigators in charting a career path.

Pharmacoepidemiology may be maturing, but many exciting opportunities and challenges lie ahead as the field continues to grow and respond to unforeseeable future events. It is our hope that this book can serve as a useful introduction and resource for students of pharmacoepidemiology, both those enrolled in formal classes and those learning in "the real world," who will respond to the challenges that they encounter. Of course, we are always students of our own discipline, and the process of developing this textbook has been educational for us. We hope that this book will also be stimulating and educational for you.

Brian L. Strom, M.D., M.P.H.
Stephen E. Kimmel, M.D., M.S.C.E.
Sean Hennessy, Pharm.D., Ph.D.

Acknowledgements

There are many individuals and institutions to whom we owe thanks for their contributions to our efforts in preparing this book. Over the years, our pharmacoepidemiology work has been supported mostly by numerous grants from government, foundations, and industry. While none of this support was specifically intended to support the development of this book, without this assistance, we would not have been able to support our careers in pharmacoepidemiology. We would like to thank our publisher, John Wiley & Sons, Ltd., for their assistance and insights, both in support of this book, and in support of the field's journal, *Pharmacoepidemiology and Drug Safety*.

Rita Schinnar's contributions to this book were instrumental in helping to shorten several of the chapters that were merged together from *Pharmacoepidemiology, 5th edition*, and providing excellent editorial assistance with all the other chapters, as well as contributing a chapter. She also coordinated the entire process of contacting the authors and pulling the book together. Finally, we would like to thank all of the authors for the work that they did in helping to revise their book chapters for this textbook and provide case examples, key points, and suggested readings.

BLS would like to thank Steve Kimmel and Sean Hennessy for joining him as co-editors in this edition. Steve did the bulk of the work on the first edition of this textbook, and Steve and Sean joined BLS as co-editors for the 5th edition of *Pharmacoepidemiology*. These are two very special and talented men. It has been BLS's pleasure to help to train them, now too many years ago, help them cultivate their own careers, and see them blossom into star senior pharmacoepidemiologists in their own right, now extremely effective and successful. It is wonderful to be able to share with them this book, which has been an important part of BLS's life and career.

BLS would also like to thank his parents for the support and education that were critical to his being able to be successful in his career. BLS would also like to thank Paul D. Stolley, M.D., M.P.H. and the late Kenneth L. Melmon, M.D., for their direction, guidance, and inspiration in the formative years of his career. He would also like to thank his trainees, from whom he learns at least as much as he teaches. Last, but certainly not least, BLS would like to thank his family—Lani, Shayna, and Jordi—for accepting the time demands of the book, for tolerating his endless hours working at home (on its earlier editions, for the kids), and for their ever present love and support.

SEK expresses his sincere gratitude to BLS for his 20 years as a mentor and colleague and for the chance to work on this book, to his parents for providing the foundation for all of his work, and to his family—Alison, David, Benjamin, and Jonathan—for all their support and patience.

SH also thanks BLS, his longtime friend and career mentor, and all of his students, mentees, and collaborators. Finally, he thanks his parents, Michael and Catherine; and his family—Kristin, Landis, and Bridget—for their love and support.

PART I
Introduction to Pharmacoepidemiology

CHAPTER 1
What is Pharmacoepidemiology?

Brian L. Strom

Perelman School of Medicine at the University of Pennsylvania, Philadelphia, PA, USA

"A desire to take medicine is, perhaps, the great feature which distinguishes man from other animals."

Sir William Osler, 1891

Introduction

In recent decades, modern medicine has been blessed with a pharmaceutical armamentarium that is much more powerful than what it had before. Although this has given health care providers the ability to provide better medical care for their patients, it has also resulted in the ability to do much greater harm. It has also generated an enormous number of product liability suits against pharmaceutical manufacturers, some appropriate and others inappropriate. In fact, the history of drug regulation parallels the history of major adverse drug reaction "disasters." Each change in pharmaceutical law was a political reaction to an epidemic of adverse drug reactions. A 1998 study estimated that 100 000 Americans die each year from adverse drug reactions (ADRs), and 1.5 million US hospitalizations each year result from ADRs; yet, 20–70% of ADRs may be preventable. The harm that drugs can cause has also led to the development of the field of pharmacoepidemiology, which is the focus of this book. More recently, the field has expanded its focus to include many issues other than adverse reactions, as well.

To clarify what is, and what is not, included within the discipline of pharmacoepidemiology, this chapter will begin by defining pharmacoepidemiology, differentiating it from other related fields. The history of drug regulation will then be briefly and selectively reviewed, focusing on the US experience as an example, demonstrating how it has led to the development of this new field. Next, the current regulatory process for the approval of new drugs will be reviewed, in order to place the use of pharmacoepidemiology and postmarketing drug surveillance into proper perspective. Finally, the potential scientific and clinical contributions of pharmacoepidemiology will be discussed.

Definition of pharmacoepidemiology

Pharmacoepidemiology is the study of the use, and effects, of drugs and other medical devices in large numbers of people. The term pharmacoepidemiology obviously contains two components: "pharmaco" and "epidemiology." In order to better appreciate and understand what is and what is not included in this new field, it is useful to compare its scope to that of other related fields. The scope of pharmacoepidemiology will first be compared to that of clinical pharmacology, and then to that of epidemiology.

Pharmacoepidemiology versus clinical pharmacology

Pharmacology is the study of the effects of drugs. *Clinical pharmacology* is the study of the effects of drugs in humans (see also Chapter 4). Pharmacoepidemiology

---

Textbook of Pharmacoepidemiology, Second Edition. Edited by Brian L. Strom, Stephen E. Kimmel, and Sean Hennessy.
© 2013 John Wiley & Sons, Ltd. Published 2013 by John Wiley & Sons, Ltd.

obviously can be considered, therefore, to fall within clinical pharmacology. In attempting to optimize the use of drugs, one central principle of clinical pharmacology is that therapy should be individualized, or tailored, to the needs of the specific patient at hand. This individualization of therapy requires the determination of a risk/benefit ratio specific to the patient at hand. Doing so requires a prescriber to be aware of the potential beneficial and harmful effects of the drug in question and to know how elements of the patient's clinical status might modify the probability of a good therapeutic outcome. For example, consider a patient with a serious infection, serious liver impairment, and mild impairment of his or her renal function. In considering whether to use gentamicin to treat his infection, it is not sufficient to know that gentamicin has a small probability of causing renal disease. A good clinician should realize that a patient who has impaired liver function is at a greater risk of suffering from this adverse effect than one with normal liver function. Pharmacoepidemiology can be useful in providing information about the beneficial and harmful effects of any drug, thus permitting a better assessment of the risk/benefit balance for the use of any particular drug in any particular patient.

Clinical pharmacology is traditionally divided into two basic areas: pharmacokinetics and pharmacodynamics. *Pharmacokinetics* is the study of the relationship between the dose administered of a drug and the serum or blood level achieved. It deals with drug absorption, distribution, metabolism, and excretion. *Pharmacodynamics* is the study of the relationship between drug level and drug effect. Together, these two fields allow one to predict the effect one might observe in a patient from administering a certain drug regimen. Pharmacoepidemiology encompasses elements of both of these fields, exploring the effects achieved by administering a drug regimen. It does not normally involve or require the measurement of drug levels. However, pharmacoepidemiology can be used to shed light on the pharmacokinetics of a drug when used in clinical practice, such as exploring whether aminophylline is more likely to cause nausea when administered to a patient simultaneously taking cimetidine. However, to date this is a relatively novel application of the field.

Specifically, the field of pharmacoepidemiology has primarily concerned itself with the study of adverse drug effects. Adverse reactions have traditionally been separated into those which are the result of an exaggerated but otherwise usual pharmacologic effect of the drug, sometimes called *Type A reactions*, versus those which are aberrant effects, so called *Type B reactions*. Type A reactions tend to be common, dose-related, predictable, and less serious. They can usually be treated by simply reducing the dose of the drug. They tend to occur in individuals who have one of three characteristics. First, the individuals may have received more of a drug than is customarily required. Second, they may have received a conventional amount of the drug, but they may metabolize or excrete the drug unusually slowly, leading to drug levels that are too high (see also Chapter 4). Third, they may have normal drug levels, but for some reason are overly sensitive to them (see Chapter 14).

In contrast, Type B reactions tend to be uncommon, not related to dose, unpredictable, and potentially more serious. They usually require cessation of the drug. They may be due to what are known as hypersensitivity reactions or immunologic reactions. Alternatively, Type B reactions may be some other idiosyncratic reaction to the drug, either due to some inherited susceptibility (e.g., glucose-6-phosphate dehydrogenase deficiency; see Chapter 14) or due to some other mechanism. Regardless, Type B reactions are the most difficult to predict or even detect, and represent the major focus of many pharmacoepidemiologic studies of adverse drug reactions.

One typical approach to studying adverse drug reactions has been the collection of spontaneous reports of drug-related morbidity or mortality (see Chapter 7), sometimes called pharmacovigilance (although other times that term is used to refer to all of pharmacoepidemiology). However, determining causation in case reports of adverse reactions can be problematic (see Chapter 13), as can attempts to compare the effects of drugs in the same class. This has led academic investigators, industry, FDA, and the legal community to turn to the field of epidemiology. Specifically, *studies of adverse effects* have been supplemented with *studies of adverse events*. In the former, investigators examine case reports of purported adverse drug reactions and attempt to make a subjective clinical judgment on an *individual* basis about whether the adverse outcome was actually caused by the antecedent drug exposure. In the latter, controlled studies are performed examining whether the adverse outcome under study occurs more often in an exposed *population* than in an unexposed population. This marriage of the fields of clinical pharmacology and epidemiology has resulted in the development of a new field: pharmacoepidemiology.

Pharmacoepidemiology versus epidemiology

Epidemiology is the study of the distribution and determinants of diseases in populations. Since pharmacoepidemiology is the study of the use of and effects of drugs and other medical devices in large numbers of people, it obviously falls within epidemiology, as well. Epidemiology is also traditionally subdivided into two basic areas. The field began as the study of infectious diseases in large populations, i.e., epidemics. It has since been expanded to encompass the study of chronic diseases. The field of pharmacoepidemiology uses the techniques of chronic disease epidemiology to study the use of and the effects of drugs. Although application of the methods of pharmacoepidemiology can be useful in performing the clinical trials of drugs that are conducted before marketing, the major application of these methods is after drug marketing. This has primarily been in the context of postmarketing drug surveillance, although in recent years the interests of pharmacoepidemiologists have broadened considerably. Now, as will be made clearer in subsequent chapters, pharmacoepidemiology is considered of importance in the whole life cycle of a drug, from the time when it is first discovered or synthesized through when it is no longer sold as a drug.

Thus, pharmacoepidemiology is a relatively new applied field, bridging between clinical pharmacology and epidemiology. From clinical pharmacology, pharmacoepidemiology borrows its focus of inquiry. From epidemiology, pharmacoepidemiology borrows its methods of inquiry. In other words,

it applies the methods of epidemiology to the content area of clinical pharmacology. In the process, multiple special logistical approaches have been developed and multiple special methodological issues have arisen. These are the primary foci of this book.

Historical background

Early legislation

The history of drug regulation in the US is similar to that in most developed countries, and reflects the growing involvement of governments in attempting to assure that only safe and effective drug products were available and that appropriate manufacturing and marketing practices were used. The initial US law, the Pure Food and Drug Act, was passed in 1906, in response to excessive adulteration and misbranding of the food and drugs available at that time. There were no restrictions on sales or requirements for proof of the efficacy or safety of marketed drugs. Rather, the law simply gave the federal government the power to remove from the market any product that was adulterated or misbranded. The burden of proof was on the federal government.

In 1937, over 100 people died from renal failure as a result of the marketing by the Massengill Company of elixir of sulfanilimide dissolved in diethylene glycol. In response, Congress passed the 1938 Food, Drug, and Cosmetic Act. Preclinical toxicity testing was required for the first time. In addition, manufacturers were required to gather clinical data about drug safety and to submit these data to FDA before drug marketing. The FDA had 60 days to object to marketing or else it would proceed. No proof of efficacy was required.

Little attention was paid to adverse drug reactions until the early 1950s, when it was discovered that chloramphenicol could cause aplastic anemia. In 1952, the first textbook of adverse drug reactions was published. In the same year, the AMA Council on Pharmacy and Chemistry established the first official registry of adverse drug effects, to collect cases of drug-induced blood dyscrasias. In 1960, the FDA began to collect reports of adverse drug reactions and sponsored new hospital-based drug monitoring programs. The Johns Hopkins Hospital and the Boston Collaborative Drug Surveillance Program developed the use of in-hospital monitors to perform cohort studies to explore the short-term effects of drugs used in hospitals. This approach was later transported to the University of Florida-Shands Teaching Hospital, as well.

In the winter of 1961, the world experienced the infamous "thalidomide disaster." Thalidomide was marketed as a mild hypnotic, and had no obvious advantage over other drugs in its class. Shortly after its marketing, a dramatic increase was seen in the frequency of a previously rare birth defect, phocomelia–the absence of limbs or parts of limbs, sometimes with the presence instead of flippers. Epidemiologic studies established its cause to be *in utero* exposure to thalidomide. In the United Kingdom, this resulted in the establishment in 1968 of the Committee on Safety of Medicines. Later, the World Health Organization established a bureau to collect and collate information from this and other similar national drug monitoring organizations (see Chapter 7).

The US had never permitted the marketing of thalidomide and, so, was fortunately spared this epidemic. However, the "thalidomide disaster" was so dramatic that it resulted in regulatory change in the US as well. Specifically, in 1962 the Kefauver-Harris Amendments were passed. These amendments strengthened the requirements for proof of drug safety, requiring extensive preclinical pharmacologic and toxicologic testing before a drug could be tested in man. The data from these studies were required to be submitted to FDA in an Investigational New Drug (IND) Application before clinical studies could begin. Three explicit phases of clinical testing were defined, which are described in more detail below. In addition, a new requirement was added to the clinical testing, for "substantial evidence that the drug will have the effect it purports or is represented to have." "Substantial evidence" was defined as "adequate and well-controlled investigations, including clinical investigations." Functionally, this has generally been interpreted as requiring randomized clinical trials to document drug efficacy before marketing. This new procedure also delayed drug marketing until the FDA explicitly gave approval. With some modifications, these are the requirements still in place in the US today. In addition, the amendments required the review of all drugs approved between 1938 and 1962, to determine if they too were efficacious. The resulting DESI (Drug Efficacy Study Implementation) process, conducted by the National Academy of Sciences' National Research Council with support from a contract from FDA, was not completed until years later, and resulted in the removal from the US market of many ineffective drugs and drug combinations. The result of all these changes was a great prolongation of the approval process, with attendant increases in the cost of drug development, the so-called drug lag. However, the drugs that are marketed are presumably much safer and more effective.

Drug crises and resulting regulatory actions

Despite the more stringent process for drug regulation, subsequent years have seen a series of major adverse drug reactions. Subacute myelo-optic-neuropathy (SMON) was found in Japan to be caused by clioquinol, a drug marketed in the early 1930s but not discovered to cause this severe neurological reaction until 1970. In the 1970s, clear cell adenocarcinoma of the cervix and vagina and other genital malformations were found to be due to *in utero* exposure to diethylstilbestrol two decades earlier. The mid-1970s saw the UK discovery of the oculomucocutaneous syndrome caused by practolol, five years after drug marketing. In 1980, the drug ticrynafen was noted to cause deaths from liver disease. In 1982, benoxaprofen was noted to do the same. Subsequently the use of zomepirac, another nonsteroidal anti-inflammatory drug, was noted to be associated with an increased risk of anaphylactoid reactions. Serious blood dyscrasias were linked to phenylbutazone. Small intestinal perforations were noted to be caused by a particular slow release formulation of indomethacin. Bendectin®, a combination product indicated to treat nausea and vomiting in pregnancy, was removed from the market because of litigation claiming it was a teratogen, despite the absence of valid scientific evidence to justify this claim (see "Studies of drug induced birth defects" in Chapter 22). Acute flank pain and reversible acute renal failure were noted to be caused by suprofen. Isotretinoin was almost removed from the US market because of the birth defects it causes. The Eosinophilia-Myalgia syndrome was linked to a particular brand of L-tryptophan. Triazolam, thought by the Netherlands in 1979 to be subject to a disproportionate number of central nervous system side effects, was discovered by the rest of the world to be problematic in the early 1990s. Silicone breast implants, inserted by the millions in the US for cosmetic purposes, were accused of causing cancer, rheumatologic disease, and many other problems, and restricted from use except for breast reconstruction after mastectomy. Human insulin was marketed as one of the first of the new biotechnology drugs, but soon thereafter was accused of causing a disproportionate amount of hypoglycemia. Fluoxetine was marketed as a major new important and commercially successful psychiatric product, but then lost a large part of its market due to accusations about its association with suicidal ideation. An epidemic of deaths from asthma in New Zealand was traced to fenoterol, and later data suggested that similar, although smaller, risks might be present with other beta-agonist inhalers. The possibility was raised of cancer from depot-medroxyprogesterone, resulting in initial refusal to allow its marketing for this purpose in the US, multiple studies, and ultimate approval. Arrhythmias were linked to the use of the antihistamines terfenadine and astemizole. Hypertension, seizures, and strokes were noted from postpartum use of bromocriptine. Multiple different adverse reactions were linked to temafloxacin. Other examples include liver toxicity from amoxicillin-clavulanic acid; liver toxicity from bromfenac; cancer, myocardial infarction, and gastrointestinal bleeding from calcium channel blockers; arrhythmias with cisapride interactions; primary pulmonary hypertension and cardiac valvular disease from dexfenfluramine and fenfluramine; gastrointestinal bleeding, postoperative bleeding, deaths, and many other adverse reactions associated with ketorolac; multiple drug interactions

with mibefradil; thrombosis from newer oral contraceptives; myocardial infarction from sildenafil; seizures with tramadol; anaphylactic reactions from vitamin K; liver toxicity from troglitazone; and intussusception from rotavirus vaccine.

Later drug crises have occurred due to allegations of ischemic colitis from alosetron; rhabdomyolysis from cerivastatin; bronchospasm from rapacuronium; torsades de pointes from ziprasidone; hemorrhagic stroke from phenylpropanolamine; arthralgia, myalgia, and neurologic conditions from Lyme vaccine; multiple joint and other symptoms from anthrax vaccine; myocarditis and myocardial infarction from smallpox vaccine; and heart attack and stroke from rofecoxib.

Major adverse drug reactions continue to plague new drugs, and in fact are as common if not more common in the last several decades. In total, 36 different oral prescription drug products have been removed from the US market, since 1980 alone (alosetron-2000, aprotinin-2007, astemizole-1999, benoxaprofen-1982, bromfenac-1998, cerivastatin-2001, cisapride-2000, dexfenfluramine-1997, efalizumab-2009, encainide-1991, etretinate-1998, fenfluramine-1998, flosequinan-1993, grepafloxin-1999, levomethadyl-2003, lumiracoxib-2007, mibefradil-1998, natalizumab-2005, nomifensine-1986, palladone-2005, pamoline-2005, pergolide-2010, phenylpropanolamine-2000, propoxyphene-2010, rapacuronium-2001, rimonabant-2010, rofecoxib-2004, sibutramine-2010, suprofen-1987, tegaserod-2007, terfenadine-1998, temafloxacin-1992, ticrynafen-1980, troglitazone-2000, valdecoxib-2007, zomepirac 1983). The licensed vaccines against rotavirus and Lyme were also withdrawn because of safety concerns (see "Special methodological issues in pharmacoepidemiology studies of vaccine safety" in Chapter 22). Further, between 1990 and 2004, at least 15 noncardiac drugs including astemizole, cisapride, droperidol, grepafloxacin, halofantrine, pimozide, propoxyphene, rofecoxib, sertindole, sibutramine terfenadine, terodiline, thioridazine, vevacetylmethadol, and ziprasidone, were subject to significant regulatory actions because of cardiac concerns.

Since 1993, trying to deal with drug safety problems, FDA morphed its extant spontaneous reporting system into the MedWatch program of collecting spontaneous reports of adverse reactions (see Chapter 7), as part of that issuing monthly notifications of label changes. Compared to the 20–25 safety-related label changes that were being made every month by mid-1999, between 19 and 57 safety-related label changes (boxed warnings, warnings, contraindications, precautions, adverse events) were made every month in 2009.

According to a study by the US Government Accountability Office, 51% of approved drugs have serious adverse effects not detected before approval. Further, there is recognition that the initial dose recommended for a newly marketed drug is often incorrect, and needs monitoring and modification after marketing.

In some of the examples above, the drug was never convincingly linked to the adverse reaction, yet many of these accusations led to the removal of the drug involved from the market. Interestingly, however, this withdrawal was not necessarily executed in all of the different countries in which each drug was marketed. Most of these adverse discoveries have led to litigation, as well, and a few have even led to criminal charges against the pharmaceutical manufacturer and/or some of its employees (see Chapter 6).

Legislative actions resulting from drug crises

Through the 1980s, there was concern that an underfunded FDA was approving drugs too slowly, and that the US suffered, compared to Europe, from a "drug lag." To provide additional resources to FDA to help expedite the drug review and approval process, Congress passed in 1992 the Prescription Drug User Fee Act (PDUFA), allowing the FDA to charge manufacturers a fee for reviewing New Drug Applications. This legislation was reauthorized by Congress several times: PDUFA II–the Food and Drug Modernization Act of 1997; PDUFA III–the Public Health Security and Bioterrorism Preparedness and Response Act of 2002; PDUFA IV, the Food and Drug Administration Amendments (FDAAA-PL 110-85) of 2007; and PDUFA V, the Food and Drug Administration Safety and Innovation Act of 2012. The goals for PDUFA have been to

enable the FDA to complete review of over 90% of priority drug applications in 6 months, and complete review of over 90% of standard drug applications in 12 months (under PDUFA I) or 10 months (under PDUFA II, III, and IV). In addition to reauthorizing the collection of user fees from the pharmaceutical industry, PDUFA II allowed the FDA to accept a single well-controlled clinical study under certain conditions, to reduce drug development time. The result was a system where more than 550 new drugs were approved by FDA in the 1990s.

However, whereas 1400 FDA employees in 1998 worked with the drug approval process, only 52 monitored safety; FDA spent only $2.4 million in extramural safety research. This state of affairs has coincided with the growing numbers of drug crises cited above. With successive reauthorizations of PDUFA, this changed markedly. PDUFA III for the first time allowed the FDA to use a small portion of the user fees for postmarketing drug safety monitoring, to address safety concerns.

However, there now was growing concern, in Congress and the US public, that perhaps FDA was approving drugs too *fast*. There were also calls for the development of an independent drug safety board, with wider mission than FDA's regulatory mission, to complement the latter. Such a board could investigate drug safety crises, looking for ways to prevent them, and deal with issues such as improper physician prescribing of drugs, the need for training, and the development of new approaches to the field of pharmacoepidemiology.

Recurrent concerns about FDA's management of postmarketing drug safety issues led to a systematic review of the entire drug risk assessment process. In 2006, the US General Accountability Office issued its report of a review of the organizational structure and effectiveness of FDA's postmarketing drug safety decision-making, followed in 2007 by the Institute of Medicine's independent assessment. Important weaknesses in the current system included failure of FDA's Office of New Drugs and Office of Drug Safety to communicate with each other on safety issues, failure of FDA to track ongoing postmarketing studies, ambiguous role of FDA's Office of Drug Safety in scientific advisory committees, limited authority by FDA to require the pharmaceutical industry to perform studies to obtain needed data, culture problems at FDA where recommendations by the FDA's drug safety staff were not followed, and conflict of interest involving advisory committee members. This Institute of Medicine report was influential in shaping PDUFA IV.

Indeed, with the passage of PDUFA IV, FDA authority was substantially increased, with the ability to require postmarketing studies and levy heavy fines if these requirements were not met. Further, its resources were substantially increased, with specific mandates to: (i) fund epidemiology best practices and data acquisition ($7 million in fiscal 2008, increasing to $9.5 million in fiscal 2012); (ii) fund new drug trade name review ($5.3 million in fiscal 2008, rising to $6.5 million in fiscal 2012); and (iii) fund risk management and communication ($4 million in fiscal 2008, rising to $5 million in fiscal 2012) (see also "Comparative effectiveness research" in Chapter 22). In another use of the new PDUFA funds, the FDA plans to develop and implement agency-wide and special-purpose postmarket IT systems, including the MedWatch Plus Portal, the FDA Adverse Event Reporting System, the Sentinel System (a virtual national medical product safety system–see Chapter 22), and the Phonetic and Orthographic Computer Analysis System to find similarities in spelling or sound between proposed proprietary drug names that might increase the risk of confusion and medication errors.

Intellectual development of pharmacoepidemiology emerging from drug crises

Several developments of the 1960s can be thought to have marked the beginning of the field of pharmacoepidemiology. The Kefauver-Harris Amendments that were introduced in 1962 required formal safety studies for new drug applications. The DESI program that was undertaken by the FDA as part of the Kefauver-Harris Amendments required formal efficacy studies for old drugs that were approved earlier. These requirements created demand for new expertise and new methods. In addition, the mid-1960s saw the publication of a series of drug utilization studies. These studies provided the first descriptive information on how physicians use drugs, and began a series of investigations of the frequency and determinants of poor prescribing (see also "Evaluating and improving physician prescribing" in Chapter 22).

In part in response to concerns about adverse drug effects, the early 1970s saw the development of the Drug Epidemiology Unit, now the Slone Epidemiology Center, which extended the hospital-based approach of the Boston Collaborative Drug Surveillance Program by collecting lifetime drug exposure histories from hospitalized patients and using these to perform hospital-based case-control studies. The year 1976 saw the formation of the Joint Commission on Prescription Drug Use, an interdisciplinary committee of experts charged with reviewing the state of the art of pharmacoepidemiology at that time, as well as providing recommendations for the future. The Computerized Online Medicaid Analysis and Surveillance System (COMPASS®) was first developed in 1977, using Medicaid billing data to perform pharmacoepidemiologic studies (see Chapter 9). The Drug Surveillance Research Unit, now called the Drug Safety Research Trust, was developed in the United Kingdom in 1980, with its innovative system of Prescription Event Monitoring. Each of these represented major contributions to the field of pharmacoepidemiology. These and newer approaches are reviewed in Part II of this book.

In the examples of drug crises mentioned above, these were serious but uncommon drug effects, and these experiences have led to an accelerated search for new methods to study drug effects in large numbers of patients. This led to a shift from adverse effect studies to adverse event studies, with concomitant increasing use of new data resources and new methods to study adverse reactions. The American Society for Clinical Pharmacology and Therapeutics issued, in 1990, a position paper on the use of purported postmarketing drug surveillance studies for promotional purposes, and the International Society for Pharmacoepidemiology (ISPE) issued, in 1996, Guidelines for Good Epidemiology Practices for Drug, Device, and Vaccine

Research in the United States, which were updated in 2007. Since the late 1990s, pharmacoepidemiologic research has also been increasingly burdened by concerns about patient confidentiality (see also Chapter 15).

There is also increasing recognition that most of the risk from most drugs to most patients occurs from known reactions to old drugs. Attempting to address concerns about underuse, overuse, and adverse events of medical products and medical errors that may cause serious impairment to patient health, a new program of Centers for Education and Research on Therapeutics (CERTs) was authorized under the FDA Modernization Act of 1997 (as part of the same legislation that reauthorized PDUFA II). Starting in 1999 and incrementally adding more centers in 2002, 2006, and 2007, the Agency for Healthcare Research and Quality (AHRQ) that was selected to administer this program has been funding up to 14 Centers for Education and Research and Therapeutics (see "Comparative effectiveness research" in Chapter 22), although this has since been reduced to six centers.

The research and education activities sponsored by AHRQ through the CERTs program since the late 1990s take place in academic centers. These CERTs centers conduct research on therapeutics, exploring new uses of drugs, ways to improve the effective uses of drugs, and the risks associated with new uses or combinations of drugs. They also develop educational modules and materials for disseminating the research findings about medical products. With the development of direct-to-consumer advertising of drugs since the mid 1980s in the US, the CERTs' role in educating the public and health care professionals by providing evidence-based information has become especially important.

Another impetus for research on drugs resulted from one of the mandates (in Sec. 1013) of the Medicare Prescription Drug, Improvement, and Modernization Act of 2003 to provide beneficiaries with scientific information on the outcomes, comparative clinical effectiveness, and appropriateness of health care items and services. In response, AHRQ created in 2005 the DEcIDE (Developing Evidence to Inform Decisions about Effectiveness) Network to support in academic settings the conduct of studies on effectiveness, safety, and usefulness of drugs and other treatments and services.

Another major new initiative of relevance to pharmacoepidemiology is risk management. There is increasing recognition that the risk/benefit balance of some drugs can only be considered acceptable with active management of their use, to maximize their efficacy and/or minimize their risk. In response, in the late 1990s, there were new initiatives underway, ranging from FDA requirements for risk management plans, to a FDA Drug Safety and Risk Management Advisory Committee, and issuing risk minimization and management guidances in 2005 (see Chapters 6 and 22).

Another initiative related to pharmacoepidemiology is the Patient Safety movement. In the Institute of Medicine's report, "To Err is Human: Building a Safer Health System," the authors note that: (a) "even apparently single events or errors are due most often to the convergence of multiple contributing factors," (b) "preventing errors and improving safety for patients requires a systems approach in order to modify the conditions that contribute to errors," and (c) "the problem is not bad people; the problem is that the system needs to be made safer." In this framework, the concern is not about substandard or negligent care, but rather, is about errors made by even the best trained, brightest, and most competent professional health caregivers and/or patients. From this perspective, the important research questions ask about the conditions under which people make errors, the types of errors being made, and the types of systems that can be put into place to prevent errors altogether when possible. Errors that are not prevented must be identified and corrected efficiently and quickly, before they inflict harm. Turning specifically to medications, from 2.4 to 6.5% of hospitalized patients suffer ADEs, prolonging hospital stays by 2 days, and increase costs by $2000–2600 per patient. Over 7000 US deaths were attributed to medication errors in 1993. Although these estimates have been disputed, the overall importance of reducing these errors has not been questioned. In recognition of this problem, AHRQ launched a major new grant program of over 100 projects, at its peak with over $50 million/year of funding. While only a portion of this is dedicated to medication errors, they are clearly a focus of interest and relevance to many (see "Medication errors" in Chapter 22.)

The 1990s and especially the 2000s have seen another shift in the field, away from its exclusive emphasis on drug utilization and adverse reactions, to the inclusion of other interests as well, such as the use of pharmacoepidemiology to study beneficial drug effects, the application of health economics to the study of drug effects, quality-of-life studies, meta-analysis, etc. These new foci are discussed in more detail in Part III of this book.

Also, with the publication of the results from the Women's Health Initiative indicating that combination hormone replacement therapy causes an increased risk of myocardial infarction rather than a decreased risk, there has been increased concern about reliance solely on nonexperimental methods to study drug safety after marketing. This has led to increased use of massive randomized clinical trials as part of postmarketing surveillance. This is especially important because often the surrogate markers used for drug development cannot necessary be relied upon to map completely to true clinical outcomes.

Finally, with the advent of the Obama administration in the US, there has been enormous interest in comparative effectiveness research (CER). CER was defined in 2009 by the Federal Coordinating Council for Comparative Effectiveness Research as

> the conduct and synthesis of research comparing the benefits and harms of different interventions and strategies to prevent, diagnose, treat and monitor health conditions in "real world" settings. The purpose of this research is to improve health outcomes by developing and disseminating evidence-based information to patients, clinicians, and other decision-makers, responding to their expressed needs, about which interventions are most effective for which patients under specific circumstances.

By this definition, CER includes three key elements: (1) evidence synthesis, (2) evidence generation, and (3) evidence dissemination. Typically, CER is conducted through observational studies of either large administrative or medical record databases (see Chapter 9), or large naturalistic clinical trials (see Chapter 16). The UK has been focusing on CER for years, with its National Institute for Health and Clinical Excellence (NICE), an independent organization responsible for providing national guidance on promoting good health and preventing and treating ill health. However, the Obama administration included $1.1 billion for CER in its federal stimulus package, and has plans for hundreds of millions of dollars of support per year thereafter. While CER does not overlap completely with pharmacoepidemiology, the scientific approaches are very close. Pharmacoepidemiologists evaluate the use and effects of medications. CER investigators compare, in the real world, the safety and benefits of one treatment compared to another. CER extends beyond pharmacoepidemiology in that CER can include more than just drugs; pharmacoepidemiology extends beyond CER in that it includes studies comparing exposed to unexposed patients, not just alternative exposures. However, to date, most work done in CER has been done in pharmacoepidemiology. See Chapter 22 for more discussion of CER.

The current drug approval process

Drug approval in the US

Since the mid-1990s, there has been a decline in the number of novel drugs approved per year, while the cost of bringing a drug to market has risen sharply. The total cost of drug development to the pharmaceutical industry increased from $24 billion in 1999, to $32 billion in 2002, and to $65.2 billion on research and development in 2008. The cost to discover and develop a drug that successfully reached the market rose from over $800 million in 2004 to an estimated $1.3 billion to 1.7 billion currently. In addition to the sizeable costs of research and development, a substantial part of this total cost is determined also by the regulatory requirement to test new drugs during several premarketing and postmarketing phases, as will be reviewed next.

The current drug approval process in the US and most other developed countries includes preclinical animal testing followed by three phases of clinical testing. Phase I testing is usually conducted in just a few normal volunteers, and represents the initial trials of the drug in humans. Phase I trials are generally conducted by clinical pharmacologists, to determine the metabolism of the drug in humans, a safe dosage range in humans, and to exclude any extremely common toxic reactions which are unique to humans.

Phase II testing is also generally conducted by clinical pharmacologists, on a small number of patients who have the target disease. Phase II testing is usually the first time patients are exposed to the drug. Exceptions are drugs that are so toxic that it would not normally be considered ethical to expose healthy individuals to them, like cytotoxic drugs. For these, patients are used for Phase I testing as well. The goals of Phase II testing are to obtain more information on the pharmacokinetics of the drug and on any relatively common adverse reactions, and to obtain initial information on the possible efficacy of the drug. Specifically, Phase II is used to determine the daily dosage and regimen to be tested more rigorously in Phase III.

Phase III testing is performed by clinician-investigators in a much larger number of patients, in order to rigorously evaluate a drug's efficacy and to provide more information on its toxicity. At least one of the Phase III studies needs to be a randomized clinical trial (see Chapter 16). To meet FDA standards, at least one of the randomized clinical trials usually needs to be conducted in the US. Generally between 500 and 3000 patients are exposed to a drug during Phase III, even if drug efficacy can be demonstrated with much smaller numbers, in order to be able to detect less common adverse reactions. For example, a study including 3000 patients would allow one to be 95% certain of detecting any adverse reactions that occur in at least one exposed patient out of 1000. At the other extreme, a total of 500 patients would allow one to be 95% certain of detecting any adverse reactions that occur in six or more patients out of every 1000 exposed. Adverse reactions that occur less commonly than these are less likely to be detected in these premarketing studies. The sample sizes needed to detect drug effects are discussed in more detail in Chapter 3. Nowadays, with the increased focus on drug safety, premarketing dossiers are sometimes being extended well beyond 3000 patients. However, as one can tell from the sample size calculations in Chapter 3 and Appendix A, by itself these larger numbers gain little additional information about adverse drug reactions, unless one were to increase to perhaps 30 000 patients, well beyond the scope of most premarketing studies.

Finally, Phase IV testing is the evaluation of the effects of drugs after general marketing. The bulk of this book is devoted to such efforts.

Drug approval in other countries

Outside the US, national systems for the regulation and approval of new drugs vary greatly, even among developed countries and especially between developed and developing countries. While in most developed countries, at least, the general process of drug development is very analogous to that in the US, the implementation varies widely. A WHO comparative analysis of drug regulation in ten countries found that not all countries even have a written national drug policy document. Regulation of medicines in some countries is centralized in a single agency that performs the gamut of functions involving product registration, licensing, product review, approval for clinical trials, postmarketing surveillance, and inspection of manufacturing practice.. In other countries, regulatory functions are distributed among different agencies. In the Netherlands, for example, the Ministry of Health, Welfare & Sports performs the functions of licensing; the Healthcare Inspectorate checks on general manufacturing practice; and the Medicines Evaluation Board performs the functions of product assessment and registration and adverse drug reaction monitoring. Another dimension on which countries may vary is the degree of autonomy of regulatory decisions from political influence. Drug regulation in most countries is performed by a department within the executive branch. In other countries (e.g., the Netherlands) this function is performed by a commission or board, independent of interference by other government authorities. All the countries examined by the WHO require registration of pharmaceutical products, but they differ on the documentation requirements for evidence of safety and efficacy. Some countries carry out independent assessments while others, especially many developing countries, rely on WHO assessments or other sources. With the exception of Cyprus, the remaining 9 countries surveyed by the WHO were found to regulate the conduct of clinical trials, but with varying rates of participation of health care professionals in reporting adverse drug reactions. Countries also differ on the extent of emphasis on quantitative or qualitative analysis for assessing pre- and postmarketing data.

Further, within Europe, each country has its own regulatory agency, e.g., the United Kingdom's Medicines and Healthcare Products Regulatory Agency (MHRA), formed in 2003 as a merger of the Medicines Control Agency (MCA) and the Medical Devices Agency (MDA). In addition, since January 1998, some drug registration and approval within the European Union has shifted away from the national licensing authorities of the EU members to that of the centralized authority of the European Medicines Evaluation Agency (EMEA), which was established in 1993. To facilitate this centralized approval process, the EMEA pushed for harmonization of drug approvals. While the goals of harmonization are to create a single pharmaceutical market in Europe and to shorten approval times, concerns were voiced that harmonized safety standards would lower the stricter standards that were favored by some countries such as Sweden, for example, and would compromise patient safety. Now called the European Medicines Agency (EMA), the EMA is a decentralized body of the European Union, responsible for the scientific evaluation and supervision of medicines. These functions are performed by the EMA's Committee for Medicinal Products for Human Use (CHMP). EMA authorization to market a drug is valid in all European Union countries, but individual national medicines agencies are responsible for monitoring the safety of approved drugs and sharing this information with EMA.

Potential contributions of pharmacoepidemiology

The potential contributions of pharmacoepidemiology are now well recognized, even though the field is still relatively new. However, some contributions are already apparent (see Table 1.1). In fact, in the 1970s the FDA requested postmarketing research at the time of approval for about one-third of drugs, compared to over 70% in the 1990s. Now, since the passage of the Food, and Drug Administration Amendments Act of 2007 (FDAAA-PL 110-85) noted above, FDA has the right to require such studies be completed. In this section of this chapter, we will first review the potential for pharmacoepidemiologic studies to supplement the information available prior to marketing, and then review the new types of information obtainable from postmarketing pharmacoepidemiologic studies but not obtainable prior to drug marketing. Finally, we will review the general, and probably most important, potential contributions such studies can make. In each case, the relevant

Table 1.1 Potential contributions of pharmacoepidemiology.

(A) Information which supplements the information available from premarketing studies—better quantitation of the incidence of known adverse and beneficial effects
  a. Higher precision
  b. In patients not studied prior to marketing, e.g., the elderly, children, in pregnant women
  c. As modified by other drugs and other illnesses
  d. Relative to other drugs used for the same indications

(B) New types of information not available from premarketing studies
  1. Discovery of previously undetected adverse and beneficial effects
    a. Uncommon effects
    b. Delayed effects
  2. Patterns of drug utilization
  3. The effects of drug overdoses
  4. The economic implications of drug use

(C) General contributions of pharmacoepidemiology
  1. Reassurances about drug safety
  2. Fulfillment of ethical and legal obligations

information available from premarketing studies will be briefly examined first, to clarify how postmarketing studies can supplement this information.

Supplementary information

Premarketing studies of drug effects are necessarily limited in size. After marketing, nonexperimental epidemiologic studies can be performed, evaluating the effects of drugs administered as part of ongoing medical care. These allow the cost-effective accumulation of much larger numbers of patients than those studied prior to marketing, resulting in a more precise measurement of the incidence of adverse and beneficial drug effects (see Chapter 3). For example, at the time of drug marketing, prazosin was known to cause a dose-dependent first dose syncope, but the FDA requested the manufacturer to conduct a postmarketing surveillance study of the drug in the US to quantitate its incidence more precisely. In recent years, there has even been an attempt, in selected special cases, to release selected critically important drugs more quickly, by taking advantage of the work that can be performed after marketing. Probably the best-known example was zidovudine. As noted above, the increased sample size available after postmarketing also permits a more precise determination of the correct dose to be used.

Premarketing studies also tend to be very artificial. Important subgroups of patients are not typically included in studies conducted before drug marketing, usually for ethical reasons. Examples include the elderly, children, and pregnant women. Studies of the effects of drugs in these populations generally must await studies conducted after drug marketing.

Additionally, for reasons of statistical efficiency, premarketing clinical trials generally seek subjects who are as homogeneous as possible, in order to reduce unexplained variability in the outcome variables measured and increase the probability of detecting a difference between the study groups, if one truly exists. For these reasons, certain patients are often excluded, including those with other illnesses or those who are receiving other drugs. Postmarketing studies can explore how factors such as other illnesses and other drugs might modify the effects of the drugs, as well as looking at the effects of differences in drug regimen, adherence,

etc. For example, after marketing, the ophthalmic preparation of timolol was noted to cause many serious episodes of heart block and asthma, resulting in over ten deaths. These effects were not detected prior to marketing, as patients with underlying cardiovascular or respiratory disease were excluded from the premarketing studies.

Finally, to obtain approval to market a drug, a manufacturer needs to evaluate its overall safety and efficacy, but does not need to evaluate its safety and efficacy relative to any other drugs available for the same indication. To the contrary, with the exception of illnesses that could not ethically be treated with placebos, such as serious infections and malignancies, it is generally considered preferable, or even mandatory, to have studies with placebo controls. There are a number of reasons for this preference. First, it is easier to show that a new drug is more effective than a placebo than to show it is more effective than another effective drug. Second, one cannot actually prove that a new drug is as effective as a standard drug. A study showing a new drug is no worse than another effective drug does not provide assurance that it is better than a placebo; one simply could have failed to detect that it was in fact worse than the standard drug. One could require a demonstration that a new drug is more effective than another effective drug, but this is a standard that does not and should not have to be met. Yet, optimal medical care requires information on the effects of a drug relative to the alternatives available for the same indication. This information must often await studies conducted after drug marketing. Indeed, as noted, this is a major component of the very new focus on comparative effectiveness research (see Chapter 22).

New types of information not available from premarketing studies

As mentioned above, premarketing studies are necessarily limited in size (see Chapter 3). The additional sample size available in postmarketing studies permits the study of drug effects that may be uncommon, but important, such as drug-induced agranulocytosis.

Premarketing studies are also necessarily limited in time; they must come to an end, or the drug could never be marketed. In contrast, postmarketing studies permit the study of delayed drug effects, such as the unusual clear cell adenocarcinoma of the vagina and cervix, which occurred two decades later in women exposed *in utero* to diethylstilbestrol.

The patterns of physician prescribing and patient drug utilization often cannot be predicted prior to marketing, despite pharmaceutical manufacturers' best attempts to predict when planning for drug marketing. Studies of how a drug is actually being used, and determinants of changes in these usage patterns, can only be performed after drug marketing (see "Studies of drug utilization" and "Evaluating and improving physician prescribing" in Chapter 22).

In most cases, premarketing studies are performed using selected patients who are closely observed. Rarely are there any significant overdoses in this population. Thus, the study of the effects of a drug when ingested in extremely high doses is rarely possible before drug marketing. Again, this must await postmarketing pharmacoepidemiologic studies.

Finally, it is only in the past decade or two that our society has become more sensitive to the costs of medical care, and the techniques of health economics been applied to evaluate the cost implications of drug use. It is clear that the exploration of the costs of drug use requires consideration of more than just the costs of the drugs themselves. The costs of a drug's adverse effects may be substantially higher than the cost of the drug itself, if these adverse effects result in additional medical care and possibly even hospitalizations. Conversely, a drug's beneficial effects could reduce the need for medical care, resulting in savings that can be much larger than the cost of the drug itself. As with studies of drug utilization, the economic implications of drug use can be predicted prior to marketing, but can only be rigorously studied after marketing (see Chapter 17).

General contributions of pharmacoepidemiology

Lastly, it is important to review the general contributions that can be made by pharmacoepidemiology. As an academic or a clinician, one is most interested in the new information about drug effects and drug costs that can be gained from pharmacoepidemiology. Certainly, these are the findings that receive the greatest public and political attention. However, often no new information is obtained, particularly about new adverse drug effects. This is not a disappointing outcome, but in fact, a very reassuring one, and this reassurance about drug safety is one of the most important contributions that can be made by pharmacoepidemiologic studies. Related to this is the reassurance that the sponsor of the study, whether manufacturer or regulator, is fulfilling its organizational duty ethically and responsibly by looking for any undiscovered problems which may be there. In an era of product liability litigation, this is an important assurance. One cannot change whether a drug causes an adverse reaction, and the fact that it does will hopefully eventually become evident. What can be changed is the perception about whether a manufacturer did everything possible to detect it and was not negligent in its behavior.

Key points

- *Pharmacoepidemiology* is the study of the use of and the effects of drugs and other medical devices in large numbers of people. It uses the methods of epidemiology to study the content area of clinical pharmacology.
- The history of pharmacoepidemiology is a history of increasingly frequent accusations about adverse drug reactions, often arising out of the spontaneous reporting system, followed by formal studies proving or disproving those associations.
- The drug approval process is inherently limited, so it cannot detect before marketing adverse effects that are uncommon, delayed, unique to high risk populations, due to misuse of the drugs by prescribers or patients, etc.
- Pharmacoepidemiology can contribute information about drug safety and effectiveness that is not available from premarketing studies.

Further reading

Califf RM (2002) The need for a national infrastructure to improve the rational use of therapeutics. *Pharmacoepidemiol Drug Saf* **11**: 319–27.

Caranasos GJ, Stewart RB, Cluff LE (1974) Drug-induced illness leading to hospitalization. *JAMA* **228**: 713–17.

Cluff LE, Thornton GF, Seidl LG (1964) Studies on the epidemiology of adverse drug reactions. I. Methods of surveillance. *JAMA* **188**: 976–83.

Crane J, Pearce N, Flatt A, Burgess C, Jackson R, Kwong T, *et al.* (1989) Prescribed fenoterol and death from asthma in New Zealand, 1981–83: case–control study. *Lancet* **1**: 917–22.

Erslev AJ, Wintrobe MM (1962) Detection and prevention of drug induced blood dyscrasias. *JAMA* **181**: 114–19.

Geiling EMK, Cannon PR (1938) Pathogenic effects of elixir of sulfanilimide (diethylene glycol) poisoning. *JAMA* **111**: 919–26.

Herbst AL, Ulfelder H, Poskanzer DC (1971) Adenocarcinoma of the vagina: association of maternal stilbestrol therapy with tumor appearance in young women. *N Engl J Med* **284**: 878–81.

ISPE (2008) Guidelines for good pharmacoepidemiology practices (GPP). *Pharmacoepidemiol Drug Saf.* **17**: 200–8.

Joint Commission on Prescription Drug Use (1980) *Final Report.* Washington, DC.

Kimmel SE, Keane MG, Crary JL, Jones J, Kinman JL, Beare J, *et al.* (1999) Detailed examination of fenfluramine-phentermine users with valve abnormalities identified in Fargo, North Dakota. *Am J Cardiol* **84**: 304–8.

Kono R (1980) Trends and lessons of SMON research. In: Soda T, ed., *Drug-Induced Sufferings.* Princeton, NJ: Excerpta Medica, p. 11.

Lazarou J, Pomeranz BH, Corey PN (1998) Incidence of adverse drug reactions in hospitalized patients: a meta-analysis of prospective studies. *JAMA* **279**: 1200–5.

Lenz W (1966) Malformations caused by drugs in pregnancy. *Am J Dis Child* **112**: 99–106.

Meyler L (1952) *Side Effects of Drugs.* Amsterdam: Elsevier.

Miller RR, Greenblatt DJ (1976) *Drug Effects in Hospitalized Patients.* New York: John Wiley & Sons, Inc.

Rawlins MD, Thompson JW (1977) Pathogenesis of adverse drug reactions. In: Davies DM, ed., *Textbook of Adverse Drug Reactions.* Oxford: Oxford University Press, p. 44.

Strom BL (1990) Members of the ASCPT Pharmacoepidemiology Section. Position paper on the use of purported postmarketing drug surveillance studies for promotional purposes. *Clin Pharmacol Ther* **48**: 598.

Strom BL, Berlin JA, Kinman JL, Spitz PW, Hennessy S, Feldman H, *et al.* (1996) Parenteral ketorolac and risk of gastrointestinal and operative site bleeding: a postmarketing surveillance study. *JAMA* **275**: 376–82.

Wallerstein RO, Condit PK, Kasper CK, Brown JW, Morrison FR (1969) Statewide study of chloramphenicol therapy and fatal aplastic anemia. *JAMA* **208**: 2045–50.

Wright P (1975) Untoward effects associated with practolol administration. Oculomucocutaneous syndrome. *BMJ* **1**: 595–8.

CHAPTER 2

Study Designs Available for Pharmacoepidemiologic Studies

Brian L. Strom

Perelman School of Medicine at the University of Pennsylvania, Philadelphia, PA, USA

Pharmacoepidemiology applies the methods of epidemiology to the content area of clinical pharmacology. Therefore, in order to understand the approaches and methodological issues specific to the field of pharmacoepidemiology, the basic principles of the field of epidemiology must be understood as well. To this end, this chapter will begin with an overview of the scientific method in general. This will be followed by a discussion of the different types of errors one can make in designing a study. Next, the chapter will review the "Criteria for the causal nature of an association," which is how one can decide whether an association demonstrated in a particular study is, in fact, a causal association. Finally, the specific study designs available for epidemiologic studies, or in fact for any clinical studies, will be reviewed. The next chapter discusses a specific methodological issue which needs to be addressed in any study, but which is of particular importance for pharmacoepidemiologic studies: the issue of sample size. These two chapters are intended to be an introduction to the field of epidemiology for the neophyte. More information on these principles can be obtained from any textbook of epidemiology or clinical epidemiology. Finally, Chapter 4 will review basic principles of clinical pharmacology, the content area of pharmacoepidemiology.

Overview of the scientific method

The scientific method to investigate a research question involves a three-stage process (see Figure 2.1). In the first stage, one selects a group of subjects for study. These subjects may be patients or animals or biologic cells and are the sources for data sought by the study to answer a question of interest. Second, one uses the information obtained in this sample of study subjects to generalize and draw a conclusion about a population in general. This conclusion is referred to as an association. Third, one generalizes again, drawing a conclusion about scientific theory or causation. Each will be discussed in turn.

Any given study is performed on a selection of individuals, who represent the *study subjects*. These study subjects should theoretically represent a random sample of some defined population. For example, one might perform a randomized clinical trial of the efficacy of enalapril in lowering blood pressure, randomly allocating a total of 40 middle aged hypertensive men to receive either enalapril or placebo and observing their blood pressure six weeks later. One might expect to see the blood pressure of the 20 men treated with the active drug decrease more than the blood pressure of the 20 men treated with a placebo. In this example, the 40 study subjects would represent the study sample,

Textbook of Pharmacoepidemiology, Second Edition. Edited by Brian L. Strom, Stephen E. Kimmel, and Sean Hennessy.

© 2013 John Wiley & Sons, Ltd. Published 2013 by John Wiley & Sons, Ltd.

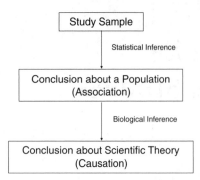

Figure 2.1 Overview of the scientific method.

theoretically a random sample of middle-aged hypertensive men. In reality, the study sample is almost never a true random sample of the underlying target population, because it is logistically impossible to identify every individual who belongs in the target population and then randomly choose from among them. However, the study sample is usually treated as if it were a random sample of the target population.

At this point, one would be tempted to make a generalization that enalapril lowers blood pressure in middle-aged hypertensive men. However, one must explore whether this observation could have occurred simply by chance, i.e., due to random variation. If the observed outcome in the study was simply a chance occurrence, then the same observation might not have been seen if one had chosen a different sample of 40 study subjects. Perhaps more importantly, it might not exist if one were able to study the entire theoretical population of all middle-aged hypertensive men. In order to evaluate this possibility, one can perform a statistical test, which allows an investigator to quantitate the probability that the observed outcome in this study (i.e., the difference seen between the two study groups) could have happened simply by chance. There are explicit rules and procedures for how one should properly make this determination: the science of statistics. If the results of any study under consideration demonstrate a "statistically significant difference" (i.e., ruling out the probability of a chance occurrence), then one is said to have an *association*. The process of assessing whether

random variation could have led to a study's findings is referred to as *statistical inference*, and represents the major role for statistical testing in the scientific method.

If there is no statistically significant difference, then the process in Figure 2.1 stops. If there is an association, then one is tempted to generalize the results of the study even further, to state that enalapril is an antihypertensive drug, in general. This is referred to as *scientific or biological inference*, and the result is a conclusion about *causation*, that the drug really does lower blood pressure in a population of treated patients. To draw this type of conclusion, however, requires one to generalize to populations other than that included in the study, including types of people who were not represented in the study sample, such as women, children, and the elderly. Although it may be apparent in this example that this is in fact appropriate, that may well not always be the case. Unlike statistical inference, there are no precise quantitative rules for biological inference. Rather, one needs to examine the data at hand in light of all other relevant data in the rest of the scientific literature, and make a subjective judgment. To assist in making that judgment, however, one can use the "Criteria for the Causal Nature of an Association," described below. First, however, we will place causal associations into a proper perspective, by describing the different types of errors that can be made in performing a study and the different types of associations that each results in.

Types of errors that one can make in performing a study

There are four basic types of associations that can be observed in a study (Table 2.1). The basic purpose of research is to differentiate among them.

First, of course, one could have no association.

Second, one could have an *artifactual association*, i.e., a spurious or false association. This can occur by either of two mechanisms: chance or bias. Chance is unsystematic, or random, variation. The purpose of statistical testing in science is to evaluate this, estimating the probability that the result

Table 2.1 Types of associations between factors under study.

---

1. None (independent)
2. Artifactual (spurious or false)
   a. Chance (unsystematic variation)
   b. Bias (systematic variation)
3. Indirect (confounded)
4. Causal (direct or true)

---

observed in a study could have happened purely by chance.

The other possible mechanism for creating an artifactual association is bias. Epidemiologists' use of the term bias is different from that of the lay public. To an epidemiologist, *bias* is systematic variation, a consistent manner in which two study groups are treated or evaluated differently. This consistent difference can create an apparent association where one actually does not exist. Of course, it also can mask a true association.

There are many different types of potential biases. For example, consider an interview study in which the research assistant is aware of the investigator's hypothesis. Attempting to please the boss, the research assistant might probe more carefully during interviews with one study group than during interviews with the other. This difference in how carefully the interviewer probes could create an apparent but false association, which is referred to as interviewer bias. Another example would be a study of drug-induced birth defects that compares children with birth defects to children without birth defects. A mother of a child with birth defect, when interviewed about any drugs she took during her pregnancy, may be likely to remember drug ingestion during pregnancy with greater accuracy than a mother of a healthy child, because of the unfortunate experience she has undergone. The improved recall in the mothers of the children with birth defects may result in false apparent associations between drug exposure and birth defects. This systematic difference in recall is referred to as recall bias.

Note that biases, once present, cannot be corrected. They represent errors in the study design

that can result in incorrect results in the study. It is important to note that a *statistically significant result is no protection against a bias*; one can have a very precise measurement of an incorrect answer! The only protection against biases is proper study design. (See Chapter 21 for more discussion about biases in pharmacoepidemiologic studies.)

Third, one can have an indirect, or confounded, association. A *confounding variable*, or *confounder*, is a variable, other than the risk factor and other than the outcome under study, which is related independently to both the risk factor and the outcome and which may create an apparent association or mask a real one. For example, a study of risk factors for lung cancer could find a very strong association between having yellow fingertips and developing lung cancer. This is obviously not a causal association, but an indirect association, confounded by cigarette smoking. Specifically, cigarette smoking causes both yellow fingertips and lung cancer. Although this example is transparent, most examples of confounding are not. In designing a study, one must consider every variable that can be associated with the risk factor under study or the outcome variable under study, in order to plan to deal with it as a potential confounding variable. Preferably, one will be able to specifically control for the variable, using one of the techniques listed in Table 2.2. (See Chapter 21 for more discussion about confounding in pharmacoepidemiologic studies.)

Fourth, and finally, there are true, causal associations.

Thus, there are three possible types of errors that can be produced in a study: random error, bias, and confounding. The probability of random error can

Table 2.2 Approaches to controlling confounding.

---

1. Random allocation
2. Subject selection
   a. Exclusion
   b. Matching
3. Data analysis
   a. Stratification
   b. Mathematical modeling

---

be quantitated using statistics. Bias needs to be prevented by designing the study properly. Confounding can be controlled either in the design of the study or in its analysis. If all three types of errors can be excluded, then one is left with a true, causal association.

Criteria for the causal nature of an association

The "Criteria for the causal nature of an association" were first put forth by Sir Austin Bradford Hill, but have been described in various forms since, each with some modification. Probably the best known description of them was in the first Surgeon General's Report on Smoking and Health, published in 1964. These criteria are presented in Table 2.3, in no particular order. No one of them is absolutely necessary for an association to be a causal association. Analogously, no one of them is sufficient for an association to be considered a causal association. Essentially, the more criteria that are present, the more likely it is that an association is a causal association. The fewer criteria that are met, the less likely it is that an association is a causal association. Each will be discussed in turn.

The first criterion listed in Table 2.3 is *coherence with existing information* or *biological plausibility*. This refers to whether the association makes sense, in light of other types of information available in the literature. These other types of information could include data from other human studies, data from studies of other related questions, data from animal studies, or data from *in vitro* studies, as well as

Table 2.3 Criteria for the causal nature of an association.

1. Coherence with existing information (biological plausibility)
2. Consistency of the association
3. Time sequence
4. Specificity of the association
5. Strength of the association
   a. Quantitative strength
   b. Dose-response relationship
   c. Study design

scientific or pathophysiologic theory. To use the example provided above, it clearly was not biologically plausible that yellow fingertips could cause lung cancer, and this provided the clue that confounding was present. Using the example of the association between cigarettes and lung cancer, cigarette smoke is a known carcinogen, based on animal data. In humans, it is known to cause cancers of the head and neck, the pancreas, and the bladder. Cigarette smoke also goes down into the lungs, directly exposing the tissues in question. Thus, it certainly is biologically plausible that cigarettes could *cause* lung cancer. It is much more reassuring if an association found in a particular study makes sense, based on previously available information, and this makes one more comfortable that it might be a causal association. Clearly, however, one could not require that this criterion always be met, or one would never have a major breakthrough in science.

The second criterion listed in Table 2.3 is the *consistency of the association*. A hallmark of science is reproducibility: if a finding is real, one should be able to reproduce it in a different setting. This could include different geographic settings, different study designs, different populations, etc. For example, in the case of cigarettes and lung cancer, the association has now been reproduced in many different studies, in different geographic locations, using different study designs. The need for reproducibility is such that one should never believe a finding reported only once: there may have been an error committed in the study, which is not apparent to either the investigator or the reader.

The third criterion listed is that of *time sequence*–a cause must precede an effect. Although this may seem obvious, there are study designs from which this cannot be determined. For example, if one were to perform a survey in a classroom of 200 medical students, asking each if he or she were currently taking diazepam and also whether he or she were anxious, one would find a strong association between the use of diazepam and anxiety, but this does not mean that diazepam causes anxiety! Although this is obvious, as it is not a biologically plausible interpretation, one cannot differentiate from this type of cross-sectional study which variable came first and which came second. In the example of cigarettes and lung cancer, obviously the cigarette smoking usually precedes the lung cancer, as a patient would not survive long enough to smoke much if the opposite were the case.

The fourth criterion listed in Table 2.3 is *specificity*. This refers to the question of whether the cause ever occurs without the presumed effect and whether the effect ever occurs without the presumed cause. This criterion is almost never met in biology, with the occasional exception of infectious diseases. Measles never occurs without the measles virus, but even in this example, not everyone who becomes infected with the measles virus develops clinical measles. Certainly, not everyone who smokes develops lung cancer, and not everyone who develops lung cancer was a smoker. This is one of the major points the tobacco industry stresses when it attempts to make the claim that cigarette smoking has not been proven to cause lung cancer. Some authors even omit this as a criterion, as it is so rarely met. When it is met, however, it provides extremely strong support for a conclusion that an association is causal.

The fifth criterion listed in Table 2.3 is the *strength of the association*. This includes three concepts: its quantitative strength, dose-response, and the study design. Each will be discussed in turn.

The *quantitative strength* of an association refers to the effect size. To evaluate this, one asks whether the magnitude of the observed difference between the two study groups is large. A quantitatively large association can only be created by a causal association or a large error, which should be apparent in evaluating the methods of a study. A quantitatively small association may still be causal, but it could be created by a subtle error, which would not be apparent in evaluating the study. Conventionally, epidemiologists consider an association with a relative risk of less than 2.0 a weak association. Certainly, the association between cigarette smoking and lung cancer is a strong association: studies show relative risks ranging between 10.0 and 30.0.

A dose–response relationship is an extremely important and commonly used concept in clinical pharmacology and is used similarly in epidemiology. A *dose–response relationship* exists when an increase in the intensity of an exposure results in an increased risk of the disease under study. Equivalent to this is a *duration–response relationship*, which exists when a longer exposure causes an increased risk of the disease. The presence of either a dose–response relationship or a duration–response relationship strongly implies that an association is, in fact, a causal association. Certainly in the example of cigarette smoking and lung cancer, it has been shown repeatedly that an increase in either the number of cigarettes smoked each day or in the number of years of smoking increases the risk of developing lung cancer.

Finally, *study design* refers to two concepts: whether the study was well designed, and which study design was used in the studies in question. The former refers to whether the study was subject to one of the three errors described earlier in this chapter, namely random error, bias, and confounding. Table 2.4 presents the study designs typically used for epidemiologic studies, or in fact for any clinical studies. They are organized in a hierarchical fashion. As one advances from the designs at the bottom of the table to those at the top of the table, studies get progressively harder to perform, but are progressively more convincing. In other words, associations shown by studies using designs at the top of the list are more likely to be causal associations than associations shown by studies using designs at the bottom of the list. The association between cigarette smoking and lung cancer has been reproduced in multiple well-designed studies, using analyses of secular trends, case-control studies, and cohort studies. However, it has not been shown using a randomized clinical trial, which is the "cadillac" of study designs, as will be discussed below. This is the other major defense used by the tobacco industry. Of course, it would not be ethical or logistically feasible to randomly allocate individuals to smoke or not to smoke and expect this to be followed for 20 years to observe the outcome in each group.

The issue of causation is discussed more in Chapter 7 as it relates to the process of spontaneous reporting of adverse drug reactions, and in Chapter 13 as it relates to determining causation in case reports.

Table 2.4 Advantages and disadvantages of epidemiologic study designs.

Study Design	Advantages	Disadvantages
Randomized clinical trial (Experimental study)	Most convincing design	Most expensive
	Only design which controls for unknown or unmeasurable confounders	Artificial Logistically most difficult
		Ethical objections
Cohort study	Can study multiple outcomes	Possibly biased outcome data
	Can study uncommon exposures	More expensive
	Selection bias less likely	If done prospectively, may take years to complete
	Unbiased exposure data	
	Incidence data available	
Case-control study	Can study multiple exposures	Control selection problematic
	Can study uncommon diseases	Possibly biased exposure data
	Logistically easier and faster	
	Less expensive	
Analyses of secular trends	Can provide rapid answers	No control of confounding
Case series	Easy quantitation of incidence	No control group, so cannot be used for hypothesis testing
Case reports	Cheap and easy method for generating hypotheses	Cannot be used for hypothesis testing

Epidemiologic study designs

In order to clarify the concept of study design further, each of the designs in Table 2.4 will be discussed in turn, starting at the bottom of the list and working upwards.

Case reports

Case reports are simply reports of events observed in single patients. As used in pharmacoepidemiology, a case report describes a single patient who was exposed to a drug and experiences a particular, usually adverse, outcome. For example, one might see a published case report about a young woman who was taking oral contraceptives and who suffered a pulmonary embolism.

Case reports are useful for raising hypotheses about drug effects, to be tested with more rigorous study designs. However, in a case report one cannot know if the patient reported is either typical of those with the exposure or typical of those with the disease. Certainly, one cannot usually determine whether the adverse outcome was due to the drug exposure or would have happened anyway. As such, it is very rare that a case report can be used to make a statement about causation. One exception to this would be when the outcome is so rare and so characteristic of the exposure that one knows that it was likely to be due to the exposure, even if the history of exposure were unclear. An example of this is clear cell vaginal adenocarcinoma occurring in young women exposed *in utero* to diethylstilbestrol. Another exception would be when the disease course is very predictable and the treatment causes a clearly apparent change in this disease course. An example would be the ability of penicillin to cure streptococcal endocarditis, a disease that is nearly uniformly fatal in the absence of treatment. Case reports can be particularly useful to document causation when the treatment causes a change in disease course which is reversible, such that the patient returns to his or her untreated state when the exposure is withdrawn, can be treated again, and when the change returns upon repeat treatment. Consider a patient who is suffering from an overdose of methadone, a long-acting narcotic, and is comatose. If this patient is then treated with naloxone, a narcotic antagonist, and immediately awakens, this would be very suggestive that the drug indeed is efficacious as a narcotic antagonist. As the naloxone wears off the patient would become comatose again, and then if he or she were given another dose of naloxone the patient would awaken again. This, especially if repeated a few times, would represent strong evidence that the drug is indeed effective as a narcotic antagonist. This type of challenge–rechallenge situation is relatively uncommon, however, as physicians generally will avoid exposing a patient to a drug if the patient experienced an adverse reaction to it in the past. This issue is discussed in more detail in Chapters 7 and 13.

Case series

Case series are collections of patients, all of whom have a single exposure, whose clinical outcomes are then evaluated and described. Often they are from a single hospital or medical practice. Alternatively, case series can be collections of patients with a single outcome, looking at their antecedent exposures. For example, one might observe 100 consecutive women under the age of 50 who suffer from a pulmonary embolism, and note that 30 of them had been taking oral contraceptives.

After drug marketing, case series are most useful for two related purposes. First, they can be useful for quantifying the incidence of an adverse reaction. Second, they can be useful for being certain that any particular adverse effect of concern does not occur in a population which is larger than that studied prior to drug marketing. The so-called

"Phase IV" postmarketing surveillance study of prazosin was conducted for the former reason, to quantitate the incidence of first dose syncope from prazosin. The "Phase IV" postmarketing surveillance study of cimetidine was conducted for the latter reason. Metiamide was an H-2 blocker, which was withdrawn after marketing outside the US because it caused agranulocytosis. Since cimetidine is chemically related to metiamide there was a concern that cimetidine might also cause agranulocytosis. In both examples, the manufacturer asked its sales representatives to recruit physicians to participate in the study. Each participating physician then enrolled the next series of patients for whom the drug was prescribed.

In this type of study, one can be more certain that the patients are probably typical of those with the exposure or with the disease, depending on the focus of the study. However, in the absence of a control group, one cannot be certain which features in the description of the patients are unique to the exposure, or outcome. As an example, one might have a case series from a particular hospital of 100 individuals with a certain disease, and note that all were men over the age of 60. This might lead one to conclude that this disease seems to be associated with being a man over the age of 60. However, it would be clear that this would be an incorrect conclusion once one noted that the hospital this case series was drawn from was a Veterans Administration hospital, where most patients are men over the age of 60. In the previous example of pulmonary embolism and oral contraceptives, 30% of the women with pulmonary embolism had been using oral contraceptives. However, this information is not sufficient to determine whether this is higher, the same as, or even lower than would have been expected. For this reason, case series are also not very useful in determining causation, but provide clinical descriptions of a disease or of patients who receive an exposure.

Analyses of secular trends

Analyses of secular trends, also called "ecological studies," examine trends in an exposure that is a presumed cause and trends in a disease that is a presumed effect and test whether the trends coincide. These trends can be examined over time or across geographic boundaries. In other words, one could analyze data from a single region and examine how the trend changes over time, or one could analyze data from a single time period and compare how the data differ from region to region or country to country. Vital statistics are often used for these studies. As an example, one might look at sales data for oral contraceptives and compare them to death rates from venous thromboembolism, using recorded vital statistics. When such a study was actually performed, mortality rates from venous thromboembolism were seen to increase in parallel with increasing oral contraceptive sales, but only in women of reproductive age, not in older women or in men of any age.

Analyses of secular trends are useful for rapidly providing evidence for or against a hypothesis. However, these studies lack data on individuals; they utilize only aggregated group data (e.g., annual sales data in a given geographic region in relation to annual cause-specific mortality in the same region). As such, they are unable to control for confounding variables. Thus, among exposures whose trends coincide with that of the disease, analyses of secular trends are unable to differentiate which factor is likely to be the true cause. For example, lung cancer mortality rates in the US have been increasing in women, such that lung cancer is now the leading cause of cancer mortality in women. This is certainly consistent with the increasing rates of cigarette smoking observed in women until the mid-1960s, and so appears to be supportive of the association between cigarette smoking and lung cancer. However, it would also be consistent with an association between certain occupational exposures and lung cancer, as more women in the US are now working outside the home.

Case-control studies

Case-control studies are studies that compare cases with a disease to controls without the disease, looking for differences in antecedent exposures. As an example, one could select cases of young women with venous thromboembolism and compare them to controls without venous thromboembolism,

looking for differences in antecedent oral contraceptive use. Several such studies have been performed, generally demonstrating a strong association between the use of oral contraceptives and venous thromboembolism.

Case-control studies can be particularly useful when one wants to study multiple possible causes of a single disease, as one can use the same cases and controls to examine any number of exposures as potential risk factors. This design is also particularly useful when one is studying a relatively rare disease, as it guarantees a sufficient number of cases with the disease. Using case-control studies, one can study rare diseases with markedly smaller sample sizes than those needed for cohort studies (see Chapter 3). For example, the classic study of diethylstilbestrol and clear cell vaginal adenocarcinoma required only 8 cases and 40 controls, rather than the many thousands of exposed subjects that would have been required for a cohort study of this question.

Case-control studies generally obtain their information on exposures retrospectively, i.e., by recreating events that happened in the past. Information on past exposure to potential risk factors is generally obtained by abstracting medical records or by administering questionnaires or interviews. As such, case-control studies are subject to limitations in the validity of retrospectively collected exposure information. In addition, the proper selection of controls can be a challenging task, and appropriate control selection can lead to a selection bias, which may lead to incorrect conclusions. Nevertheless, when case-control studies are done well, subsequent well-done cohort studies or randomized clinical trials, if any, will generally confirm their results. As such, the case-control design is a very useful approach for pharmacoepidemiologic studies.

Cohort studies

Cohort studies are studies that identify subsets of a defined population and follow them over time, looking for differences in their outcome. Cohort studies generally are used to compare exposed patients to unexposed patients, although they can also be used to compare one exposure to another.

For example, one could compare women of reproductive age who use oral contraceptives to users of other contraceptive methods, looking for the differences in the frequency of venous thromboembolism. When such studies were performed, they in fact confirmed the relationship between oral contraceptives and thromboembolism, which had been noted using analyses of secular trends and case-control studies. Cohort studies can be performed either prospectively, that is simultaneous with the events under study, or retrospectively, that is after the outcomes under study had already occurred, by recreating those past events using medical records, questionnaires, or interviews.

The major difference between cohort and case-control studies is the basis upon which patients are recruited into the study (see Figure 2.2). Patients are recruited into case-control studies based on the presence or absence of a disease, and their antecedent exposures are then studied. Patients are recruited into cohort studies based on the presence or absence of an exposure, and their subsequent disease course is then studied.

Cohort studies have the major advantage of being free of the major problem that plagues case-control studies: the difficult process of selecting an undiseased control group. In addition, prospective cohort studies are free of the problem of the questionable validity of retrospectively collected data. For these reasons, an association demonstrated by a cohort study is more likely to be a causal association than one demonstrated by a case-control study. Furthermore, cohort studies are particularly useful when one is studying multiple possible outcomes from a single exposure, especially a relatively uncommon exposure. Thus, they are particularly useful in postmarketing drug surveillance studies, which are looking at any possible effect of a newly marketed drug. However, cohort studies can require extremely large sample sizes to study relatively uncommon outcomes (see Chapter 3). In addition, prospective cohort studies can require a prolonged time period to study delayed drug effects.

Analysis of case-control and cohort studies

As can be seen in Figure 2.2, both case-control and cohort studies are intended to provide the same basic information; the difference is how this information is collected. The key statistic reported from these studies is the relative risk. The *relative risk* is the ratio of the incidence rate of an outcome in the exposed group to the incidence rate of the outcome in the unexposed group. A relative risk of greater than 1.0 means that exposed subjects have a *greater* risk of the disease under study than unexposed subjects, or that the exposure appears to cause the disease. A relative risk less than 1.0 means that exposed subjects have a *lower* risk of the disease than unexposed subjects, or that the exposure seems to protect against the disease. A relative risk of 1.0 means that exposed subjects and unexposed subjects have the same risk of developing the disease, or that the exposure and the disease appear unrelated.

One can calculate a relative risk directly from the results of a cohort study. However, in a case-control study one cannot determine the size of either the exposed population or the unexposed population that the diseased cases and undiseased controls were drawn from. The results of a case-control study do not provide information on the incidence rates of the disease in exposed and unexposed individuals. Therefore, relative risks cannot be calculated directly from a case-control study. Instead, in reporting the results of a case-control study one generally reports the *odds ratio*, which is a close estimate of the relative risk when the disease under study is relatively rare. Since case-control studies

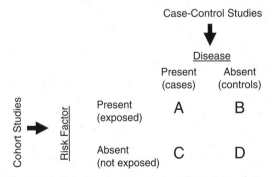

Figure 2.2 Cohort and case-control studies provide similar information, but approach data collection from opposite directions. (Reprinted with permission from Strom BL (1986) Medical databases in post-marketing drug surveillance. *Trends in Pharmacological Sciences* **7**: 377–80.)

are generally used to study rare diseases, there generally is very close agreement between the odds ratio and the relative risk, and the results from case-control studies are often loosely referred to as relative risks, although they are in fact odds ratios.

Both relative risks and odds ratios can be reported with *p-values*. These p-values allow one to determine if the relative risk is statistically significantly different from 1.0, that is whether the differences between the two study groups are likely to be due to random variation or are likely to represent real associations.

Alternatively, and probably preferably, relative risks and odds ratios can be reported with *confidence intervals*, which are an indication of the range of relative risks within which the true relative risk for the entire theoretical population is most likely to lie. As an approximation, a 95% confidence interval around a relative risk means that we can be 95% confident that the true relative risk lies in the range between the lower and upper limits of this interval. If a 95% confidence interval around a relative risk excludes 1.0, then the finding is statistically significant with a p-value of less than 0.05. A confidence interval provides much more information than a p-value, however. As an example, a study that yields a relative risk (95% confidence interval) of 1.0 (0.9–1.1) is clearly showing that an association is very unlikely. A study that yields a relative risk (95% confidence interval) of 1.0 (0.1–100) provides little evidence for or against an association. Yet, both could be reported as a relative risk of 1.0 and a p-value greater than 0.05. As another example, a study that yields a relative risk (95% confidence interval) of 10.0 (9.8–10.2) precisely quantifies a tenfold increase in risk that is also statistically significant. A study that yields a relative risk (95% confidence interval) of 10.0 (1.1–100) says little, other than an increased risk is likely. Yet, both could be reported as a relative risk of 10.0 (p < 0.05). As a final example, a study yielding a relative risk (95% confidence interval) of 3.0 (0.98–5.0) is strongly suggestive of an association, whereas a study reporting a relative risk (95% confidence interval) of 3.0 (0.1–30) would not be. Yet, both could be reported as a relative risk of 3.0 (p > 0.05).

Finally, another statistic that one can calculate from a cohort study is the *excess risk*, also called the risk difference or, sometimes, the attributable risk. Whereas the relative risk is the ratio of the incidence rates in the exposed group versus the unexposed groups, the excess risk is the arithmetic difference between the incidence rates. The relative risk is more important in considering questions of causation. The excess risk is more important in considering the public health impact of an association, as it represents the increased rate of disease due to the exposure. For example, oral contraceptives are strongly associated with the development of myocardial infarction in young women. However, the risk of myocardial infarction in nonsmoking women in their 20s is so low, that even a five-fold increase in that risk would still not be of public health importance. In contrast, women in their 40s are at higher risk, especially if they are cigarette smokers as well. Thus, oral contraceptives should not be as readily used in these women.

As with relative risks, excess risks cannot be calculated from case-control studies, as incidence rates are not available. As with the other statistics, p-values can be calculated to determine whether the differences between the two study groups could have occurred just by chance. Confidence intervals can be calculated around excess risks as well, and would be interpreted analogously.

Randomized clinical trials

Finally, *experimental studies* are studies in which the investigator controls the therapy that is to be received by each participant. Generally, an investigator uses that control to randomly allocate patients between or among the study groups, performing a *randomized clinical trial*. For example, one could theoretically randomly allocate sexually active women to use either oral contraceptives or no contraceptive, examining whether they differ in their incidence of subsequent venous thromboembolism. The major strength of this approach is random assignment, which is the only way to make it likely that the study groups are comparable in potential confounding variables that are either unknown or unmeasurable. For this reason, associations demonstrated in randomized clinical trials are more likely to be causal associations than those demonstrated using one of the other study designs reviewed above.

However, even randomized clinical trials are not without their problems. The randomized clinical trial outlined above, allocating women to receive contraceptives or no contraceptives, demonstrates the major potential problems inherent in the use of this study design. It would obviously be impossible to perform, ethically and logistically. In addition, randomized clinical trials are expensive and artificial. Inasmuch as they have already been performed prior to marketing to demonstrate each drug's efficacy, they tend to be unnecessary after marketing. They are likely to be used in pharmacoepidemiologic studies mainly for supplementary studies of drug efficacy. However, they remain the "gold standard" by which the other designs must be judged. Indeed, with the publication of the results from the Women's Health Initiative indicating that combination hormone replacement therapy causes an increased risk of myocardial infarction rather than a decreased risk, there has been increased concern about reliance solely on nonexperimental methods to study drug safety after marketing, and we are beginning to see the use of massive randomized clinical trials as part of postmarketing surveillance (see Chapter 16).

Discussion

Thus, a series of different study designs are available (Table 2.4), each with respective advantages and disadvantages. Case reports, case series, analyses of secular trends, case-control studies, and cohort studies have been referred to collectively as *observational study designs* or *nonexperimental study designs*, in order to differentiate them from experimental studies. In nonexperimental study designs the investigator does not control the therapy, but simply observes and evaluates the results of ongoing medical care. Case reports, case series, and analyses of secular trends have also been referred to as *descriptive studies*. Case-control studies, cohort studies, and randomized clinical trials all have control groups, and have been referred to as *analytic studies*. The analytic study designs can be classified

Table 2.5 Epidemiologic study designs.

A. Classified by how subjects are recruited into the study
  1. Case-control (case-history, case-referent, retrospective, trohoc) studies
  2. Cohort (follow-up, prospective) studies
    a. Experimental studies (clinical trials, intervention studies)
B. Classified by how data are collected for the study
  1. Retrospective (historical, nonconcurrent, retrolective) studies
  2. Prospective (prolective) studies
  3. Cross-sectional studies

in two major ways, by how subjects are selected into the study and by how data are collected for the study (see Table 2.5). From the perspective of how subjects are recruited into the study, case-control studies can be contrasted with cohort studies. Specifically, case-control studies select subjects into the study based on the presence or absence of a disease, while cohort studies select subjects into the study based on the presence or absence of an exposure. From this perspective, randomized clinical trials can be viewed as a subset of cohort studies, a type of cohort study in which the investigator controls the allocation of treatment, rather than simply observing ongoing medical care. From the perspective of timing, data can be collected *prospectively*, that is simultaneously with the events under study, or *retrospectively*, that is after the events under study had already developed. In the latter situation, one re-creates events that happened in the past using medical records, questionnaires, or interviews. Data can also be collected using *cross-sectional studies*, studies that have no time sense, as they examine only one point in time. In principle, either cohort or case-control studies can be performed using any of these time frames, although prospective case-control studies are unusual. Randomized clinical trials must be prospective, as this is the only way an investigator can control the therapy received.

The terms presented in this chapter, which are those that will be used throughout the book, are probably the terms used by a majority of epidemiologists. Unfortunately, however, other terms have been used for most of these study designs, as well.

Table 2.5 also presents several of the synonyms that have been used in the medical literature. The same term is sometimes used by different authors to describe different concepts. For example, in this book we are reserving the use of the terms "retrospective study" and "prospective study" to refer to a time sense. As is apparent from Table 2.5, however, in the past some authors used the term "retrospective study" to refer to a case-control study and used the term "prospective study" to refer to a cohort study, confusing the two concepts inherent in the classification schemes presented in the table. Other authors use the term "retrospective study" to refer to any nonexperimental study, while others appear to use the term to refer to any study they do not like, as a term of derision! Unfortunately, when reading a scientific paper, there is no way of determining which usage the author intended. What is more important than the terminology, however, are the concepts underlying the terms. Understanding these concepts, the reader can choose to use whatever terminology he or she is comfortable with.

Conclusion

From the material presented in this chapter, it is hopefully now apparent that each study design has an appropriate role in scientific progress. In general, science proceeds from the bottom of Table 2.4 upward, from case reports and case series that are useful for suggesting an association, to analyses of trends and case-control studies that are useful for exploring these associations. Finally, if a study question warrants the investment and can tolerate the delay until results become available, then cohort studies and randomized clinical trials can be undertaken to assess these associations more definitively.

For example, regarding the question of whether oral contraceptives cause venous thromboembolism, an association was first suggested by case reports and case series, then was explored in more detail by analyses of trends and a series of case-control studies. Later, because of the importance of oral contraceptives, the number of women

using them, and the fact that users were predominantly healthy women, the investment was made in two long-term, large-scale cohort studies. This question might even be worth the investment of a randomized clinical trial, except it would not be feasible or ethical. In contrast, when thalidomide was marketed, it was not a major breakthrough; other hypnotics were already available. Case reports of phocomelia in exposed patients were followed by case-control studies and analyses of secular trends. Inasmuch as the adverse effect was so terrible and the drug was not of unique importance, the drug was then withdrawn, without the delay that would have been necessary if cohort studies and/or randomized clinical trials had been awaited. Ultimately, a retrospective cohort study was performed, comparing those exposed during the critical time period to those exposed at other times.

In general, however, clinical, regulatory, commercial, and legal decisions need to be made based on the best evidence available at the time of the decision. To quote Sir Austin Bradford Hill (1965):

> All scientific work is incomplete–whether it be observational or experimental. All scientific work is liable to be upset or modified by advancing knowledge. That does not confer upon us a freedom to ignore the knowledge we already have, or to postpone the action that it appears to demand at a given time.

> Who knows, asked Robert Browning, but the world may end tonight? True, but on available evidence most of us make ready to commute on the 8:30 next day.

Key points

• Many different types of potential biases can create artifactual associations in a scientific study. Among them are: interviewer bias, recall bias, and confounding.
• Four basic types of association can be observed in studies that examine whether there is an association between an exposure and an outcome: no association, artifactual association (from chance or

bias), indirect association (from confounding), or true association.

• A series of criteria can be used to assess the causal nature of an association, to assist in making a subjective judgment about whether a given association is likely to be causal. These are: biological plausibility, consistency, time sequence, specificity, and quantitative strength.

• Study design options, in hierarchical order of progressively harder to perform but more convincing, are: case reports, case series, analyses of secular trends, case-control studies, retrospective cohort studies, prospective cohort studies, and randomized clinical trials.

• Associations between an exposure and an outcome are reported with relative risk ratios (in cohort studies), odds ratios (in case-control studies), confidence intervals, and p-values. Sometimes also as attributable (excess) risk.

Further reading

Bassetti WHC, Woodward M (2004) *Epidemiology: Study Design and Data Analysis*. 2nd ed. Boca Raton, Florida: Chapman & Hall/CRC.

Bhopal RS (2008) *Concepts of Epidemiology: Integrating the Ideas, Theories, Principles and Methods of Epidemiology*. 2nd ed. New York: Oxford University Press.

Fletcher RH, Fletcher SW (2005) *Clinical Epidemiology: The Essentials*. 4th ed. Lippincott Williams & Wilkins.

Friedman G (2003) *Primer of Epidemiology*. 5th ed. New York: McGraw Hill.

Gordis L (2009) *Epidemiology*. 4th ed. Philadelphia, PA: Saunders.

Hennekens CH, Buring JE (1987) *Epidemiology in Medicine*. Boston, MA: Little Brown.

Hill AB (1965) The environment and disease: association or causation? *Proc R Soc Med* **58**: 295–300.

Hulley SB, Cummings SR, Browner WS, Grady D, Newman TB (2006) *Designing Clinical Research: An Epidemiologic Approach*. 3rd ed. Baltimore, MD: Lippincott Williams & Wilkins.

Katz DL (2001) *Clinical Epidemiology and Evidence-based Medicine: Fundamental Principles of Clinical Reasoning and Research*. Thousand Oaks, CA: Sage Publications.

Kelsey JL, Whittemore AS, Evans AS (1996) *Methods in Observational Epidemiology*. 2nd ed. New York: Oxford University Press.

Lilienfeld DE, Stolley P (1994) *Foundations of Epidemiology*. 3rd ed. New York: Oxford University Press.

MacMahon B (1997) *Epidemiology: Principles and Methods*. 2nd ed. Hagerstown MD, Lippincott-Raven.

Mausner JS, Kramer S (1985) *Epidemiology: An Introductory Text*. 2nd ed. Philadelphia, PA: Saunders.

Rothman KJ (2002) *Epidemiology: An Introduction*. New York: Oxford University Press.

Rothman KJ, Greenland S, Lash TL (2008) *Modern Epidemiology*. 3rd ed. Philadelphia, PA: Lippincott Williams & Wilkins.

Sackett DL, Haynes RB, Tugwell P (1991) *Clinical Epidemiology: A Basic Science for Clinical Medicine*. 2nd ed. Boston, MA: Little Brown.

Sackett DL (1979) Bias in analytic research. *J Chronic Dis* **32**: 51–63.

Strom BL (1986) Medical databases in post-marketing drug surveillance. *Trends in Pharmacological Sciences* **7**: 377–80.

Szklo M, Nieto FJ (2006) *Epidemiology: Beyond the Basics*. Sudbury, MA: Jones & Bartlett.

US Public Health Service (1964) *Smoking and Health. Report of the Advisory Committee to the Surgeon General of the Public Health Service*. Washington DC: Government Printing Office, p. 20.

Weiss NS (1996) *Clinical Epidemiology: The Study of the Outcome of Illness*. 2nd ed. New York: Oxford University Press.

Weiss NS, Koepsall T, Koepsell TD (2004) *Epidemiologic Methods: Studying the Occurrence of Illness*. New York: Oxford University Press.

CHAPTER 3

Sample Size Considerations for Pharmacoepidemiologic Studies

Brian L. Strom

Perelman School of Medicine at the University of Pennsylvania, Philadelphia, PA, USA

Introduction

Chapter 1 pointed out that between 500 and 3000 subjects are usually exposed to a drug prior to marketing, in order to be 95% certain of detecting adverse effects that occur in between 1 and 6 in 1000 exposed individuals. While this seems like a reasonable goal, it poses some important problems that must be taken into account when planning pharmacoepidemiologic studies. Specifically, such studies must generally include a sufficient number of subjects to add significantly to the premarketing experience, and this requirement for large sample sizes raises logistical obstacles to cost-effective studies. This central special need for large sample sizes is what has led to the innovative approaches to collecting pharmacoepidemiologic data that are described in Part II of this book.

The approach to considering the implications of a study's sample size is somewhat different depending on whether a study is already completed or is being planned. After a study is completed, if a real finding was statistically significant, then the study had a sufficient sample size to detect it, by definition. If a finding was not statistically significant, then one can use either of two approaches. First, one can examine the resulting confidence intervals in order to determine the smallest differences between the two study groups that the study had sufficient sample size to exclude. Alternatively, one can approach the question in a manner similar to

the way one would approach it if one were planning the study *de novo*. Nomograms can be used to assist a reader in interpreting negative clinical trials in this way.

In contrast, in this chapter we will discuss in more detail how to determine a proper study sample size, from the perspective of one who is designing a study *de novo*. Specifically, we will begin by discussing how one calculates the minimum sample size necessary for a pharmacoepidemiologic study, to avoid the problem of a study with a sample size that is too small. We will first present the approach for cohort studies, then for case-control studies, and then for case series. For each design, one or more tables will be presented to assist the reader in carrying out these calculations.

Sample size calculations for cohort studies

The sample size required for a cohort study depends on what you are expecting from the study. To calculate sample sizes for a cohort study, one needs to specify five variables (see Table 3.1).

The first variable to specify is the *alpha* (α) *or type I error* that one is willing to tolerate in the study. Type I error is the probability of concluding there is a difference between the groups being compared when in fact a difference does not exist. Using diagnostic tests as an analogy, a type I error is a false positive

Textbook of Pharmacoepidemiology, Second Edition. Edited by Brian L. Strom, Stephen E. Kimmel, and Sean Hennessy.

Table 3.1 Information needed to calculate a study's sample size.

For cohort studies	For case–control studies
1. α or type I error considered tolerable, and whether it is one-tailed or two-tailed	1. α or type I error considered tolerable, and whether it is one-tailed or two tailed
2. β or type II error considered tolerable	2. β or type II error considered tolerable
3. Minimum relative risk to be detected	3. Minimum relative risk to be detected
4. Incidence of the disease in the unexposed control group	4. Prevalence of the exposure in the undiseased control group
5. Ratio of unexposed controls to exposed study subjects	5. Ratio of undiseased controls to diseased study subjects

study finding. The more tolerant one is willing to be of type I error, the smaller the sample size required. The less tolerant one is willing to be of type I error, the smaller one would set alpha, and the larger the sample size that would be required. Conventionally the alpha is set at 0.05, although this certainly does not have to be the case. Note that alpha needs to be specified as either one-tailed or two-tailed. If only one of the study groups could conceivably be more likely to develop the disease and one is interested in detecting this result only, then one would specify alpha to be one-tailed. If either of the study groups may be likely to develop the disease, and either result would be of interest, then one would specify alpha to be two-tailed. To decide whether alpha should be one-tailed or two-tailed, an investigator should consider what his or her reaction would be to a result that is statistically significant in a direction opposite to the one expected. For example, what if one observed that a drug increased the frequency of dying from coronary artery disease instead of decreasing it, as expected? If the investigator's response to this would be: "Boy, what a surprise, but I believe it," then a two-tailed test should be performed. If the investigator's response would be: "I don't believe it, and I will interpret this simply as a study that does not show the expected decrease in coronary artery disease in the group treated with the study drug," then a one-tailed test should be performed. The more conservative option is the two-tailed test, assuming that the results could turn out in either direction. This is the option usually, although not always, used.

The second variable that needs to be specified to calculate sample size for a cohort study is the *beta* (β) *or type II error* that one is willing to tolerate in the study. A type II error is the probability of concluding there is no difference between the groups being compared when in fact a difference does exist. In other words, a type II error is the probability of missing a real difference. Using diagnostic tests as an analogy, a type II error is a false negative study finding. The complement of beta is the power of a study, i.e., the probability of detecting a difference if a difference really exists. *Power* is calculated as $(1 - \beta)$. Again, the more tolerant one is willing to be of Type II errors, i.e., the higher the beta, the smaller the sample size required. The beta is conventionally set at 0.1 (i.e., 90% power) or 0.2 (i.e., 80% power), although again this need not be the case. Beta is always one-tailed.

The third variable one needs to specify to calculate sample size is the *minimum effect size* one wants to be able to detect. For a cohort study, this is expressed as a relative risk. The smaller the relative risk that one wants to detect, the larger the sample size required. Note that the relative risk often used by investigators in this calculation is the relative risk the investigator is expecting from the study. This is *not correct*, as it will lead to inadequate power to detect relative risks that are smaller than expected, but still clinically important to the investigator. In other words, if one chooses a sample size that is designed to detect a relative risk of 2.5, one should be comfortable with the thought that, if the actual relative risk turns out to be 2.2, one may not be able to detect it as a statistically significant finding.

In a cohort study one selects subjects based on the presence or absence of an exposure of interest and then investigates the incidence of the disease of interest in each of the study groups. Therefore, the fourth variable one needs to specify is the expected *incidence of the outcome* of interest in the unexposed control group. Again, the more you ask of a study, the larger the sample size needed. Specifically, the rarer the outcome of interest, the larger the sample size needed.

The fifth variable one needs to specify is the *number of unexposed control subjects to be included in the study for each exposed study subject*. A study has the most statistical power for a given number of study subjects if it has the same number of controls as exposed subjects. However, sometimes the number of exposed subjects is limited and, therefore, inadequate to provide sufficient power to detect a relative risk of interest. In that case, additional power can be gained by increasing the number of controls alone. Doubling the number of controls, that is including two controls for each exposed subject, results in a modest increase in the statistical power, but it does not double it. Including three controls for each exposed subject increases the power further. However, the increment in power achieved by increasing the ratio of control subjects to exposed subjects from $2:1$ to $3:1$ is smaller than the increment in power achieved by increasing the ratio from $1:1$ to $2:1$. Each additional increase in the size of the control group increases the power of the study further, but with progressively smaller gains in statistical power. Thus, there is rarely a reason to include greater than three or four controls per study subject. For example, one could design a study with an alpha of 0.05 to detect a relative risk of 2.0 for an outcome variable that occurs in the control group with an incidence rate of 0.01. A study with 2319 exposed individuals and 2319 controls would yield a power of 0.80, or an 80% chance of detecting a difference of that magnitude. With the same 2319 exposed subjects, ratios of control subjects to exposed subjects of $1:1$, $2:1$, $3:1$, $4:1$, $5:1$, $10:1$, and $50:1$ would result in statistical powers of 0.80, 0.887, 0.913, 0.926, 0.933, 0.947, and 0.956, respectively.

It is important to differentiate between the number of controls (as was discussed and illustrated above) and the number of control groups. It is not uncommon, especially in case-control studies, where the selection of a proper control group can be difficult, to choose more than one control group (for example, a group of hospital controls and a group of community controls). This is done for reasons of validity, not for statistical power, and it is important that these multiple control groups not be aggregated in the analysis. In this situation, the goal is to assure that the comparison of the exposed subjects to each of the different control groups yields the same answer, not to increase the available sample size. Accordingly, the comparison of each control group to the exposed subjects should be treated as a separate study, requiring a separate sample size calculation.

Once these five variables have been specified, the sample size needed for a given study can be calculated. Different formulas have been used for this calculation, each of which gives slightly different results. The formula that is probably the most often used is modified from Schlesselman [1974]:

$$N = \frac{1}{[p(1-R)]^2} \left[Z_{1-\alpha} \sqrt{\left(1 + \frac{1}{K}\right) U(1-U)} + Z_{1-\beta} \sqrt{pR(1-Rp) + \frac{p(1-p)}{K}} \right]^2$$

where p is the incidence of the disease in the unexposed, R is the minimum relative risk to be detected, α is the Type I error rate which is acceptable, β is the Type II error rate which is acceptable, $Z_{1-\alpha}$ and $Z_{1-\beta}$ refer to the unit normal deviates corresponding to α and β, K is the ratio of number of unexposed control subjects to the number of exposed subjects, and

$$U = \frac{Kp + pR}{K+1}.$$

$Z_{1-\alpha}$ is replaced by $Z_{1-\alpha/2}$ if one is planning to analyze the study using a two-tailed alpha. Note that K does not need to be an integer.

A series of tables are presented in the Appendix, calculated using this formula. In Tables A1 through

A4 we have assumed an alpha (two-tailed) of 0.05, a beta of 0.1 (90% power), and control-to-exposed ratios of 1 : 1, 2 : 1, 3 : 1, and 4 : 1, respectively. Tables A5 through A8 are similar, except they assume a beta of 0.2 (80% power). Each table presents the number of exposed subjects needed to detect any of several specified relative risks, for outcome variables that occur at any of several specified incidence rates. The total study size will be the sum of exposed subjects (as listed in the table) plus the controls.

For example, what if one wanted to investigate a new nonsteroidal anti-inflammatory drug that is about to be marketed, but premarketing data raised questions about possible hepatotoxicity? This would presumably be studied using a cohort study design and, depending upon the values chosen for alpha, beta, the incidence of the disease in the unexposed population, the relative risk one wants to be able to detect, and the ratio of control to exposed subjects, the sample sizes needed could differ markedly (see Table 3.2). For example, what if your goal was to study hepatitis that occurs, say, in 0.1% of all unexposed individuals? If one wanted to design a study with one control per exposed subject to detect a relative risk of 2.0 for this outcome variable, assuming an alpha (two-tailed) of 0.05 and a beta of 0.1, one could look in Table A1 and see that it would require 31 483 exposed subjects, as well as an equal number of unexposed controls. If one were less concerned with missing a real finding, even if it was there, one could change beta to 0.2, and the required sample size would drop to 23,518 (see Table 3.2 and Table A5). If one wanted to minimize the number of exposed subjects needed for the study, one could include up to four controls for each exposed subject (Table 3.2 and Table A8). This would result in a sample size of 13 402, with four times as many controls, a total of 67,010 subjects. Finally, if one considers it inconceivable that this new drug could *protect* against liver disease and one is not interested in that outcome, then one might use a one-tailed alpha, resulting in a somewhat lower sample size of 10,728, again with four times as many controls. Much smaller sample sizes are needed to detect relative risks of 4.0 or greater; these are also presented in Table 3.2.

In contrast, what if one's goal was to study elevated liver function tests, which, say, occur in 1% of an unexposed population? If one wants to detect a relative risk of 2 for this more common outcome variable, only 3104 subjects would be needed in each group, assuming a two-tailed alpha of 0.05, a beta of 0.1, and one control per exposed subject. Alternatively, if one wanted to detect the same relative risk for an outcome variable that occurred as infrequently as 0.0001, perhaps cholestatic jaundice, one would need 315 268 subjects in each study group.

Obviously, cohort studies can require very large sample sizes to study uncommon diseases. A study of uncommon diseases is often better performed using a case-control study design, as described in the previous chapter.

Sample size calculations for case-control studies

The approach to calculating sample sizes for case-control studies is similar to the approach for cohort studies. Again, there are five variables that need to be specified, the values of which depend on what the investigator expects from the study (see Table 3.1). Three of these are *alpha*, or the type I error one is willing to tolerate; *beta*, or the type II error one is willing to tolerate; and the *minimum odds ratio* (an approximation of the relative risk) one wants to be able to detect. These are discussed in the section on cohort studies, above.

In addition, in a case-control study one selects subjects based on the presence or absence of the disease of interest, and then investigates the prevalence of the exposure of interest in each study group. This is in contrast to a cohort study, in which one selects subjects based on the presence or absence of an exposure, and then studies whether or not the disease of interest develops in each group. Therefore, the fourth variable to be specified for a case-control study is the expected *prevalence of the exposure* in the undiseased control group, rather than the incidence of the disease of interest in the unexposed control group of a cohort study.

Table 3.2 Examples of sample sizes needed for a cohort study.

Disease	Incidence rate assumed in unexposed	α	β	Relative risk to be detected	Control: exposed ratio	Sample size needed in exposed group	Sample size needed in control group
Abnormal liver function tests	0.01	0.05 (2-tailed)	0.1	2	1	3104	3104
	0.01	0.05 (2-tailed)	0.2	2	1	2319	2319
	0.01	0.05 (2-tailed)	0.2	2	4	1323	5292
	0.01	0.05 (1-tailed)	0.2	2	4	1059	4236
	0.01	0.05 (2-tailed)	0.1	4	1	568	568
	0.01	0.05 (2-tailed)	0.2	4	1	425	425
	0.01	0.05 (2-tailed)	0.2	4	4	221	884
	0.01	0.05 (1-tailed)	0.2	4	4	179	716
Hepatitis	0.001	0.05 (2-tailed)	0.1	2	1	31483	31483
	0.001	0.05 (2-tailed)	0.2	2	1	23518	23518
	0.001	0.05 (2-tailed)	0.2	2	4	13402	53608
	0.001	0.05 (1-tailed)	0.2	2	4	10728	42912
	0.001	0.05 (2-tailed)	0.1	4	1	5823	5823
	0.001	0.05 (2-tailed)	0.2	4	1	4350	4350
	0.001	0.05 (2-tailed)	0.2	4	4	2253	9012
	0.001	0.05 (1-tailed)	0.2	4	4	1829	7316
Cholestatic jaundice	0.0001	0.05 (2-tailed)	0.1	2	1	315268	315268
	0.0001	0.05 (2-tailed)	0.2	2	1	235500	235500
	0.0001	0.05 (2-tailed)	0.2	2	4	134194	536776
	0.0001	0.05 (1-tailed)	0.2	2	4	107418	429672
	0.0001	0.05 (2-tailed)	0.1	4	1	58376	58376
	0.0001	0.05 (2-tailed)	0.2	4	1	43606	43606
	0.0001	0.05 (2-tailed)	0.2	4	4	22572	90288
	0.0001	0.05 (1-tailed)	0.2	4	4	18331	73324

Finally, analogous to the consideration in cohort studies of the ratio of the number of unexposed control subjects to the number of exposed study subjects, one needs to consider in a case-control study the *ratio of the number of undiseased control subjects to the number of diseased study subjects.* The principles in deciding upon the appropriate ratio to use are similar in both study designs. Again, there is rarely a reason to include a ratio greater than 3 : 1 or 4 : 1. For example, if one were to design a study with a two-tailed alpha of 0.05 to detect a relative risk of 2.0 for an exposure which occurs in 5% of the undiseased control group, a study with 516 diseased individuals and 516 controls would yield a power of 0.80, or an 80% chance of detecting a difference of that size. Studies with the same 516 diseased subjects and ratios of controls to cases of 1 : 1, 2 : 1, 3 : 1, 4 : 1, 5 : 1, 10 : 1, and 50 : 1 would result in statistical powers of 0.80, 0.889, 0.916, 0.929, 0.936, 0.949, and 0.959, respectively.

The formula for calculating sample sizes for a case-control study is similar to that for cohort studies (modified from Schlesselman, 1974):

$$N = \frac{1}{(p - V)^2} \left[Z_{1-\alpha} \sqrt{\left(1 + \frac{1}{K}\right) U(1 - U)} \right. $$
$$\left. + Z_{(1-\beta)} \sqrt{p(1 - p)/K + V(1 - V)} \right]^2$$

where R, α, β, $Z_{1-\alpha}$, and $Z_{1-\beta}$ are as above, p is the prevalence of the exposure in the control group, and K is the ratio of undiseased control subjects to diseased cases,

$$U = \left(\frac{p}{K + 1} K + \frac{R}{1 + p(R - 1)} \right)$$

and

$$V = \frac{pR}{1 + p(R - 1)}.$$

Again, a series of tables that provide sample sizes for case-control studies is presented in the Appendix. In Tables A9 through A12, we have assumed an alpha (two-tailed) of 0.05, a beta of 0.1 (90% power), and control-to-case ratios of 1 : 1, 2 : 1, 3 : 1, and 4 : 1, respectively. Tables A13 through A16 are similar, except they assume a beta of 0.2 (80% power). Each table presents the number of diseased subjects needed to detect any of a number of specified relative risks, for a number of specified exposure rates.

For example, what if again one wanted to investigate a new nonsteroidal anti-inflammatory drug that is about to be marketed but premarketing data raised questions about possible hepatotoxicity? This time, however, one is attempting to use a case-control study design. Again, depending upon the values chosen of alpha, beta, and so on, the sample sizes needed could differ markedly (see Table 3.3). For example, what if one wanted to

design a study with one control per diseased subject, assuming an alpha (two-tailed) of 0.05 and a beta of 0.1? The sample size needed to detect a relative risk of 2.0 for any disease would vary, depending on the prevalence of use of the drug being studied. If one optimistically assumed the drug will be used nearly as commonly as ibuprofen, by perhaps 1% of the population, then one could look in Table A9 and see that it would require 3210 diseased subjects and an equal number of undiseased controls. If one were less concerned with missing a real association, even if it existed, one could opt for a beta of 0.2, and the required sample size would drop to 2398 (see Table 3.3 and Table A13). If one wanted to minimize the number of diseased subjects needed for the study, one could include up to four controls for each diseased subject (Table 3.3 and Table A16). This would result in a sample size of 1370, with four times as many controls. Finally, if one considers it inconceivable that this new drug could *protect* against liver disease, then one might use a one-tailed alpha, resulting in a somewhat lower sample size of 1096, again with four times as many controls. Much smaller sample sizes are needed to detect relative risks of 4.0 or greater, as presented in Table 3.3.

In contrast, what if one's estimates of the new drug's sales were more conservative? If one wanted to detect a relative risk of 2.0 assuming sales to 0.1% of the population, perhaps similar to tolmetin, then 31 588 subjects would be needed in each group, assuming a two-tailed alpha of 0.05, a beta of 0.1, and one control per diseased subject. In contrast, if one estimated the drug would be used in only 0.01% of the population (i.e., in controls without the study disease of interest), perhaps like phenylbutazone, one would need 315 373 subjects in each study group.

Obviously, case-control studies can require very large sample sizes to study relatively uncommonly used drugs. In addition, each disease of interest requires a separate case group and, thereby, a separate study. As such, as described in the prior chapter, studies of uncommonly used drugs and newly marketed drugs are usually better done using cohort study designs, whereas studies of rare diseases are better done using case-control designs.

Table 3.3 Examples of sample sizes needed for a case–control study.

Hypothetical drug	Prevalence rate assumed in undiseased	α	β	Odds ratio to be detected	Control: case ratio	Sample size needed in case group	Sample size needed in control group
Ibuprofen	0.01	0.05 (2-tailed)	0.1	2	1	3210	3210
	0.01	0.05 (2-tailed)	0.2	2	1	2398	2398
	0.01	0.05 (2-tailed)	0.2	2	4	1370	5480
	0.01	0.05 (1-tailed)	0.2	2	4	1096	4384
	0.01	0.05 (2-tailed)	0.1	4	1	601	601
	0.01	0.05 (2-tailed)	0.2	4	1	449	449
	0.01	0.05 (2-tailed)	0.2	4	4	234	936
	0.01	0.05 (1-tailed)	0.2	4	4	190	760
Tolmetin	0.001	0.05 (2-tailed)	0.1	2	1	31588	31588
	0.001	0.05 (2-tailed)	0.2	2	1	23596	23596
	0.001	0.05 (2-tailed)	0.2	2	4	13449	53796
	0.001	0.05 (1-tailed)	0.2	2	4	10765	43060
	0.001	0.05 (2-tailed)	0.1	4	1	5856	5856
	0.001	0.05 (2-tailed)	0.2	4	1	4375	4375
	0.001	0.05 (2-tailed)	0.2	4	4	2266	9064
	0.001	0.05 (1-tailed)	0.2	4	4	1840	7360
Phenylbutazone	0.0001	0.05 (2-tailed)	0.1	2	1	315373	315373
	0.0001	0.05 (2-tailed)	0.2	2	1	235579	235579
	0.0001	0.05 (2-tailed)	0.2	2	4	134240	536960
	0.0001	0.05 (1-tailed)	0.2	2	4	107455	429820
	0.0001	0.05 (2-tailed)	0.1	4	1	58409	58409
	0.0001	0.05 (2-tailed)	0.2	4	1	43631	43631
	0.0001	0.05 (2-tailed)	0.2	4	4	22585	90340
	0.0001	0.05 (1-tailed)	0.2	4	4	18342	73368

Sample size calculations for case series

As described in Chapter 2, the utility of case series in pharmacoepidemiology is limited, as the absence of a control group makes causal inference difficult. Despite this, however, this is a design that has been used repeatedly. There are scientific questions that can be addressed using this design, and the collection of a control group equivalent in size to the case series would add considerable cost to the study. Case series are usually used in pharmacoepidemiology to quantitate better the incidence of a particular disease in patients exposed to a newly marketed drug. For example, in the "Phase 4" post-marketing drug surveillance study conducted for prazosin, the investigators collected a case series of 10 000 newly exposed subjects recruited through the manufacturer's sales force, to quantitate better the incidence of first dose syncope, which was a well-recognized adverse effect of this drug. Case series are usually used to determine whether a disease occurs more frequently than some predetermined incidence in exposed patients. Most often, the predetermined incidence of interest is zero, and one is looking for any occurrences of an extremely rare illness. As another example, when cimetidine was first marketed, there was a concern over whether it could cause agranulocytosis, since it was closely related chemically to metiamide, another H-2 blocker, which had been removed from the market in Europe because it caused agranulocytosis. This study also collected 10 000 subjects. It found only two cases of neutropenia, one in a patient also receiving chemotherapy. There were no cases of agranulocytosis.

To establish drug safety, a study must include a sufficient number of subjects to detect an elevated incidence of a disease, if it exists. Generally, this is calculated by assuming the frequency of the event in question is vanishingly small, so that the occurrence of the event follows a Poisson distribution, and then one generally calculates 95% confidence intervals around the observed results.

Table A17 in the Appendix presents a table useful for making this calculation. In order to apply this table, one first calculates the incidence rate observed from the study's results, that is the number of subjects who develop the disease of interest during the specified time interval, divided by the total number of individuals in the population at risk. For example, if three cases of liver disease were observed in a population of 1000 patients exposed to a new nonsteroidal anti-inflammatory drug during a specified period of time, the incidence would be 0.003. The number of subjects who develop the disease is the "Observed Number on Which Estimate is Based (n)" in Table A17. In this example, it is three. The lower boundary of the 95% confidence interval for the incidence rate is then the corresponding "Lower Limit Factor (L)"

multiplied by the observed incidence rate. In the example above, it would be $0.206 \times 0.003 = 0.000618$. Analogously, the upper boundary would be the product of the corresponding "Upper Limit Factor (U)" multiplied by the observed incidence rate. In the above example, this would be $2.92 \times 0.003 = 0.00876$. In other words, the incidence rate (95% confidence interval) would be 0.003 (0.000618 − 0.00876). Thus, the best estimate of the incidence rate would be 30 per 10 000, but there is a 95% chance that it lies between 6.18 per 10 000 and 87.6 per 10 000.

In addition, a helpful simple guide is the so-called "rule of threes," useful in the common situation where no events of a particular kind are observed. Specifically, if no events of a particular type (i.e., the events of interest to the study) are observed in a study of X individuals, then one can be 95% certain that the event occurs no more often than 3/X. For example, if 500 patients are studied prior to marketing a drug, then one can be 95% certain that any event which does not occur in any of those patients may occur with a frequency of 3 or less in 500 exposed subjects, or that it has an incidence rate of less than 0.006. If 3000 subjects are exposed prior to drug marketing, then one can be 95% certain that any event which does not occur in this population may occur no more than three in 3000 subjects, or the event has an incidence rate of less than 0.001. Finally, if 10 000 subjects are studied in a postmarketing drug surveillance study, then one can be 95% certain that any events which are not observed may occur no more than three in 10 000 exposed individuals, or that they have an incidence rate of less than 0.0003. In other words, events not detected in the study may occur less often than one in 3333 subjects in the general population.

Discussion

The above discussions about sample size determinations in cohort and case-control studies assume one is able to obtain information on each of the five variables that factor into these sample size calculations. Is this in fact realistic? Four of the variables are, in fact, totally in the control of the investigator, subject to his or her specification: alpha, beta, the ratio of control subjects to study subjects, and the minimum relative risk to be detected. Only one of the variables requires data derived from other sources. For cohort studies, this is the expected incidence of the disease in the unexposed control group. For case-control studies, this is the expected prevalence of the exposure in the undiseased control group. In considering this needed information, it is important to realize that the entire process of sample size calculation is approximate, despite its mathematical sophistication. There is certainly no compelling reason why an alpha should be 0.05, as opposed to 0.06 or 0.04. The other variables specified by the investigator are similarly arbitrary. As such, only an approximate estimate is needed for this missing variable. Often the needed information is readily available from some existing data source, for example vital statistics or commercial drug utilization data sources. If not, one can search the medical literature for one or more studies that have collected these data for a defined population, either deliberately or as a by-product of their data collecting effort, and assume that the population you will study will be similar. If this is not an appropriate assumption, or if no such data exist in the medical literature, one is left with two alternatives. The first, and better, alternative is to conduct a small pilot study within your population, in order to measure the information you need. The second is simply to guess. In the second case, one should consider what a reasonable higher guess and a reasonable lower guess might be, as well, to see if your sample size should be increased to take into account the imprecision of your estimate.

Finally, what if one is studying multiple outcome variables (in a cohort study) or multiple exposure variables (in a case-control study), each of which differs in the frequency you expect in the control group? In that situation, an investigator might base the study's sample size on the variable that leads to the largest requirement, and note that the study will have even more power for the other outcome (or exposure) variables. Regardless, it is usually better to have a somewhat larger than expected sample size than the minimum, to allow some leeway if any of the underlying assumptions were wrong. This also will permit subgroup analyses with adequate power. In fact, if there are important subgroup analyses that represent *a priori* hypotheses that one wants to be able to evaluate, one should perform separate sample size calculations for those subgroups. In this situation, one should use the incidence of disease or prevalence of exposure that occurs in the subgroups, not that which occurs in the general population.

Note that sample size calculation is often an iterative process. There is nothing wrong with performing an initial calculation, realizing that it generates an unrealistic sample size, and then modifying the underlying assumptions accordingly. What is important is that the investigator examines his or her final assumptions closely, asking whether, given the compromises made, the study is still worth undertaking.

Note that the discussion above was restricted to sample size calculations for dichotomous variables, i.e., variables with only two options: a study subject either has a disease or does not have a disease. Information was not presented on sample size calculations for continuous outcome variables, i.e., variables that have some measurement, such as height, weight, blood pressure, or serum cholesterol. Overall, the use of a continuous variable as an outcome variable, unless the measurement is extremely imprecise, will result in a marked increase in the power of a study. Details about this are omitted because epidemiologic studies unfortunately do not usually have the luxury of using such variables. Readers who are interested in more information on this can consult a textbook of sample size calculations.

All of the previous discussions have focused on calculating a minimum necessary sample size. This is the usual concern. However, two other issues specific to pharmacoepidemiology are important to consider as well. First, one of the main advantages of postmarketing pharmacoepidemiologic studies is the increased sensitivity to rare adverse reactions that can be achieved, by including a sample size larger than that used prior to marketing. Since between 500 and 3000 patients are usually studied before marketing, most pharmacoepidemiologic cohort studies are designed to include at least 10 000 exposed subjects. The total population from which these 10 000 exposed subjects would be recruited would need to be very much larger, of course. Case-control studies can be much smaller, but generally need to recruit cases and controls from a source population of equivalent size as for cohort studies. These are not completely arbitrary figures, but are based on the principles described above, applied to the questions which remain of great importance to address in a postmarketing setting. Nevertheless, these figures should not be rigidly accepted but should be reconsidered for each specific study. Some studies will require fewer subjects, many will require more. To accumulate these sample sizes while performing cost-effective studies, several special techniques have been developed, which are described in Part II of this book.

Second, because of the development of these new techniques and the development of large automated data systems (see Chapter 9), pharmacoepidemiologic studies have the potential for the relatively unusual problem of *too large* a sample size. It is even more important than usual, therefore, when interpreting the results of studies that use these data systems to examine their findings, differentiating clearly between statistical significance and clinical significance. With a very large sample size, one can find statistically significant differences that are clinically trivial. In addition, it must be kept in mind that subtle findings, even if statistically and clinically important, could easily have been created by biases or confounders (see Chapter 2). Subtle findings should not be ignored, but should be interpreted with caution.

Key points

• Premarketing studies of drugs are inherently limited in size, meaning larger studies are needed after marketing in order to detect less common drug effects.
• For a cohort study, the needed sample size is determined by specifying the Type I error one is willing to tolerate, the Type II error one is willing to tolerate, the smallest relative risk which one wants to be able to detect, the expected incidence of the outcome of interest in the unexposed control group, and the ratio of the number of unexposed control subjects to be included in the study to the number of exposed study subjects.
• For a case-control study, the needed sample size is determined by specifying the Type I error one is willing to tolerate, the Type II error one is willing to tolerate, the smallest odds ratio which one wants to be able to detect, the expected prevalence of the exposure of interest in the undiseased control group, and the ratio of the number of undiseased control subjects to be included in the study to the number of exposed study subjects.
• As a rule of thumb, if no events of a particular type are observed in a study of X individuals, then one can be 95% certain that the event occurs no more often than $3/X$.

References and further readings

Cohen J (1977) *Statistical Power Analysis for the Social Sciences.* New York: Academic Press.

Gifford LM, Aeugle ME, Myerson RM, Tannenbaum PJ (1980) Cimetidine postmarket outpatient surveillance program. *JAMA* **243**: 1532–5.

Graham RM, Thornell IR, Gain JM, Bagnoli C, Oates HF, Stokes GS. Prazosin (1976) The first dose phenomenon. *BMJ* **2**: 1293–4.

Haenszel W, Loveland DB, Sirken MG (1962) Lung cancer mortality as related to residence and smoking history. I. White males. *J Natl Cancer Inst* **28**: 947–1001.

Joint Commission on Prescription Drug Use (1980) Final Report. Washington, DC.

Makuch RW, Johnson MF (1986) Some issues in the design and interpretation of "negative" clinical trials. *Arch Intern Med* **146**: 986–9.

Schlesselman JJ (1974) Sample size requirements in cohort and case–control studies of disease. *Am J Epidemiol* **99**: 381–4.

Stolley PD, Strom BL (1986) Sample size calculations for clinical pharmacology studies. *Clin Pharmacol Ther* **39**: 489–90.

Young MJ, Bresnitz EA, Strom BL (1983) Sample size nomograms for interpreting negative clinical studies. *Ann Intern Med* **99**: 248–51.

CHAPTER 4

Basic Principles of Clinical Pharmacology Relevant to Pharmacoepidemiologic Studies

Jeffrey S. Barrett and Athena F. Zuppa
Perelman School of Medicine at the University of Pennsylvania, Philadelphia, PA, USA

Pharmacology deals with the study of drugs while *clinical pharmacology* deals with the study of drugs in humans. More specifically, clinical pharmacology evaluates the characteristics, effects, properties, reactions, and uses of drugs, particularly their therapeutic value in humans, including their toxicology, safety, pharmacodynamics, and pharmacokinetics. While the foundation of the discipline is underpinned by basic pharmacology (the study of the interactions that occur between a living organism and exogenous chemicals that alter normal biochemical function), the important emphasis of clinical pharmacology is the application of pharmacologic principles and methods in the care of patients. From the discovery of new target molecules and molecular targets to the evaluation of clinical utility in specific populations, clinical pharmacology bridges the gap between laboratory science and medical practice. The main objective is to promote the safe and effective use of drugs, maximizing the beneficial drug effects while minimizing harmful side effects. It is important that caregivers are skilled in the areas of drug information, medication safety, and other aspects of pharmacy practice related to clinical pharmacology. Clinical pharmacology is an important bridging discipline that includes knowledge about the relationships between: dose and exposure at the site of action (pharmacokinetics); exposure at the site of action

and clinical response (pharmacodynamics); and between clinical response and outcomes. In the process, it defines the therapeutic window (the dosage of a medication between the minimum amount that gives a desired effect and the minimum amount that gives more adverse effects than desired effects) of a drug in various patient populations. Likewise, clinical pharmacology also guides dose modifications in various patient subpopulations (e.g., pediatrics, pregnancy, elderly, and organ impairment) and/or dose adjustments for various lifestyle factors (e.g., food, time of day, drug interactions).

The discovery and development of new medicines is reliant upon clinical pharmacologic research. Scientists in academic, regulatory, and industrial settings participate in this research as part of the overall drug development process. The output from clinical pharmacologic investigation appears in the drug monograph or package insert of all new medicines and forms the basis of how drug dosing information is communicated to healthcare providers.

Clinical pharmacology and pharmacoepidemiology

Pharmacoepidemiology is the study of the use and effects of drugs in large numbers of people.

Textbook of Pharmacoepidemiology, Second Edition. Edited by Brian L. Strom, Stephen E. Kimmel, and Sean Hennessy.
© 2013 John Wiley & Sons, Ltd. Published 2013 by John Wiley & Sons, Ltd.

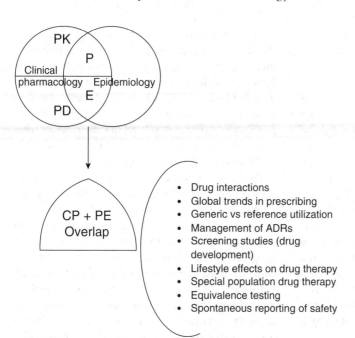

Pharmacoepidemiology borrows from both clinical pharmacology and epidemiology. Thus, pharmacoepidemiology can also be called a bridging science spanning both clinical pharmacology and epidemiology. Part of the task of clinical pharmacology is to provide a risk-benefit assessment for the effect of drugs in patients.

- Drug interactions
- Global trends in prescribing
- Generic vs reference utilization
- Management of ADRs
- Screening studies (drug development)
- Lifestyle effects on drug therapy
- Special population drug therapy
- Equivalence testing
- Spontaneous reporting of safety

Figure 4.1 Relationship between clinical pharmacology and pharmacoepidemiology, illustrating the overlapping areas of interest.

To accomplish this, pharmacoepidemiology borrows from both clinical pharmacology and epidemiology. Thus, pharmacoepidemiology can also be called a bridging science. Part of the task of clinical pharmacology is to provide risk-benefit assessment for the effect of drugs in patients. Studies that estimate the probability and magnitude of beneficial effects in populations, or the probability and magnitude of adverse effects in populations, will benefit from epidemiologic methodology. Pharmacoepidemiology then can also be defined as the application of epidemiologic methods to the content area of clinical pharmacology. Figure 4.1 illustrates the relationship between clinical pharmacology and pharmacoepidemiology as well as some of the specific research areas reliant on both disciplines.

Basics of clinical pharmacology

Clinical pharmacology encompasses drug composition, drug properties, interactions, toxicology, and effects (both desirable and undesirable) that can be used in pharmacotherapy of diseases. Underlying

the discipline of clinical pharmacology are the fields of pharmacokinetics and pharmacodynamics, and each of these disciplines can be further defined by specific subprocesses (absorption, distribution, metabolism, elimination). Clinical pharmacology is essential to our understanding of how drugs work as well as how to guide their administration. Pharmacotherapy can be challenging because of physiologic factors that may alter drug kinetics (age, size, etc.), pathophysiologic differences that may alter pharmacodynamics, disease etiologies in studied patients that may differ from those present in the general population, and other factors that may result in great variation in safety and efficacy outcomes. The challenge is more difficult in the critically ill given the paucity of well-controlled clinical trials in vulnerable populations.

Pharmacokinetics

Pharmacokinetics refers to the study of the absorption and distribution of an administered drug, the chemical changes of the substance in the body (metabolism), and the effects and routes of excretion of the metabolites of the drug (elimination).

Absorption

Absorption is the process of drug transfer from its site of administration to the blood stream. The rate and efficiency of absorption depend on the route of administration. For intravenous administration, absorption is complete; the total dose reaches the systemic circulation. Drugs administered enterally may be absorbed by either passive diffusion or active transport. The *bioavailability* (F) of a drug is the fraction of the administered dose that reaches the systemic circulation. If a drug is administered intravenously, then bioavailability is 100% and F = 1.0. When drugs are administered by routes other than intravenous, the bioavailability is usually less. Bioavailability is reduced by incomplete absorption, first-pass metabolism (defined below), and distribution into other tissues.

Volume of distribution

The *apparent volume of distribution* (Vd) is a hypothetical volume of fluid through which a drug is dispersed. A drug rarely disperses solely into the water compartments of the body. Instead, the majority of drugs disperse to several compartments, including adipose tissue and plasma proteins. The total volume into which a drug disperses if it were only fluid is called the apparent volume of distribution. This volume is not a physiologic space, rather a conceptual parameter. It relates the total amount of drug in the body to the concentration of drug (C) in the blood or plasma: Vd = Drug/C.

Figure 4.2 represents the fate of a drug after intravenous administration. After administration, maximal plasma concentration is achieved, and the drug is distributed. The plasma concentration then decreases over time. This initial alpha (α) phase of drug distribution indicates the decline in plasma concentration due to the distribution of the drug. Once a drug is distributed, it undergoes metabolism and elimination. The second beta (β) phase indicates the decline in plasma concentration due to drug metabolism and clearance. The terms A and B are intercepts with the vertical axis. The extrapolation of the β phase defines B. The dotted line is generated by subtracting the extrapolated line from the original concentration line. This second line defines α and A. The plasma concentration can be

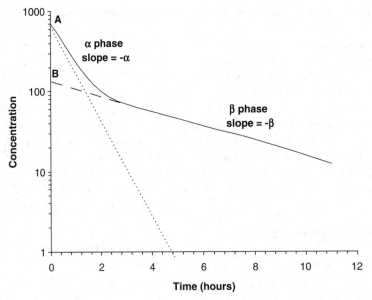

Figure 4.2 Semi-logarithmic plot of concentration vs. time after an intravenous administration of a drug that follows two-compartment pharmacokinetics.

estimated using the formula: $C = Ae^{-\alpha t} + Be^{-\beta t}$. The distribution and elimination half lives can be determined by: $t_{1/2\alpha} = 0.693/\alpha$ and $t_{1/2\beta} = 0.693/\beta$, respectively.

For drugs in which distribution is homogenous across the various physiologic spaces, the distinction between the alpha and beta phase may be subtle and essentially a single phase best describes the decline in drug concentration.

Metabolism

The *metabolism* of drugs is catalyzed by enzymes, and most reactions follow Michaelis Menten kinetics: $V(\text{rate of drug metabolism}) = [((V_{max})(C)/K_m) + (C)]$, where C is the drug concentration, V_{max} is the maximum rate of metabolism in units of amount of product over time, typically $\mu\text{mol/min}$, and K_m is the Michaelis Menten constant (substrate concentration at which the rate of conversion is half of V_{max}) also in units of concentration. In most situations, the drug concentration is much less than K_m and the equation simplifies to: $V = (V_{max})(C)/K_m$. In this case, the rate of drug metabolism is directly proportional to the concentration of free drug, and follows first order kinetic theory. A constant percentage of the drug is metabolized per unit time, and the absolute amount of drug eliminated per unit time is proportional to the amount of drug in the body.

Most drugs used in the clinical setting are eliminated in this manner. A few drugs, such as aspirin, ethanol, and phenytoin, are used in higher doses, resulting in higher plasma concentrations. In these situations, C is much greater than K_m, and the Michaelis Menten equation reduces to: $V(\text{rate of drug metabolism}) = (V_{max})(C)/(C) = V_{max}$. The enzyme system becomes saturated by a high free-drug concentration, and the rate of metabolism is constant over time. This is called zero-order kinetics, and a constant amount of drug is metabolized per unit time. For drugs that follow zero-order elimination, a large increase in serum concentration can result from a small increase in dose.

The liver is the principal organ of drug metabolism. Other organs that display considerable metabolic activity include the gastrointestinal tract,

lungs, skin, and kidneys. Following oral administration, many drugs are absorbed intact from the small intestine and transported to the liver via the portal system, where they are metabolized. This process is called first pass metabolism, and may greatly limit the bioavailability of orally administered drugs. In general, all metabolic reactions can be classified as either phase I or phase II biotransformations. Phase I reactions usually convert the parent drug to a polar metabolite by introducing or unmasking a more polar site. If phase I metabolites are sufficiently polar, they may be readily excreted. However, many phase I metabolites undergo a subsequent reaction in which endogenous substances such as glucuronic acid, sulfuric acid, or an amino acid combine with the metabolite to form a highly polar conjugate. Many drugs undergo these sequential reactions.

Phase I reactions are usually catalyzed by enzymes of the cytochrome P450 system. These drug-metabolizing enzymes are located in the lipophilic membranes of the endoplasmic reticulum of the liver and other tissues. Three gene families, CYP1, CYP2, and CYP3, are responsible for most drug biotransformations. The CYP3A subfamily accounts for greater than 50% of phase I drug metabolism, predominantly by the CYP3A4 subtype. CYP3A4 is responsible for the metabolism of drugs commonly used in the intensive care setting, including acetaminophen, cyclosporine, methadone, midazolam, and tacrolimus. Most other drug biotransformations are performed by CYP2D6 (e.g., clozapine, codeine, flecainide, haloperidol, oxycodone), CYP2C9 (e.g., phenytoin, S-warfarin), CYP2C19 (e.g., diazepam, omeprazole, propranolol), CYP2E1 (e.g., acetaminophen, enflurane, halothane), and CYP1A2 (e.g., acetaminophen, theophylline, warfarin).

Biotransformation reactions may be enhanced or impaired by multiple factors, including age, enzyme induction or inhibition, pharmacogenetics, and the effects of other disease states. Approximately 95% of the metabolism occurs via conjugation to glucuronide (50–60%) and sulfate (25–35%). Most of the remainder of acetaminophen is metabolized via the cytochrome P450 forming N-acetyl-p-benzoquinone imine (NAPQI) thought to be responsible for hepatotoxicity. This minor but important pathway is catalyzed by CYP 2E1, and to a lesser extent, CYP 1A2 and CYP 3A4. NAPQI is detoxified by reacting with either glutathione directly or through a glutathione transferase catalyzed reaction. When hepatic synthesis of glutathione is overwhelmed, manifestations of toxicity appear, producing centrilobular necrosis. In the presence of a potent CYP 2E1 inhibitor, disulfiram, a 69% reduction in the urinary excretion of these 2E1 metabolic products is observed, supporting the major role for 2E1 in the formation of NAPQI. CYP 2E1 is unique among the CYP gene families in an ability to produce reactive oxygen radicals through a reduction of O2 and is the only CYP system strongly induced (drug molecule initiates or enhances the expression of an enzyme) by alcohol which is itself a substrate (a molecule upon which an enzyme acts). In addition to alcohol, isoniazid acts as inducer and a substrate. Ketoconazole and other imidazole compounds are inducers but not substrates. Barbiturates and phenytoin, which are nonspecific inducers, have no role as CYP 2E1 inducers, nor are they substrates for that system. Phenytoin in fact may be hepato-protective because it is an inducer of the glucuronidation metabolic pathway for acetaminophen, thus shunting metabolism away from NAPQI production.

Elimination

Elimination is the process by which drug is removed or "cleared" from the body. Clearance (CL) is the amount of blood from which all drug is removed per unit time (volume/time). The primary organs responsible for drug clearance are the kidneys and liver. The total body clearance is equal to the sum of individual clearances from all mechanisms. Typically, this is partitioned into renal and nonrenal clearance. Most elimination by the kidneys is accomplished by glomerular filtration. The amount of drug filtered is determined by glomerular integrity, the size and charge of the drug, water solubility, and the extent of protein binding. Highly protein-bound drugs are not readily filtered. Therefore, estimation of the glomerular filtration rate (GFR) has traditionally served as an approximation of renal function.

In addition to glomerular filtration, drugs may be eliminated from the kidneys via active secretion. Secretion occurs predominantly at the proximal tubule of the nephron, where active transport systems secrete primarily organic acids and bases. Organic acids include most cephalosporins, loop diuretics, methotrexate, nonsteroidal anti-inflammatories, penicillins, and thiazide diuretics. Organic bases include ranitidine and morphine. As drugs move toward the distal convoluting tubule, concentration increases. High urine flow rates decrease drug concentration in the distal tubule, decreasing the likelihood of diffusion from the lumen. For both weak acids and bases, the nonionized form is reabsorbed more readily. Altering pH can minimize reabsorption, by placing a charge on the drug and preventing diffusion. For example, salicylate is a weak acid. In case of salicylate toxicity, urine alkalinization places a charge on the molecule, and increases its elimination. The liver also contributes to elimination through metabolism or excretion into the bile. After drug is secreted in bile, it may then be either excreted into the feces or reabsorbed via enterohepatic recirculation. The *half-life of elimination* is the time it takes to clear half of the drug from plasma. It is directly proportional to the Vd, and inversely proportional to CL: $t_{1/2\beta} = (0.693)(Vd)/CL$.

Special populations

The term "special populations" as applied to drug development refers to discussions in the early 1990s by industry, academic, and regulatory scientists struggling with the then current practice that early drug development was focused predominantly on young, Caucasian, male populations. Representatives from the US, Europe, and Japan jointly issued regulatory requirements for drug testing and labeling in "special populations" (namely the elderly) in 1993. In later discussions, this generalization was expanded to include four major demographic segments (women, elderly, pediatric, and major ethnic groups); despite the size of each of these subpopulations, pharmaceutical research had been limited. More importantly, these "special populations" represent diverse sub-populations of patients in whom dosing guidance is often needed and likewise targeted clinical pharmacologic research is essential.

Elderly

Physical signs consistent with aging include wrinkles, change of hair color to gray or white, hair loss, lessened hearing, diminished eyesight, slower reaction times, and decreased agility. We are generally more concerned with how aging affects physiologic processes that dictate drug pharmacokinetics and pharmacodynamics. Advancing age is characterized by impairment in the function of the many regulatory processes that provide functional integration between cells and organs. Cardiac structure and function, renal and gastrointestinal systems, and body composition are the physiologic systems most often implicated when pharmacokinetic or pharmacodynamic differences are observed between an elderly and young population. Table 4.1

lists the primary physiologic factors affected by aging.

With respect to absorption, the impact of age is unclear and many conflicting results exist. While many studies have not shown significant age-related differences in absorption rates, the absorption of vitamin B_{12}, iron, and calcium is slower through reduced active transport mechanisms. A reduction in first-pass metabolism is associated with aging, most likely due to a reduction in liver mass and blood flow. Likewise, drugs undergoing significant first-pass metabolism experience an increase in bioavailability with age. This is the case for propranolol and labetalol. Conversely prodrugs requiring activation in the liver (e.g., ACE inhibitors enalapril and perindopril) are likely to experience reduction in this phase and therefore reduced exposure to the active species.

Based on age-related changes in body composition, polar drugs that are primarily water soluble often exhibit smaller volumes of distribution,

Table 4.1 Physiologic systems affected during aging that influence drug pharmacokinetic and/or pharmacodynamic behavior.

Physiologic system	Impact of aging
Cardiac structure and function	• Reduced elasticity and compliance of the aorta and great arteries (higher systolic arterial pressure, increased impedance to left ventricular hypertrophy and interstitial fibrosis)
	• Decrease in rate of myocardial relaxation
	• Left ventricle stiffens and takes longer to relax and fill in diastole
	• Isotonic contraction is prolonged and velocity of shortening reduced
	• Reduction in intrinsic heart rate and increased sinoatrial node conduction time
Renal system	• Renal mass decreases (reduction in number of nephrons)
	• Reduced blood flow in the afferent arterioles in the cortex
	• Renal plasma flow and glomerular filtration rate decline
	• Decrease in ability to concentrate the urine during water deprivation
	• Impaired response to water loading
Gastrointestinal system	• Secretion of hydrochloric acid and pepsin is decreased under basal conditions
	• Reduced absorption of several substances in the small intestine including sugar, calcium and iron
	• Decrease in lipase and trypsin secretion in the pancreas
	• Progressive reduction in liver volume and liver blood flow
Body composition	• Progressive reduction in total body water and lean body mass, resulting in a relative increase in body fat

resulting in higher plasma concentrations in older patients. This is the case for agents including ethanol, theophylline, digoxin, and gentamicin. Conversely, nonpolar compounds are often lipid soluble and exhibit larger volumes of distribution in older patients. The impact of the larger Vd is prolongation of half-life with age. This is the case for drugs such as chlormethiazole and thiopentone. Conflicting results have been reported with respect to age effects on protein binding, making generalizations difficult.

Several drug classes including water-soluble antibiotics, diuretics, water-soluble beta-adrenoceptor blockers, and nonsteroidal anti-inflammatory drugs exhibit changes in clearance with age because of declining renal function. With respect to hepatic metabolism, studies have shown that significant reductions in clearance with age are observed for phase I pathways in the liver.

From the standpoint of a clinical trial, age categories are necessary to define the inclusion and exclusion criteria for the population targeted for enrollment. Pharmaceutical sponsors are increasingly encouraged to include a broader range of ages in their pivotal trials or specifically target an elderly subpopulation in a separate study, consistent with FDA guidance. The FDA guideline for studies in the elderly is directed principally toward new molecular entities likely to have significant use in the elderly, either because the disease intended to be treated is characteristically a disease of aging (e.g., Alzheimer's disease) or because the population to be treated is known to include substantial numbers of geriatric patients (e.g., hypertension).

Pediatrics

As children develop and grow changes in body composition, development of metabolizing enzymes, and maturation of renal and liver function, all affect drug disposition.

Renal

Renal function in the premature and full-term neonate, both glomerular filtration and tubular secretion, is significantly reduced, as compared to older children. Maturation of renal function is a dynamic process that begins during fetal life and is complete by early childhood. Maturation of tubular function

is slower than that of glomerular filtration. The glomerular filtration rate is approximately 2 to 4 mL/minute/1.73 m² in full term neonates, but it may be as low as 0.6 to 0.8 mL/minute/1.73 m² in preterm neonates. The glomerular filtration rate increases rapidly during the first two weeks of life and continues to rise until adult values are reached at 8–12 months of age. For drugs that are renally eliminated, impaired renal function decreases clearance, increasing the half-life. Therefore, for drugs that are primarily eliminated by the kidney, dosing should be performed in an age-appropriate fashion that takes into account both maturational changes in kidney function.

Hepatic

Hepatic biotransformation reactions are substantially reduced in the neonatal period. At birth, the cytochrome p450 system is 28% that of the adult. The expression of phase I enzymes such as the P-450 cytochromes changes markedly during development. CYP3A7, the predominant CYP isoform expressed in fetal liver, peaks shortly after birth and then declines rapidly to levels that are undetectable in most adults. Within hours after birth, CYP2E1 activity increases, and CYP2D6 becomes detectable soon thereafter. CYP3A4 and CYP2C appear during the first week of life, whereas CYP1A2 is the last hepatic CYP to appear, at one to three months of life. The ontogeny of phase II enzymes is less well established than the ontogeny of reactions involving phase I enzymes. Available data indicate that the individual isoforms of glucuronosyltransferase (UGT) have unique maturational profiles with pharmacokinetic consequences. For example, the glucuronidation of acetaminophen (a substrate for UGT1A6 and, to a lesser extent, UGT1A9) is decreased in newborns and young children as compared with adolescents and adults. Glucuronidation of morphine (a UGT2B7 substrate) can be detected in premature infants as young as 24 weeks of gestational age.

Gastrointestinal

Overall, the rate at which most drugs are absorbed is slower in neonates and young infants than in older children. As a result, the time required to achieve maximal plasma levels is longer in the very young. The effect of age on enteral absorption is not uniform and difficult to predict. Gastric emptying and intestinal motility are the primary determinants of the rate at which drugs are presented to and dispersed along the mucosal surface of the small intestine. At birth, the coordination of antral contractions improves, resulting in a marked increase in gastric emptying during the first week of life. Similarly, intestinal motor activity matures throughout early infancy, with consequent increases in the frequency, amplitude, and duration of propagating contractions. Changes in the intraluminal pH in different segments of the gastrointestinal tract can directly affect both the stability and the degree of ionization of a drug, thus influencing the relative amount of drug available for absorption. During the neonatal period, intragastric pH is relatively elevated (>4). Thus, oral administration of acid-labile compounds such as penicillin G produces greater bioavailability in neonates than in older infants and children. In contrast, drugs that are weak acids, such as phenobarbital, may require larger oral doses in the very young in order to achieve therapeutic plasma levels. Other factors that impact the rate of absorption include age-associated development of villi, splanchnic blood flow, changes in intestinal microflora, and intestinal surface area.

Body composition

Age-dependent changes in body composition alter the physiologic spaces into which a drug may be distributed. The percent of total body water drops from about 85% in premature infants to 75% in full-term infants to 60% in the adult. Extracellular water decreases from 45% in the infant to 25% in the adult. Total body fat in the premature infant can be as low as 1%, as compared to 15% in the normal, term infant. Many drugs are less bound to plasma proteins in the neonate and infant than in the older child. Limited data in neonates suggest that the passive diffusion of drugs into the central nervous system is age dependent, as reflected by the progressive increase in the ratios of brain phenobarbital to plasma phenobarbital from 28 to 39 weeks of gestational age, demonstrating the increased transport of phenobarbital into the brain.

Pregnancy

The FDA classifies drugs into five categories of safety for use during pregnancy (normal pregnancy, labor, and delivery). Few well-controlled studies of therapeutic drugs have been conducted in pregnant women. Most information about drug safety during pregnancy is derived from animal studies and uncontrolled assessments (e.g., postmarketing reports).

Observational studies have documented that pregnant women take a variety of medicines during pregnancy. While changes in drug exposure during pregnancy are well documented, a mechanistic understanding of these effects is not clear. The few studies conducted suggest that bioavailability is not altered during pregnancy, though increased plasma volume and protein binding changes can affect the

Table 4.2 FDA categories of drug safety during pregnancy.

Category	Description
A	Controlled human studies show no fetal risks; these drugs are the safest.
B	Animal studies show no risk to the fetus and no controlled human studies have been conducted, or animal studies show a risk to the fetus but well-controlled human studies do not.
C	No adequate animal or human studies have been conducted, or adverse fetal effects have been shown in animals but no human data are available.
D	Evidence of human fetal risk exists, but benefits may outweigh risks in certain situations (e.g., life-threatening disorders, serious disorders for which safer drugs cannot be used or are ineffective).
X	Proven fetal risks outweigh any possible benefit.

apparent volume of distribution of some drugs. Likewise, changes in volume of distribution and clearance during pregnancy can cause increases or decreases in the terminal elimination half-life. Renal excretion of unchanged drugs is increased during pregnancy and hence these agents may require dose increases with pregnancy. Likewise, the metabolism of drugs via select P450-mediated pathways (3A4, 2D6, and 2C9) and UGT isoenzymes are increased during pregnancy, necessitating increased dosages of drugs metabolized by these pathways. In contrast, CYP1A2 and CYP2C19 activity is decreased during pregnancy, suggesting dosing reductions for agents metabolized via these pathways. The effect of pregnancy on transport proteins is unknown. Data are limited; more clinical studies to determine the effect of pregnancy on the pharmacokinetics and pharmacodynamics of drugs commonly used in pregnancy are sorely needed.

Organ impairment

Renal dysfunction
Renal failure can influence the pharmacokinetics of drugs. In renal failure, the binding of acidic drugs to albumin is decreased, because of competition with accumulated organic acids and uremia-induced structural changes in albumin which decrease drug binding affinity, altering the Vd. Drugs that are more than 30% eliminated unchanged in the urine are likely to have significantly diminished CL in the presence of renal insufficiency.

Hepatic dysfunction
Drugs that undergo extensive first-pass metabolism may have a significantly higher oral bioavailability in patients with liver failure than in normal subjects. Gut hypomotility may delay the peak response to enterally administered drugs in these patients. Hypoalbuminemia or altered glycoprotein levels may affect the fractional protein binding of acidic or basic drugs, respectively. Altered plasma protein concentrations may affect the extent of tissue distribution of drugs that normally are highly protein-bound. The presence of significant edema and ascites may alter the Vd of highly water-soluble

agents, such as aminoglycoside antibiotics. The capacity of the liver to metabolize drugs depends on hepatic blood flow and liver enzyme activity, both of which can be affected by liver disease. In addition, some P450 isoforms are more susceptible than others to liver disease, impairing drug metabolism.

Cardiac dysfunction
Circulatory failure, or shock, can alter the pharmacokinetics of drugs frequently used in the intensive care setting. Drug absorption may be impaired because of bowel wall edema. Passive hepatic congestion may impede first-pass metabolism, resulting in higher plasma concentrations. Peripheral edema inhibits absorption by intramuscular parenteral routes. The balance of tissue hypoperfusion versus increased total body water with edema may unpredictably alter Vd. In addition, liver hypoperfusion may alter drug-metabolizing enzyme function, especially flow-dependent drugs such as lidocaine.

Drug interactions
Patients are often treated with more than one (often many) drug, increasing the chance of a drug–drug interaction. Pharmacokinetic interactions can alter absorption, distribution, metabolism, and clearance. Drug interactions can affect absorption through formation of drug–drug complexes, alterations in gastric pH, and changes in gastrointestinal motility. This can have a substantial impact on the bioavailability of enterally administered agents. The volume of distribution may be altered with competitive plasma protein binding and subsequent changes in free drug concentrations.

Biotransformation reactions vary greatly among individuals and are susceptible to drug-drug interactions. Induction is the process by which enzyme activity is increased by exposure to a certain drug, resulting in an increase in metabolism of other drugs and lower plasma concentrations. Common inducers include barbiturates, carbamezapine, isoniazid, and rifampin. In contrast, inhibition is the process by which enzyme activity is decreased by exposure to a certain drug, resulting in a decrease in metabolism of other drugs, and subsequent higher plasma concentrations. Common enzyme inhibitors include ciprofloxacin, fluconazole, metronidazole, quinidine, and valproic acid. Inducers and inhibitors of phase II enzymes have been less extensively characterized, but some clinical applications of this information have emerged, including the use of phenobarbital to induce glucuronyl transferase activity in icteric neonates. Water-soluble drugs are eliminated unchanged in the kidneys. The clearance of drugs that are excreted entirely by glomerular filtration is unlikely to be affected by other drugs. Organic acids and bases are renally secreted, and can compete with one another for elimination, resulting in unpredictable drug disposition.

Pharmacodynamics

Pharmacodynamics characterizes what the drug does to the body (i.e., the effects or response to drug therapy). Pharmacodynamic modeling constructs quantitative relationships of measured, physiological parameters before and after drug administration, with effects defined as the changes in a physiological parameter relative to its pre-dose or baseline value. Baseline refers to un-dosed state and may be complicated in certain situations due to diurnal variations. Efficacy can be defined numerically as the expected sum of all beneficial effects following treatment. In this case, we refer to clinical and not necessarily economic benefits. Similarly, toxicity can be characterized either by the time course of a specific toxic event or the composite of toxic responses attributed to a common toxicity.

Overview

Pharmacodynamic response to drug therapy, i.e., the concentration-effect relationship, evolves only after active drug molecules reach their intended site(s) of action. Hence, the link between pharmacokinetic and pharmacodynamic processes is implicit. Likewise, the respective factors that influence various subprocesses (absorption, distribution, tolerance, etc.) are relevant and may necessitate separate study. Differences among drug entities in

pharmacodynamic time course can be considered as being direct or indirect. A direct effect is directly proportional to concentration at the site of measurement, usually the plasma. An indirect effect exhibits some type of temporal delay, either because of differences between site of action and measurement or because the effect results only after other physiologic or pharmacologic conditions are satisfied.

Direct effect relationships are easily observed with some cardiovascular agents, whose site of action is the vascular space. Pharmacologic effects such as blood pressure, ACE-inhibition, and inhibition of platelet aggregation can be characterized by direct response relationships. Such relationships can usually be defined by three typical patterns—linear, hyperbolic (E_{max}), and sigmoid Emax functions. These are shown in Figure 4.3.

In each case, the plasma concentration and drug concentration at the effect site are proportional. Likewise, the concentration–effect relationship is assumed to be independent of time.

Other drugs exhibit an indirect relationship between concentration and response. In this case, the concentration–effect relationship is time-dependent. One explanation for such effects is hysteresis. Hysteresis refers to the phenomenon where there is a time-lapse between the cause and its effect. With respect to pharmacodynamics, this most often indicates a situation in which there is a delay in equilibrium between plasma drug concentration and the concentration of active substance at the effect site (e.g., thiopental, fentanyl). Three conditions are predominantly responsible for hysteresis: the biophase (actual site of drug action) is not in the central compartment (i.e., plasma or blood compartment); the mechanism of action involves protein synthesis; and/or active metabolites are present. One can conceptualize a hypothetical effect compartment (a physical space where drug concentrations are directly correlated with drug actions) such that the relationships defined in Figure 4.4 are only observed when the effect site concentrations (Ce) are used as opposed to the plasma concentrations (Cp). In this situation, a hysteresis loop is observed when plotting Ce versus Cp.

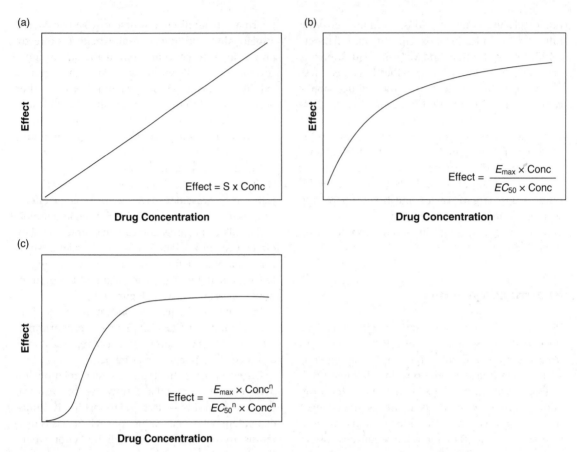

Figure 4.3 Representative pharmacodynamic relationships for drugs which exhibit direct responses: linear, hyperbolic and Sigmoid-E_{max} relationships shown. S is the slope of the linear response; E_{max} refers to the maximum effect observed; EC_{50} refers to the concentration at which 50% of the maximal response is acheved, and n is the degree of sigmoidicity or shape factor (sometimes referred to as the Hill coefficient).

More complicated models (indirect-response models) have been used to express the same observations but typically necessitate a greater understanding of the underlying physiologic process (e.g., cell trafficking, enzyme recruitment, etc.). The salient point is that pharmacodynamic characterization and likewise dosing guidance derived from such investigation stands to be more informative than drug concentrations alone.

Likewise, pharmacodynamics may be the discriminating characteristic that defines dose adjustment in special populations. This is the case for the observed markedly enhanced sensitivity in infants compared with older children and adults with respect to immunosuppressive effects of cyclosporine, and calcium channel blocking effects on the PR interval in the elderly.

Pharmacogenomics

Pharmacogenomics is the study of how an individual's genetic inheritance affects the body's response to drugs. Pharmacogenomics holds the promise that drugs might one day be tailored to individuals and adapted to each person's own genetic makeup. Environment, diet, age, lifestyle, and state of health all can influence a person's response to medicines, but understanding an individual's genetic composition is thought to be the key to creating

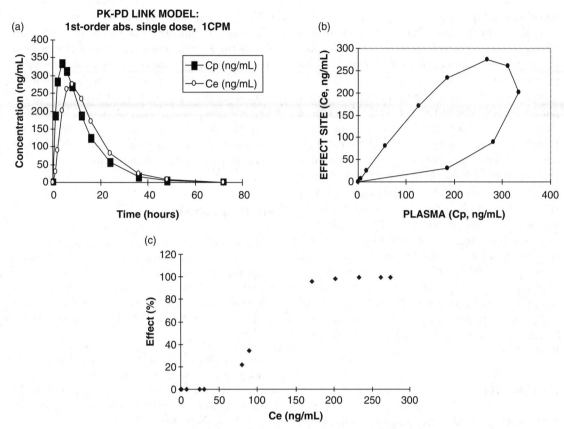

Figure 4.4 Concentration-time, hysteresis, and effect-concentration plots (clockwise order) illustrating the use of an effect compartment to explain observed hysteresis.

personalized drugs with greater efficacy and safety. Pharmacogenomics combines traditional pharmaceutical sciences, such as biochemistry, with comprehensive knowledge of genes, proteins, and single nucleotide polymorphisms. Genetic variations, or SNPs (single nucleotide polymorphisms), in the human genome can be a diagnostic tool to predict a person's drug response. For SNPs to be used in this way, a person's DNA must be sequenced for the presence of specific SNPs. SNP screenings will benefit drug development; those people whose pharmacogenomic screening shows that the drug being tested would be harmful or ineffective for them would be excluded from clinical trials. Prescreening clinical trial subjects might also allow clinical trials to be smaller, faster, and

therefore less expensive. Finally, the ability to assess an individual's reaction to a drug before it is prescribed will increase confidence in prescribing the drug and the patient's confidence in taking the drug, which in turn should encourage the development of new drugs tested in a like manner.

Conclusion

Clinical pharmacology serves an important role in the development of new drugs and the management of pharmacotherapy. In the context of pharmacoepidemiologic investigations, clinical pharmacology also provides a fundamental backbone for understanding the expected associations between drug therapy and clinical benefit as well as potential toxicity. The pharmacoepidemiologist must also have intimate knowledge of clinical pharmacology as the impact (clinical and economic) of a new drug once available to the marketplace can often be forecast based on how the agent's clinical pharmacologic attributes compare to existing therapies. The connection between utilization, compliance, the complexities of multimodal therapy, and the associations of drug behavior with disease- or population-specific indices must be defined relative to the known clinical pharmacologic principles that govern how drugs behave in humans. In an era when more holistic approaches for the care of patients are sought to maintain a healthy overall well-being and avoid chronic and severe disease, clinical strategies are likely to engage more preventative approaches. Likewise, clinical pharmacology and pharmacoepidemiology will be essential disciplines that discriminate strategies that are truly beneficial from those that are not, or are even harmful.

Key points

• There is a great need for caregivers to be skilled in the areas of drug information, medication safety, and other aspects of pharmacy practice related to clinical pharmacology.
• Clinical pharmacology defines the therapeutic window (the dosage of a medication between the minimum amount that gives a desired effect and the minimum amount that gives more adverse effects than desired effects) of a drug in various patient populations and guides dose modifications in various patient subpopulations (e.g., pediatrics, pregnancy, elderly, and organ impairment) and/or dose adjustments for various lifestyle factors (e.g., food, time of day, drug interactions).
• Clinical pharmacology comprises all aspects of the scientific study of medicinal drugs in humans. It can be divided into pharmacokinetics (the relationship between the dose of a drug administered and the serum or blood level achieved) and pharmacodynamics (the study of the relationship between drug level and effect).

• There are many factors that affect an individual's response to a drug. These factors include sex, age, health conditions, concomitant medications, and genetic makeup. An important goal of pharmacoepidemiology is to use population research methods to characterize factors that influence individual drug response.
• Factors that influence individual drug response may do so via pharmacokinetic mechanisms, pharmacodynamic mechanisms, or both.

Further reading

Avorn J (2007) In defense of pharmacoepidemiology– embracing the yin and yang of drug research. *N Engl J Med* **357** (22): 2219–21.

De Vries TP (1993) Presenting clinical pharmacology and therapeutics: a problem based approach for choosing and prescribing drugs. *Br J Clin Pharmacol* **35** (6): 581–6.

Etminan M, Gill S, *et al.* (2006) Challenges and opportunities for pharmacoepidemiology in drug-therapy decision making. *J Clin Pharmacol* **46** (1): 6–9.

Etminan M, Samii A (2004) Pharmacoepidemiology I: a review of pharmacoepidemiologic study designs. *Pharmacotherapy* **24** (8): 964–9.

Evans SJ (2012) An agenda for UK clinical pharmacology Pharmacoepidemiology. *Br J Clin Pharmacol* **73** (6): 973–8.

Guess HA (1991) Pharmacoepidemiology in pre-approval clinical trial safety monitoring. *J Clin Epidemiol* **44** (8): 851–7.

Hartzema AG (1992) Pharmacoepidemiology–its relevance to clinical practice. *J Clin Pharm Ther* **17** (2): 73–4.

Jones JK (1992) Clinical pharmacology and pharmacoepidemiology: synergistic interactions. *Int J Clin Pharmacol Ther Toxicol* **30** (11): 421–4.

Leake CD (1948) Current pharmacology; general principles in practical clinical application. *J Am Med Assoc* **138** (10): 730–7.

Lehmann DF (2000) Observation and experiment on the cusp of collaboration: a parallel examination of clinical pharmacology and pharmacoepidemiology. *J Clin Pharmacol* **40** (9): 939–45.

Lehmann DF (2001) Improving family ties: an examination of the complementary disciplines of pharmacoepidemiology and clinical pharmacology. *Pharmacoepidemiol Drug Saf* **10** (1): 63–8.

Luo X, Cappelleri JC, *et al.* (2007) A systematic review on the application of pharmacoepidemiology in assessing prescription drug-related adverse events in pediatrics. *Curr Med Res Opin* **23** (5): 1015–24.

Royer RJ (1992) Clinical pharmacology and pharmacoepidemiology: future challenges for the European Community. *Int J Clin Pharmacol Ther Toxicol* **30** (11): 449–52.

Suissa S. (1991) Statistical methods in pharmacoepidemiology. Principles in managing error. *Drug Saf* **6** (5): 381–9.

Theodore WH (1990) Basic principles of clinical pharmacology. *Neurol Clin* **8** (1): 1–13.

Tilson HH (1990) Major advances in international pharmacoepidemiology. *Ann Epidemiol* **1** (2): 205–12.

CHAPTER 5

When Should One Perform Pharmacoepidemiologic Studies?

Brian L. Strom

Perelman School of Medicine at the University of Pennsylvania, Philadelphia, PA, USA

As discussed in the previous chapters, pharmacoepidemiologic studies apply the techniques of epidemiology to the content area of clinical pharmacology. This chapter will review when pharmacoepidemiologic studies should be performed. It will begin with a discussion of the various reasons why one might perform pharmacoepidemiologic studies. Central to many of these is one's willingness to tolerate risk. Whether one's perspective is that of a manufacturer, regulator, academician, or clinician, one needs to consider the risk of adverse reactions which one considers tolerable. Thus, this chapter will continue with a discussion of the difference between safety and risk. It will conclude with a discussion of the determinants of one's tolerance of risk.

Reasons to perform pharmacoepidemiologic studies

The decision to conduct a pharmacoepidemiologic study can be viewed as similar to the regulatory decision about whether to approve a drug for marketing or the clinical decision about whether to prescribe a drug. In each case, decision-making involves weighing the costs and risks of a therapy against its benefits.

The main costs of a pharmacoepidemiologic study are obviously the costs (monetary, effort, time) of conducting the study itself. These costs clearly will vary, depending on the questions posed and the approach chosen to answer them. Generally, the cost per patient in a postmarketing study, with the exception of postmarketing randomized clinical trials, is likely to be at least an order of magnitude less than the cost of a premarketing study. Other costs to consider are the opportunity costs of other research that might be left undone if this research is performed.

One risk of conducting a pharmacoepidemiologic study is the possibility that it could identify an adverse outcome as associated with the drug under investigation when in fact the drug does not cause this adverse outcome. Another risk is that it could provide false reassurances about a drug's safety. Both these risks can be minimized by appropriate study designs, skilled researchers, and appropriate and responsible interpretation of the results obtained.

The benefits of pharmacoepidemiologic studies could be conceptualized in four different categories: regulatory, marketing, clinical, and legal (see Table 5.1). Each will be of importance to different organizations and individuals involved in deciding whether to initiate a study. Any given study will usually be performed for several of these reasons. Each will be discussed in turn.

Regulatory

Perhaps the most obvious and compelling reason to perform a postmarketing pharmacoepidemiologic

Textbook of Pharmacoepidemiology, Second Edition. Edited by Brian L. Strom, Stephen E. Kimmel, and Sean Hennessy.
© 2013 John Wiley & Sons, Ltd. Published 2013 by John Wiley & Sons, Ltd.

Table 5.1 Reasons to perform pharmacoepidemiologic studies.

A. Regulatory
   1. Required
   2. To obtain earlier approval for marketing
   3. As a response to question by regulatory agency
   4. To assist application for approval for marketing elsewhere
B. Marketing
   1. To assist market penetration by documenting the safety of the drug
   2. To increase name recognition
   3. To assist in re-positioning the drug
      a. Different outcomes, e.g., quality of life and economic
      b. Different types of patients, e.g., the elderly
      c. New indications
      d. Less restrictive labeling
   4. To protect the drug from accusations about adverse effects
C. Legal
   1. In anticipation of future product liability litigation
D. Clinical
   1. Hypothesis testing
      a. Problem hypothesized on the basis of drug structure
      b. Problem suspected on the basis of preclinical or premarketing human data
      c. Problem suspected on the basis of spontaneous reports
      d. Need to better quantitate the frequency of adverse reactions
   2. Hypothesis generating–need depends on whether:
      a. it is a new chemical entity
      b. the safety profile of the class
      c. the relative safety of the drug within its class
      d. the formulation
      e. the disease to be treated, including
         i. its duration
         ii. its prevalence
         iii. its severity
         iv. whether alternative therapies are available

---

study is regulatory: a plan for a postmarketing pharmacoepidemiologic study is required before the drug will be approved for marketing. Requirements for postmarketing research have become progressively more frequent in recent years. For example, in the 1970s the FDA required postmarketing research at the time of approval for about one-third of drugs, a requirement which increased to over 70% in the 1990s. Many of these required studies have been randomized clinical trials, designed to clarify residual questions about a drug's efficacy. Others focus on questions of drug toxicity. Often it is unclear whether the pharmacoepidemiologic study was undertaken in response to a regulatory requirement or in response to merely a "suggestion" by the regulator, but the effect is essentially the same. Early examples of studies conducted to address regulatory questions include the "Phase IV" cohort studies performed of cimetidine and prazosin. These are discussed more in Chapters 1 and 2. Now that FDA has the authority to require such studies, such requirements are likely to get even more common.

Sometimes a manufacturer may offer to perform a pharmacoepidemiologic study with the hope that the regulatory agency might thereby approve the drug's earlier marketing. If the agency believed that any new serious problem would be detected rapidly and reliably after marketing, it could feel more comfortable about releasing the drug sooner. Although it is difficult to assess the impact of volunteered postmarketing studies on regulatory decisions, the very large economic impact of an earlier approval has motivated some manufacturers to initiate such studies. In addition, in recent years regulatory authorities have occasionally released a particularly important drug after essentially only Phase II testing, with the understanding that additional data would be gathered during postmarketing testing. For example, zidovudine was released for marketing after only limited testing, and only later were additional data gathered on both safety and efficacy, data which indicated, among other things, that the doses initially recommended were too large.

Some postmarketing studies of drugs arise in response to case reports of adverse reactions reported to the regulatory agency. One response to such a report might be to suggest a labeling change. Often a more appropriate response, clinically and commercially, would be to propose a pharmacoepidemiologic study. This study would explore whether this adverse event in fact occurs more often in those exposed to the drug than would have been expected in the absence of the drug and, if so, how large is the increased risk of the disease. As an example, a Medicaid database was used to study hypersensitivity reactions to tolmetin, following reports about this problem to the FDA's Spontaneous Reporting System.

Finally, drugs are obviously marketed at different times in different countries. A postmarketing pharmacoepidemiologic study conducted in a country which marketed a drug relatively early could be useful in demonstrating the safety of the drug to regulatory agencies in countries which have not yet permitted the marketing of the drug. This is becoming increasingly feasible, as both the industry and the field of pharmacoepidemiology are becoming more international, and regulators are collaborating more.

Marketing

As will be discussed below, pharmacoepidemiologic studies are performed primarily to obtain the answers to clinical questions. However, it is clear that a major underlying reason for some pharmacoepidemiologic studies is the potential marketing impact of those answers. In fact, some companies make the marketing branch of the company responsible for pharmacoepidemiology, rather than the medical branch.

Because of the known limitations in the information available about the effects of a drug at the time of its initial marketing, many physicians are appropriately hesitant to prescribe a drug until a substantial amount of experience in its use has been gathered. A formal postmarketing surveillance study can speed that process, as well as clarifying any advantages or disadvantages a drug has compared to its competitors.

A pharmacoepidemiologic study can also be useful to improve product name recognition. The fact that a study is underway will often be known to prescribers, as will its results once it is publicly presented and published. This increased name recognition will presumably help sales. An increase in a product's name recognition is likely to result particularly from pharmacoepidemiologic studies that recruit subjects for the study via prescribers. However, while this technique can be useful in

selected situations, it is extremely expensive and less likely to be productive of scientifically useful information than most other alternatives available. In particular, the conduct of a purely marketing exercise under the guise of a postmarketing surveillance study, not designed to collect useful scientific information, is to be condemned. It is misleading and could endanger the performance of future scientifically useful studies, by resulting in prescribers who are disillusioned and, thereby, reluctant to participate in future studies.

Pharmacoepidemiologic studies can also be useful to re-position a drug that is already on the market, i.e., to develop new markets for the drug. One could explore different types of outcomes resulting from the use of the drug for the approved indication, for example the impact of the drug on the cost of medical care (see Chapter 17) and on patients' quality-of-life (see Chapter 18). One could also explore the use of the drug for the approved indication in types of patients other than those included in premarketing studies, for example in children or in the elderly. By exploring unintended beneficial effects, or even drug efficacy, one could obtain clues to and supporting information for new indications for drug use. Finally, whether because of questions about efficacy or questions about toxicity, drugs are sometimes approved for initial marketing with restrictive labeling. For example, bretylium was initially approved for marketing in the US only for the treatment of life-threatening arrhythmias. Approval for more widespread use requires additional data. These data can often be obtained from pharmacoepidemiologic studies.

Finally, and perhaps most importantly, pharmacoepidemiologic studies can be useful to protect the major investment made in developing and testing a new drug. When a question arises about a drug's toxicity, it often needs an immediate answer, or else the drug may lose market share or even be removed from the market. Immediate answers are often unavailable, unless the manufacturer had the foresight to perform pharmacoepidemiologic studies in anticipation of this problem. Sometimes these problems can be specifically foreseen and addressed. More commonly, they are not.

However, the availability of an existing cohort of exposed patients and a control group will often allow a much more rapid answer than would have been possible if the study had to be conducted *de novo*. One example of this is provided by the experience of Pfizer Pharmaceuticals, when the question arose about whether piroxicam (Feldene) was more likely to cause deaths in the elderly from gastrointestinal bleeding than the other non-steroidal anti-inflammatory drugs. Although Pfizer did not fund studies in anticipation of such a question, it was fortunate that several pharmacoepidemiologic research groups had data available on this question because of other studies that they had performed. McNeil was not as fortunate when questions were raised about anaphylactic reactions caused by zomepirac. If the data they eventually were able to have had been available at the time of the crisis, they might not have removed the drug from the market. Later, Syntex recognized the potential benefit, and the risk, associated with the marketing of parenteral ketorolac, and chose to initiate a postmarketing surveillance cohort study at the time of the drug's launch. Indeed, the drug was accused of multiple different adverse outcomes, and it was only the existence of this study, and its subsequently published results, that saved the drug in its major markets.

Legal

Postmarketing surveillance studies can theoretically be useful as legal prophylaxis, in anticipation of eventually having to defend against product liability suits (see Chapter 6). One often hears the phrase "What you don't know, won't hurt you." However, in pharmacoepidemiology this view is shortsighted and, in fact, very wrong. All drugs cause adverse effects; the regulatory decision to approve a drug and the clinical decision to prescribe a drug both depend on a judgment about the relative balance between the benefits of a drug and its risks. From a legal perspective, to win a product liability suit using a legal theory of negligence, a plaintiff must prove causation, damages, and negligence. A pharmaceutical manufacturer that is a defendant in such a suit cannot change whether its drug causes an adverse effect. If the drug does, this will presumably be detected at some point. The manufacturer also cannot change whether the plaintiff suffered legal damages from the adverse effect, that is whether the plaintiff suffered a disability or incurred expenses resulting from a need for medical attention. However, even if the drug did cause the adverse outcome in question, a manufacturer certainly can document that it was performing state-of-the-art studies to attempt to detect whatever toxic effects the drug had. In addition, such studies could make easier the defense of totally groundless suits, in which a drug is blamed for producing adverse reactions it does not cause.

Clinical

Hypothesis testing

The major reason for most pharmacoepidemiologic studies is hypothesis testing. The hypotheses to be tested can be based on the structure or the chemical class of a drug. For example, the cimetidine study mentioned above was conducted because cimetidine was chemically related to metiamide, which had been removed from the market in Europe because it caused agranulocytosis. Alternatively, hypotheses can also be based on premarketing or postmarketing animal or clinical findings. For example, the hypotheses can come from spontaneous reports of adverse events experienced by patients taking the drug in question. The tolmetin, piroxicam, zomepirac, and ketorolac questions mentioned above are all examples of this. Finally, an adverse effect may clearly be due to a drug, but a study may be needed to quantitate its frequency. An example would be the postmarketing surveillance study of prazosin, performed to quantitate the frequency of first dose syncope. Of course, the hypotheses to be tested can involve beneficial drug effects as well as harmful drug effects, subject to some important methodological limitations.

Hypothesis generating

Hypothesis generating studies are intended to screen for previously unknown and unsuspected drug effects. In principle, all drugs could, and perhaps should, be subjected to such studies. However, some drugs may require these studies more than others. This has been the focus of a formal study, which surveyed experts in pharmacoepidemiology.

For example, it is generally agreed that new chemical entities are more in need of study than so-called "me too" drugs. This is because the lack of experience with related drugs makes it more likely that the new drug has possibly important unsuspected effects.

The safety profile of the class of drugs should also be important to the decision about whether to conduct a formal screening postmarketing surveillance study for a new drug. Previous experience with other drugs in the same class can be a useful predictor of what the experience with the new drug in question is likely to be. For example, with the finding that troglitazone had an increased risk of liver disease, that became a concern as well with the later thiazolidinediones, i.e., pioglitazone and rosiglitazone. Similarly, with the finding that rofecoxib was associated with myocardial infarction, that became a concern as well with celecoxib.

The relative safety of the drug within its class can also be helpful. A drug that has been studied in large numbers of patients before marketing and appears safe relative to other drugs within its class is less likely to need supplementary postmarketing surveillance studies. An extension of this approach, of course, is comparative effectiveness research (see Chapter 22).

The formulation of the drug can be considered a determinant of the need for formal screening pharmacoepidemiologic studies. A drug that will, because of its formulation, be used mainly in institutions, where there is close supervision, may be less likely to need such a study. When a drug is used under these conditions, any serious adverse effect is likely to be detected, even without any formal study.

The disease to be treated is an important determinant of whether a drug needs additional postmarketing surveillance studies. Drugs used to treat chronic illnesses are likely to be used for a long period of time. As such, it is important to know their long-term effects. This cannot be addressed adequately in the relatively brief time available for each premarketing study. Also, drugs used to treat

common diseases are important to study, as many patients are likely to be exposed to these drugs. Drugs used to treat mild or self-limited diseases also need careful study, because serious toxicity is less acceptable. This is especially true for drugs used by healthy individuals, such as contraceptives. On the other hand, when one is using a drug to treat individuals who are very ill, one is more tolerant of toxicity, assuming the drug is efficacious.

Finally, it is also important to know whether alternative therapies are available. If a new drug is not a major therapeutic advance, since it will be used to treat patients who would have been treated with the old drug, one needs to be more certain of its relative advantages and disadvantages. The presence of significant adverse effects, or the absence of beneficial effects, is less likely to be tolerated for a drug that does not represent a major therapeutic advance.

Safety versus risk

Clinical pharmacologists are used to thinking about drug "safety": the statutory standard that must be met before a drug is approved for marketing in the US is that it needs to be proven to be "safe and effective under conditions of intended use." It is important, however, to differentiate safety from risk. Virtually nothing is without some risks. Even staying in bed is associated with a risk of acquiring bed sores! Certainly no drug is completely safe. Yet, the unfortunate misperception by the public persists that drugs mostly are and should be without any risk at all. Use of a "safe" drug, however, still carries some risk. It would be better to think in terms of *degrees of safety*. Specifically, a drug "is safe if its risks are judged to be acceptable." Measuring risk is an objective but probabilistic pursuit. A judgment about safety is a personal and/or social value judgment about the acceptability of that risk. Thus, assessing safety requires two extremely different kinds of activities: measuring risk and judging the acceptability of those risks. The former is the focus of much of pharmacoepidemiology and most of this book. The latter is the focus of the following discussion.

Table 5.2 Factors affecting the acceptability of risks.

A. Features of the adverse outcome
   1. Severity
   2. Reversibility
   3. Frequency
   4. "Dread disease"
   5. Immediate versus delayed
   6. Occurs in all people versus just in sensitive people
   7. Known with certainty or not

B. Characteristics of the exposure
   1. Essential versus optional
   2. Present versus absent
   3. Alternatives available
   4. Risk assumed voluntarily
   5. Drug use will be as intended versus misuse is likely

C. Perceptions of the evaluator

Risk tolerance

Whether or not to conduct a postmarketing surveillance pharmacoepidemiologic study also depends on one's willingness to tolerate risk. From a manufacturer's perspective, one can consider this risk in terms of the risk of a potential regulatory or legal problem that may arise. Whether one's perspective is that of a manufacturer, regulator, academician, or clinician, one needs to consider the risk of adverse reactions that one is willing to accept as tolerable. There are several factors that can affect one's willingness to tolerate the risk of adverse effects from drugs (see Table 5.2). Some of these factors are related to the adverse outcome being studied. Others are related to the exposure and the setting in which the adverse outcome occurs.

Features of the adverse outcome

The severity and reversibility of the adverse reaction in question are of paramount importance to its tolerability. An adverse reaction that is severe is much less tolerable than one that is mild, even at the same incidence. This is especially true for adverse reactions that result in permanent harm, for example birth defects.

Another critical factor that affects the tolerability of an adverse outcome is the frequency of the adverse outcome in those who are exposed. Notably, this is *not* a question of the relative risk of the

disease due to the exposure, but a question of the excess risk (see Chapter 2). Use of tampons is extraordinarily strongly linked to toxic shock: prior studies have shown relative risks between 10 and 20. However, toxic shock is sufficiently uncommon, that even a 10–20-fold increase in the risk of the disease still contributes an extraordinarily small risk of the toxic shock syndrome in those who use tampons.

In addition, the particular disease caused by the drug is important to one's tolerance of its risks. Certain diseases are considered by the public to be so-called "dread diseases," diseases that generate more fear and emotion than other diseases. Examples are AIDS and cancer. It is less likely that the risk of a drug will be considered acceptable if it causes one of these diseases.

Another relevant factor is whether the adverse outcome is immediate or delayed. Most individuals are less concerned about delayed risks than immediate risks. This is one of the factors that have probably slowed the success of anti-smoking efforts. In part this is a function of denial; delayed risks seem as if they may never occur. In addition, an economic concept of "discounting" plays a role here. An adverse event in the future is less bad than the same event today, and a beneficial effect today is better than the same beneficial effect in the future. Something else may occur between now and then, which could make that delayed effect irrelevant or, at least, mitigate its impact. Thus, a delayed adverse event may be worth incurring if it can bring about beneficial effects today.

It is also important whether the adverse outcome is a Type A reaction or a Type B reaction. As described in Chapter 1, Type A reactions are the result of an exaggerated but otherwise usual pharmacological effect of a drug. Type A reactions tend to be common, but they are dose-related, predictable, and less serious. In contrast, Type B reactions are aberrant effects of a drug. Type B reactions tend to be uncommon, are not related to dose, and are potentially more serious. They may be due to hypersensitivity reactions, immunologic reactions, or some other idiosyncratic reaction to the drug. Regardless, Type B reactions are the more difficult to predict or even detect. If one can predict an adverse effect, then one can attempt to prevent it. For example, in order to prevent aminophylline-induced arrhythmias and seizures, one can begin therapy at lower doses and follow serum levels carefully. For this reason, all other things being equal, Type B reactions are usually considered less tolerable.

Finally, the acceptability of a risk also varies according to how well established it is. The same adverse effect is obviously less tolerable if one knows with certainty that it is caused by a drug than if it is only a remote possibility.

Characteristics of the exposure

The acceptability of a risk is very different, depending upon whether an exposure is essential or optional. Major adverse effects are much more acceptable when one is using a therapy that can save or prolong life, such as chemotherapy for malignancies. On the other hand, therapy for self-limited illnesses must have a low risk to be acceptable. Pharmaceutical products intended for use in healthy individuals, such as vaccines and contraceptives, must be exceedingly low in risk to be considered acceptable.

The acceptability of a risk is also dependent on whether the risk is from the presence of a treatment or its absence. One could conceptualize deaths from a disease that can be treated by a drug that is not yet on the market as an adverse effect from the absence of treatment. For example, the six-year delay in introducing beta-blockers into the US market has been blamed for resulting in more deaths than all recent adverse drug reactions combined. As a society, we are much more willing to accept risks of this type than risks from the use of a drug that has been marketed prematurely. Physicians are taught *primum non nocere*–first do no harm. This is somewhat analogous to our willingness to allow patients with terminal illnesses to die from these illnesses without intervention, while it would be considered unethical and probably illegal to perform euthanasia. In general, we are much more tolerant of sins of omission than sins of commission.

Whether any alternative treatments are available is another determinant of the acceptability of risks. If a drug is the only available treatment for a disease, particularly a serious disease, then greater risks

will be considered acceptable. This was the reason zidovudine was allowed to be marketed for treatment of AIDS, despite its toxicity and the limited testing which had been performed. Analogously, studies of toxic shock syndrome associated with the use of tampons were of public health importance, despite the infrequency of the disease, because consumers could choose among other available tampons that were shown to carry different risks.

Whether a risk is assumed voluntarily is also important to its acceptability. We are willing to accept the risk of death in automobile accidents more than the much smaller risk of death in airline accidents, because we control and understand the former and accept the attendant risk voluntarily. Some people even accept the enormous risks of death from tobacco-related disease, but would object strongly to being given a drug that was a small fraction as toxic. In general, it is agreed that patients should be made aware of possibly toxic effects of drugs that they are prescribed. When a risk is higher than it is with the usual therapeutic use of a drug, as with an invasive procedure or an investigational drug, one usually asks the patient for formal informed consent. The fact that fetuses cannot make voluntary choices about whether or not to take a drug contributes to the unacceptability of drug-induced birth defects.

Finally, from a societal perspective, one also needs to be concerned about whether a drug will be and is used as intended or whether misuse is likely. Misuse, in and of itself, can represent a risk of the drug. For example, a drug is considered less acceptable if it is addicting and, so, is likely to be abused. In addition, the potential for over-prescribing by physicians can also decrease the acceptability of the drug. For example, in the controversy about birth defects from isotretinoin, there was no question that the drug was a powerful teratogen, and that it was a very effective therapy for serious cystic acne refractory to other treatments. There also was no question about its effectiveness for less severe acne. However, that effectiveness led to its widespread use, including in individuals who could have been treated with less toxic therapies, and a larger number of pregnancy exposures, abortions, and birth defects than otherwise would have occurred.

Perceptions of the evaluator

Finally, much depends ultimately upon the perceptions of the individuals who are making the decision about whether a risk is acceptable. In the US, there have been more than a million deaths from traffic accidents over the past 30 years; tobacco-related diseases kill the equivalent of three jumbo jet loads every day; and 3000 children are born each year with embryopathy from their mothers' use of alcohol in pregnancy. Yet, these deaths are accepted with little concern, while the uncommon

Table 5.3 Annual risks of death from some selected hazards.

Hazard	Annual death rate (per 100,000 exposed individuals)
Heart disease (US, 1985)	261.4
Sport parachuting	190
Cancer (US, 1985)	170.5
Cigarette smoking (age 35)	167
Hang gliding (UK)	150
Motorcycling (US)	100
Power boat racing (US)	80
Cerebrovascular disease (US, 1985)	51.0
Scuba diving (US)	42
Scuba diving (UK)	22
Influenza (UK)	20
Passenger in motor vehicle (US)	16.7
Suicide (US, 1985)	11.2
Homicide (US, 1985)	7.5
Cave exploration (US)	4.5
Oral contraceptive user (age 25–34)	4.3
Pedestrian (US)	3.8
Bicycling (US)	1.1
Tornados (US)	0.2
Lightning (US)	0.05

Source: data derived from O'Brien (1986), Silverberg and Lubera (1988), and Urquhart and Heilmann (1984).

risk of an airplane crash or being struck by lightning generate fear. The decision about whether to allow isotretinoin to remain on the market hinged on whether the efficacy of the drug for a small number of people who had a disease which was disfiguring but not life-threatening was worth the birth defects that would result in some other individuals. There is no way to remove this subjective component from the decision about the acceptability of risks. Indeed, much more research is needed to elucidate patients' preferences in these matters. However, this subjective component is part of what makes informed consent so important. Most people feel that the final subjective judgment about whether an individual should assume the risk of ingesting a drug should be made by that individual, after education by their physician. However, as an attempt to assist that judgment, it is useful to have some quantitative information about the risks inherent in some other activities. Some such information is presented in Table 5.3.

Conclusion

This chapter reviewed when pharmacoepidemiologic studies should be performed. After beginning with a discussion of the various reasons why one might perform pharmacoepidemiologic studies, it reviewed the difference between safety and risk. It concluded with a discussion of the determinants of one's tolerance of risk. Now that it is hopefully clear when one might want to perform a pharmacoepidemiologic study, the next sections of this book will provide perspectives on pharmacoepidemiology from some of the different fields that use it.

Key points

• The decision to conduct a pharmacoepidemiologic study can be viewed as similar to the regulatory decision about whether to approve a drug for marketing or the clinical decision about whether to prescribe a drug. In each case, decision making involves weighing the costs and risks of a therapy against its benefits.

• The main costs of a pharmacoepidemiologic study are: the costs (monetary, effort, time) of conducting the study itself, the opportunity costs of other research that might be left undone if this research is performed, the possibility that it could identify an adverse outcome as associated with the drug under investigation when in fact the drug does not cause this adverse outcome, and that it could provide false reassurances about a drug's safety.

• The benefits of pharmacoepidemiologic studies could be conceptualized in four different categories: regulatory, marketing, legal, and clinical. Each will be of importance to different organizations and individuals involved in deciding whether to initiate a study. Any given study will usually be performed for several of these reasons.

• There are several factors that can affect one's willingness to tolerate the risk of adverse effects from drugs. Some of these factors are related to the adverse outcome being studied. Others are related to the exposure and the setting in which the adverse outcome occurs.

Further reading

Binns TB (1987) Therapeutic risks in perspective. *Lancet* **2**: 208–9.

Bortnichak EA, Sachs RM (1986) Piroxicam in recent epidemiologic studies. *Am J Med* **81**: 44–8.

Feldman HI, Kinman JL, Berlin JA, Hennessy S, Kimmel SE, Farrar J *et al.* (1997) Parenteral ketorolac: the risk for acute renal failure. *Ann Intern Med* **126**: 193–9.

Hennessy S, Kinman JL, Berlin JA, Feldman HI, Carson JL, Kimmel SE *et al.* (1997) Lack of hepatotoxic effects of parenteral ketorolac in the hospital setting. *Arch Intern Med* **157**: 2510–14.

Humphries TJ, Myerson RM, Gifford LM *et al.* (1984) A unique postmarket outpatient surveillance program of cimetidine: report on phase II and final summary. *Am J Gastroenterol* **79**: 593–6.

Joint Commission on Prescription Drug Use (1980) *Final Report*. Washington, DC.

Lowrance WW (1976) *Of Acceptable Risk*. Los Altos, CA: William Kaufmann.

Marwick C (1988) FDA ponders approaches to curbing adverse effects of drug used against cystic acne. *JAMA* **259**: 3225.

Mattison N, Richard BW (1987) Postapproval research requested by the FDA at the time of NCE approval, 1970–1984. *Drug Inf J* **21**: 309–29.

O'Brien B (1986) *"What Are My Chances Doctor?"–A Review of Clinical Risks*. London: Office of Health Economics.

Rogers AS, Porta M, Tilson HH (1990) Guidelines for decision making in postmarketing surveillance of drugs. *J Clin Res Pharmacol* **4**: 241–51.

Rossi AC, Knapp DE (1982) Tolmetin-induced anaphylactoid reactions. *N Engl J Med* **307**: 499–500.

Silverberg E, Lubera JA (1988) Cancer statistics. *CA Cancer J Clin* **38**: 5–22.

Stallones RA (1982) A review of the epidemiologic studies of toxic shock syndrome. *Ann Intern Med* **96**: 917–20.

Strom BL, and members of the ASCPT Pharmacoepidemiology Section (1990) Position paper on the use of purported postmarketing drug surveillance studies for promotional purposes. *Clin Pharmacol Ther* **48**: 598.

Strom BL, Berlin JA, Kinman JL, Spitz RW, Hennessy S, Feldman H *et al.* (1996) Parenteral ketorolac and risk of gastrointestinal and operative site bleeding: a postmarketing surveillance study. *JAMA* **275**: 376–82.

Strom BL, Carson JL, Morse ML, West SL, Soper KA (1987) The effect of indication on hypersensitivity reactions associated with zomepirac sodium and other nonsteroidal antiinflammatory drugs. *Arthritis Rheum* **30**: 1142–8.

Strom BL, Carson JL, Schinnar R, Sim E, Morse ML (1988) The effect of indication on the risk of hypersensitivity reactions associated with tolmetin sodium vs. other nonsteroidal antiinflammatory drugs. *J Rheumatol* **15**: 695–9.

Urquhart J, Heilmann K (1984) *Risk Watch–The Odds of Life*. New York: Facts on File.

Young FE (1988) The role of the FDA in the effort against AIDS. *Public Health Rep* **103**: 242–5.

CHAPTER 6

Views from Academia, Industry, Regulatory Agencies, and the Legal System

The following individuals contributed to writing sections of this chapter:

Jerry Avorn[1], Jingping Mo[2], Robert F. Reynolds[2], Gerald J. Dal Pan[3], Peter Arlett[4], and Aaron S. Kesselheim[1]

[1] *Harvard Medical School and Brigham and Women's Hospital, Boston, MA, USA*
[2] *Epidemiology, Worldwide Research & Development, Pfizer Inc., New York, NY, USA*
[3] *Office of Surveillance and Epidemiology, Center for Drug Evaluation and Research, US Food and Drug Administration, Silver Spring, MD, USA*
[4] *Pharmacovigilance and Risk Management, European Medicines Agency, London, UK*

The view from academia

Introduction

Every year prescribers and patients have more medications at their disposal, each with its own efficacy, side effects, and cost. But when a new drug is introduced, its benefit-to-risk relationship is often understood in only a preliminary way, as is its cost-effectiveness. This provides a limited perspective on how it ideally should be used. High-profile withdrawals of drugs for safety reasons, along with prominent warnings about widely-used medications that remain on the market, have caused physicians, patients, and policy-makers to become more aware of drug safety concerns. At the same time, health care systems all over the globe are struggling with how to provide the most appropriate care in the face of rising costs and increasingly tight fiscal constraints. Pharmacoepidemiology can serve as a key tool for helping to address all of these concerns. These issues are growing throughout the heath care system, and particularly in academic medical centers.

Once a drug is approved for marketing, its prescription, its use by patients, and its outcomes often move into a kind of "automatic pilot" status. Until recently, scant attention has been paid to systematic surveillance of these actions, except for the atypical settings of some integrated health care delivery systems. The prevailing view has been that after the US Food and Drug Administration or comparable national authority approves a drug, it is used at the discretion of the clinician, with little formal follow-up of the appropriateness or consequences of such decisions. Further, many regulatory agencies purposely (and often by statute) do not base their approval decisions on a medication's clinical or economic value compared to similar products; often superiority over placebo is sufficient for a drug to be approved. In addition, it is generally no one's responsibility (other than the harried prescriber) to determine how faithfully patients are adhering to the prescribed regimen. It is only recently that more attention has been paid to assessing the outcomes of medication use on a population level, considering what its useful and

Textbook of Pharmacoepidemiology, Second Edition. Edited by Brian L. Strom, Stephen E. Kimmel, and Sean Hennessy.
© 2013 John Wiley & Sons, Ltd. Published 2013 by John Wiley & Sons, Ltd.

harmful outcomes are when it is taken by hundreds, thousands, or even millions of patients rather than by single individuals in a clinical trial or in routine practice. There is growing recognition that some adverse events can be identified and their risk quantified only by observing its use in large numbers of patients. The best perspective on the impact of a medication on the health of the public requires measuring those outcomes in the health care system itself, rather than one person at a time. It is here that the insights of pharmacoepidemiology are playing an increasingly central role.

Medications that seem acceptably safe on approval may prove to have important risks that were under-appreciated at the time of approval. In typical practice, physicians often make prescribing decisions that do not reflect the best evidence-base or guideline recommendations, and even this evidence base is often thinner than it should be because head-to-head comparisons of drug effectiveness or safety—either trial-based or observational—have not been done. As a result, inadequate information is available to inform decisions about which drugs work best, or most cost-effectively, for specific indications. Finally, even if all of the above goes well, patients frequently fail to take their medications as directed.

Pharmacoepidemiology is the core discipline required for a rigorous understanding of each of these areas, and to guide the development and evaluation of programs to address them.

The drug approval process

Each national health care system must grapple with the following inherent paradox of pharmacology: A new therapy must be evaluated for approval when the available data on its benefits and harms is still modest. Yet waiting until "all the evidence is in" can pose its own public health threat if this prevents an important new treatment from being used by patients who need it. Since any medication that is effective is bound to have some adverse effect in some organ system in some patients, any approval must by definition be based on a judgment that a drug's efficacy is "worth it" in light of the known and unknown risks of the treatment. However, the trials conducted by a given drug manufacturer to win approval are often powered (see Chapter 3) to demonstrate success for that single product in achieving a prespecified therapeutic endpoint. Especially when this is demonstration of superiority over placebo, and/or when the required endpoint is reaching a surrogate outcome (e.g., a change in a laboratory test such as hemoglobin A1c or low density lipoprotein (LDL) cholesterol), the number of subjects required for these exercises is often inadequate to reveal important safety problems, if present. This is exacerbated by the extensive exclusion criteria for study participation, and the often-brief duration of these trials.

As a result, additional methods often need to be applied even to pre-approval data to aggregate adverse events from multiple study populations to provide the power needed to assess safety. Meta-analysis (see Chapter 19) of adverse effects data from multiple pre-approval trials represents the first opportunity to use these tools to inform the appropriate use of medications. This makes it possible to combine findings from different smaller studies—many of them conducted before the drug in question was approved—to produce evidence of potential harm for drugs such as rofecoxib (cardiovascular harm), rosiglitazone (myocardial infarction), or the selective serotonin reuptake inhibitors (SSRIs) used in children (suicidality).

Prescribing practices

Once a drug has entered the health care delivery system, prescribing often falls short of existing knowledge—another issue that can be elucidated using the tools of pharmacoepidemiology. First, and often neglected, is the issue of *underprescribing*. Studies of many important chronic diseases such as hypertension, hypercholesterolemia, and diabetes reveal that many patients with these conditions have not been diagnosed as such by their physicians, and when they have, they are often not prescribed an adequate regimen to control their risks, or even any regimen at all (see "Evaluating and improving physician prescribing" in Chapter 22). Even utilizing a database that includes only drug utilization information, pharmacoepidemiology makes it possible to achieve a good first approximation of the problem of under-treatment by measuring the age- and gender-adjusted prevalence of use of medications to manage specific chronic conditions by a given physician, or a given practice or health system. When patterns of use are combined with other research on physician characteristics and decision-making, it becomes possible to identify more clearly when and how prescribing falls short, insights which can then be used to shape programs to improve care.

When medications are used, physicians frequently do not prescribe regimens that are optimal based on the available clinical evidence, or they choose more expensive drugs when comparable generic preparations would work as well and be much more affordable. Pharmacoepidemiology makes it possible to assess the distribution of drugs used for a given indication by doctor, practice, or system, even if only drug utilization datasets are available, though it is necessary to take into account whether a given prescriber is a specialist who may see in referral most of the refractory patients cared for by colleagues.

If diagnostic data are also available, as they increasingly are in many health care systems, a more sophisticated approach can also take into account contraindications and compelling indications related to specific drug choices, to refine the assessment of the appropriateness of prescribing in an entire health care system, or for individual clinicians (see Chapter 22). Numerous studies have documented these shortfalls in several domains of care.

Moving deeper an additional level in database detail, more sophisticated health records systems are becoming available each year that integrate pharmacy data with information from clinical laboratories or from the visit itself to measure the adequacy of use of cholesterol-lowering agents, diabetes drugs, or antihypertensives. This makes it possible to assess the effectiveness of prescribing outcomes for a given physician (or practice or system), by measuring how well target metrics such as normotension or goal LDL cholesterol or hemoglobin A1c are being achieved. In all these analyses, pharmacoepidemiology makes it possible to evaluate the appropriateness of medication use in selected populations, even if it cannot with certainty determine whether a given prescription in a particular patient was the best choice.

Evaluation of patients' use of drugs in the health care system

Underuse of needed drugs by patients is one of the most common medication-related problems, and one that can be readily identified by pharmacoepidemiology. Although less striking than obvious drug-induced adverse events, under-use is probably responsible for at least as much morbidity and mortality, if not more. To be fully understood, this requires the kind of denominator-grounded population orientation of a pharmacoepidemiologic perspective, which is still lacking in many health care systems. The clinical trialist or the treating physician focuses on patients who are assigned to receive a drug in a study, or who are prescribed a drug in practice, respectively. But by expanding the view to the larger population of people of which those study subjects or patients make up a subsample, the pharmacoepidemiologist can also take into account all those people with a particular diagnosis who are *not* taking a given drug or drug class, perhaps because their clinician did not prescribe treatment, or because the patient did not have access to the medication, or had stopped treatment because of side effects.

The fidelity with which a patient fills a prescribed medication (see Chapter 20) has been described as *compliance, adherence,* and *persistence.* The field of modern adherence research (see Chapter 20) is relatively new, because assessing patients' use of prescribed medications on a large scale required computerized pharmacy claims datasets to make such measurements efficiently. Until around 1990, this was an under-studied area, and most physicians assumed that after they wrote a prescription, a patient filled it and took it more or less as directed. But once the methods of pharmacoepidemiology made it possible to readily measure the prescription-filling behavior of large numbers of people, it became clear that this simple assumption was often false.

Datasets based on the complete paid-claims files of drug benefit programs provided the first means of studying adherence in defined populations. When such datasets are analyzed, a grim fact emerges: averaging across studies, about half of all medications prescribed for the treatment of chronic conditions such as hypercholesterolemia, elevated blood pressure, osteoporosis, glaucoma etc., are not taken. This causes a massive and still underappreciated shortfall—at both the clinical and public health levels—in the benefit that these regimens could generate in preventing myocardial infarction, strokes, fractures, or visual loss, respectively.

Because many assessments of underuse are based on pharmacy-generated data on filled prescriptions, it is sometimes difficult to know whether non-use of an indicated drug was the result of a failure of the patient to fill a prescription, or the failure of the physician to write it. The advent of electronic prescribing is making it possible to define this problem more precisely. As bad as the problem of low refill rates is, these newer analyses have made it clear that the situation is even worse. One large study found that a fourth of initial prescriptions written electronically were never picked up at the pharmacy. As a result, the approximately 50% rate of nonadherence seen over time in pharmacoepidemiologic datasets based on filled prescriptions is a best-case scenario, as it does not even take into account the additional millions of regimens that are not even initiated by the patient.

These findings about adherence have implications for other aspects of pharmacoepidemiologic studies. First, they raise important concerns about the validity of large databases (such as the UK General Practice Research Database) that define drug exposure in terms of what a doctor prescribed, as opposed to what the patient actually obtained from the pharmacy (see Chapter 9). Second, the very high rates of non-use in typical practice settings cast doubt on randomized trial-based assumptions about the clinical benefit, public health impact, and cost-effectiveness of many regimens in widespread use. This issue points up the value of the "real-world" analyses performed by pharmacoepidemiologists using data from typical practice settings (see "Comparative effectiveness research" in Chapter 22).

Many pharmacoepidemiologic studies have attempted to identify risk factors for poor adherence, with the goal of helping prescribers to spot proactively which patients are likely to be nonadherent. Yet this literature has identified remarkably few such predictors. High drug cost has been one, especially in patients without adequate pharmacy benefit insurance. Such studies have also demonstrated that insured patients prescribed a higher-cost medication adhere less well to their regimens than those prescribed a lower-cost generic in the same therapeutic class. Another consistent risk factor has been race, suggesting an important problem in physician-patient communication and/or trust for nonwhite patients. But other variables such as physician characteristics or patient age, level of education, or morbidity, have not consistently been found to be associated with poor medication adherence, making the management of this common problem even more difficult.

Assessment of the quality and outcomes of medication use in populations

A growing application of the tools of pharmacoepidemiology is the assessment of the outcomes of medication use in typical "real-world" populations. This perspective is based on the difference between *efficacy,* the effect of a medication in the rigorous but idealized setting of a clinical trial, compared to its *effectiveness,* a measure of its outcomes in typical practice settings (see "Comparative effectiveness research" in Chapter 22). These often differ. For example, one important conventional randomized trial demonstrated convincingly that addition of spironolactone to the regimen of patients with congestive heart failure substantially improved their clinical status and reduced mortality. However, a population-based analysis later found that when these findings were applied in routine practice by typical physicians treating a much larger number of typical patients, there was a significant increase in hyperkalemia-associated morbidity and mortality.

Other "lost in translation" analyses show that, despite overwhelming randomized trial evidence demonstrating the efficacy of warfarin use in preventing stroke in patients with atrial fibrillation, population-based studies of older patients living in nursing homes revealed a surprisingly low prevalence of use of this therapy. Such underuse was found to be associated with physicians' recent experience with adverse events caused by the drug, as well as by their perceptions and attitudes about risks and benefits. This kind of real-world population research can lay the foundation for enlightened interventions to address such non-use, by taking on its underlying causes.

Pharmacoepidemiologic methods can also be used to track the diffusion of new medication classes into practice, as well as the reaction of practitioners in various settings to new information about drug risks, as in the case of warnings about the cardiovascular toxicity of rosiglitazone.

Policy analysis

Usually, policy changes are implemented in the health care system with no systematic plans for their evaluation, and no follow-up studies of their impact; this can be hyperbolically but poignantly characterized as a form of large-scale sloppy human experimentation without informed consent. Such changes in benefit design are often applied to medication use. However, even if a policy is changed in a way that does not anticipate an evaluation, population-based observational studies after the fact can still yield important conclusions concerning its effects, both good and bad.

One large US employer introduced a change in its drug benefit plan that reduced or eliminated patient co-payment requirements for cholesterol-lowering drugs and an expensive anti-platelet agent. While this new policy seemed intuitively appealing, no plan had been put in place to determine whether the additional costs incurred by the employer would result in patient benefit. A pharmacoepidemiologic analysis compared adherence rates to these medications by employees of that company with rates for comparable people insured by similar employers with less generous drug benefit plans, and found that the change in benefit design significantly improved adherence.

Not all such policy interventions are as well-conceived. Hard-pressed governmental programs such as Medicaid must often resort to prior-approval requirements for certain costly drugs, which require prescribers to seek permission from the program before a given medication is dispensed. Sometimes the criteria that determine whether permission is granted are evidence-based and plausible; other times they are not. The methods of pharmacoepidemiology are increasingly used to assess the clinical and economic consequences of such policies.

Interventional pharmacoepidemiology

Once the tools of pharmacoepidemiology make it possible to define patterns of suboptimal use such as poor drug choices, under-use, overuse, and problematic dosing, such surveillance can be employed to identify problems amenable to interventions to improve utilization. Although epidemiology is traditionally seen as a merely observational discipline, it can also be used for what might be called "interventional epidemiology"—in this case, using the tools of pharmacoepidemiology to define baseline medication use, to direct the implementation of programs to improve such use, and then to employ the same rigorous ascertainment of practice patterns and clinical events to evaluate the effectiveness of those interventions.

One example of such interventional pharmacoepidemiology has been the development, testing, and widespread deployment of the form of educational outreach known as "academic detailing," discussed in greater detail in "Evaluating and improving physician prescribing" in Chapter 22. This approach was designed to build on observational data showing that prescribing patterns often appear to be shaped by the promotional efforts of drug manufacturers more strongly than by evidence-based guidelines. This is in large part because drug companies are much more effective in communicating their messages about what clinicians should prescribe than are academics. Much of industry's successful behavior change results from the activities of pharmaceutical sales representatives, known as "detailers," who go to the physician's office and engage in interactive conversations with the clinician that are specifically designed to change prescribing behavior. By contrast, most traditional continuing medical education offered by the academic world is far more passive: the physician is expected to come to a central location to attend a didactic presentation, usually with little interaction or feedback, and no clear-cut behavioral goal.

In the early 1980s, the academic detailing approach was developed, which used the engaging interactive outreach of the pharmaceutical industry, but put it in the service of transmitting messages based solely on evidence-based recommendations of optimal prescribing, developed by academic physicians. Building on pharmacoepidemiologic assessment of overall prescribing patterns in a given area, the method was then tested in several population-based randomized trials in which it was shown to be effective in improving prescribing, as well as in reducing unnecessary medication expenditures.

The first academic detailing programs represent some of the earliest uses of population-based medication use datasets (in this case, from US Medicaid programs) to define medication use by large and well-defined populations of practitioners and patients. The availability of complete data on actual claims from the pharmacy datasets made possible a rigorous assessment of the interventions' efficacy as well as of their cost-effectiveness. Based on these initial observations, such programs have been subjected to over 60 subsequent randomized trials, and are now in widespread use globally.

Economic assessment of medication-related issues

Using population-based datasets that contain information on expenditures as well as utilization, makes it possible to assess the economic impact of such prescribing issues as well (see Chapter 17). One application of pharmacoepidemiology to the economic assessment of medications builds on its capacity to model the effects of clinical trials well beyond their often-brief duration. For example, although statins usually must be taken for a lifetime, many randomized trials demonstrating their benefits have lasted for a much shorter time, often under two years. Epidemiologic methods make it possible to project the likely trajectories of simulated study subjects in both the experimental and control arms of a study. Based on differences observed during the trial itself, and some assumptions about their durability—assumptions that should be both transparent and conservative—it becomes possible to estimate the lifelong benefits, risks, and costs of use of such treatments.

The academic medical center

The academic medical center represents a special case of inquiry for pharmacoepidemiology, and one where it can make particularly useful contributions. These centers are the home base for many researchers in the field, and such settings are more likely than many routine practices to have available the electronic datasets that make such analyses possible. Although the patients cared for in the acute hospital setting comprise a temporary and highly selected population, data on the medications they receive and the outcomes that result can nonetheless form a useful substrate for the perspectives and tools of pharmacoepidemiology.

The application of population-based approaches can then make it possible to subject problematic prescribing in an academic medical center to data-guided interventions, particularly if a computer-based order-entry system is being used (see "Evaluating and improving physician prescribing" in Chapter 22). Until recently, this was possible only in advanced comprehensive health care organizations. But in any institution in which prescriptions are written on a computerized order-entry system, prompts can be installed to propose more evidence-based medication use. In addition, academic detailing programs or other interventions can then be deployed to address specific prescribing problems, and evaluated using the same order-entry data. For academic medical centers that evolve in the coming years to become the hubs of comprehensive accountable care organizations, the availability of such data and investigator teams will make it possible to use these epidemiologic tools to study—and improve—the patterns of use and outcomes of medications across the entire inpatient-outpatient continuum of care.

Consortia of academic medical center programs for pharmacoepidemiologic research

As the field of pharmacoepidemiology matures, new collaborations are emerging to enhance the capacity of the health care delivery system and of academic centers to address important questions in medication use. Such collaborations can bring together large groups of patients for study, increasing the size of populations available for research, as well as their diversity and representativeness. Equally importantly, such consortia can bring together the expertise of several groups whose skills may be complementary in addressing the difficult methodological issues inherent in observational studies of drug use and outcomes. The European Medicines Agency has created ENCePP, the European Network of Centres for Pharmacoepidemiology and Pharmacovigilance. The project has developed an inventory of European research centers and data sources in pharmacoepidemiology and pharmacovigilance, and provides a public index of such resources. ENCePP has also developed an electronic register of studies that provides a publicly accessible means of identifying all registered ongoing projects in pharmacoepidemiology and pharmacovigilance. In order to be registered and receive formal ENCePP approval, study investigators must agree to a Code of Conduct, which sets forth a set of principles for such studies concerning methodological practices and transparency; they must also agree to adhere to a checklist of methodological standards. ENCePP will also make study designs and data available publicly, to enable others to scrutinize methods and even re-analyze study data. This should help to increase the standards for pharmacoepidemiologic research globally.

In the United States, the federal Agency for HealthCare Research and Quality (AHRQ) has established the DEcIDE network (Developing Evidence to Inform Decisions about Effectiveness), to help inform policy-makers about the comparative effectiveness and safety of alternative treatment approaches (see also Chapter 22 on comparative effectiveness research). It has established a particular focus on methodological issues, since they play such a critical role in the validity and generalizability of nonrandomized comparative effectiveness studies. Other examples are the Sentinel Initiative of the FDA, mandated to perform postmarketing surveillance of adverse events (see Chapter 22), and the HMO Research Network (see Chapter 9).

A major milestone in the real-world application of pharmacoepidemiologic methods in the US healthcare system was the establishment in 2010 of the Patient-Centered Outcomes Research Institute (PCORI). A product of the healthcare reform program enacted the same year, PCORI was designed to be a stable source of ongoing funding for comparative effectiveness research, which will include the study of medications, often by means of observational studies. (See also Chapter 22.)

The future

The continuing evolution of health care systems in both the industrialized and the developing worlds will bring about a growing role for pharmacoepidemiology in multiple settings. Many new medications have novel efficacy but also daunting risks of toxicity, and often enormous costs. Health care systems all over the world face pressures to provide only those interventions that have the best efficacy and safety, but also at the most affordable price. To accomplish this will require relying on more than manufacturers' assessments of the utility, safety, or economic value of their own products, and more than clinicians' received wisdom or traditional prescribing habits. Nor will the interest of some insurers in promoting use of the most inexpensive medications necessarily lead to optimal outcomes clinically, economically, or ethically. Pharmacoepidemiology (and its related discipline, pharmacoeconomics) can provide the tools for rigorous assessment of the good and harm that specific medications provide, and hold the promise of applying science to therapeutic decisions that are still too dominated by other forces.

Summary points for the view from academia

• Pharmacoepidemiology has a growing role in providing insights into therapeutic decisions as health care transactions are increasingly captured digitally. Such data are analyzed by increasingly powerful software and hardware, combined with emerging sophisticated epidemiologic methods.

• Beyond defining the benefits and risks of therapeutics, these tools can point to how best to maximize benefits, reduce risks, and contain costs.

Case Example 6.1: The view from academia: The role of academia in developing, implementing, and evaluating innovative programs to improve medication use

Background

• Practitioners have difficulty keeping up with important new findings about drug risks and benefits. As a result, there is a knowledge gap between what is known and what is practiced.

• Pharmacoepidemiology can play a more prominent role in defining prescribing patterns and identifying opportunities for improving them.

• Commercial purveyors of information (e.g., pharmaceutical manufacturers) employ more sophisticated means of communicating with prescribers and changing their behavior, compared to academics.

Question

• How can faculty in Academic Medical Centers (AMCs) improve the use of therapeutics to maximize patient benefit and minimize the likelihood of harm?

• Can the effective tools of communication and promotion used by the drug industry be re-deployed to "market" the recommendations of evidence-based medicine?

Approach

• AMC faculty have expertise in analyzing population-based data to identify patterns of medication use. They also have a broad grasp of the overall clinical literature; train future practitioners and researchers; develop and evaluate therapies; deliver care to patients; and include thought leaders who influence national policy.

• Such expertise can be used to improve medication use.

• Programs of "academic detailing" devised by AMC faculty can adopt the effective outreach methods of pharmaceutical companies for noncommercial purposes by visiting physicians in their offices to promote optimal prescribing practices.

Results

• Many randomized controlled trials have demonstrated that this approach is effective in providing prescribers with better information about benefits, risks and appropriate use of therapeutics, and changing their prescribing.

Strengths

• This approach enables AMC faculty to combine the analytic tools of pharmacoepidemiology with evidence-based medicine expertise and social marketing methods to create interventions that bridge the gap between therapeutics knowledge and practice.

• Such programs can help offset their costs by improving outcomes and reducing use of therapies that are not cost-effective.

Limitations

• Requires cooperation among stakeholders with different goals and perspectives within a fragmented health care system.

• Lack of cooperation among different payors can reduce incentives to operate such programs and sustain their costs.

Key points

• As health care organizations become more centered on enhancing outcomes and value rather than on maximizing volume, opportunities are increasing for AMC faculty to "push out" innovative user-friendly educational programs to improve medication use.

• Pharmacoepidemiology can play a central role in such work, by defining patterns of medication use, assessing risks and benefits, and evaluating changes in prescribing and outcomes in populations of patients.

- Health care organizations face pressing needs to develop data repositories and local expertise in the analysis of medication use and outcomes. Academic Medical Centers (AMCs) can set the example by organizing their own data and providing access to it to improve quality and therapeutic strategies.
- AMCs can leverage their combined missions of education, health care delivery, and research to move national practice towards better use of therapeutics.
- AMC faculty are well suited to translate medical research findings on drug benefits, risks, and cost-effectiveness into educational outreach programs that can be acted upon by policy-makers, practitioners and the public.

The view from industry

Introduction

Epidemiology is recognized as a key component of risk management and safety assessment activities during pre- and post-approval drug development. In addition to risk management, epidemiology contributes to several other important functions within a biopharmaceutical company, including product planning, portfolio development, and the commercialization of drugs. The use of epidemiology to support the commercialization and appropriate marketing of drugs, including health economics and quality-of-life measures, are discussed elsewhere in this book (see Chapters 17 and 18). The most visible contribution of epidemiology in the biopharmaceutical industry is arguably drug safety evaluation, including the contextualization of safety signals and examination of specific research hypotheses. To meet these aims, epidemiologists design and implement background epidemiologic studies among indicated populations, risk management interventions and evaluations, and post-approval safety studies. Additionally, epidemiologists contribute strategy, content, and expertise to global risk management plans (RMP), pediatric investigation plans (PIP), and orphan drug applications, and are key contributors in interactions with regulatory authorities.

Regulatory and industry focus on risk management and epidemiology

Safety has been a central theme in biopharmaceutical regulation since the first Food and Drug Act of 1906, which prohibited the manufacture and sale of mislabeled or adulterated drugs. It was not until 1938, however, that manufacturers and marketers were required to demonstrate the safety of drugs as a result of more than a 100 deaths from an adulterated sulfanilamide preparation. Amendments in 1962 extended the requirement to both efficacy and safety after birth defects were found to be associated with the use of thalidomide. In the intervening years, the FDA handled risk management type activities on a case-by-case basis, such as requiring manufacturers to communicate to prescribers and patients via Dear Healthcare Professional Letters or Patient Package Inserts, respectively. The first restricted distribution product came in 1990 with clozapine, in which patients could not receive a prescription until safe-use conditions, i.e., no agranulocytosis, were demonstrated. Public pressure to speed drug approvals for HIV and cancer drugs led to the Prescription Drug User Fee Act (PDUFA). Ten years later, the concern that speed might come at the expense of fully evaluating safety led to the inclusion of a risk management framework for safety assessment in PDUFA III of 2002. For the first time, dedicated funding was provided to the FDA for risk management resources. In response to this regulation, the FDA issued three guidances in 2005 on: (1) Premarketing Risk Assessment, (2) Pharmacovigilance and Pharmacoepidemiology, and (3) Risk Minimization Action Plans (RiskMAPs). By 2007, at least 16 products had RiskMAPs, which could include any combination of enhanced education, reminder systems, or performance-linked access, i.e., restricted distribution, to minimize risks and maintain a positive benefit-risk profile in appropriate patient populations.

After a number of widely used drugs were withdrawn in 2004 and 2005 for safety reasons, the public questioned the effectiveness of the FDA's methods to assess and approve drugs. The Institute of Medicine (IOM) was tasked with evaluating the US drug safety system and making recommendations for improvements to risk assessment, safety surveillance, and the safer use of drugs. The IOM focused on the US FDA's structure and function, but also assessed the role of the biopharmaceutical industry, academia, the healthcare system, the legislature, patients, and the public. It recommended that FDA receive additional funding and staff; improve communications on drug safety, including a larger role for the drug safety staff; and most importantly, be given additional authority and enforcement tools.

As a result of the IOM report and other stakeholder research and advocacy, Congress passed the Food and Drug Administration Amendment Act FDAAA 2007 (PL 110-85). FDAAA further strengthened the FDA's oversight of risk management activities (see Chapter 22). Previously, Risk-MAPs and post-approval commitment studies were defined agreements between industry and the Agency. Although the FDA frequently required such studies of Sponsors of new drugs, its legal authority to require and enforce completion of these activities post-approval was perceived by many to be limited. With FDAAA, the FDA was granted the ability to mandate post-approval studies (postmarketing requirements, or PMR) and risk mitigation evaluation strategies ("REMS") by imposing substantial fines for noncompliance or denial/revocation of drug approval. FDAAA also allowed for voluntarily postmarketing commitments (PMC), i.e., studies that may not necessarily be required but could provide important public health information.

Europe had legislation passed in 2005, The Rules Governing Medicinal Products in the European Union-Volume 9A, which similarly expanded the requirements for industry, and included detailed guidance on development and maintenance of pharmacovigilance and risk management systems within companies. New EU pharmacovigilance legislation published in December 2010 (Regulation (EU) 1235/2010 and Directive 2010/84/EU) replaced Volume 9A, effective July 2012. The new legislation represents a major overhaul of the requirements specified in Volume 9a. A set of modules on Good Pharmacovigilance Practices (GVP) under development are intended to facilitate implementation of the new EU pharmacovigilance

legislation within companies. The most relevant module to epidemiologists within the biopharmaceutical industry is module VIII, Post-authorization Safety Studies (PASS). In general, there will now be more oversight of post approval safety studies. For example, under the new requirements, the draft protocols for most PASS requested by EU authorities, will need to be submitted for endorsement to a new committee making recommendations to the European Medicines Agency Committee for Medicinal Products for Human Use (CHMP), the Pharmacovigilance Risk Assessment Committee (PRAC). Amendments to the protocol will also need to be submitted prior to implementation, as will final study reports and abstracts. PRAC may make recommendations concerning the terms of the MA based on the results of safety studies.

While the methods of epidemiology have become increasingly important to safety assessment and risk management over the last three decades, US and EU regulations have further solidified epidemiology's role in informing the benefit-risk of medicines throughout the development lifecycle.

Epidemiology in drug safety evaluation

Background

The safety profile of any drug reflects an evolving body of knowledge extending from preclinical investigations through the post-approval life cycle of the product. Drug manufacturers traditionally relied on two major sources for information on the safety of drugs: the clinical trials supporting the New Drug Application (NDA) and, once the drug is marketed, spontaneous reports received throughout the world (see Chapter 7). Clinical trials and spontaneous reports are useful and have a unique place in assessing drug safety. However, both sources have limitations that can be addressed, in part, by the proper use of observational epidemiology. Epidemiologic studies complement these two sources of data to provide a more comprehensive and pragmatic picture of the safety profile of a drug as it is used in clinical practice.

Contributions of preapproval epidemiology

Before evaluation of a potential medicine can begin, extensive preclinical research is conducted, involving lengthy *in vitro* and *in vivo* testing. Preclinical safety studies evaluate and identify potential toxic effects of the drug, which include assessing whether a medicine is carcinogenic, mutagenic, or teratogenic. Although the information generated from preclinical studies provides guidance on the selection of a safe starting dose for the first administration-to-human study, the limited predictability of animal studies to the toxicity of drugs in human is well recognized. However, these studies can provide important information about hypothetical drug risks.

Randomized clinical trials provide abundant data about identified and hypothetical risks, but still have several limitations. Preapproval randomized clinical trials typically involve highly selected subjects, followed for a short period of time, and in the aggregate include at most a few thousand patients. These studies are sufficiently large to provide evidence of a beneficial clinical effect, exclude large increases in risk of common adverse events, and to identify the most common and acutely occurring adverse events. However, they are rarely large enough to detect small differences in the risk of common adverse events or to reliably estimate the risk of rare events. Typically, these trials have a total patient sample size up to several thousand. See Chapter 3 for more discussion of the sample sizes needed for studies. While clinical trials are not intended or designed to address all potential safety issues related to a particular drug, like preclinical studies, they often give rise to signals that cannot be adequately addressed from trial data alone.

Preapproval epidemiology complements safety data from preclinical and clinical studies and provides a context for signals arising from clinical trials. Comprehensive reviews of the epidemiologic literature are complemented by epidemiologic studies to establish among patients expected to use the new medication (i.e., indicated populations) the background epidemiology (e.g., incidence, prevalence, mortality) of the indication; expected prevalence/incidence of risk factors, comorbidities and complications; patterns of health care utilization and prescribing of currently approved treatments; and background rates of mortality and serious nonfatal events. Epidemiologists use this information to complete epidemiologic sections of key regulatory documents such as risk management and pediatric investigation plans and orphan drug applications.

Epidemiologic studies conducted before or during the clinical development program are also useful to place the incidence of adverse events observed in clinical trials in perspective. Data are often lacking on the expected rates of events in the population likely to be treated. These background epidemiologic data can be a key component for internal decision making such as trial design, data monitoring committee decisions to stop/continue trials, decisions to move/not move to next phase of development, risk management and mitigation planning, and regulatory approvals.

In addition to summarizing the existing relevant literature and designing and executing background epidemiologic studies, industry epidemiologists are often involved in safety signal evaluation, observational analyses of RCT data (e.g., as-treated or observed versus expected analyses), and designing post-approval epidemiologic studies during development. Planning for successful post-approval epidemiologic studies often begins well before approval. During the preapproval phase, epidemiologists may conduct feasibility assessments for planned post-approval studies, start post-approval studies (e.g., identifying key external partners such as contract research organizations and scientific steering committee members for the design and conduct of the study), and contribute to regulatory submissions, responses and negotiations (e.g., responding to regulatory inquiries related to epidemiology, participate in regulatory meetings).

Contributions of post-approval epidemiology

The need for a post-approval epidemiologic study can be known and devised preapproval or can arise once a new drug is marketed. Post-approval signals may come from clinical trial extension data, spontaneous reports, published case-series, or signal detection of electronic healthcare data. Post-approval, epidemiologists execute post-approval commitments (e.g., epidemiologic studies, enhanced surveillance studies, other registries, REMS evaluations, PIP observational studies, etc.); conduct studies evaluating the effectiveness of risk mitigation activities; perform signal detection in existing cohorts (e.g., via claims or electronic patient record data); and design and implement new studies as additional signals arise (e.g., from spontaneous reports, signal detection or other sources). Epidemiologists also communicate scientific findings through oral and poster presentations at scientific conferences and in peer-reviewed publications.

Spontaneous reporting systems are the most commonly used pharmacovigilance method to generate signals on new or rare adverse events not discovered in clinical trials. However, there are several important limitations in interpreting spontaneous report data (also see Chapters 7 and 13). Because of the lack of complete numerator (number of cases) and the need to estimate the denominator (total number of patients actually exposed to the drug) data, it is not possible to determine the incidence of a particular event from spontaneous reports. Further evaluation of an apparent association between a drug and an adverse reaction usually requires post-approval epidemiologic studies.

Likewise, the nature of preapproval clinical trials often necessitates further safety evaluation through post-approval epidemiology. In addition to the limited sample size and length of follow-up of preapproval RCTs, with respect to drug safety, an additional limitation of these studies is the common strict inclusion/exclusion criteria. Patients included in pre-approval clinical studies may be the healthiest segment of that patient population. Special groups such as the elderly, pregnant women, or children are frequently excluded from trials. Patients in clinical trials also tend to be treated for well-defined indications, have limited and well-monitored concomitant drug use, and are closely followed for early signs and symptoms of adverse events which may be reversed with proper treatment.

In contrast, once a drug is marketed, it is used in a "real-world" clinical context. Patients using the drug may have multiple comorbidities for which they are being treated simultaneously. Patients may also be taking over-the-counter medications, "natural" remedies, or illicit drugs unbeknownst to the prescribing physician. The interactions of various drugs and treatments may result in a particular drug having a different safety profile in a postmarketing setting compared to the controlled premarketing environment.

Because of the logistical complexity, high cost, and low external validity, large controlled trials have not been widely used for the postmarketing evaluation of drugs. Regulators and the medical community have communicated a desire for safety data from the populations that actually use the drugs in "real-world" clinical practice. This has led to a greater emphasis on the use of observational methods to understand the safety profile of new medications after they are marketed.

Purely observational epidemiologic studies may not always be the most appropriate method of evaluating safety signals or comparing the safety profile of different medications, especially when there are concerns of confounding by indication. Confounding by indication occurs when the risk of an adverse event is related to the indication for medication use such those actually exposed are at higher (or lower) risk of the adverse event than those unexposed, even in the absence of the medication. As with any other form of confounding, one can, in theory, control for its effects if the severity of the underlying illness (i.e., any conditions specified as labeled indications or contraindications, or included in the precautions or warnings) can be validly measured (see also Chapters 12 and 21). Confounding by indication is more of an issue when a particular property of the drug is very likely to affect the type of patient it is used by or prescribed to. In these cases, studies using randomization to treatment may be necessary. The Large Simplified Trial (LST) is a design used by epidemiologists when confounding is a large concern but real world follow-up is critical (see Chapter 16). Randomization of treatment assignment is a key feature of an LST, which controls for confounding of outcome by known and unknown factors. Further, the large study size provides the power needed to evaluate small risks, both absolute and relative. By maintaining simplicity in study procedures, including the study's inclusion/exclusion criteria, patients' use of concomitant medications, and the frequency of patient monitoring, the study approximates real life practice (see Case Example 6.2)

Epidemiology in evaluation of risk mitigation interventions

Epidemiology not only plays an important role in evaluation of the drug safety profile pre- and post-approval but also makes significant contributions to the evaluation of the effectiveness of risk mitigation intervention measures (see also "Risk management" in Chapter 22). In the last five years, this component of biopharmaceutical risk management has grown considerably. Guidances such as the US FDA's Risk Minimization Action Plan (RiskMAP) issued in 2005 and associated with PDUFA III outlined the tools that industry could use to help reduce known or hypothetical risks when traditional minimization approaches (i.e., the product label) were insufficient. These tools generally fall into three categories: enhanced education, e.g., patient labeling or prescriber training programs; reminder systems, e.g., patient consent forms or specialized packaging; or performance-linked access systems, e.g., requiring documentation of laboratory tests before each prescription or restricting distribution only to those who are certified prescribers. A critical addition to this guidance that was particularly relevant to epidemiologists within industry was the suggestion to perform assessments of the effectiveness of these risk minimization tools and to submit these to the Agency for review.

The same year in Europe, Volume 9A of "The Rules Governing Medicinal Products in the European Union—Guidelines on Pharmacovigilance for Medicinal Products for Human Use" outlined the requirement to submit risk management plans for all new medicinal products, or new indications/dosage forms of existing products, or when requested by a competent authority. These risk management plans have an explicit section dedicated to "Ensuring the effectiveness of risk minimization activities/Assessment of risk minimization." Thus, in addition to requiring the filing of risk management plans, this legislation gives the EMA or any competent authority the right to require risk minimization activities such as restricted distribution or other evaluation of risk mitigation effectiveness. Under the EU pharmacovigilance legislation effective in 2012, studies that evaluate the effectiveness of risk management measures will now also be considered PASS.

Risk evaluation and mitigation strategies (REMS)

Under FDAAA, the FDA can require a sponsor to submit a proposed risk evaluation and mitigation strategies (REMS) as part of its initial application if the FDA finds that a REMS is necessary to ensure the benefits of the drug or biological product outweigh the risks. The FDA may also require a REMS post approval based upon "new safety information." FDAAA has defined this as any information obtained during the initial review process, as a result of post-approval studies, or spontaneous reports. The REMS requirement is an expansion of RiskMAPs described in the Risk Management Guidances issued by the FDA in 2005. Conceptually the tools have remained similar, but the emphasis has shifted to medication guides, the mandatory patient information that is required to be distributed with each prescription for drugs under a REMS. Medication guides are intended to directly inform patients about the most important risks in lay language, in contrast to the lengthy and comprehensive information contained in product labels intended for prescribers. In addition, REMS can include communication plans or elements to assure safe use (ETASU), which correspond to the activities utilized in the "performance-linked access systems."

When determining whether to require a REMS, the REMS statute states that the FDA must consider the estimated size of the target use population, the seriousness of the treated condition, the expected treatment benefit, the treatment duration, the severity of known or potential adverse events, and whether or not the drug is a new molecular entity. All drugs and biologics may be eligible for REMS designations. Sponsor-Agency agreement on the necessity and scope of potential REMS is an element to be resolved during the drug or REMS approval process. Moreover, the possibility of a REMS remains throughout a product's lifecycle, and the FDA may impose civil monetary penalties for violations or noncompliance.

In September 2009, the FDA published a draft guidance for REMS, providing a framework for REMS submissions. All REMS for patent-protected products must include a timetable for submission of the REMS assessments, typically at 18 months, three years, and seven years following REMS approval. FDA may waive the seven-year requirement. Currently, the vast majority (~75%) of REMS only require a medication guide and assessment. Medication guides are thus viewed as the primary tool in enhanced risk mitigation efforts, despite several studies suggesting dubious effectiveness. The results of REMS assessments should provide further important insight to this much-needed area of research.

Epidemiologists play a critical role in the design and implementation of these assessments because of their expertise in observational study design, survey design, data analysis, and program evaluation. For example, using an automated healthcare or claims database, assessments may measure compliance with monitoring guidelines or measure whether a contraindicated population is prescribed the drug. Assessments may also examine the frequency of occurrence of an adverse event of interest before and after implementation of the risk minimization tool. Most commonly, however, assessments measure prescriber, pharmacist, or patient comprehension of risk information, and require the epidemiologist to design cross-sectional surveys specific for each recipient, drug, and associated unique risk profile, given that standardized or validated questionnaires that measure drug-specific medication guide-comprehension do not exist.

The implementation of the REMS legislation has highlighted a number of difficulties. The mandated assessment timelines associated with REMS may be difficult to achieve for many reasons: the need to develop and pilot knowledge/comprehension surveys unique to each drug covered under a REMS; to design, implement, and assess complex safe use programs; the scarcity of patients treated with the drug of interest; or difficulties in identifying them through automated channels. The fractured healthcare and prescription delivery system in the United States presents a barrier to efficient distribution of medication guides and educational materials, and certainly to the implementation of many safe use elements.

In addition, as of publication, there is no FDA guidance that provides detailed information on the preferred methods to assess the effectiveness of risk mitigation activities. There is little information in the peer-reviewed literature to provide a scientific basis for the utility of medication guides, or to provide information on what constitutes an "effective" risk mitigation program, on what constitutes an "important" or "meaningful" change in knowledge/comprehension, or what is the minimally acceptable level of comprehension. The lack of regulatory or scientific guidance currently leaves the industry and regulators in a position of exploration and building iterative knowledge about the preferred methods for behavioral risk intervention, including how they vary across and within patient populations. Better information in this area is especially critical when the ideal measurement of the true effectiveness of a risk mitigation program—a decrease in or elimination of the adverse event of interest associated with a drug—may be difficult to measure, or infer that it is a result of the intervention. Knowledge in these areas is expected to mature as more companies and the regulatory agencies garner additional experience.

Risk mitigation evaluation is thus an emerging area for epidemiologists in industry. Specialized expertise in survey design and implementation, observational study experience using both primary and secondary data collection methods, program and behavioral risk intervention evaluation, and data analysis are clearly critical to successful evaluation of risk mitigation activities now required by legislation in the US and EU.

Collaborations in research efforts and drug safety initiatives

Pharmacoepidemiology is a constantly evolving field, with changes in areas such as pharmacogenomics (Chapter 17) and comparative effectiveness research (Chapter 22) occurring rapidly. Nonetheless, there are some emerging topics that are important specifically for those involved in or with industry. The most important is the increased collaboration across all disciplines, including collaboration between biopharmaceutical companies to further pharmacoepidemiologic research approaches and sources, and to enhance the study of drug safety in general. The goal of these cross-sector collaborations is to combine data to increase scientific/logistical efficiency and sample size, and to pool scarce resources. These collaborations tend to be either (a) disease area- or subpopulation-specific, or (b) broad drug safety initiatives.

In the sphere of disease area- or subpopulation-specific collaborations, there are several ongoing and successful examples. One is the Highly Active Antiretroviral Therapy Oversight Committee (HAART OC), comprised of manufacturers of anti-retroviral medications for the treatment of HIV/AIDS, US and European regulatory agencies, academics, and patient advocates. HAART OC has collectively sponsored observational studies to fulfill multicompany post-approval commitments to assess the risk of cardiovascular morbidity and mortality of these drugs, as well as to construct validated case definitions of clinical phenomena such as lipodystrophy. Similar consortia exist to study the risk of birth defects potentially associated with anti-epileptic drug (AED) use during pregnancy in North America (the North American AED pregnancy Registry) and Internationally (EURAP, the European Registry of AEDs in Pregnancy, which now includes countries beyond Europe).

Alternatively, some cross-sector partnerships are disease-based rather than drug-based, such as the new JIA CORE (US) or PharmaChild (EU) initiatives to better characterize the safety profile of new and existing immunomodulatory drugs used in JIA; or the well-established Cystic Fibrosis Foundation Patient Registry in the US that has been continuously collecting data for over 40 years.

While great efficiency is gained by combining efforts, all approaches present unique logistical, legal, ethical, and regulatory challenges. The structure and governance of these consortia demand

flexibility to meet various scientific and regulatory needs to fulfill an individual company's post-approval study requirements. Furthermore, as these are long-term endeavors, they require adaptability and scalability since safety questions and treatment paradigms often shift considerably over time.

In addition to disease area specific collaborations, epidemiologists in the biopharmaceutical industry are active contributors to drug safety initiatives in the US and EU designed to advance the field of pharmacoepidemiology, including the Observational Medical Outcomes Partnership (OMOP) and the FDA Sentinel Initiative (see Chapter 22) in the US; the European Network of Centres for Pharmacoepidemiology and Pharmacovigilance (ENCePP), and the Pharmacoepidemiological Research on Outcomes of Therapeutics by a European Consortium (PROTECT), one of the projects of Innovative Medicine Initiative (IMI) in Europe.

Conclusions

Epidemiology makes a significant contribution to the development and marketing of safe and effective biopharmaceutical products worldwide. It facilitates the regulatory process and provides a rational basis for drug safety evaluation, particularly in the post-approval phase, and evaluation of risk mitigation interventions. Like any other discipline, it must be properly understood and appropriately utilized. Industry has an opportunity to contribute to the development of the field and the responsibility to do so in a manner that expands resources while assuring scientific validity. With the passage of the 2007 FDAAA and the 2010 EU pharmacovigilance legislation effective in 2012, the need for scientists with training and research experience in pharmacoepidemiology has never been greater. To best support drug safety evaluation epidemiologic strategies must: (1) begin early in development, (2) continue throughout the lifecycle of the drug, (3) evolve as new safety information becomes available, and (4) be innovative, requiring epidemiologists to be aware of new methods and methods specific to the disease area.

Summary points for the view from industry

• The safety profile of any drug reflects an evolving body of knowledge extending from preclinical investigations to the first use of the agent in humans and through the post-approval life cycle of the product.

• Results from clinical trials, spontaneous reports, epidemiologic studies, and where relevant, preclinical datasets, should all be evaluated for their potential to address safety questions, with close consideration given to the unique strengths and limitations of the study designs and data collection methods used.

• Epidemiology plays a central role in drug safety assessment and risk management activities within the pharmaceutical industry, whether through studies of the natural history of disease, disease progression/treatment pathways, and mortality and morbidity patterns, or in the design and implementation of post-approval safety studies or risk minimization programs.

• Pharmacoepidemiology is a constantly evolving field, with increased collaborations between bio-pharmaceutical companies and cross-sector partnerships.

Case Example 6.2: The view from industry: An innovative study design to assess a medicine's postapproval safety

Background

• Geodon (ziprasidone), an atypical antipsychotic, was approved for the treatment of schizophrenia by the US FDA in 2001.

• A comparative clinical study of six antipsychotics conducted by the sponsor demonstrated that ziprasidone's QTc interval at steady state was 10 milliseconds greater than that of haloperidol, quetiapine, olanzapine and risperidone and approximately 10 milliseconds less than that of thioridazine; further, the results were similar in the presence of a metabolic inhibitor.

• No serious cardiac events related to QTc prolongation were observed in the NDA clinical database.

• Patients with schizophrenia have higher background rates of mortality and cardiovascular outcomes, regardless of treatment type.

• Unknown whether modest QTc prolongation results in an increased risk of serious cardiac events.

• Sponsor proposed and designed an innovative study to assess the postapproval cardiovascular safety of Geodon in clinical practice settings.

Question

• Is modest QTc prolongation associated with an increased risk of death and serious cardiovascular events as medicines are used in the "real world"?

Approach

• Randomized, large simple trial to compare the cardiovascular safety of ziprasidone to olanzapine (ZODIAC, or Ziprasidone Observational Study of Cardiac Outcomes).

Results

• Recruited 18 154 patients from 18 countries in Asia, Europe, Latin America, and North America.

• Broad entry criteria based on approved labeling,

• Random assignment to ziprasidone or olanzapine.

• No additional study monitoring or tests required after randomization.

• Patients followed up during usual care over 12 months regardless of how long the patient stayed on randomized medication.

• No difference between the ziprasidone and olanzapine treatment arms with respect to nonsuicide mortality (RR = 1.02, 95% CI: 0.79–1.39). The risk of all-cause hospitalization was 39% higher among patients randomized to ziprasidone versus olanzapine (RR = 1.39, 95% CI: 1.29–1.50).

Strengths

- Random allocation eliminates confounding by indication and other biases
- Large sample size allows for evaluation of small risks
- Study criteria reflects "real world" normal practice, maximizing generalizability

Limitations

- Minimal data collection limits ability to address multiple research questions
- Subjective endpoints may be difficult to study using this design
- Large simple trials are resource and time-intensive

Key points

- Large simple trials, when conducted as randomized, prospective epidemiology studies, are appropriate for evaluating potentially small to moderate risks.
- Large simple trials permit the study of drug safety in a real world clinical practice setting while controlling for confounding by indication.

The view from regulatory agencies

Note

The views expressed herein are those of the authors, and not necessarily of the US Food and Drug Administration or the European Medicines Agency.

Introduction

The role of regulatory agencies in the regulation of medicines is broad, spanning the lifecycle of a medicine, from the first human studies through the entire marketing period. While the range of individual activities is wide, the fundamental purposes of drug regulation include overseeing clinical research and the protection of human subjects in the prelicensing phase, granting access to medicines via licensing, monitoring the safety of medicines in the postlicensing phase, monitoring pharmaceutical advertising and promotion in the postlicensing phase, and insuring the quality of medicines. The regulator's approach is one with a public-health focus, based in science, and executed in the context of applicable laws and regulations. Within that framework, pharmacoepidemiology is playing a growing role.

At its core, pharmacoepidemiology seeks to describe the use and effects of medicines in a population. For a drug regulator, this is clearly a relevant science, one which contributes robust data upon which to make sound decisions regarding licensing, postlicensing safety monitoring, and increasingly, in managing the known risks of marketed medicines.

For the regulator, three aspects of pharmacoepidemiology are particularly important at this time. First, as the scope of pharmacoepidemiology broadens, it is used increasingly throughout the lifecycle of a medicine. The roles of pharmacoepidemiology vary across the lifecycle, but at all times seek to understand the impact of medicines and their use in the population.

Second, the synthesis of data from multiple sources, many of which may rely heavily on pharmacoepidemiology, is critical for sound regulatory decisions. Synthesizing the data is challenging, but it is critical for the regulator to weigh all sources of evidence and arrive at a regulatory action that is based on a clear and transparent integration of all available data.

Third, building capacity and collaboration in pharmacoepidemiology is essential, both within and outside of regulatory agencies, in order for regulators, industry, and academia to meet the demand for high quality pharmacoepidemiologic investigations.

The scope of pharmacoepidemiology throughout the product lifecycle

In the past two decades, the role of pharmacoepidemiology, from the regulator's perspective, has grown beyond post-approval risk assessment to encompass assessing the need for medicines, planning certain aspects of drug development programs, evaluating pre-approval clinical safety data, planning post-approval safety studies, monitoring post-approval safety, assessing actual use patterns of a medicine, and measuring the impact of regulatory actions. Each of these aspects is discussed in more detail below.

Assessing the need for medicines

Pharmacoepidemiology, and clinical epidemiology more broadly, can be used in drug development long before a medicine is licensed or even tested in humans. Population-based databases can be used to characterize the frequency and distribution of specific diseases, so that relevant populations can be included in the developmental clinical trials. Healthcare databases can be used to estimate the frequency of comorbid conditions in the setting of the specific underlying disease to be treated, so that relevant background rates can be derived to place potential adverse events that arise during development in context. This is especially useful for clinical events that are seen more frequently in patients with the disease for which the new treatment is being tested, but which could also represent an adverse drug reaction. This situation, known as confounding by indication, is a well-known methodological problem in nonrandomized pharmacoepidemiologic studies (see also Chapter 2), but can also complicate the interpretation of adverse events in clinical trials, especially if the trial is not designed or powered to analyze these events. In these situations, careful understanding of background rates can be important.

Characterizing the frequency of specific diseases can also be important in the development of medicines for rare diseases. For example, orphan drug programs are designed to provide incentives to pharmaceutical manufacturers who develop medicines for rare conditions, known as "orphan drugs." In the United States, an orphan drug designation is given to a drug or biologic that has shown promise as a therapy intended to treat disease affecting fewer than 200 000 persons in the United States. In the European Union (EU), a prevalence of 5 per 10 000 persons in the EU is used. When all rare diseases are taken together, their public health impact is significant; approximately 25 million people in North America are affected by these diseases.

Pharmacoepidemiology is central to the designation of a product as an orphan drug product, as determination of prevalence is the basis for such designation. Methods for determining prevalence can include administrative healthcare databases, electronic medical record systems, registries, and surveys. Most of these methods would not cover the entire jurisdiction for which the orphan designation applies. Thus, some form of extrapolation must be performed to determine if the relevant population prevalence has been exceeded. For estimates of population prevalence near the threshold, care must be taken to ensure that the most rigorous methods have been used. In this setting, regulators must ensure that the prevalence of the condition or disease does not exceed the threshold. The closer the estimated prevalence is to the threshold, the greater the precision needed to characterize the prevalence.

A review of 25 years' experience with the orphan drug program in the United States indicated that 1892 orphan designations had been granted. The median prevalence of the condition being treated was 39 000; the most common patient prevalence was 10 000 or fewer patients. Relatively few prevalence estimates were near the 200 000 threshold.

Planning drug development programs

Regulators understand that there are not adequate therapies for certain serious or life-threatening diseases, and that development programs that require definitive evidence of an effect on irreversible morbidity or mortality may be very long and delay access of effective therapies to patients. To allow patient access as rapidly as is feasible, and to assure that definitive evidence of effectiveness is obtained, the concept of "accelerated approval" has been developed. Under this framework, FDA may grant marketing approval for a new drug product on the basis of adequate and well-controlled clinical trials establishing that the drug product has an effect on a surrogate endpoint that is reasonably likely, based on epidemiologic, therapeutic, pathophysiologic, or other evidence, to predict clinical benefit, or on the basis of an effect on a clinical endpoint other than survival or irreversible morbidity. A key regulatory tool in the EU to fulfill unmet medical needs is the conditional marketing authorization which has reduced data requirements linked to a one-year time-limited authorization where the authorizations renewal is linked to further data submission. Under the applicable regulations, manufacturers must study the drug further once it is approved, to verify and describe its clinical benefit, where there is uncertainty as to the relation of the surrogate endpoint to clinical benefit, or of the observed clinical benefit to ultimate outcome. At the time of approval, postmarketing studies would usually already be underway.

Understanding the relationship between a surrogate endpoint and a disease outcome is an opportunity for pharmacoepidemiologists to contribute to drug development. The hallmark of a surrogate marker is that it is reasonably likely to predict a clinical outcome of interest, even if it is not itself a direct measure of that clinical outcome. For example, in the field of oncology, improved overall survival is an outcome of clinical interest. Although this outcome measure can be reliably measured in clinical trials, it can take a long time to generate the data needed to demonstrate an improvement in overall survival. To accelerate drug development, alternative outcome measures, which do not require such lengthy trials but which are believed to predict overall survival, can be used. Such surrogate measures could include disease-free survival, objective response rate, complete response rate, and progression free survival. However, these measures have not been validated as surrogates for overall survival in all settings. In addition, these outcomes are less precisely measured than overall survival. The pharmacoepidemiologist can play a role in establishing the relationship between this type of surrogate marker and a clinical outcome of interest.

Pre-approval review of clinical safety data

The traditional role of pharmacoepidemiology, from a regulatory standpoint, has been the assessment of the safety of medicines in the postlicensing period. The limitations of prelicensing clinical trials in defining the full scope of adverse drug reactions are well known. Clinical trials are relatively small in size, compared to the size of the population of patients who will ultimately take the medicine once it is marketed. Patients who participate in clinical trials may have fewer comorbidities and take fewer concomitant medications than those treated in actual practice. Prelicensing clinical trials generally provide relatively few data, or no data at all, in certain populations such as children, the elderly, and pregnant women. These groups, however, are often treated with the medicines in the course of clinical practice.

The analytic methods of clinical trials are best suited for data arising from randomized, comparative trials. Many clinical trials of medicines intended for chronic or long-term use, including those trials in pre-approval drug development programs, may have single-arm, open-label extensions after participants have completed the randomized portion of the trial. For data generated from this portion of the clinical trial, the techniques of observational pharmacoepidemiology may be appropriate. In addition to tallying the frequencies of specific adverse events, data from long-term extension studies can be examined to characterize patterns of adverse event onset over time. If appropriate, analyses based on person-time can be performed. In this setting, the interpretations of adverse events must take into account the prior treatment received during the randomized portion of the trial, the duration of treatment, the underlying frequency of medical outcomes in the population with the disease being treated, and other factors. Pharmacoepidemiology can inform this approach. The same approach can be applied to protocols designed to grant expanded access to a medicine before it is approved, such as may occur during a "treatment protocol" in the United States. Such protocols are typically single-arm, open-label studies.

Planning for post-approval safety studies

At the time a medicine is approved, it is well known that there are uncertainties and unknowns regarding the safety profile of the medicine. In many cases, the nature of the safety issues that will unfold postapproval cannot be predicted at the time the product is brought to market. In some cases, however, a careful review of the clinical data at the time of approval can lead to a proactive approach to obtaining more safety information.

An example of a proactive approach is the strategy the US FDA has developed to require sponsors of anti-diabetic agents to characterize as fully as possible the cardiovascular risks of these medicines. The strategy starts prior to approval, when data from clinical trials are examined to determine the cardiovascular risk of the new medicine to that of comparative agents. A relative risk estimate is calculated. If the upper limit of the 95% confidence limits of this estimate exceeds 1.8, the product will require a large cardiovascular outcomes clinical trial prior to approval. If the upper bound of the 95% confidence limit falls between 1.3 and 1.8, the product can be marketed, provided that all other criteria for approval are met, and the manufacturer will be required to conduct a post-approval clinical trial to determine the frequency of adverse cardiovascular outcomes relative to other anti-diabetic agents. If the upper limit of the 95% confidence interval is below 1.3, and the product otherwise qualifies for approval, no further cardiovascular study is needed. This strategy provides a tiered approach, spanning the pre- and post-approval periods, to assessing the cardiovascular risks of anti-diabetic agents, and accounts for the level of uncertainty in the pre-approval data.

Monitoring post-approval safety

For the regulator, the postlicensing assessment of the safety of medicines involves both a pro-active approach and, of necessity, a reactive approach. Proactive strategies involve carefully identifying important gaps in the safety profile of a medicine, and designing observational studies or clinical trials to address the unanswered questions. The approach to studying the cardiovascular risk of anti-diabetic agents, noted above, is an example of a proactive step taken at the time of approval. However, the identification of knowledge gaps can come anywhere in the life cycle of a medicine, and can be based on data from clinical trials or observational studies of the medicine, or safety findings

from other medicines in the same class. In these cases, careful review of the available data can allow the regulator, working with industry, to develop a proactive approach to drug safety issues in the postapproval period. In the EU the planning of post-approval studies is formalized as the Pharmacovigilance Plan, part of the EU Risk Management Plan where identification of risks and of knowledge gaps is based on the Safety Specification.

Reactive approaches are also needed in regulatory pharmacoepidemiology because the adverse effects of medicines can become recognized at any time, including several years, after approval. To the extent that regulators can use proactive pharmacoepidemiologic approaches, reactive approaches can be minimized. But not all drug safety issues can be predicted, so regulators will continue to need reactive approaches. These approaches require efficient review of the existing data, careful and timely assessment of the need for immediate or near-term regulatory action, and interaction with the product's manufacturer to plan further study. Reactive approaches become necessary, for example, when a new safety issue is identified from spontaneously reported suspected adverse drug reactions (see Chapters 7 and 13), or when drug safety findings are published by independent groups, and neither the regulator nor the manufacturer is aware of them. Reactive approaches may also be needed when events such as manufacturing-related product recalls result in a large number of adverse event reports that need to be reviewed in a short period of time.

The specific scientific approach to an individual postapproval safety issue is beyond the scope of this chapter. From the regulator's point of view, scientific undertakings to address new safety issues in the postapproval setting must be designed in ways that address the specific questions that regulators have, so that the results of these scientific undertakings can appropriately inform regulatory actions. As a regulator will use scientific information to reach sometimes urgent regulatory decisions that impact directly on the use of a medicine and therefore on product safety, the scientific investigations must be those that answer the question as accurately as possible in as little time as possible.

Assessing actual use patterns of a medicine

Regulators are interested not only in whether a medicine meets the relevant regulatory standards for approval, but also in how a medicine is actually used in clinical practice. Understanding the actual use of a medicine in practice allows regulators to assess the degree to which the medicine is used in ways that are consistent with the safe use of the medicine. To do so, regulators can use a variety of pharmacoepidemiologic resources, including administrative claims data, electronic medical records, or other public health databases.

Assessing impact of regulatory actions

Because of its public health focus, drug regulation must ensure that its actions lead to the intended public health outcomes. For serious safety issues, it is sometimes not enough simply to add a warning to a product label. The impact of this regulatory action must be assessed. Because many regulatory actions recommend certain conditions of use for a medicine, it is possible to measure adherence to these conditions, rather than directly measuring the health outcome of interest. As formal risk management programs become increasingly used to manage specific serious risks of medicines, scientifically rigorous assessments of these programs will be needed to insure that the goals of the program are being met (see "Risk management" in Chapter 22). Pharmacoepidemiology is critical to these endeavors, as it can relate drug usage both to patient characteristics and patterns of use of other medicines as well as to patient outcomes. The case below illustrates the measurement of adherence to labeled recommendations regarding contraindicated medicines.

Integrating data from multiple sources

Central to the role of a drug regulator is determining the benefit-risk balance of a medicine and, to date, pharmacoepidemiology has been particularly central to determining the risk part of this balance. The entirety of the pharmacoepidemiologic armamentarium is involved. Case reports, case series, nonrandomized epidemiologic studies, clinical trials, and meta-analyses are amongst the most common techniques used. These topics are covered extensively in this book (see Chapters 2, 5, 13, 16 and 19), and their technical aspects will not be discussed here. While the regulator must be familiar with these techniques, the regulator's approach to pharmacoepidemiology must be one that integrates findings from various data sources that have been analyzed with various techniques. Other sources of data, such as clinical pharmacology findings (see Chapter 4) and the results of animal toxicology studies, may also contribute to the overall body of data. Indeed, the ability to integrate findings from diverse data sources depends, in large part, on a thorough understanding of the data and the methods of analysis. Beyond the technical issues, the regulator is faced with determining the significance of the data at hand, and what regulatory action, if any, must be taken.

There is no one single approach to synthesizing data from multiple data sources. Rather, a careful and structured approach must be taken in each case. Considerations include the risk being studied, the magnitude of the effect seen, the sources of the data used, the control for bias and confounding in each study, the robustness of each finding, biological plausibility, and prior findings.

Standard hierarchies of evidence have been published, though these are not always relevant for the drug regulator in making a decision about the safety of a medicine. For example, case reports and case series, which are usually accorded the lowest status in an evidence hierarchy (see Chapter 2), may be the only practical way to determine that rare, serious adverse events are associated with a medicine. Thus, strict reliance on clinical trials to determine that a certain medicine is associated with aplastic anemia or acute liver failure would be misguided. In other situations, a safety outcome might be sufficiently uncommon, or occur with such long latency, that it might not be feasible to study it in clinical trials. If the outcome may nonetheless be seen in patients with the condition for which the medicine is given, case reports will not be helpful. In these situations, carefully designed observational studies would be appropriate.

Recently, there has been renewed attention to the role of synthesizing evidence from many sources, and to the notion that the traditional hierarchies of evidence may not always be appropriate for assessment of drug safety. Because of their rigid, step-wise approach to evidence, hierarchies are not well-suited to integrating diverse sources of information. To make the issue more challenging, data from experimental settings (i.e., clinical trials) may yield one estimate of effect, while observational data may yield a quantitatively different estimate. These differences in effect size between study settings may be sufficient to result in different interpretations of the risk-benefit balance. In practice, however, data on a safety issue do come from diverse sources. The challenge for regulators, who must use the data to make public health decisions, is to integrate the available information optimally. This may be particularly challenging when trying to integrate and balance clinical trial results relating to benefit and pharmacoepidemiologic study results relating to risk.

Building capacity and collaboration in pharmacoepidemiology

Pharmacoepidemiology is a complex field, and relies on epidemiology, clinical pharmacology, pharmacy, medicine, statistics, and other disciplines, for its full execution (see also Chapters 2, 4, 14, 17, 19 and 21). Acquiring expertise in pharmacoepidemiology thus requires an environment that provides access to experts in all the relevant disciplines. Furthermore, this discipline relies on population-based healthcare data, which experts in the above fields may not have. As more and more drug safety questions arise that require expertise in pharmacoepidemiologic and appropriate data, it is crucial that there be sufficient capacity, in the form of well-trained pharmacoepidemiologists, and that there also be appropriate venues for collaboration. Regulators can play a role in reaching these goals.

To strengthen the post-approval monitoring of medicines, the European Medicines Agency (EMA) developed The European Network of Centres for Pharmacoepidemiology and Pharmacovigilance (ENCePP). EMA identified available expertise and research experience in the fields of pharmacovigilance and pharmacoepidemiology across Europe, and developed a network of centers with the capacity to perform post-authorization studies focusing on safety and benefit-risk. The "ENCePP Database of Research Resources," launched in early 2010, is a publically availabe searchable, electronic index of European research resources in pharmacovigilance and pharmacoepidemiology. The database covers both centers and networks, as well as data sources in the European Union. The "ENCePP Code of Conduct," also released in 2010, provides a set of rules and principles for pharmacovigilance and pharmacoepidemiologic studies, with regard to best practices and transparency. A parallel "Checklist of Methodological Standards for ENCePP Study Protocols" allows researchers to be aware of and consider important methodological considerations. The ENCePP "e-Register of Studies," also released in 2010, provides an important transparency, tracking, and results dissemination tool focused on pharmacoepidemiologic studies. The ENCePP project illustrates one way that a regulatory agency can be involved in building capacity.

The US FDA, as one of its commitments under the re-authorization of the Prescription Drug User Fee Act in 2007, was tasked with developing a guidance document, with input from academia, industry, and others, "that addresses epidemiologic best practices and provides guidance on carrying out scientifically sound observational studies using quality data resources." This task illustrates another mechanism through which regulatory agencies can promote the field of pharmacoepidemiology.

In addition to providing guidance on best practices for pharmacoepidemiologic studies, FDA has funded formal pharmacoepidemiologic studies. One early effort in this area was funding the development and use of the Computerized On-Line Medicaid Pharmaceutical Analysis and Surveillance System (COMPASS), a computerized database of inpatient and outpatient medical claims and outpatient pharmacy claims of participants in the Medicaid program, a health benefit program in the US for certain low-income individuals and families who meet defined eligibility criteria. As additional large, population-based databases have become available for pharmacoepidemiologic studies, FDA's funding has focused on funding experts in pharmacoepidemiology who have access to relevant data and who collaborate with FDA epidemiologists on drug safety questions of mutual interest, and on funding studies using many of the data sources described elsewhere in this book.

Because pharmacoepidemiology depends on many areas of expertise, fostering collaboration is another potential role that regulators can play. Through a project funded by the Innovative Medicines Initiative (IMI) in March 2010, the EMA, along with the national drug regulatory agencies from Denmark, Spain, and the United Kingdom, have partnered with a number of public and private organizations, academic organizations, and pharmaceutical companies to form IMI PROTECT (Pharmacoepidemiological Research on Outcomes of Therapeutics by a European Consortium), a consortium dedicated to strengthening the methods used to monitor the benefits and risks of medicines. Topic areas covered by PROTECT include enhancing data collection from consumers; improving early and proactive signal detection from spontaneous reports, electronic health records, and clinical trials; developing, testing, and disseminating methodological standards for the design, conduct, and analysis of pharmacoepidemiologic studies; developing methods for continuous benefit-risk monitoring of medicines; and testing and validating various methods developed in PROTECT.

In the US, the Agency for Healthcare Research and Quality, one of FDA's sister agencies in the Department of Health and Human Services, consults with FDA on funding and running the Centers for Education and Research on Therapeutics (CERTs), a national initiative to conduct research and provide education that advances the optimal use of therapeutics (see also Chapter 1). Until 2011, the program consisted of 14 academic research centers focusing on a particular population or therapeutic area, a Coordinating Center, a Steering Committee, and partnerships with public and private organizations. Only six centers received funding starting in 2011.

FDA's Sentinel Initiative (see Chapter 22) also represents an example of a program sponsored by a regulatory agency that seeks to advance pharmacoepidemiology though a collaborative effort. The goal of the Sentinel Initiative is to create a sustainable, linked system of electronic healthcare databases to investigate safety questions about FDA-regulated medical products. The use of healthcare data in this way raises many questions of public interest, including questions of governance, privacy, data standards, and public disclosure of results. In view of these issues, FDA has sought extensive stakeholder input as it works with outside organizations to develop Sentinel. In addition to the logistical issues above, the fundamental premise of Sentinel—that data from many sources can be used to address a drug safety question—implies that a collaborative effort is needed for the success of this project.

Conclusion

In conclusion, pharmacoepidemiology is a critical discipline in the activities of a drug regulatory agency. Key issues for regulators at this time include optimally using pharmacoepidemiology across the lifecycle of a product; developing clear, robust, and transparent methods of integrating data from multiple sources to arrive at sound, evidence-based conclusions; and promoting the building of capacity in the field of pharmacoepidemiology. These efforts are interdependent and depend not only on the efforts of regulatory agencies, but also on collaborations with academia and industry.

Summary points for the view from regulatory agencies

• Drug regulation has a public-health focus, is based in science, and is executed in the context of applicable laws and regulations.
• Pharmacoepidemiology is playing an increasingly important role in drug regulation.
• Pharmacoepidemiology is important across the lifecycle of a medicine.
• Synthesis of data from multiple sources is critical for sound regulatory decisions.
• Building capacity and collaboration in pharmacoepidemiology is essential.

Case Example 6.3: The view from regulatory agencies: Duration of use of metoclopramide

Background

The use of long-term treatment with metoclopramide is a known risk factor for tardive dyskinesia. The product label in the United States recommended a treatment duration of no longer than 12 weeks.

Issue

The extent of use beyond the recommended 12 weeks of treatment had not been quantified.

Approach

Prescription claims data were used to estimate duration of therapy and the extent of therapy beyond the maximum time period of 12 weeks evaluated in the clinical trials and recommended in the label.

Results

During the study period, almost 80% of approximately 200 000 persons who had received a prescription for metoclopramide had only one episode of therapy. The length of the longest episode for most patients (85%) varied from 1 to 90 days, yet 15% of the patients appeared to have received prescriptions for metoclopramide for a period longer than 90 days. Cumulative therapy for longer than 90 days was recorded for almost 20% of the patients. These data indicate that a substantial percentage of patients were taking metoclopramide for longer than the recommended duration of treatment. The manufacturer was subsequently required to add an additional warning to the product's label, cautioning against prolonged use.

Strengths

The data were drawn from a reasonably large population.

Limitations

The data did not include information on diagnoses, so the outcome of tardive dyskinesia could not be ascertained.

Key points

- Drug safety problems can emerge not only from problematic drugs, but problematic drug use
- Studies of the appropriateness of drug use in populations can identify poor drug use and lead to regulatory intervention

---

The view from the legal system

Introduction

Pharmacoepidemiologists in their daily work encounter many different aspects of the law. Three of the most important intersections of pharmacoepidemiology and the law involve product liability law, contract law, and intellectual property law. The basic legal rules in these subject areas, and practical and ethical implications for pharmacoepidemiology, will be discussed in turn.

1 Tort law and product liability lawsuits

Individuals harmed by a drug may seek damages from its manufacturer. A basic understanding of product liability law is essential for pharmacoepidemiologists, even for those who might never find themselves in a courtroom, because such lawsuits also exert substantial influence on the field itself. Tort litigation brought by government agencies and individual patients can help uncover previously unavailable data on adverse effects, questionable practices by manufacturers, and flaws in drug regulatory systems.

(a) The legal theory of product liability

Product liability law is a variation of tort law that covers the principles under which consumers harmed by products sold in interstate commerce may seek redress for their injuries. Originally, consumers were required to prove four elements to make out a claim for negligence against manufacturers for creating a dangerous product: (1) that defendants had a duty to exercise reasonable care; (2) that defendants' conduct diverged from customary practices that would be followed by other manufacturers or members of the industry; (3) that there was a causal link between the defendants' lack of care and the outcome at issue; and (4) that the preceding three factors led to damages.

However, some products contained a high enough inherent risk of harm that courts decided they should be held to a different legal standard. Starting in the early 1960s, judges started applying the theory of strict liability to certain product liability cases, which merely requires demonstration that the dangerous product caused the injury. As distinguished from negligence, the question of whether the defendants followed customary practices or exercised reasonable precautions is moot. For example, the product could have a "manufacturing defect," meaning that the product did not comply with the manufacturer's own standards, or a "design defect," meaning that the product was designed in a way that conferred inherently unreasonable risk for the consumer. However, courts also generally agreed that if the manufacturer of a dangerous product adequately warned about the known risks of its product, those warnings were sufficient to insulate the manufacturer from liability. Thus, strict product liability also allowed plaintiffs to bring causes of action against manufacturers based on a third principle: a "warning defect" (also called a "failure to warn").

In the pharmaceutical field, product liability cases alleging a manufacturing defect are rare, in part because of strict regulatory oversight of drug manufacturing plants. Also, cases based on a design defect theory are also difficult to win because most courts agree that all prescription drugs have some inherent risks that must be weighed against their substantial benefits. Rather, the most common bases for litigation over pharmaceutical products are warning defects about the adverse event at issue. The ultimate disposition of failure to warn cases turns on the question of whether the warning is reasonable.

(b) Failure-to-warn claims

A failure-to-warn product liability action includes three main contentions: (i) knowledge of the drug risk by the manufacturer, (ii) improper warning of the drug risk, and (iii) causation of damages.

(i) Knowledge

The plaintiff must demonstrate that a pharmaceutical manufacturer knew, or should have known, of the risk. A manufacturer of a pharmaceutical product generally cannot be held accountable for risks about which it could not have known. For example, in one case, a plaintiff brought a lawsuit claiming that her oral contraceptive medication led to her having a cerebrovascular accident. The jury found that the particular risk the plaintiff claimed could not have been known at the time the drug was prescribed, based in part on the testimony of the expert pharmacoepidemiologist who reported that "new techniques to measure these clotting effects had not then been developed" at the time of the injury. According to the court, "The warnings contained in the package inserts were adequate or that the statements contained therein were a fair representation of the medical and scientific knowledge available at the time the drug was taken by the plaintiff."

Knowledge can be actual or constructive. *Actual knowledge* is defined as literal awareness. Actual knowledge can be demonstrated by a showing that the manufacturer was cognizant of reasonable information suggesting a particular risk that it did not pass on to consumers. In the case of selective serotonin reuptake inhibitors (SSRIs), used to treat depression, various manufacturers were found to have conducted clinical trials that showed an increased risk of suicidal ideation in adolescent patients taking the drug. Plaintiffs brought lawsuits charging that these findings were delayed for lengthy periods of time, not released, or the concerns not fairly represented.

Constructive knowledge is sometimes called "legal knowledge," because it is knowledge that the law assumes should be present, even if it is not. This knowledge could have been acquired by the exercise of reasonable care. For example, the cholesterol-lowering drug cerivastatin (Baycol®) was removed from the market in 2001 after it was linked to cases of rhabdomyolysis, a potentially fatal kidney disease. The manufacturer, Bayer, was found to possess several reports from as early as 1999 suggesting a 10-fold risk of rhabdomyolysis relative to other medications in its class, but it allegedly did not process these reports and pass them along to patients or regulators. In some lawsuits, Bayer was charged with having constructive knowledge of these concerns by 1999, because the company should have processed the reports and acted on them by that time. A common legal standard used in these situations is what a reasonably prudent company with expertise in this area would have done.

(ii) Warning

If a manufacturer has the duty to provide a warning about adverse events associated with its product, then the next question is whether an adequate warning was provided. A proper warning is relevant, timely, and accurate. For example, a relevant warning about an adverse effect is commensurate with the scope and extent of dangers associated with the drug. Warnings must not be subject to undue delay. A manufacturer must keep up with emerging scientific data and patient reports, and warn of new side effects discovered after initial approval. In the case of rosiglitazone (Avandia®), a 2007 meta-analysis linked the drug to life-threatening cardiovascular adverse events. However, after a review of internal company documents, a US Senate Finance Committee report suggested that the manufacturer knew about these risks but delayed publicly warning about them and sought to limit their dissemination. Thus, a primary question in lawsuits arising from use of rosiglitazone is whether these tactics inappropriately delayed reasonable warnings about the adverse effect. Finally, warnings must be of appropriately urgent tone. In the case of rofecoxib (Vioxx®), lawsuits alleged that the warning was insufficiently urgent because the risk of cardiovascular events was described in vague terms and placed in the less prominent "precautions" section of the label.

The plaintiff must also demonstrate that the inadequate warnings about the adverse effect were relevant to the plaintiff's receiving the drug. If a defendant can demonstrate that even an adequate warning would have made no difference in the decision to prescribe the drug, or to monitor the patient postprescription, the case may be dismissed for lack of a proximate cause.

According to the "learned intermediary" rule, pharmaceutical manufacturers fulfill their duties to warn by providing an accurate and adequate warning to the prescribing physician. If the manufacturer imparts an appropriate warning that physicians can sufficiently grasp, then the manufacturer can be insulated from liability. Therefore, warnings do not have to be offered about risks that should be obvious or are generally known to skilled medical practitioners. However, when the information given to physicians omits, underemphasizes, misstates, or obfuscates dangers, this deficiency is legally transferred to the patient, who maintains a right of redress against the manufacturer if those dangers materialize and cause injury.

In some special situations, pharmaceutical manufacturers may lose the ability to invoke the learned intermediary defense. If a manufacturer markets its product very aggressively and without sufficient attention to certain risks, courts may rule that it has essentially undone the physician-patient prescribing relationship. Direct-to-consumer advertising (DTCA) is one modality that can undercut the assumption that patients are largely ignorant of prescription drug risks and manufacturers lack means of interacting with patients other than through physicians. The New Jersey Supreme Court has ruled that DTCA created a limited exception to the learned intermediary defense, and in 2007 the West Virginia Supreme Court rejected the learned intermediary defense in its entirety on this basis. Nonetheless, in most jurisdictions, the learned intermediary rule still stands.

(iii) Causation

Legal causation usually requires a clear causal chain from event to outcome, in an individual. The legal standard for causation is therefore challenged by product liability cases, where probabilistic evidence links drugs to injuries. Courts struggle with the question of legal causation in these cases on two distinct levels: general and specific causation.

General causation addresses whether a product is capable of causing a particular injury in the population of patients like the plaintiff. The basic common law standard to prove general causation is that a particular product "more likely than not" caused the damages. Some courts have held that legal causation must be demonstrated by more than an association and a mere possibility of causation, even though causal hypotheses based on such considerations are common in the scientific literature. A few courts have even gone further and defined "more likely than not" as having a relative risk of greater than 2.0, no matter how tight the confidence intervals are around a statistically significant finding of association between 1.0 and 2.0. Presumably this is based on the calculation of attributable risk in the exposed group exceeding 50%, when the relative risk exceeds 2.0. This standard has been replicated in the Federal Judicial Center's "Reference Manual on Scientific Evidence" and employed in some cases to exclude epidemiologic evidence with weaker associations.

However, all courts do not adhere rigidly to the relative risk = 2.0 rule for general causation. Both clinical trials and epidemiologic studies of the product at issue can establish general causation between a pharmaceutical product and an outcome. Animal studies, meta-analyses, case reports/case series, and secondary source materials (such as internal company documents) have also been used in court to help support establishing a causal link. Since pharmacoepidemiologic studies tend to assess the presence of an association, rather than directly addressing causation, courts sometimes apply the Bradford Hill criteria to build the bridge between an association and general causation (see Table 6.1).

To demonstrate *specific causation*, a plaintiff must show that the product in question caused the alleged injury in the individual plaintiff. In some cases, like instantaneous allergic reactions, the causal link is clear. For more subacute or later-onset responses, however, specific causation may be hard to demonstrate. For example, in one case against Merck brought by a plaintiff who suffered a myocardial infarction shortly after starting rofecoxib, the manufacturer argued that the outcome was attributable to the plaintiff's prior existing coronary artery disease. The plaintiff countered with the fact that he was in a state of stable cardiovascular health prior to initiation of rofecoxib and that he simultaneously developed two coronary artery clots after the drug's initiation (a rare presentation for ischemic heart disease). While the trial court held for the plaintiff, the decision was reversed on appeal; the appeals court ruled, "although plaintiffs were not required to establish specific causation in terms of medical certainty, nor to conclusively exclude every other reasonable hypothesis, because [the plaintiff's] preexisting cardiovascular disease was another plausible cause of his death, the plaintiffs were required to offer evidence excluding that cause with *reasonable certainty*."

(c) Pharmacoepidemiologic expertise and *Daubert*

In product liability cases, pharmacoepidemiologists serve as expert witness, helping explain data about drugs and determine whether risk information was acted upon appropriately. Experts usually describe the current state of knowledge about the adverse event at issue, and may analyze available data to present before the court.

As federal Circuit Court Judge Richard Posner has explained, "the courtroom is not the place for scientific guesswork, even of the inspired sort." Pharmacoepidemiologists seeking to present expert evidence in litigation will routinely face judicial inquiry to determine whether they are fit to serve in that role. Traditionally, the judge evaluated whether expert witnesses lack qualifications or espouse scientific theories out of step with accepted knowledge. In the 1993 case of *Daubert v. Merrell Dow*, the US Supreme Court outlined a number of markers for reviewing the appropriateness of expert witness testimony, including whether the

Table 6.1 Bradford Hill criteria.

1. Strength of association
2. Consistency and replication of findings
3. Specificity with respect to both the substance and injury at issue
4. Temporal relationship
5. Biological gradient and evidence of a dose-response relationship
6. Plausibility
7. Coherence
8. Experimental removal of exposure
9. Consideration of alternative explanation

theory was current and whether it had been tested or subjected to peer review and publication. A subsequent case applied these rules and further refined them in evaluating a debate over the admissibility of expert testimony suggesting that polychlorinated biphenyls (PCBs) can cause lung cancer. The research was excluded because the experts did not validate their conclusions—the epidemiologic studies did not report a statistically significant causal link between PCBs and lung cancer, lacked proper controls, and examined substances other than PCBs. In the US, some state courts have embraced the *Daubert* guidelines, which have also been taken up by revised Federal Rules of Evidence; others adhere to a more basic doctrine that excludes testimony containing theories that do not enjoy "general acceptance in the relevant scientific community."

(d) Intersection between drug regulation and product liability litigation

In most countries, when the government regulatory authority charged with overseeing sales of pharmaceutical products approves a drug for widespread use, the drug comes with an official drug label. The label presents a description of drug's efficacy, including the trials performed in the premarket period, as well as safety concerns that have emerged during this period of testing. At the time of drug approval, the label represents the regulatory authority's best judgment about risks that warrant disclosure and how to describe those risks.

In the US, the label takes on particular legal significance as well. The FDA requires the manufacturer to mention important warnings that are in the official label when marketing its product, but does not require manufacturers to mention warnings that are not in the label. Recently, there has been controversy over the intersection between the drug label and product liability lawsuits. For example, in one case, a man was prescribed the antidepressant sertraline (Zoloft®) and immediately started experiencing agitation, confusion, and suicidal thinking, ultimately leading him to take his own life one week later. The plaintiffs claimed that the manufacturer failed to warn appropriately about the risks of suicidal behaviors. The manufacturer contended that such a claim could not be

brought because the FDA had not included such a warning in the official label. That is, the claim was "preempted" by the FDA's regulatory action. However, this view was overturned by the US Supreme Court in the seminal case of *Wyeth v. Levine*, which held, "It has remained a central premise of drug regulation that the manufacturer bears responsibility for the content of its label at all times." The brand-name drug manufacturer can therefore strengthen the label at its own discretion by adding warnings to it without first notifying the FDA and receiving approval to do so. Notably, if the FDA does review all the data surrounding a particular safety issue and makes a specific statement that a strong warning is not necessary, such an action can still preempt a failure-to-warn lawsuit. The Supreme Court has also held that the responsibility to proactively update the label does not extend to generic drug manufacturers, which only must have labels that match their brand-name counterparts.

2 Pharmacoepidemiology and contract law

Many studies in the field of pharmacoepidemiology emerge from collaborations between individuals at different institutions. Cooperative work can allow more complex research to be performed and help advance the field of pharmacoepidemiology. One type of collaborative work of particular public health importance is contract research. Contract research is undertaken by an individual, academic, or nonprofit investigator supported by a sponsor (usually an industry or governmental agency). The contract classically represents the full outline of the agreement between the parties. In countless cases, contract research in pharmacoepidemiology has led to important public health findings and changes in health care delivery.

However, contract research may pose various potential concerns, generally centering around: (i) trial design, (ii) access to data and data analysis, and (iii) publication of results. Investigators should be wary of performing contract research in which the sponsor has the right to unduly influence the design of the trial. Many sponsors prefer to retain control of the data and insert their own statistical analyses. They argue that such efforts guard against "investigators [who] want to take the data beyond where the data should go," while investigators argue that this arrangement provides the company with an opportunity to "provide the spin on the data that favors them." Examples from both government and industry abound. In the case of rosiglitazone, a clinical trial organized by the manufacturer sought to compare the product against other treatment options for diabetes, and an independent academic steering committee was organized to oversee the data analysis. Company documents suggest that the clinical trial database was exclusively controlled by the company, which provided limited access to the investigators. When members of the steering committee questioned the presentation of the results, their concerns were largely overlooked.

There have also been numerous conflicts over so-called "gag clauses" that prevent contract investigators from publishing their ultimate results. For example, after a University of Toronto physician identified safety issues related to an experimental drug used to treat iron overload in transfusion-dependent patients with thalassemia, she was not granted permission to publish her results. When she ultimately exposed her findings, she was the subject of a breach of contract lawsuit from the

sponsor on the basis that her research contract provided that the published work-product was "secret and confidential" and could not be disclosed except with the manufacturer's "prior written consent."

For researchers based in academic medical centers, institutional research administration offices usually handle the details of contract negotiation with research sponsors. However, surveys of academic medical centers have found that academic institutions routinely engage in industry-sponsored research without sufficient protection for investigators. For example, improper contracts can pass through such offices that allow contract provisions permitting the research sponsor to insert its own statistical analyses and draft the manuscript, while prohibiting investigators from sharing data with third parties after a trial had ended.

Whether or not they receive support from research administration offices, pharmacoepidemiologists must thoroughly evaluate contracts guiding research for inappropriate language regarding control of design of the trial, access to data, and reporting of results (see Table 6.2). Problematic language includes overly broad confidentiality clauses, clauses that define and assign ownership of intellectual property, and clauses that require

Table 6.2 Potentially objectionable language in research contracts for pharmacoepidemiologists.

Category	Contractual terms	Critique
Control over investigator work product	"____ shall provide confidential information to CONSULTANT for the purpose of conducting the CONSULTANT'S professional services. All information whether written or verbal provided by, or developed for ____, and all data collected during the performance of this Agreement is deemed to be the Confidential Information of ____."	Broad definition of "confidential information" seems to cover all information. Researcher's work product becomes sponsor's confidential information.
Gag clauses	"No information regarding this Agreement or the interest of ____ or Client in the subject matter hereof shall be disclosed to any third party without the prior written consent of ____"	Prevents disclosure of existence of the contract as a financial source in publication.
Opportunity to influence outcome	Client "shall not present or publish, nor submit for publication, any work resulting from the Services without ____ prior written approval."	Contract allows sponsor to quash publication unless it approves analyses.

All examples adapted from actual contracts offered to engage in sponsored research.

approval from a sponsor prior to publication. It may be reasonable to allow sponsors a limited amount of time to review proposed publications for inadvertent release of proprietary company information or to contribute suggestions based on their expertise. However, researchers have an ethical obligation to ensure that contracts do not unreasonably delay the publication of potentially important results. Poorly written contracts can lead to inappropriate secrecy of results, which can have public health ramifications, as well as result in litigation against researcher.

3 Pharmacoepidemiology and intellectual property law

A patent is a formal grant of market exclusivity authorized by the federal government, lasting for 20 years. Patents can be issued for any process, machine, manufacture, or composition of matter. To be worthy of a patent, an innovation must be useful, novel, and nonobvious. These criteria ensure that patents cannot be awarded for inventions that already exist, or small improvements on those inventions that are obvious to a person of ordinary skill in the field.

A patent is classically thought of as a "quid pro quo" between inventors and society. The goal of a patent is to encourage inventors to invest in the development of their ideas, because it gives them a competition-free period in which to market a successful invention. At the same time, in filing for a patent, an inventor must fully disclose the content of the claimed invention in a patent document. The government provides its police power to protect an inventor's intellectual property for a set length of time and, in exchange, the inventor makes his invention available to the public and fully describes it, so that others can use it and potentially improve on it in creating subsequent innovation.

Patents have become increasingly visible in the practice of pharmacoepidemiology. Most fall into the "process" category, such as methods of analyzing claims data and comparing outcomes to identify adverse events. In recent years, numerous patents have been obtained on methods and techniques used in pharmacoepidemiology, including investigating characteristics of drug use and adverse events. The US Supreme Court has held that patentable processes may not include fundamental principles such as "laws of nature, natural phenomena, or abstract ideas," or purely mental process. On the other hand, applications of laws of nature to a particular process may still be patentable. For example, a well-known case involved a patent over a method of curing synthetic rubber that used the Arrhenius Equation to calculate the optimal cure time. The process was found to be patentable because the formula was a part of a larger inventive process for curing rubber.

There are important ethical and legal concerns related to patenting processes that provide exclusive control over various aspects of the conduct of pharmacoepidemiology and pharmacovigilance research. In one case, an HIV researcher at Stanford has faced a patent-infringement lawsuit over a publicly-available database he created to help guide antiretroviral therapy based on the resistance characteristics of the disease, because searching this database may involve a similar process to one previously patented (but never implemented) by a for-profit company.

Recently, the US Supreme Court laid down a new, strict standard for patentability of processes, excluding those that simply describe a correlation or instruct people to "gather data from which they may draw an inference." A patentable process must involve an inventive and novel application of a law of nature beyond "well-understood, routine, conventional activity, previously engaged in by those in the field." One way to operationalize this definition is using the machine-or-transformation test. That is, a process is likely to be patentable if it can be tied to a particular machine or apparatus, or if it transforms an object into a different state or thing. Notably, as pertaining to pharmacoepidemiologic patents, gathering data may not constitute a "transformation" because every algorithm inherently requires the gathering of data inputs.

4 Conclusion

Legal issues intersect with the practice of pharmacoepidemiology in a number of ways. Pharmacoepidemiologists may be involved in product liability cases brought by individuals against drug manufacturers, either as expert witnesses or on the basis of academic work they undertake. These cases traditionally involve a claim of a failure to warn, which requires proof that the manufacturer knew of the safety issue, that any provided warnings were insufficient, and that the injury received was directly caused by use of the drug. Manufacturers can invoke a "learned intermediary" defense to deflect responsibility onto the treating physician. Pharmacoepidemiologists may also be involved in contract research, but should carefully consider contractual requirements related to ownership of the work product and withholding publication. Finally, pharmacoepidemiologists may decide to try to patent their research methods, but should weigh the risks and benefits of this form of intellectual property.

Summary points for the view from the legal system

• Product liability is the term for the set of principles under which consumers harmed by products sold in interstate commerce seek redress for their injuries.

• A product liability case against a manufacturer alleging failure to warn about a drug risk includes three main contentions: (1) actual or constructive knowledge of the risk, (2) lack of a warning, or a warning that is not relevant, timely, and accurate, and (3) causation of damages.

• Product liability cases involve two types of causation: general causation, which addresses whether the product can cause the alleged injury in patients like the plaintiff, and specific causation, which addresses whether the product caused the alleged injury in the individual plaintiff. The standard for general causation is usually that the product "more

likely than not" caused the damages, which some courts have interpreted as a relative risk of greater than 2.0. The Bradford Hill criteria can build the bridge between an association and general causation.

• Pharmaceutical manufacturers can fulfill their duties to warn by providing accurate and adequate warnings to the prescribing physician (the "learned intermediary" defense). Warnings do not have to be offered about obvious risks or risks generally known to skilled medical practitioners.

• A regulatory authority's drug label represents its best judgment about risks that warrant disclosure and how to describe those risks. In the US, the drug label does not preempt manufacturers' responsibility to monitor emerging data about adverse effects and update the label as needed.

• Contract research is central to effective pharmacoepidemiologic collaborations but problematic contract terms includes overly broad confidentiality clauses, clauses that define and assign ownership of intellectual property, and clauses that require approval from a sponsor prior to publication.

• Patents offer 20-year period of government-enforced market exclusivity for novel and non-obvious processes or products. A patentable process must involve an inventive and novel application of a natural law or correlation. For example, a natural correlation may be patentable if it can be tied to a particular machine, or if it can transform an object into a different state.

• Patented processes that provide exclusive control over the conduct of pharmacoepidemiology and pharmacovigilance research can hurt the public health if they prevent sharing of data or technologies necessary for research into drug outcomes and effects.

Case Example[1] 6.4: The view from the legal system

Background

• An inventor seeks to patent a method of using adverse event data regarding vaccine administration to inform subsequent health care delivery. The patent claims, "A method of determining whether an immunization schedule affects the incidence or severity of a chronic immune-mediated disorder in a treatment group of mammals, relative to a control group of mammals, which comprises immunizing mammals in the treatment group of mammals

---

[1] Derived from *Classen Immunotherapies v. Biogen Idec* (Fed. Cir., 2008).

with one or more doses of one or more immunogens, according to said immunization schedule, and comparing the incidence, prevalence, frequency, or severity of said chronic immune-mediated disorder or the level of a marker of such a disorder, in the treatment group, with that in the control group." Patentable methods may not include fundamental principles such as "laws of nature, natural phenomena, or abstract ideas," or purely mental processes. By contrast, applications of laws of nature to a particular process may still be patentable.

Question

- Is the inventor's patent valid, or does it improperly claim a "natural law"?

Approach

- The recent Supreme Court case of *Mayo Collaborative Services v. Prometheus Laboratories* holds that processes cannot be patentable if they restate a basic scientific discovery and then instruct physicians to gather data from which they may draw an inference. That is, a patentable method cannot amount to "nothing significantly more than an instruction to doctors to apply the applicable laws when treating their patients."

Results

- Under the *Prometheus* reasoning, the method described above likely would not reach the level of a patentable invention. The inventor here has uncovered a potentially important correlation between immunization schedules and patient outcomes, but these natural correlations are not patentable by themselves.

Strengths

- The *Prometheus* principle prevents patents from being issued on certain fundamental discoveries related to pharmacoepidemiology. Patents in this field that are sufficiently broad could prevent others from conducting necessary research into drug outcomes and effects.

Limitations:

- Excluding certain discoveries from the possibility of patenting has led some observers to worry about the implications for private investment. The prospect of patents on new pharmacoepidemiologic methods and discoveries may be essential for recouping the costs of innovation.

- Government patent offices, which are often underfunded and understaffed, will now face the task of distinguishing the development and characterization of patentable methods from other methods that simply describe natural correlations.

Key points

- A patentable process needs to involve an inventive and novel application of a law of nature or natural correlation beyond "well-understood, routine, conventional activity, previously engaged in by those in the field."

Further reading

The view from academia

Avorn J (2005) *Powerful Medicines: The Benefits, Risks, and Costs of Prescription Drugs*. New York: Knopf.

Avorn J (2011) Teaching clinicians about drugs—50 years later, whose job is it? *N Engl J Med* **364**: 1185–7.

Avorn J, Soumerai SB (1983) Improving drug-therapy decisions through educational outreach. A randomized controlled trial of academically based "detailing." *N Engl J Med* **308**: 1457–63.

Choudhry NK *et al.* (2011) Post-myocardial infarction free Rx event and economic evaluation (MI FREEE) trial. Full coverage for preventive medications after myocardial infarction. *N Engl J Med* **365**: 2088–97.

Clancy C, Collins FS (2010) Patient-Centered Outcomes Research Institute: the intersection of science and health care. *Sci Transl Med* **2**: 37.

Cutrona SL *et al.* (2010) Physician effectiveness in interventions to improve cardiovascular medication adherence: a systematic review. *J Gen Intern Med* **25**: 1090–6.

Fischer MA, Choudhry NK, Winkelmayer WC (2007) Impact of Medicaid prior authorization on angiotensin-receptor blockers: can policy promote rational prescribing? *Health Aff (Millwood)* **26**: 800–7.

Fischer MA, Avorn J (2004) Economic implications of evidence-based prescribing for hypertension: can better care cost less? *JAMA* **291**: 1850–6.

Fischer MA, Morris CA, Winkelmayer WC, Avorn J (2007) Nononcologic use of human recombinant erythropoietin therapy in hospitalized patients. *Arch Intern Med* **167**: 840–6.

Fischer MA, Stedman MR, Lii J, Vogeli C, Shrank WH, Brookhart MA, Weissman JS (2010) Primary medication non-adherence: analysis of 195, 930 electronic prescriptions. *J Gen Intern Med* **25**: 284–90.

Jackevicius CA, Li P, Tu JV (2008) Prevalence, predictors, and outcomes of primary nonadherence after acute myocardial infarction. *Circulation* **117**: 1028–36.

Jackevicius CA *et al.* (2008) Cardiovascular outcomes after a change in prescription policy for clopidogrel. *N Engl J Med* **359**: 1802–10.

Juurlink DN *et al.* (2004) Rates of hyperkalemia after publication of the Randomized Aldactone Evaluation Study. *N Engl J Med* **351**: 543–51.

O'Brien MA *et al.* (2007) Educational outreach visits: effects on professional practice and health care outcomes. *Cochrane Database Syst Rev* Oct 17 (4): CD000409.

Shah ND et al. (2010) Responding to an FDA warning—geographic variation in the use of rosiglitazone. *N Engl J Med* **363**: 2081–4.

Shrank WH *et al.* (2006) The implications of choice: prescribing generic or preferred pharmaceuticals improves medication adherence for chronic conditions. *Arch Intern Med* **166**: 332–7.

Solomon DH, Finkelstein JS, Katz JN, Mogun H, Avorn J (2003) Underuse of osteoporosis medications in elderly patients with fractures. *Am J Med* **115**: 398–400.

Solomon DH, Van Houten L, Glynn RJ, Baden L, Curtis K, Schrager H, Avorn J (2001) Academic detailing to improve use of broad-spectrum antibiotics at an academic medical center. *Arch Intern Med* **161**: 1897–1902.

The view from industry

Berger MS, Berger BA (2006) *FDA Overview*.http://www.emedicinehealth.com/fda_overview/article_em.htm (accessed June 2011).

Directive 2010/84/EU. http://eurlex.europa.eu/LexUriServ/LexUriServ.do?uri=OJ:L:2010:348:0074:0099:EN:PDF (accessed May 2012)

European Network of Centres for Pharmacoepidemiology and Pharmacovigilance (ENCePP). http://www.encepp.eu/ (accessed June 2011).

FDA (2011) *Guidance for Industry Postmarketing Studies and Clinical Trials*. http://www.fda.gov/downloads/Drugs/GuidanceComplianceRegulatoryInformation/Guidances/UCM172001.pdf (accessed May 2012).

FDA (2005) *Guidance for Industry: Development and Use of Risk Minimization Action Plans*. http://www.fda.gov/downloads/Drugs/GuidanceComplianceRegulatory

Information/Guidances/ucm071616.pdf (accessed June 2011).

FDA (2007) *Food and Drug Administration Amendments Act of 2007*. http://www.fda.gov/RegulatoryInformation/Legislation/FederalFoodDrugandCosmeticActFDCAct/SignificantAmendmentstotheFDCAct/FoodandDrugAdministrationAmendmentsActof2007/FullTextofFDAAALaw/default.htm (accessed June 2011).

FDA (2009) *Draft Guidance for Industry: Format and Content of Proposed Risk Evaluation and Mitigation Strategies (REMS), REMS Assessments, and Proposed REMS Modifications*. http://www.fda.gov/downloads/Drugs/GuidanceComplianceRegulatoryInformation/Guidances/UCM184128.pdf (accessed June 2011).

FDA. *Approved Risk Evaluation and Mitigation Strategies (REMS)*. http://www.fda.gov/Drugs/DrugSafety/PostmarketDrugSafetyInformation for PatientsandProviders/ucm111350.htm (accessed June 2011).

Institute of Medicine (2006) *The Future of Drug Safety: Promoting and Protecting the Health of the Public,* http://www.iom.edu/Reports/2006/The-Future-of-Drug-Safety-Promoting-and-Protecting-the-Healthof-the-Public.aspx (accessed June 2011).

International Society for Pharmacoepidemiology (2008) Guidelines for good pharmacoepidemiology practices (GPP). *Pharmacoepidemiol Drug Saf* **17**: 200–8.

Observational Medical Outcomes Partnership. http://omop.fnih.org/ (accessed June 2011).

Pharmacoepidemiological Research on Outcomes of Therapeutics by a European Consortium. http://www.imi-protect.eu/ (accessed June 2011).

Regulation (EU) 1235/2010. http://eurlex.europa.eu/LexUriServ/LexUriServ.do?uri=OJ:L:2010:348:0001:0016:EN:PDF (accessed May 2012)

Smith MY, Sobel RE, Wallace CA (2010) Monitoring the long-term safety of therapies for children with juvenile idiopathic arthritis: time for a consolidated patient registry. *Arthritis Care Res (Hoboken)* **62**: 800–4.

Strom BL, Eng SM, Faich G, Reynolds RF, D'Agostino RB, Ruskin J, *et al.* (2011) Comparative mortality associated with ziprasidone and olanzapine in real-world use among 18,154 patients with schizophrenia: the ziprasidone observational study of cardiac outcomes (ZODIAC). appi. *Am J Psychiatry* **168**: 193–201.

Strom BL, Faich GA, Reynolds RF, Eng SM, D'Agostino RB, Ruskin JN, *et al.* (2008) The Ziprasidone Observational Study of Cardiac Outcomes (ZODIAC): design and baseline subject characteristics. *J Clin Psychiatry* **69**: 114–21.

Tomson T, Battino D, Craig J, Hernandez-Diaz S, Holmes LB, Lindhout D, *et al.* (2010) Pregnancy registries: differences, similarities, and possible harmonization. *Epilepsia* **51**: 909–15.

Worm SW, Sabin C, Weber R, Reiss P, El-Sadr W, Dabis F, *et al.* (2010) Risk of myocardial infarction in patients with HIV infection exposed to specific individual antiretroviral drugs from the 3 major drug classes: the data collection on adverse events of anti-HIV drugs (D: A: D) study. *J Infect Dis* **201**: 318–30.

The view from regulatory agencies

Braun MM, Farag-El-Massah S, Xu K, and Cote TR (2010) Emergence of orphan drugs in the United States; a quantitative assessment of the first 25 years. *Nat Rev Drug Discov* **9**: 519–22.

FDA (2009) FDA requires boxed warning and risk mitigation strategy for metoclopramide-containing drugs: Agency warns against chronic use of these products to treat gastrointestinal disorders, February 26, 2009, available at http://www.fda.gov/NewsEvents/Newsroom/PressAnnouncements/2009/ucm149533.htm

Kaplan S, Staffa JA, Dal Pan GJ (2007) Duration of therapy with metoclopramide: a prescription claims data study. *Pharmacoepidemiol Drug Saf* Aug; **16** (8): 878–81.

McKee AE, Farrell AT, Pazdur R, Woodcock J (2010) The role of the US Food and Drug Administration review process: Clinical trials endpoints in oncology. *The Oncologist* **15** (suppl 1): 13–18.

Rawlins M (2008) *De Testimonio*: on the evidence for decisions about the use of therapeutic interventions. *Lancet.* **372**: 2152–61.

Schieppati A, Henter JI, Daina E, Aperia A (2008) Why rare diseases are an important medical and social issue. *Lancet* **371**: 2039–41.

US Department of Health and Human Services. US Food and Drug Administration (2008) Guidance for Industry: Diabetes Mellitus—Evaluating Cardiovascular Risk in New Anitdiabetic Therapies to Treat Type 2 Diabetes. December 2008.

US Department of Health and Human Services. US Food and Drug Administration (2008) The Sentinel Initiative—National Strategy for Monitoring Medical Product Safety. May 2008, Available at http://www.fda.gov/downloads/Safety/FDAsSentinelInitiative/UCM124701.pdf

van Staa TP, Smeeth L, Persson I, Parkinson J, Leufkens HG, (2008) Evaluating drug toxicity signals: is a hierarchical classification of evidence useful or harmful? *Pharmacoepidemiol Drug Safety* **17**: 475–84.

Drug safety and tort law

Angell M (1997) *Science on Trial: The Clash of Medical Evidence and the Law in the Breast Implant Case.* New York: W. W. Norton & Co.

Avorn J (2004) *Powerful Medicines: The Benefits, Risks and Costs of Prescription Drugs.* New York, NY: Alfred A Knopf.

Brennan TA (1988) Causal chains and statistical links: the role of scientific uncertainty in hazardous-substance litigation. *Cornell Law Review* **73**: 469–533.

Federal Judicial Center (2000) *Reference manual on scientific evidence* (2nd edn). Available at http://www.fjc.gov/public/pdf.nsf/lookup/sciman00.pdf/$file/sciman00.pdf

Green MD (1996) *Bendectin and Birth Defects: The Challenges of Mass Toxic Substances Litigation.* Philadelphia, PA: University of Pennsylvania Press.

Hill AB (1965) The environment and disease: association or causation? *Proceedings of the Royal Society of Medicine* **58**: 295–300.

Kesselheim AS, Avorn J (2007) The role of litigation in defining drug risks. *JAMA* **297**: 308–11.

Kessler DA, Vladeck DC (2008) A critical examination of the FDA's efforts to preempt failure-to-warn claims. *Georgetown Law Journal* **96**: 461–95.

Shapo MS (2008) *Experimenting with the Consumer: The Mass Testing of Risky Products on the American Public.* Westport, CT: Praeger.

Contract-related issues in pharmacoepidemiology

Bodenheimer T (2000) Uneasy alliance—clinical investigators and the pharmaceutical industry. *New Engl J Med* **342**: 1539–44.

Eichler HG, Kong SX, Grégoire JP (2006) Outcomes research collaborations between third-party payers, academia, and pharmaceutical manufacturers: What can we learn from clinical research? *European Journal of Health Economics* **7** (2): 129–35.

Kong SX, Wertheimer AI (1998) Outcomes research: collaboration among academic researchers, managed care organizations, and pharmaceutical manufacturers. *American Journal of Managed Care* **4** (1): 28–34.

Washburn J. University Inc. (2006) *The Corporate Corruption of Higher Education.* New York: Basic Books.

Patent law and pharmacoepidemiology

Heller MA, Eisenberg RS (1998) Can patents deter innovation: the anticommons in biomedical research. *Science* **280**: 698–701.

Jaffe AB, Lerner J (2004) *Innovation and Its Discontents: How Our Broken Patent System Is Endangering Innovation and Progress, and What To Do About It.* Princeton, NJ: Princeton University Press.

Kesselheim AS, Karlawish J (2012) Biomarkers unbound — the Supreme Court's ruling on diagnostic-test patents. *New England Journal of Medicine* **366**: 2338–40.

Nard CA, Wagner RP (2007) *Patent Law: Concepts and Insights.* St. Paul, MN: Foundation Press.

National Research Council (2004) *A Patent System for the 21st Century.* (Merrill SA, Levin RC, Myers MB, eds.) Washington, DC: The National Academies Press.

Walker AM (2006) More lawyers, more bureaucrats, less information on drug safety. *Pharmacoepi Drug Safety* **15**: 394–5.

PART II
Sources of Pharmacoepidemiology Data

CHAPTER 7

Postmarketing Spontaneous Pharmacovigilance Reporting Systems

Gerald J. Dal Pan[1], Marie Lindquist[2], and Kate Gelperin[1]

[1] *Office of Surveillance and Epidemiology, Center for Drug Evaluation and Research, US Food and Drug Administration, Silver Spring, MD, USA*
[2] *Uppsala Monitoring Centre, WHO Collaborating Centre for International Drug Monitoring, Uppsala, Sweden*

The views expressed herein are those of the authors, and not necessarily of the US Food and Drug Administration

Introduction

Just about fifty years ago a concerned obstetrician from Australia sent a letter to the editor of *The Lancet* medical journal describing severe malformations in babies born to several of his patients, and posing the question: "Have any of your readers seen similar abnormalities in babies delivered of women who have taken [thalidomide] during pregnancy?" An accompanying editor's note gave the news that the drug's manufacturer (Distillers) planned to withdraw the product from marketing based on "reports from two overseas sources possibly associating thalidomide ('Distaval') with harmful effects on the fetus." Sadly, the number of babies born with thalidomide-related deformities has been estimated to exceed 10 000 worldwide before the scope and consequences of this adverse drug reaction were adequately appreciated and effectively prevented. Today, perhaps in part as a result of this tragic occurrence, drug safety surveillance and regulatory decision-makers are more vigilant in detecting safety signals and more active in alerting prescribers about serious adverse drug effects, largely through established pharmacovigilance reporting systems worldwide.

In recent years, the term "pharmacovigilance" has become widely used to denote postmarketing safety activities, and is defined by the World Health Organization (WHO) as "the science and activities relating to the detection, assessment, understanding and prevention of adverse effects or any other possible drug-related problems." (See also Chapter 13.)

Monitoring and understanding the safety of drug and therapeutic biologic products is a process that proceeds throughout the product's life cycle, spanning the period prior to first administration to humans through the entire marketing life of the product (see Chapter 1 and also "The view from regulatory agencies" in Chapter 6). Throughout the product lifecycle, astute clinical observations made at the point of care constitute an important source of information. While new technologies have enabled more thorough knowledge of a drug's actions, and computerized databases have enabled large-scale, population-based analyses of drug safety investigations (see Chapter 9), these advancements are adjuncts to, and not substitutes for, careful, well thought-out clinical observations.

Though the preapproval testing of a drug is typically rigorous, and the review of the data is thorough, there are still inevitable uncertainties about the complete safety profile of a drug when it is

Textbook of Pharmacoepidemiology, Second Edition. Edited by Brian L. Strom, Stephen E. Kimmel, and Sean Hennessy.
© 2013 John Wiley & Sons, Ltd. Published 2013 by John Wiley & Sons, Ltd.

brought to market, for several reasons. First, the number of patients treated with the drug prior to approval is limited, generally from several hundred to a few thousand. Second, patients in clinical trials tend to be carefully selected, and are thus more clinically homogeneous than patients treated in the course of clinical practice once a drug is marketed (see Chapter 16). Third, additional populations of patients, such as children or the elderly, may be treated with the product once it is marketed. In addition, marketed drug products are often used for diseases or conditions for which they are not indicated, or at doses outside of the approved range (see "Evaluating and improving physician prescribing" in Chapter 22). For these reasons, a postmarketing drug pharmacovigilance reporting system is necessary.

Description

Adverse events and adverse drug reactions

Central to an understanding of postmarketing pharmacovigilance reporting systems are the closely related, but nonetheless distinct, concepts of *adverse event* and *adverse drug reaction*. The International Conference on Harmonization of Technical Requirements for Registration of Pharmaceuticals for Human Use (ICH) E2D guideline on Post-Approval Safety Data Management: Definitions and Standards for Expedited Reporting, defines an adverse event as follows:

> An adverse event (AE) is any untoward medical occurrence in a patient administered a medicinal product and which does not necessarily have to have a causal relationship with this treatment. An adverse event can therefore be any unfavorable and unintended sign (for example, an abnormal laboratory finding), symptom, or disease temporally associated with the use of a medicinal product, whether or not considered related to this medicinal product.

The same guideline describes an adverse drug reaction as follows:

> All noxious and unintended responses to a medicinal product related to any dose should be considered adverse drug reactions.

The phrase "responses to a medicinal product" means that a causal relationship between a medicinal product and an adverse event is at least a possibility.

A reaction, in contrast to an event, is characterized by the fact that a causal relationship between the drug and the occurrence is suspected. If an event is spontaneously reported, even if the relationship is unknown or unstated, it meets the definition of an adverse drug reaction.

The principal difference between an adverse event and an adverse drug reaction is that a causal relationship is suspected for the latter, but is not required for the former. In this framework, adverse drug reactions are a subset of adverse events. In some countries, postmarketing pharmacovigilance reporting systems are focused on adverse drug reactions, while in others data on adverse events are collected. In the United States, for example, the scope of reporting requirements is "[a]ny adverse event associated with the use of a drug in humans, whether or not considered drug related . . . "

While many of the principles discussed in this chapter apply equally to adverse events and adverse drug reactions, it is important to understand the distinction between these two concepts. Specifically, some databases may contain only adverse drug reactions, while others may contain adverse events. These databases may behave differently when used for data mining. However, because many of the principles of drug safety surveillance apply to both adverse events and adverse drug reactions, we will use the term "AE/ADR" to refer to these two terms collectively in this chapter, for convenience. When needed, we will use the individual terms if a distinction between the two is required.

Overview of pharmacovigilance reporting systems

The goal of a postmarketing, or post-approval, safety program is to identify drug-related adverse events (AEs), or adverse drug reactions (ADRs), that were not identified prior to approval, to refine knowledge of the known adverse effects of a drug, and to understand better the conditions under which the safe use of a drug can be assured.

The scope of pharmacovigilance is broad. The core activity is usually the identification of previously unrecognized AEs/ADRs with the use of the drug. However, it is not sufficient simply to note that use of a drug can lead to an AE/ADR. Rather, an investigation into not only the potential causal role of the drug in the development of the AE/ADR, but also into the conditions leading to the occurrence of the AE/ADR in one person or population and not in others must be the focus of any postmarketing drug safety effort. Factors such as dose–response relationships, drug–drug interactions, drug–disease interactions, drug–food interactions, and the possibility of medication errors must be carefully considered (see also "The use of pharmacoepidemiology to study medication errors" in Chapter 22). A full understanding of the factors that can lead to an AE/ADR may yield ideas for effective interventions to minimize the severity or occurrence of the AE/ADR, and thus enhance the safe use of the drug.

The identification of a new safety issue with a medicinal product often begins with a single observation. In the postmarketing period, such observations are usually clinical observations, often made at the point of care in the course of clinical practice. A practitioner or patient notes the development of symptoms or signs that were not present, or were present in less severe form, prior to the patient's using the medicine. If this sign or symptom is not listed in the product's approved labeling, patients and healthcare professionals may not think to attribute it to the medicine. If further evaluation reveals a clinically significant process (e.g., liver injury, rhabdomyolysis, agranulocytosis), it is important to keep in mind the possibility of a side effect due to a medication in the differential diagnosis of the event. If a medication side effect is not included in the differential diagnosis, the patient may not be treated appropriately.

In the postmarketing period, the investigation of AEs/ADRs is a multidisciplinary one. The analysis of a complex AE/ADR can involve the fields of medicine, pharmacology, epidemiology, statistics, pharmacy, toxicology, and others. There are several methods of clinical postmarketing safety assessment. These include the review of case reports and case series from spontaneous reporting systems, a wide variety of types of observational epidemiologic studies, and clinical trials (see also Chapter 13). This chapter will focus on spontaneous pharmacovigilance reporting systems. No one method is *a priori* better than another in all settings. Rather, the choice of methods depends on the particular safety question to be answered.

The concept of spontaneous AE/ADR Reporting

A core aspect of pharmacovigilance is the voluntary reporting of AEs/ADRs either directly to established national or regional centers, or alternatively to pharmaceutical manufacturers, who in turn are obligated to report the information to regulators. National reporting systems are typically run by regulatory agencies (e.g., the US FDA runs the MedWatch program) or by centers designated by the health ministry or the drug regulatory authority. In a few countries, the national pharmacovigilance center is run by a university or other scientific body. In the United States for example, AEs/ADRs in individual patients are generally identified at the point of care. Patients, physicians, nurses, pharmacists, or anyone else who suspects that there may be an association between an AE/ADR and a drug or therapeutic biologic product are encouraged to, but are generally not required to, report the case to either the manufacturer or to the FDA.

This system of AE/ADR reporting is often referred to as a spontaneous reporting system; "spontaneous" because the person who initially reports the AE/ADR to either the reporting center or to the manufacturer chooses what events to report. Sometimes, spontaneous reporting systems are also labeled as "passive," based on the argument that the reporting center or the manufacturer passively receives this information, rather than actively seeking it out. However, this term does not do justice to the proactive way in which many pharmacovigilance centers seek to operate, even if resource constraints often limit the ability to interact adequately with reporters. Moreover, "spontaneous reporting" does not fit well with the reporting situation of today, when most countries have introduced or enacted legislation which mandates reporting from pharmaceutical companies. Reporting may also include canvassed or stimulated reporting of suspected reactions of particular interest (see also below, in the section "National pharmacovigilance systems").

Underlying the concept of a spontaneous postmarketing AE/ADR pharmacovigilance reporting system is the notion that clinical observations made at the point of care are often valuable pieces of information in further refining the knowledge of a drug's safety profile. This is an important, though frequently underemphasized, idea. After approval, when formal study often ends and marketing of the medicine begins, there is often no further systematic way to continue the study of a medicine's safety, or even to generate drug safety hypotheses. While scientific advances and access to new data sources (e.g., electronic healthcare records) may provide some opportunity to monitor the safety of a marketed medicine (see Chapter 9), these alternative approaches to safety signal detection remain unproven.

When healthcare professionals, patients, and consumers want to make a notification of a potentially adverse effect of a medication, it is useful for this information to be systematically organized, stored, and analyzed. A reporting system fills this need. If such information were not systematically collected, potentially valuable data about medicines would be lost. This system implies an important role for healthcare professionals in postmarketing safety assessment, as the quality of reports is always dependent on the details provided by healthcare professionals.

Because most AE/ADR reporting systems rely on voluntary reports, it is generally recognized that there is substantial underreporting of AEs/ADRs via current reporting systems. Two survey-based studies conducted in the US in the 1980s, one in Maryland and the other in Rhode Island, examined physician reporting to FDA, and concluded that fewer than 10% of AEs/ADRs were reported to FDA. These studies were conducted prior to the development of the current MedWatch program in 1993, and do not consider the contribution of reporting from sources other than physicians. Calculating the proportion of adverse event reports that a reporting system actually receives requires that the true number of AEs/ADRs in the population be known. For most AEs/ADRs, this number is not known or readily available. In some cases, however, data are available that allow an estimate of the extent of reporting to be calculated. For example, the extent of reporting to FDA of cases of hospitalized rhabdomyolysis associated with statin use was estimated using a projected estimate of the number of such cases in the United States and comparing it to the number of reports of statin-associated hospitalized rhabdomyolysis in FDA's Adverse Event Reporting System (AERS), a database that houses FDA's postmarketing adverse event reports. The projected national estimate was obtained by using incidence rates from a population-based cohort study, and applying those incidence rates to national estimates of statin use. Across four statins (atorvastatin, cerivastatin, pravastatin, and simvastatin), the estimated overall extent of adverse event reporting was 17.7%. For individual statins, the estimated extent of reporting ranged from 5.0% (atorvastatin) to 31.2% (cerivastatin). Further analysis revealed that the high proportion of reporting of cerivastatin cases was driven by reports received after the dissemination of a Dear Healthcare Professional letter notifying physicians of the risks of cerivastatin-associated rhabdomyolysis. The estimated extent of reporting was 14.8% before the letter and rose to 35.0% after. It is important to note that the results of this study apply only to reporting cases of statin-associated rhabdomyolysis. The extent of reporting for different drug-adverse pairs will be different, and cannot be estimated from the results of this study.

Once reports are received by national pharmacovigilance centers, they are entered into AE/ADR databases. These databases can then be inspected for drug safety signals, which form the basis of further study, necessary regulatory action, or both.

Report characteristics

The individual case report is the fundamental unit of a postmarketing pharmacovigilance reporting system. The extent to which such a reporting system can address specific drug safety questions depends, in large part, on the characteristics and quality of the individual reports. Specific report formats differ across jurisdictions, though many countries and regions collect information compatible with the ICH E2B format. The International Conference on Harmonization (ICH) E2B standard specifies both administrative and product identification information, as well as information on the case. The principal domains of case information in the ICH E2B standard include: (1) patient characteristics, (2) reaction(s) or event(s), (3) results of tests and procedures relevant to the investigation of the patient, (4) drug(s) information, and (5) a narrative case summary and further information.

Regardless of the specific formatting requirements across jurisdictions, there are some fundamental components of an individual safety report that are important for a thorough review.

Product identification, in as much detail as possible, is essential for an assessment of a case report. For pharmaceuticals, the identification of the active ingredient(s) is critical to product identification. However, other factors can also be important, depending on the specific safety question. For example, the formulation of the product can be important, as the pharmacokinetic and other pharmaceutical properties can differ. Additionally, if the drug safety question involves the assessment of an AE/ADR related to a product quality defect, information on both manufacturer and lot/batch number can be very important, as product quality problems typically involve specific lots from an individual manufacturer.

Reports describing medication errors, or the potential for medication errors, ideally contain information on the product involved, the sequence of events leading up to the error, the work environment in which the error occurred, and the type of error that occurred.

Characteristics of a good quality case report include adequate information on product use, patient characteristics, medical history, and concomitant treatments, and a description of the AE/ADR, including response to treatments and clinical outcome. Our experience, based on many years of reviewing case reports, is that while a substantial amount of useful clinical information can be written in a succinct narrative, most narratives are incomplete, many to the extent that they are uninterpretable. While follow-up with the reporter is sometimes feasible for drug safety analysts during case review, this has been the exception not the rule, often due to resource constraints. Incomplete and uninterpretable case reports limit the effectiveness of postmarketing pharmacovigilance reporting systems. Attempts to improve the systems will need to address the problem of poor case report quality rather than merely increasing the number of reports. Unfortunately, it is not unusual for FDA to receive potentially important spontaneous reports which cannot be evaluated because of missing key information. For instance, 13 (2%) of a total 675 reports of hypersensitivity AEs/ADRs associated with heparin administration during an investigation of tainted heparin were excluded from a recently published analysis of AERS data because the reports were "not interpretable."

Information on product use should include the start date(s), stop date(s), doses, frequency of use, and indication for use. Dosage information is important in exploring dose-event relationships. Duration of use is important for characterizing the time course of AEs/ADRs relative to initiation of product use. Indication for use is also an important piece of information, as many products are used for more than one indication (either on-label or off-label).

Patient information should include age, gender, medical history, and concomitant medication usage. The presence of factors that could confound the relationship of the drug to the AE/ADR, especially elements of the medical history and concomitant medication usage, are critical to the interpretation of individual case safety reports.

A description of the AE/ADR that allows for independent medical assessment is critical. A narrative of the event that includes the temporal relationship of drug usage to the development of the AE/ADR, the clinical and diagnostic features, the clinical course, any measures instituted to treat the AE/ADR, the response to these measures, and the clinical outcome are all essential components of a high quality case report. Results of laboratory tests, imaging, and pathology results facilitate an independent interpretation of the report. Information on de-challenge (the course of the AE/ADR when the medication is withdrawn) and re-challenge (the re-development or not of the AE/ADR when the drug is re-introduced), if available, can be invaluable.

National pharmacovigilance systems

The organization of postmarketing safety reporting systems and national pharmacovigilance systems varies around the world. The fundamental feature is that health professionals, and in some cases patients or consumers, are encouraged to send reports of AEs/ADRs to one or more specified locations. These locations can be the drug regulatory authority, an academic or hospital-based pharmacovigilance center (often working with or on behalf of a drug regulatory authority), or the drug manufacturer. The roles of these institutions vary from country to country, and depend greatly on the regulatory and national drug monitoring system in the country.

In resource-poor countries, with varying regulatory infrastructure, the focus in pharmacovigilance has been different from that in the more affluent parts of the world. Reports can result from counterfeit and substandard drugs, known ADRs and drug interactions of concern to reporters, and ADRs resulting from medical error. In some countries, responding to queries about adverse reaction incidence, diagnosis, and management are a major part of the work of pharmacovigilance centers. In developing countries, there are often deficiencies in access to up-to-date information on drug safety that need remedying. On the other hand, large donations of new drugs to combat the endemic scourges of malaria, HIV/AIDS, tuberculosis, infestations, and other diseases, along with vaccines, have led to the high priority of monitoring their use for both safety and efficacy.

However, in many resource-poor countries there is currently not enough capacity for effective safety monitoring, and the improved access to new medicines adds additional strain on already overburdened or nonexistent pharmacovigilance systems. In a recent survey of pharmacovigilance systems in low- and middle-income countries, seven of 55 responding countries indicated that they had no designated system in place, and fewer than half of the respondents had a budget for pharmacovigilance. Consequently, lack of funding was mentioned as a hindrance to the development of pharmacovigilance, together with lack of training and a culture that does not promote AE/ADR reporting. Suggested key developments included: training for health workers and pharmacovigilance program managers; active surveillance methods, sentinel sites and registries; and better collaboration between pharmacovigilance centers and public health programs, with a designated budget for pharmacovigilance included in the latter.

The World Health Organization (WHO) is now working together with major donor organizations to address the urgent need for capacity building in low- and middle-income countries. The strategy will be focused on sustainable development, covering not only the implementation of reporting systems, technical support, and training of healthcare professionals, but also improvements in governance and infrastructure to support pharmacovigilance activities.

The perceived responsibility of healthcare professionals to report AEs/ADRs often varies around the world. Because the largest gaps in drug safety knowledge are believed to be for recently approved medicines, most countries emphasize the need to report AEs/ADRs, even less serious ones, for this group of medicines. For example, in the United Kingdom, recently approved drugs containing new active ingredients are marked in the British National Formulary with a black triangle, a symbol used to denote a drug product whose active ingredient has been newly licensed for use in the UK. In some cases, drug products meeting certain additional criteria are also marked with a black triangle, even if the active ingredient has been previously approved. The aim of the black triangle program is to prompt health professionals to report all suspected adverse reactions associated with the use of these products. In New Zealand, the Intensive Medicines Monitoring Programme monitors cohorts of all patients taking selected new drugs, and specifically requests that all clinical events be reported, not just suspected adverse drug reactions. In some countries, it is mandatory for physicians and dentists to report cases of suspected adverse drug reactions to the regulatory authority. Most countries, however, do not have such specific programs or requirements, but health professionals are encouraged to report and the national reporting centers provide general advice to health professionals on what events to report.

In a majority of countries, including countries in the ICH region (Europe, Japan, and the United States), other high income countries, and 33 of 55 low- and middle-income countries responding to a 2008 survey, pharmaceutical companies that hold marketing authorizations are obligated to report adverse events or adverse drug reactions to the regulatory authority. In some countries, the event is reportable only if an attribution of causality has been made. In other countries, the event is reportable even if no attribution has been made. For example, in the United States, pharmaceutical companies are required by law to submit spontaneous reports of AEs/ADRs, regardless of attribution of causality, on an expedited basis if they are serious and unexpected. The AE/ADR is considered serious when the patient outcome is: death; life-threatening; hospitalization (initial or prolonged); disability; congenital anomaly; or, requires intervention to prevent permanent impairment or damage. Periodic reporting of other types of AEs/ADRs, such as those considered serious and expected (labeled), or nonserious, is typically required as well. The periodicity of such aggregate reports is determined by the length of time the drug has been marketed, with increased frequency for newly approved drugs, and decreased (e.g., annual) with older drugs.

While spontaneous reports of AEs/ADRs usually originate initially from the point of care, the source of reports coming into the national pharmacovigilance centers may vary from country to country.

Some countries restrict reports to those received by physicians. Other countries accept reports from pharmacists, nurses, and patients. There is a current trend towards encouraging direct patient or consumer reporting, replacing the notion held by many in the past that such reports would not be a reliable and useful source of information.

In most countries, the national pharmacovigilance center is part of the drug regulatory authority; in some, the monitoring is carried out jointly by the drug regulatory authority/Ministry of Health and an independent institution. In Germany, the Federal Institute for Drugs and Medical Devices (BfArM) maintains a joint database for recording reported adverse drug reactions, together with the Drug Commission of the German Medical Profession. According to the professional code of conduct of physicians in Germany, all adverse drug reactions should be reported to the Drug Commission. In the Netherlands, the practical responsibility for postmarketing surveillance is shared between the Medicines Evaluation Board (MEB) and the Netherlands Pharmacovigilance Centre (Lareb). The MEB handles communications with market authorization holders; the role of Lareb is to process and analyze reports from health professionals and patients.

Decentralized drug monitoring systems exist both within and outside the ICH region. In France, the French Medicines Agency coordinates the network of 31 regional centers that are connected to major university hospitals. In the United Kingdom, there are four regional centers connected to university hospitals, which have a special function of encouraging reporting in their regions. The reporting system in China involves 31 regional centers reporting to the National Center for Adverse Drug Reaction Monitoring in the State Food and Drug Administration, SFDA. In India, an improved pharmacovigilance system is being developed by the Central Drugs Standard Control Organization, under the Ministry of Health and Family Welfare. In the first year, up to 40 medical institutes planned to participate in pharmacovigilance activities, with further increases in a phased manner until, in 2013, all medical colleges will be linked to four to six regional offices.

National and international postmarketing safety databases

Once submitted to the national drug safety monitoring program, individual case safety reports are stored in computerized postmarketing safety databases. Examples of national reporting systems and databases include the "Blue Card" system (Australia), Canada Vigilance (Canada), the Canadian Adverse Events Following Immunization Surveillance System (CAEFISS) database (Canada), the French Pharmacovigilance Spontaneous Reporting System database (France), the Adverse Drug Reaction Information Management System of the Pharmaceutical and Medication Devices Agency, Ministry of Health, Labor, and Welfare (Japan), the Lareb database (Netherlands), the SWEDIS database (Sweden), the Sentinel database (United Kingdom), the Adverse Event Reporting system (AERS) database (United States), and the Vaccine Adverse Event Reporting System (VAERS) database (United States). In addition, there are two international reporting and database systems: EudraVigilance in the European Union (run by the European Medicines Agency, EMA); and VigiBase, pooling data from the approximately 100 member countries of the WHO International Drug Monitoring Programme (run by the Uppsala Monitoring Centre, UMC). VigiBase is also the system used as the national database by 28 pharmacovigilance centers around the world; reports are stored directly in VigiBase, but entered, managed, and analyzed remotely through an internet-based data management tool, VigiFlow.

To understand the results of an analysis of individual case reports from a postmarketing safety database, it is necessary to understand the unique features of the database, as each large postmarketing safety database differs from the others. It is necessary to understand if, and how, the data are coded. Many databases code drugs according to a local or national standard drug dictionary, while others use a standard international dictionary, such as the WHO Drug Dictionary Enhanced. Similarly, many databases code individual AE/ADR reporter verbatim terms which describe the AE/ADR according to a standard medical dictionary, such as the Medical Dictionary for Regulatory Activities (MedDRA). In the ICH regions, (Europe, Japan, and the United States) use of MedDRA is mandatory for coding of AEs/ADRs.

Beyond coding, several other features of the database are important to understand. First, does the database include only reports from postmarketing systems, or does it include reports from other sources, such as the medical literature or clinical trials? Second, does the database include reports only from health professionals, or does it also include reports from patients and consumers? Third, what is the range of medical products included in the database–drugs, biologicals, blood, blood products, vaccines, dietary supplements? Fourth, does the database include reports from only one country or region, or does it include reports from regions outside the jurisdiction of the regulatory authority? Fifth, does the database include both "nonserious" and "serious" AEs/ADRs; if so, what proportion of the reports have been classified by the health authority (or other database manager) as serious? Sixth, does the database include all adverse events (i.e., events which may or may not be judged to be causally related to a medicine) or does it include only adverse drug reactions (i.e., events for which a likely causal relationship has been determined prior to entering the report into the database)? Seventh, how many individual case reports are in the database? Each of these factors is important in determining the utility of a particular database in answering a specific drug safety question.

Detecting signals from a postmarketing safety database

Identifying potential associations of AEs/ADRs to drugs using only information within the database involves the detection of signals. According to the WHO, a signal is "reported information on a possible causal relationship between an adverse event and a drug, the relationship being unknown or incompletely documented previously." While there have been many definitions of a signal put forth over the years, the important underlying principle is that a signal is a hypothesis that calls for further work to be performed to evaluate that hypothesis.

Signal detection is the act of looking for or identifying signals from any source.

In the setting of a relatively small number of reports, review of groups of reports or periodic summaries of reports has been a standard method of signal detection. For example, one could look at a list of all reports in which the outcome was "death" to see if this outcome was reported more frequently for some drugs than others. Summaries based on specific organ class toxicities could be reviewed to examine if reports in one system organ class were proportionately more frequent for one drug than others. These methods depend on the ability of a drug safety specialist to recognize new or unusual patterns of case reports. While an astute specialist can identify signals using this method, this manual review is often neither practical nor reproducible for detecting signals from large postmarketing safety databases, some of which contain several million records.

In an effort to address this challenge, data mining techniques have been applied to pharmacovigilance AE/ADR databases. In broad terms, data mining refers to a process of analyzing data to find patterns. In the case of AE/ADR databases, most of these patterns would not be visible without the use of statistically based, computerized algorithms. There are a variety of specific algorithms that have been applied to safety signal detection in AE/ADR databases. A full discussion of the statistical principles underlying these methods is beyond the scope of this chapter.

The fundamental feature of data mining techniques used to analyze adverse event databases is that each is based on finding "disproportionalities" in data, that is, the finding that a given AE/ADR is reported for a particular drug more often than would be expected based on the number of reports of that AE/ADR for all other drugs in the database. Several features of these methods are worth noting.

First, the methods are transparent. While the total number of reports for a drug varies over time (and may be highest in the first few years of reporting), this temporal trend will not necessarily alter the proportion of specific reactions for the drug. Thus, a given reaction may still be found to be disproportionately reported even as the total number of reports for the drug changes.

Second, these methods rely exclusively on reports within the database; no external data are needed. For this reason, understanding the characteristics of the database, as discussed above, is important. This feature has several consequences. Because the expected number of reports of a specific AE/ADR for a given drug (and thus the disproportionality of the drug–event pair) depend on the reports within the individual database, the degree of disproportionality for a given drug–event pair may vary from one database to the next. In the extreme, a given drug–event pair may have a strong signal of disproportionality in one database, and no such signal in another. A second consequence is that as the background information for all drugs in the database changes, so does the expected number of reports of a specific AE/ADR for a given drug (and again the disproportionality of the drug–event pair).

Third, a signal of disproportionality is a measure of a statistical association within a collection of AE/ADR reports, and it is not a measure of causality. In this regard, it is important to underscore that *the use of data mining is for signal detection–that is, for hypothesis generation–and that further work is needed to evaluate the signal.*

Fourth, the absence of a signal of disproportionality in a postmarketing safety database is not evidence that an important AE/ADR is not associated with a particular drug.

Some of the data mining techniques used in pharmacovigilance have included the proportional reporting ratio, the reporting odds ratio, the Bayesian Confidence Propagation Neural Network (BCPNN), and the Empirical Bayes method (also know as the Gamma Poisson Shrinker or the Multi-item Gamma Poisson Shrinker). Data mining is sometimes done using a subset of an AE/ADR database. For example, a portion of the database limited to a specific class of drugs might be used to find relative differences in the frequencies of specific AEs/ADRs across the class.

Review of case reports

The review of individual case reports of AEs/ADRs is a complex process. (See also Chapter 13.) It typically begins by identifying one or more case reports with the outcome of interest. Because the case reports that form a case series often come from disparate sources, it is usually necessary to develop a case definition. The case definition centers on the clinical characteristics of the event of interest, without regard to the causal role of the medicine whose relationship to the adverse event is being investigated. Once a case definition is established, each report is reviewed to determine if the event meets the case definition and if the report is to be included in the case series. Depending on the specific question(s) to be answered by the case series, other exclusion criteria may also apply. For example, one would always exclude a case in which the report suggests that the patient never took the medicine of interest. In other cases, one may restrict the case series to only certain formulations of the medicine (e.g., include case reports in which an intravenous formulation, but not an oral formulation, was used, if such exclusion is appropriate for the question at hand), or to certain age groups (e.g., limit the case series to only case reports describing the suspected adverse events in pediatric patients, if such exclusion is appropriate for the question at hand), or to certain indications for use (e.g., limit the case series to case reports in which the medicine was used for a certain off-label indication, if such exclusion is appropriate to the question at hand). Exclusion criteria for a case series must be carefully considered so that potentially relevant cases are not excluded, and all available information is fully assessed. In general, if the purpose of the case series is to examine the relationship between a medicine and a suspected AE/ADR that has not been previously associated with the medicine, it is best to err on the side of inclusion to avoid missing clinically relevant, though incomplete, information about cases of interest.

Once the case series has been developed, it is next necessary to review each case report individually in order to determine if there is a plausible causal relationship between the medicine and the adverse event. At the level of the individual case report, it is often difficult to establish with certainty that the medicine caused the adverse event of interest. For example, if the AE/ADR of interest is one that is already common in the population that takes the medication, establishing a causal role for the medicine in the development of the condition is generally not feasible using individual case reports or case series. For example, the incidence of Parkinson disease is much higher in persons over age 60 years than it is in persons below that age. In this situation, review of a report describing a myocardial infarction in a 70-year-old patient on an anti-parkinsonian agent will generally not be informative in determining if the agent played a causal role in the development of the myocardial infarction, as myocardial infarction occurs commonly in this age group. Similarly, review of a case report is not likely to shed light on the causal relationship between a medicine and an AE/ADR when the AE/ADR is a manifestation of the underlying illness which the medicine is treating. For example, review of case reports of worsening asthma in patients taking an anti-asthma medication is not likely to be sufficient to establish a causal link between the worsening asthma and the medication. Review of a case series to establish a causal relationship between a drug and a AE/ADR is most straightforward when the suspected AE/ADR: (1) is rare in the population when the medication is not used, (2) is not a manifestation of the underlying disease, (3) has a strong temporal association with drug administration, and (4) is biologically plausible as a drug reaction or is generally the result of a drug reaction based on other clinical experience. Examples of AEs/ADRs that often meet these criteria are acute hepatic failure, aplastic anemia, agranulocytosis, rhabdomyolysis, serious skin reactions such as Stevens-Johnson syndrome and toxic epidermal necrolysis, and certain arrhythmias, such as torsades de pointes.

The approach to assessing the causal role of a medicine in the development of an AE/ADR has evolved over the past four decades. In general, the approach relies on a systematic review of each case report to ascertain the temporal relationship between drug intake and the development of the adverse reaction, an assessment of any coexisting diseases or medications that could confound the relationship between the medicine and the AE/ADR, the clinical course after withdrawing the drug ("de-challenge"), and the clinical course after re-introduction of the drug (re-challenge), when applicable. Naranjo and colleagues described a method based on these general principles for estimating the likelihood that a drug caused an adverse clinical event. The World Health Organization has developed a qualitative scale for categorizing causality assessments.

In the development of a case series, once the individual cases are reviewed, it is important to integrate the findings across the cases in an effort to determine patterns that may point to a relationship between the drug and the AE/ADR. For example, does the AE/ADR appear at some doses, but not at others? Does the AE/ADR appear after one or a few doses, or does it appear only after a more prolonged exposure? Is the spectrum of severity of the event homogeneous or is it heterogeneous? Are certain comorbidities or concomitant medications more likely to be present in patients with the event? In the review of a case series, there are no prespecified answers to these questions that establish or exclude the possibility that the drug led to the AE/ADR. Rather, the characteristics of the individual cases, taken together with the patterns observed in the case series itself, can lead the analyst to determine if the medication has a reasonable possibility of causing the condition of interest.

Reporting ratios

Because postmarketing safety reporting systems do not capture all cases of an event of interest, it is not possible to calculate an incidence rate for a particular drug–event pair. However, analysis of AEs/ADRs based simply on numbers of reports, even after thorough analysis of these reports, does not in itself put these reports into the context of how widely a medicine is used.

To adjust for the extent of drug utilization in a population in the analysis of AE/ADR reports, a reporting ratio can be used. A reporting ratio is defined as the number of cases of a particular AE/ADR reported to a drug safety database during a specific time period divided by some measure of drug utilization in the same time period. Across drugs, the reporting ratios measure the relative frequency of the AE/ADR reports adjusting for differences in level of drug utilization. The numerator is derived from counts of AE/ADR reports associated with the drug of interest that are recorded in the postmarketing safety database during a specified time period. In the past, the denominator typically consisted of the number of dispensed prescriptions, used as a surrogate measure of drug exposure in the population over that same time period, and often estimated from proprietary drug utilization databases. The number of dispensed prescriptions was used because data on the number of unique individuals using the drug in a specified time period was generally not available. More recently, such data have become available, and reporting ratios based on persons using the medication, and not prescriptions, are being calculated. In some cases, information is available on not only the number of persons receiving the drug or the number of prescriptions dispensed, but also on the duration of use. When such data are available, the denominator for the reporting ratio may be expressed in person-time. When using denominators based on person-time, it is important to be mindful of the assumptions of the person-time method, especially the assumption that events in the numerator occur uniformly over time. Because many AEs/ADRs do not occur uniformly over time after a drug is started, this assumption does not always hold.

Because the reporting ratio (sometimes referred to as "reporting rate") is not a measure of incidence or prevalence, it must be interpreted cautiously. For AEs/ADRs that are rare in the general population (e.g., aplastic anemia), reporting ratios are sometimes compared to the background rate (incidence or prevalence) of that event in a defined population. In other situations, individual reporting ratios of a particular AE/ADR across different drugs used for a similar indication or within the same class are calculated and the magnitude of the differences in reporting ratios is compared. Interpretation of the comparison of reporting ratios across drugs must be made with caution, since such comparisons are highly sensitive to variation in AE/ADR reporting and thus it is necessary to take into account the differential underreporting of AEs in the postmarketing safety reporting system. The underlying assumption in estimating reporting ratios for comparison across a group of drug products is that each of the respective man-ufacturer's reporting practices for the drug of inter-est are similar over the reporting period. However, this assumption may not hold true in some cases, and a comparison of reporting ratios across drugs may not be valid.

Strengths

Signal detection

The principal strength–and, arguably, the principal purpose–of a postmarketing safety reporting sys-tem is that it allows for signal detection, the fur-ther exploration of drug safety hypotheses, and appropriate regulatory decision-making and action when necessary. As noted earlier in this chapter, signals can be detected by data mining methods, review of individual case reports, or assessment of case series. In many instances, further work is needed to determine with more certainty the rela-tionship of the drug to the AE/ADR. The capability for timely and effective signal detection is a key strength of a postmarketing pharmacovigilance reporting system.

Another key strength of a well designed and effectively utilized postmarketing pharmacovigi-lance reporting system is that, in certain cases, the relationship of a drug to an AE/ADR can be estab-lished with sufficient confidence, usually by a case series, that necessary regulatory action can be taken. AEs/ADRs for which the relationship to a drug can be established with reasonable certainty are generally those that have a strong temporal association with drug administration, a low or near absent frequency in the underlying population, are not part of the underlying illness being treated, are generally the result of exposure to a drug or other toxin, and have no other likely explanation. Aplas-tic anemia, agranulocytosis, acute liver failure, rhabdomyolysis, certain arrhythmias such as tor-sades de pointes, and serious skin reactions such as Stevens-Johnson syndrome are examples of adverse events whose relationship to a drug can often be established by case series. However, rela-tive to all signals detected in a postmarketing safety reporting system, those about which a reasonably

firm conclusion can be made on the basis of AE/ADR reports alone are few in number.

Opportunity for the public to report AEs/ADRs

Postmarketing safety reporting systems allow healthcare professionals to report suspected AEs/ADRs to national pharmacovigilance centers, drug regulatory authorities, and/or manufacturers. Such systems allow for direct engagement of healthcare professionals in the drug safety monitor-ing system. The advantage of this involvement is that it allows for careful clinical observations, made at the point of care, to inform drug safety surveil-lance. Clinicians can provide succinct but detailed accounts of relevant symptoms, signs, diagnostic test results, past medical history, concomitant med-ications, and clinical course of an AE/ADR, includ-ing information on de-challenge and re-challenge. Such a synthesis of clinical information is generally not available from automated data sources. For those AEs/ADRs that are serious, rare, and often the result of a medication exposure, the ability to obtain detailed information directly from the point of care is an essential feature of postmarketing pharmacovigilance reporting systems.

Postmarketing safety reporting systems also can accept reports from consumers and patients, though this practice is not a feature of all such reporting systems. In the United States, where con-sumers and patients can report either to the manu-facturer or directly to the FDA, the percentage of reports in 2009 that originated from consumers was 46%. While consumer and patient-generated reports might not have the same level of medical detail as those provided by health professionals, subsequent follow up with health professionals may be possible in potentially important cases, so that more complete clinical information can be obtained.

Scope

The scope of a postmarketing safety reporting sys-tem is quite broad. The system can cover all medi-cines used in the populations, and it can receive reports of AEs/ADRs occurring in any member of the population. Because it need not restrict the reports it receives, it can receive AE/ADR reports throughout a medicine's marketed lifecycle. Thus, AEs/ADRs recognized late in a product's lifecycle, such as those resulting from prolonged exposure to a medicine, can, in theory, be ascertained. In practice, such ascertainment is difficult to achieve, because healthcare professionals may be less likely to ascribe an AE/ADR not known to be associated with a medicine that has been marketed for several years. In addition, patients who take a medicine for several years may also receive other treatments during that time, making it difficult to conclude that there is an association between the medicine and the AE/ADR.

Despite this broad scope, a postmarketing spontaneous reporting system can be relatively inexpensive. Most of these pharmacovigilance systems rely on voluntary reporting, and those who report AEs/ADRs are generally not paid. Thus, information collection is not expensive from the perspective of effective pharmacovigilance, given that the system has the capacity to handle all medicines and all outcomes. This is in contrast to other data used to study drug safety questions, such as data from clinical trials, registries, and electronic healthcare data, each of which is relatively expensive to operate.

Limitations

Quality of reports

Perhaps the major potential limitation of a spontaneous postmarketing safety reporting system is that it depends quite heavily on the quality of individual reports. Although data mining and other informatics methods can detect signals using coded bioinformatics terms in safety databases, each individual case report must still be carefully reviewed by a clinical analyst to determine if there is a plausible relationship between the medicine and the development of the AE/ADR. The quality of the report, as described earlier in this chapter, is critical for an informative and meaningful review of the individual case report. Report quality depends on the care, effort, and judgment of the person submitting the report, as well as the diligence of the person receiving and/or transmitting the report to the health authority. Reports without sufficient information for an independent determination of the relationship between the medicine and the AE/ADR are problematic for drug safety surveillance. However, with successful follow up, sometimes even such deficient reports can yield useful information.

Underreporting

Another well-recognized limitation of spontaneous postmarketing reporting systems is underreporting. Because most systems are voluntary, not all AEs/ADRs are reported. A consequence of underreporting of AEs/ADRs is that population-based rates of AEs/ADRs cannot be calculated, because all such occurrences in the population are not reported, and the extent of underreporting for any individual AE/ADR is not known. Reporting ratios, discussed earlier in this chapter, allow the reported number of AEs/ADRs to be put into the context of drug utilization, though this measure is not an incidence rate.

Non-uniform temporal trends in reporting

Another limitation of spontaneous reporting systems is that temporal trends in the number of AE/ADR reports for a drug–event combination may not reflect actual population-based trends for the drug–event combination. This is because multiple factors can affect the number of AE/ADR reports received for a given drug–event pair.

First, the number of reports for a medicine has been thought to peak in the second year after approval and declines thereafter, even though the drug may be used more widely. This phenomenon, known as the Weber effect, was originally described in relation to nonsteroidal anti-inflammatory medicines. A recent analysis of reporting patterns for the angiotensin II receptor blocker class of medicines revealed no discernible trend when the number of reports over time was examined. Specifically, this analysis did not confirm that the number of reports increased toward the end of the second year and declined thereafter. Rather, the analysis indicated that additional factors, such as the approval of additional indications and modifications of the firms' reporting requirements affected the total number of reports received. However, when the number of reports in a year was adjusted for the number of prescriptions dispensed in that year's period, it was found that the adjusted number of reports was highest in the first years after approval and declined thereafter. Thus, the frequency of AE/ADR reports per estimated unit of drug utilization is not likely to be constant over time.

Second, publicity about an important new AE/ADR often gives rise to a large number of reports shortly after the publicity, with a decline in the number of reports shortly thereafter. This phenomenon is known as stimulated reporting, and was observed, for example, in the reporting pattern of statin-induced hospitalized rhabdomyolysis after there was publicity of this risk. For these reasons, changes in the number of AE/ADR reports for a given drug–event pair cannot reliably be interpreted as a change in the population-based frequency of the AE/ADR.

Another limitation of a postmarketing reporting system is that it is usually not well suited to ascertaining the relationship of a medicine to an AE/ADR that is common in the treated population, especially if the condition is a manifestation of the underlying illness. In such cases, the combined effect of confounding of patient factors and indication make causality assessment of individual cases difficult.

Finally, duplicate reports of the same AE/ADR may be received by drug manufacturers and health authorities, and if undetected as duplicates, may be entered into the database as multiple occurrences of the same event. Algorithms have been developed, and various methods can be used to identify such reports; nonetheless, this issue is a potential source of bias and limits the utility of data mining or other calculations which rely on "crude" case counts which have not been "de-duplicated."

Particular applications

Case series and reporting rates
Spontaneous AE/ADR reports have at times served as a necessary and sufficient basis for regulatory

actions including product withdrawals. For instance, in August 2001 the manufacturer of cerivastatin withdrew that drug from marketing based on "a markedly increased reporting rate of fatal rhabdomyolysis" compared to the other drugs in the statin class. Additional confirmation of the unacceptably high risk of rhabdomyolysis with cerivastatin was eventually available three years later when results of a well-designed epidemiologic study were published. Clearly, that timeframe would have been far too long to delay decisive action, which in retrospect was soundly based on the signal from spontaneous reports. The timely detection of this signal would not have happened without the efforts of the point-of-care clinicians who took the time to report rhabdomyolysis when it occurred in their patients.

Data mining signals
The disproportionality measure used by the UMC is the Information Component (IC), originally introduced through the Bayesian Confidence Propagation Neural Network (BCPNN), which is a logarithmic measure of the disproportionality between the observed and expected reporting of a drug-ADR pair. A positive IC value means that a particular drug–event pair is reported more often than expected, based on all the reports in the database. The following is an example of a signal identified by data mining techniques applied to the WHO Global Individual Case Safety Report Database, VigiBase, regarding the occurrence of glaucoma with topiramate. Topiramate was approved in the US in 1996 as an anticonvulsant drug. In the second quarter of 2000, reports of topiramate and glaucoma in VigiBase reached the threshold of an "association" (i.e., the lower limit of a 95% Bayesian confidence interval for the IC exceeded zero). When potential signals are identified, the available information is reviewed by the UMC staff and an expert review panel. At the time, there were six cases reported to VigiBase. After review, a summary of the findings were circulated in the Signal document in April 2001 to all national pharmacovigilance centers in the WHO Programme. (*Note: the Signal document is a UMC publication with the purpose of communicating the results of UMC evaluations of potential signals from the*

WHO database. Previously restricted to national pharma-
covigilance centers, UMC signals from 2012 are also made
available publicly through publication in WHO Pharma-
ceuticals Newsletter.) Later the same year, the Market
Authorization Holder issued a Dear Healthcare Professional letter warning about "an ocular syndrome
that has occurred in patients receiving topiramate.
This syndrome is characterized by acute myopia
and secondary angle closure glaucoma." At the
time, there were 23 reported cases according to the
company. FDA issued a warning in the revised
labeling October 1, 2001.

Signals from developing countries

At the annual meetings of the WHO Programme
members, country representatives are invited to
share problems of current interest in their countries. The following is an example of a signal regarding iatrogenic meningitis that was investigated in a
developing country. This case was presented at a
WHO meeting in Geneva in 2005. A representative
from Sri Lanka described how the reporting of suspected AEs/ADRs may contribute significantly to
patient safety when information is analyzed and
followed-up and root causes identified. There
were 14 cases identified, with three deaths reported
due to fungal contamination of anesthetic
drugs/syringes. The date of onset ranged between
the weeks of June 27 and July 25, 2005. Case-
patients were identified following exposures in
three different health care facilities. Case-patients
did not share a common health care facility, personnel, or surgery session. Microbiology indicated
Aspergillus fumigatus as the infectious agent in three
of seven case-patients. There was evidence of the
organism in patients who received spinal anesthesia in two of the three hospitals involved. Two medications were common to six of the cases, but they
were not contaminated. A large variety of injection
devices used in the health care facilities and coming
from three manufacturers were contaminated with
Aspergillus fumigatus. Substandard storage conditions may have constituted the mode of contamination of these devices. There had been a lack of
storage facilities because of very large donations in
response to a tsunami. Two of the three syringes
implicated were tsunami donations.

The future

Spontaneous AE/ADR reporting is an important
component of drug safety surveillance. The widespread availability of electronic healthcare data
may, at first, seem to undermine the importance of
AE/ADR reporting. This is not likely to be the case.
Because careful observation at the point of care is
an essential component of pharmacovigilance,
electronic systems may be able to facilitate AE/ADR
reporting in the future, but will not replace it. It is
technologically and administratively feasible for
carefully designed systems to allow clinicians to
report AEs/ADRs directly from electronic medical
record systems. If designed properly, these systems could allow for the accurate, complete, and
efficient inclusion of laboratory, radiologic, and
other diagnostic test results, information which is
often incomplete in current AE/ADR reports. The
challenge of such a system will be to encourage
reporters to provide routinely a clinically meaningful narrative that explains concisely the clinical course of the AE/ADR and its relationship to
medication usage.

Postmarketing safety reporting systems depend
on the involvement of healthcare professionals
and, in some areas, consumers and patients as
well, for high quality AE/ADR reports. As new
medicines become available, it will be increasingly necessary to monitor postmarketing safety.
Postmarketing safety reporting systems will continue to be the cornerstone of this effort,
because of their unique advantages. As active
surveillance and the use of large healthcare
databases begin to play a role in drug safety surveillance, demonstrate their utility, and realize
their potential, they could become valuable
adjuncts to existing pharmacovigilance reporting
systems worldwide.

Key points

• Adverse events and adverse drug reactions are
closely related, but nonetheless distinct, concepts.
• Spontaneous reporting systems are based on the
notion that clinical observations made at the point

of care are often valuable pieces of information in further refining knowledge of a drug's safety.

• Spontaneous reporting systems can be used to describe adverse drug events, adverse device events, medication errors, or a combination of these.

• The characteristics and quality of individual case reports determine the extent to which the reports can address a drug safety question

• The organization of national pharmacovigilance centers can vary from one country to the next.

Case Example 7.1: Spontaneous pharmacovigilance reporting systems: Felbamate

Background:

• Felbamate is an anticonvulsant agent approved for use in the United States on July 29, 1993. Pre-approval studies showed no evidence of significant, nonreversible hematologic abnormalities.

Question

• Can spontaneous postmarketing reports identify a signal for a rare event such as aplastic anemia and can safety surveillance result in a regulatory decision and labeling change that supports the safe use of this product?

Approach

• Within about one year of approval, cases of aplastic anemia were reported to the manufacturer and to the US FDA. This finding prompted a search for and comprehensive review of all case reports of aplastic anemia in persons taking felbamate.

Results

• Twenty cases of aplastic anemia, three of them fatal, had been reported in the United States. Review of the case reports suggested a causal role for felbamate, based on a careful review of the temporal relationship of the adverse event to use of the drug, the patients' past medical history, and concomitant medication usage.

• An estimated 100 000 patients had taken felbamate during this time. While the true incidence of aplastic anemia in patients taking felbamate cannot be calculated because case ascertainment is likely incomplete, the minimum rate is 20/100 000/year, or 200/million/year.

• In contrast, the population background rate of aplastic anemia is low, about 2 per million per year. Thus, the observed cases of aplastic anemia suggest that aplastic anemia is at least 100 times more frequent in patients taking felbamate than in the general population.

Outcome

• Based on this finding, the FDA and the manufacturer recommended that patients not be treated with felbamate unless the benefits of the drug were judged to outweigh the risk of aplastic anemia.

• A subsequent review of 31 case reports of aplastic anemia in patients taking felbamate using the criteria of the International Agranulocytosis and Aplastic Anemia Study (IAAAS), established that felbamate was the only plausible cause in three cases, and the most likely cause in 11 cases. For the remaining nine cases, there was at least one other plausible cause. The authors concluded that the "most probable" incidence of aplastic anemia was estimated to be 127 per million.

Strengths

• Spontaneous reports of drug adverse events can be used to identify adverse drug reactions that are rare, serious, and generally the result of a drug or toxin exposure.

• While reporting rates cannot be used to calculate incidence rates, in certain cases a reporting rate can be compared to a background incidence rate to demonstrate that the incidence of the adverse event in patients exposed to the drug is higher than would be expected in the absence of the drug.

Limitations

• Formal incidence rates cannot be calculated from spontaneous reports.

Key points

• Because aplastic anemia is uncommon in the population and because it is generally the result of a medication or other toxin, a careful analysis of a case series can establish the relationship of a drug to aplastic anemia.

- Data mining of spontaneous reporting databases, which allows relationships and patterns to be seen in the data which would otherwise be missed, can be used to detect drug safety signals and generate hypotheses.
- Interpretation of spontaneous reports always requires careful analysis, thought, and clear communication of results, conclusions, and limitations.
- Because postmarketing safety reporting systems do not capture all cases of an event of interest, it is not possible to calculate an incidence rate for a particular drug–event pair.
- Reporting ratios help put the number of reports of a drug-adverse event pair into the context of how widely a medicine is used.
- The capability for timely and effective signal detection is a key strength of a postmarketing pharmacovigilance reporting system.

Further reading

Almenoff J, Tonning J, Gould A *et al.* (2005) Perspectives on the use of data mining in pharmacovigilance. *Drug Safety* **28** (11): 981–1007.

ICH Harmonized Tripartite Guideline (1994) Clinical Safety Data Management: Definitions and Standards for Expedited Reporting E2A. Current Step 4 version, dated October 27, 1994. Available from: http://www.ich.org/LOB/media/MEDIA436.pdf.

ICH Harmonized Tripartite Guideline (2003) Post-approval Safety Data Management: Definitions and Standards for Expedited Reporting. *The Lancet* **336**: 156–158.

Kaufman D, Kelly J, Anderson T, Harmon D, Shapiro S (1997) Evalution of case reports of aplastic anemia among patients treated with felbamate. *Epilepsia* **38** (12): 1265–69.

McAdams M, Governale L, Swartz L, Hammad T, Dal Pan G (2008) Identifying patterns of adverse event reporting for four members of the Angiotensin II receptor blockers class of drugs: Revisiting the Weber effect. *Pharmacoepidemiology and Drug Safety* **17**: 882–9.

McAdams M, Staffa J, Dal Pan G (2008) Estimating the extent of reporting to FDA: A case study of statin-associated rhabdomyolysis. *Pharmacoepidemiology and Drug Safety* **17** (3): 229–39.

McBride WG (1961) Thalidomide and congenital abnormalities. *Lancet* **2** (721): 1358.

McBride WG (2001) Specialist life–William McBride. *Eur J Obstet Gynecol Reprod Biol* **95** (1): 139–40.

McMahon A, Pratt R, Hammad T *et al.* (2010) Description of hypersensitivity adverse events following administration of heparin that was potentially contaminated with oversulfated chrondroitin sulfate in early 2008. *Pharmacoepidemiology and Drug Safety* Sep; **19** (9): 921–33.

Meyboom RHB, Hekster YA, Egberts ACG, Gribnau FWJ, Edwards IR (1997) Causal or casual? The role of causality assessment in pharmacovigilance. *Drug Safety* **17** (6): 374–89.

Nightingale S (1994) Recommendation to immediately withdraw patients from treatment with felbamate. *The Journal of the American Medical Association* **272** (13): 995.

Staffa J, Chang J, Green L (2002) Cerivastatin and reports of fatal rhabdomyolysis. *The New England Journal of Medicine* **346** (7): 539–40.

The Uppsala Monitoring Centre (2010) The use of the WHO-UMC system for standardised case causality assessment. Available from: http://www.who-umc.org/graphics/4409.pdf.

US Food and Drug Administration (2005) Guidance for Industry–E2B(M): Data Elements for Transmission of Individual Case Safety Reports. Available from: http://www.fda.gov/RegulatoryInformation/Guidances/ucm129428.htm.

US Food and Drug Administration (2005) Guidance for Industry: Good Pharmacovigilance Practices and Pharmacoepidemiologic Assessment. Available from: http://www.fda.gov/downloads/RegulatoryInformation/Guidances/UCM126834.pdf

US Food and Drug Administration (2009) 21 CFR 314.80. 4-1-2009. Available from: http://www.accessdata.fda.gov/scripts/cdrh/cfdocs/cfcfr/CFRSearch.cfm?fr=314.80.

US Food and Drug Administration (2009) The ICH Guideline on Clinical Safety Data Management: Data Elements for Transmission of Individual Case Safety Reports. 5-12-2009.

US Food and Drug Administration (2010) MedWatch: The FDA Safety Information and Adverse Events Reporting System. Available from: http://www.fda.gov/Safety/MedWatch/default.htm.

World Health Organization (2002) *The Importance of Pharmacovigilance. Safety Monitoring of Medicinal Products.* Geneva: WHO.

CHAPTER 8

Overview of Automated Databases in Pharmacoepidemiology

Brian L. Strom
Perelman School of Medicine at the University of Pennsylvania, Philadelphia, PA, USA

Introduction

Once hypotheses are generated, usually from spontaneous reporting systems (see Chapter 7), techniques are needed to test these hypotheses. Usually between 500 and 3000 patients are exposed to the drug during Phase III testing, even if drug efficacy can be demonstrated with much smaller numbers of patients. Studies of this size have the ability to detect drug effects with an incidence as low as 1 per 1000 to 6 per 1000 (see Chapter 3). Given this context, postmarketing studies of drug effects must then generally include at least 10 000 exposed persons in a cohort study, or enroll diseased patients from a population of equivalent size for a case-control study. A study of this size would be 95% certain of observing at least one case of any adverse effect that occurs with an incidence of 3 per 10 000 or greater (see Chapter 3). However, studies this large are expensive and difficult to perform. Yet, these studies often need to be conducted quickly, to address acute and serious regulatory, commercial, and/or public health crises. For these reasons, the past three decades have seen a growing use of computerized databases containing medical care data, so called "automated databases," as potential data sources for pharmacoepidemiologic studies.

Large electronic databases can often meet the need for a cost-effective and efficient means of conducting postmarketing surveillance studies. To meet the needs of pharmacoepidemiology, the ideal database would include records from inpatient and outpatient care, emergency care, mental health care, all laboratory and radiological tests, and all prescribed and over-the-counter medications, as well as alternative therapies. The population covered by the database would be large enough to permit discovery of rare events for the drug(s) in question, and the population would be stable over its lifetime. Although it is generally preferable for the population included in the database to be representative of the general population from which it is drawn, it may sometimes be advantageous to emphasize the more disadvantaged groups that may have been absent from premarketing testing. The drug(s) under investigation must of course be present in the formulary and must be prescribed in sufficient quantity to provide adequate power for analyses.

Other requirements of an ideal database are that all parts are easily linked by means of a patient's unique identifier, that the records are updated on a regular basis, and that the records are verifiable and are reliable. The ability to conduct medical chart review to confirm outcomes is also a necessity for most studies, as diagnoses entered into an electronic database may include rule-out diagnoses or interim diagnoses and recurrent/chronic, as opposed to acute, events. Information on potential confounders, such as smoking and alcohol consumption, may only be available through chart review or, more consistently, through patient

Textbook of Pharmacoepidemiology, Second Edition. Edited by Brian L. Strom, Stephen E. Kimmel, and Sean Hennessy.
© 2013 John Wiley & Sons, Ltd. Published 2013 by John Wiley & Sons, Ltd.

interviews. With appropriate permissions and confidentiality safeguards in place, access to patients is sometimes possible and useful for assessing compliance with the medication regimen as well as for obtaining information on other factors that may relate to drug effects. Information on drugs taken intermittently for symptom relief, over-the-counter drugs, and drugs not on the formulary must also be obtained directly from the patient.

These automated databases are the focus of this section of the book. Of course, no single database is ideal. In the current chapter, we will introduce these resources, presenting some of the general principles that apply to them all. In Chapter 9 of this book, we will present more detailed descriptions of those databases that have been used in a substantial amount of published research, along with the strengths and weaknesses of each.

Description

So-called automated databases have existed and been used for pharmacoepidemiologic research in North America since 1980, and are primarily administrative in origin, generated by the request for payments, or claims, for clinical services and therapies. In contrast, in Europe, medical record databases have been developed for use by researchers, and similar databases have been developed in the US more recently.

Claims and other administrative databases

Claims data (Chapter 9) arise from a person's use of the health care system (see Figure 8.1). When a patient goes to a pharmacy and gets a drug dispensed, the pharmacy bills the insurance carrier for

Claims Databases: Sources of Data

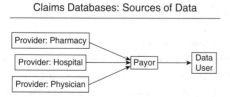

Figure 8.1 Sources of claims data.

the cost of that drug, and has to identify which medication was dispensed, the milligrams per tablet, number of tablets, etc. Analogously, if a patient goes to a hospital or to a physician for medical care, the providers of care bill the insurance carrier for the cost of the medical care, and have to justify the bill with a diagnosis. If there is a common patient identification number for both the pharmacy and the medical care claims, these elements could be linked, and analyzed as a longitudinal medical record.

Since drug identity and the amount of drug dispensed affect reimbursement, and because the filing of an incorrect claim about drugs dispensed is fraud, claims are often closely audited, e.g., by Medicaid (see Chapter 9). There have also been numerous validity checks on the drug data in claims files that showed that the drug data are of extremely high quality, i.e., confirming that the patient was dispensed exactly what the claim showed was dispensed, according to the pharmacy record. In fact, claims data of this type provide some of the best data on drug exposure in pharmacoepidemiology (see Chapter 12).

The quality of disease data in these databases is somewhat less perfect. If a patient is admitted to a hospital, the hospital charges for the care and justifies that charge by assigning International Classification of Diseases-Ninth Revision-Clinical Modification (ICD-9-CM) codes and a Diagnosis Related Group (DRG). The ICD-9-CM codes are reasonably accurate diagnoses that are used for clinical purposes, based primarily on the discharge diagnoses assigned by the patient's attending physician. (Of course, this does not guarantee that the physician's diagnosis is correct.) The amount paid by the insurer to the hospital is based on the DRG, so there is no reason to provide incorrect ICD-9-CM codes. In fact, most hospitals have mapped each set of ICD-9-CM codes into the DRG code that generates the largest payment.

In contrast, outpatient diagnoses are assigned by the practitioners themselves, or by their office staff. Once again, reimbursement does not usually depend on the actual diagnosis, but rather on the procedures administered during the outpatient medical encounter, and these procedure codes indicate the intensity of the services provided. Thus, there is no incentive for the practitioner to provide incorrect ICD-9-CM diagnosis codes, but there is also no incentive for them to be particularly careful or complete about the diagnoses provided. For these reasons, the outpatient diagnoses are the weakest link in claims databases.

Some other databases are not made up of actual claims, but derive from other administrative processes, e.g., data from US Health Maintenance Organizations (Chapter 9) or other data sources (Chapter 9). The characteristics of these data are similar in many ways to those of claims data.

Medical record databases

In contrast, medical record databases are a more recent development, arising out of the increasing use of computerization in medical care. Initially, computers were used in medicine primarily as a tool for literature searches. Then, they were used for billing. Now, however, there is increasing use of computers to record medical information itself, often replacing the paper medical record as the primary medical record. As medical practices increasingly become electronic, this opens up a unique opportunity for pharmacoepidemiology, as larger and larger numbers of patients are available in such systems. The best-known and most widely used example of this approach is the UK General Practice Research Database (GPRD), described in Chapter 9, along with the newer database, The Health Improvement Network (THIN). As general practice databases, these contain primarily outpatient data. In addition, recently there are new inpatient electronic medical record databases available.

Medical record databases have unique advantages. Importantly among them is that the validity of the diagnosis data in these databases is better than that in claims databases, as these data are being used for medical care. When performing a pharmacoepidemiologic study using these databases, there is no need to validate the data against the actual medical record, since one is analyzing the data from the actual medical record. However, there are also unique issues one needs to be concerned about, especially the uncertain completeness of the data from other physicians and sites of care. Any given practitioner provides only a piece of the care a patient receives, and inpatient and outpatient care are unlikely to be recorded in a common medical record.

Strengths

Computerized databases have several important advantages. These include their potential for providing a very large sample size. This is especially important in the field of pharmacoepidemiology, where achieving an adequate sample size is uniquely problematic. In addition, these databases are relatively inexpensive to use, especially given the available sample size, as they are by-products of existing administrative systems. Studies using these data systems do not need to incur the considerable cost of data collection, other than for those subsets of the populations for whom medical records are abstracted and/or interviews are conducted. The data can be complete, i.e., for claims databases, information is available on all medical care provided, regardless of who the provider was. As indicated above, this can be a problem though for medical records databases. In addition, these databases can be population-based, they can include outpatient drugs and diseases, and there is no opportunity for recall and interviewer bias, as they do not rely on patient recall or interviewers to obtain their data. Another advantage is that these databases can potentially be linked to external other electronic databases (e.g., death records, maternal-child records, police accident records), to expand the capabilities and scope of research. This requires using common identification elements (e.g., name and date of birth) and standardized semantics to allow communication across databases.

Weaknesses

The major weakness of such data systems is the uncertain validity of diagnosis data. This is especially true for claims databases, and for outpatient data. For these databases, access to medical record data for validation purposes is usually needed. This issue is less problematic for medical record databases. The addition of laboratory results data to these resources can assist in diagnosis validity, as well.

In addition, such databases can lack information on some potential confounding variables. For example, in claims databases there are no data on smoking, alcohol, date of menopause, etc., all of which can be of great importance to selected research questions. This argues that one either needs access to patients or access to physician records if these contain the data in question, or one needs to be selective about the research questions that one seeks to answer through these databases, avoiding questions that require data on variables which may be important potential confounders that must be controlled for.

Another major disadvantage of administrative data is the instability of the population due to job changes, employers' changes of health plans, and changes in coverage for specific employees and their family members. The opportunity for longitudinal analyses is thereby hindered by the continual enrollment and dis-enrollment of plan members. Another source of instability of the population is when patients transfer out of the system due to death or moving away. The effect of this is an inflated list with patients no longer seeking medical care. This will invalidate calculations of patient-time in studies of disease incidence, for example, because the denominator is inflated. The challenge for the investigator is to be creative in devising strategies to guard or correct for this incomplete information in the database (e.g., by performing sensitivity analysis censoring follow-up one or two years after the patient's last recorded entry in the database). Alternatively, strategies can be adopted for selecting stable populations within a particular database, and for example, by examining patterns of prescription refills for chronically used medications. Of course, the largest such data system, i.e., US Medicare, suffers much less from this problem, since it covers the elderly, so people never lose eligibility. Even there, however, patients can switch between fee-for-service plans and managed care plans, and the latter may not record all health care which is provided (see Chapter 9).

Further, by definition, such databases only include illnesses severe enough to come to medical attention. In general, this is not a problem, since illnesses that are not serious enough to come to medical attention and yet are uncommon enough for one to seek to study them in such databases, are generally not of importance.

Some results from studies that utilize these databases may not be generalizable, e.g., on health care utilization. This is especially relevant for databases created by data from a population that is atypical in some way, e.g., US Medicaid data (see Chapter 9).

Finally, as an increasing number of electronic health record databases emerge in the US, to date all are problematic in that they do not include complete data on a defined population. In the US health system, unlike other countries, patients can, and often do seek medical care from a variety of different health care providers. Thus, providers' electronic health records are inherently incomplete, and need to be linked to administrative data in order to be useful for quality research.

Particular applications

Based on these characteristics, one can identify particular situations when these databases are uniquely useful or uniquely problematic for pharmacoepidemiologic research. These databases are useful in situations: (1) when looking for uncommon outcomes because of a large sample size; (2) when a denominator is needed to calculate incidence rates; (3) when one is studying short-term drug effects (especially when the effects require specific drug or surgical therapy that can be used as validation of the diagnosis); (4) when one is studying objective, laboratory-driven diagnoses; (5) when recall or interviewer bias could influence the association; (6) when time is limited; and (7) when the budget is limited.

Uniquely problematic situations include: (1) illnesses that do not reliably come to medical attention; (2) inpatient drug exposures that are not included in some of these databases; (3) outcomes that are poorly defined by the ICD-9-CM coding system, such as Stevens-Johnson Syndrome; (4) descriptive studies, if the population studied is skewed; (5) delayed drug effects, wherein patients can lose eligibility in the interim; and (6) important confounders about which information cannot be obtained without accessing the patients, such as cigarette smoking, occupation, menarche, menopause, etc.

The future

Given the frequent use of these data resources for pharmacoepidemiologic research in the recent past, we have already learned much about their appropriate role. Inasmuch as it appears that these uses will be increasing, we are likely to continue to gain more insight in the coming years, especially with the advent in the US of FDA's Sentinel System, destined to exceed 100 million individuals (Chapter 22). However, care must be taken to ensure that all potential confounding factors of interest are available in the system or addressed in some other way, that diagnoses under study are chosen carefully, and that medical records can be obtained when needed to validate the diagnoses. In this section of the book, we review in Chapter 9 the details of several of these databases. The databases selected for detailed review have been chosen because they have been the most widely used for published research. They are also good examples of the different types of data that are available. There are multiple others like each of them (see Chapter 9) and undoubtedly many more will emerge over the ensuing years. Each has its advantages and disadvantages, but each has proven it can be useful in pharmacoepidemiologic studies.

Key points

- The past three decades have seen a growing use of computerized databases containing medical care data, so-called "automated databases," as potential data sources for pharmacoepidemiology studies.
- Claims data arise from a person's use of the health care system, and the submission of claims to insurance companies for payment. While claims data provide some of the best data on drug exposure in pharmacoepidemiology, the quality of disease data in these databases can be more problematic.
- Medical record databases are a more recent development, arising out of the increasing use of computerization in medical care. The validity of the diagnosis data in these databases is better than that in claims databases, as these data are being used for medical care. However, the completeness of the data from other physicians and sites of care is uncertain.

Further reading

Ray WA, Griffin MR (1989) Use of Medicaid data for pharmacoepidemiology. *Am J Epidemiol* **129**: 837–49.

Strom BL, Carson JL (1989) Automated data bases used for pharmacoepidemiology research. *Clinical Pharmacology and Therapeutics* **46**: 390–4.

Strom BL, Carson JL (1990) Use of automated databases for pharmacoepidemiology research. *Epidemiologic Reviews* **12**: 87–107.

CHAPTER 9
Examples of Existing Automated Databases

The following individuals contributed to writing sections of this chapter:

Sengwee Toh[1], Susan E. Andrade[2], Marsha A. Raebel[3], Denise M. Boudreau[4], Robert L. Davis[5], Katherine Haffenreffer[1], Pamala A. Pawloski[6], Richard Platt[1], Sean Hennessy[7], Cristin Palumbo Freeman[7], Francesca Cunningham[8], Yola Moride[9], Alexis Ogdie[7], Sinéad M. Langan[10], John Parkinson[11], Hassy Dattani[12], Karel Kostev[13], Joel M. Gelfand[7], Ron M.C. Herings[14], and Lars Pedersen[15]

[1]*Harvard Medical School and Harvard Pilgrim Health Care Institute, Boston, MA, USA*
[2]*Meyers Primary Care Institute and University of Massachusetts Medical School, Worcester, MA, USA*
[3]*Institute for Health Research, Kaiser Permanente Colorado and University of Colorado, Skaggs School of Pharmacy and Pharmaceutical Sciences, Aurora, CO, USA*
[4]*Group Health Research Institute, Seattle, WA, USA*
[5]*Center for Health Research, Southeast Kaiser Permanente, Atlanta, GA, USA*
[6]*HealthPartners Institute for Education and Research, Bloomington and University of Minnesota, College of Pharmacy, Minneapolis, MN, USA*
[7]*Perelman School of Medicine at the University of Pennsylvania, Philadelphia, PA, USA*
[8]*Center for Medication Safety, Hines, IL, USA*
[9]*Université de Montréal and CHUM Research Center (CRCHUM), Montreal, Quebec, Canada*
[10]*London School of Hygiene and Tropical Medicine and St John's Institute of Dermatology, London, UK*
[11]*Clinical Practice Research Datalink (CPRD), Medicines and Healthcare Products Regulatory Agency (MHRA), London, UK*
[12]*Cegedim Strategic Data Medical Research Ltd, London, UK*
[13]*Centre of Excellence Patient Data, IMS Health GmbH & Co OHG, Frankfurt/Main, Germany*
[14]*PHARMO Institute, Utrecht, The Netherlands and Erasmus University Rotterdam, Rotterdam, The Netherlands*
[15]*Aarhus University Hospital, Aarhus, Denmark*

This chapter describes five types of healthcare databases that have been useful for conducting pharmacoepidemiologic research. These databases run the gamut from regional to national in scope and from private to national governmental sponsorship. We follow the same format for each, outlining the description, strengths, and weaknesses of each. In order, the databases covered include: health maintenance organizations/ health plans, US Government claims databases, Canadian provincial databases, medical record databases, and the pharmacy-based medical record linkage systems in the Netherlands and Nordic Countries.

US Health maintenance organizations/health plans

Introduction

Health maintenance organizations (HMOs), often also referred to as health plans, are an important resource. We use the term HMO here to refer to health care delivery systems that assume

Textbook of Pharmacoepidemiology, Second Edition. Edited by Brian L. Strom, Stephen E. Kimmel, and Sean Hennessy.
© 2013 John Wiley & Sons, Ltd. Published 2013 by John Wiley & Sons, Ltd.

responsibility for covering and administering preventive and therapeutic medical services to a defined population, in contrast to insurance systems which only pay for the care provided by others. Their salient features for research typically include most of the following: (1) responsibility for the care for a defined population, (2) information about diagnoses and procedures resulting from care delivered in both ambulatory and inpatient settings, access to full inpatient and outpatient medical records, and outpatient pharmacy dispensing data, and (3) the ability to interact with providers and members/patients. HMOs with these attributes are well positioned to make extensive use of routinely collected electronic data, including both administrative and claims and electronic health record data. Researchers are also able to supplement this information with full text record review, and to obtain additional information from providers or patients.

Description

Data resources
Administrative and clinical datasets maintained by HMOs and used for clinical care, payment, and operational purposes, are used for many epidemiologic studies. The principal sources of information are administrative and claims data, and electronic medical records (EMRs).

Administrative and claims data

Demographic data and membership status
HMOs maintain information on date of birth, sex, race/ethnicity (not always, but the collection of which is increasing), historical and current residence, dates of enrollment and termination of membership, and change in benefit plans of their members. This membership data can be used to identify individuals with incident drug use, and to follow-up and censor individuals should they leave the health plan. Linkage of these data to the state's death record system or the National Death Index allows more complete capture of mortality; additional linkage to census data (geocoding) provides

group-level measures of race/ethnicity and socioeconomic status.

Outpatient drug exposure
HMOs often offer pharmacy benefits to members, providing a strong financial incentive for members to receive their drugs through a mechanism that results in a claim for reimbursement or a dispensing record. For health plans with integrated pharmacies, the pharmacy dispensing information is obtained directly from the dispensing record. Each drug claim or dispensing record contains a unique National Drug Code (NDC) that identifies the active ingredient(s), dose, and formulation, as well as the route of administration, amount dispensed, days of supply, and prescriber. Information about copayment amounts is also typically available. Injectable drugs administered in special clinics or office visits can be identified by either the dispensing record or a special designation, such as the Health Care Financing Agency Common Procedure Coding System (HCPCS) codes, for the visit during which the drug was administered. However, ascertainment of drug exposure using these automated dispensing records may be incomplete. Currently, information on drugs that are used during hospitalizations is usually not available at most HMOs. Over-the-counter medication use is generally not captured. At many HMOs, prescribing, a measure of clinicians' intent, can be identified through orders in EMRs. Many EMRs also capture a diagnosis code linked to a prescription.

Diagnoses
Diagnoses associated with hospitalizations or ambulatory visits can be identified from automated claims or health plans' EMRs. Most diagnoses are recorded in International Classification of Diseases, 9th revision, Clinical Modification (ICD-9-CM) codes.

Procedures/special examinations
Hospital and ambulatory procedures (laboratory tests, radiology examinations, endoscopy examinations, surgeries, and others) are coded according to the ICD-9-CM, Current Procedural Terminology (CPT), HCPCS, or plan-specific systems.

Electronic medical records (EMRs)

EMRs contain information that can substantially enhance pharmacoepidemiologic studies. EMRs use a controlled medical terminology (e.g., based upon ICD-9-CM and CPT systems) to document patient assessments and procedures. Further, they support clinician order entry for pharmacy, laboratory, radiology, referrals, and provider-to-provider messaging. Finally, clinical notes, diagnoses, orders, and test results are archived, allowing their use for research. Additionally, data including race/ethnicity, and other variables (e.g., smoking status, body mass index, and alcohol use) are increasingly available.

EMRs based in HMOs are especially valuable since their information can be linked to the administrative and claims data described above and therefore represent a comprehensive picture of an individual patient's care over time. Absent the HMO setting, EMR data are typically limited to care provided in a location or locations that share a practice's (or hospital's or network's) EMR. For EMR systems that are not based in HMOs or that do not have the capability to link to claims data, there is usually no way to identify eligible person-time, to obtain information about prescribing or dispensing of medications provided outside the practice, or to know about care from other providers, even when the EMR is network-based.

Full text records

HMOs typically have access to traditional paper outpatient and inpatient medical records for their enrolled members if needed for years prior to when their EMRs began.

Additional HMO research databases and registries

Health plan-based research centers have developed a variety of databases that support research, including many disease-specific disease registries. These additional databases and registries can leverage administrative, claims, and EMR data. Such embedded registries can provide efficient approaches for studying questions related to the natural history of disease conditions, the effectiveness or adverse effects of medical products, and treatment patterns.

Multi-HMO collaborations

There are a number of advantages of bringing together different HMOs that serve demographically and geographically diverse populations. A network of HMOs allows for assessment of treatment heterogeneity in specific subgroups, and improves the generalizability of findings. The practice and geographic variations within a network of health plans or delivery systems provide abundant opportunities for natural experiments. Additionally, such a network is well suited for studies that use a cluster randomization design, at the level of health plans, practices, or individual providers, to evaluate treatment strategies that assess changes in treatment strategies which cannot be evaluated through purely observational methods. The health plans' routinely collected data makes such studies especially efficient and economical, while providing highly relevant real-world data on comparative clinical effectiveness and safety.

Strengths

The potential for large and diverse defined populations, the varied delivery models and practice patterns, together with automated claims and EMR data, access to providers, and in many plans to full text medical records, and ability to work with the health plans' members are all valuable assets for research requiring large, diverse populations and delivery systems. Large cohorts can be identified to measure the incidence of rare events or with specific exposures, for instance exposure to certain drugs or vaccines. Health plans' access to medical records for confirmation of clinical events is often essential—although, when the predictive values of codes are high, medical record review may not always be necessary. The increasing richness of the computerized clinical data offers an advantage over many other data sources. Lastly, the research centers' ability to contact their health plan enrollees for participation in studies is extremely valuable for clinical research. This ability to contact members facilitates enrollment of patients in clinical trials (see Chapter 16) and pharmacogenomic research projects (see Chapter 14), and also enables the conduct of studies which include patient interviews or questionnaires to provide information on patient behaviors (e.g., physical activity, over-the-counter medication use), beliefs, and information not captured in the administrative and clinical HMO databases.

Coordination and data development infrastructure enables both observational and interventional studies to be conducted efficiently across health plans, using a distributed data processing model for such studies. Creation of institutional review board (IRB) reliance agreements among health plans further reduces the barriers.

Weaknesses

One of the most important limitation of HMO data sources is the absence of population groups that are uninsured. These missing groups are typically highly enriched with individuals who do not qualify for insurance because they are unemployed. A consequence of this is that HMO populations can be less diverse than the population as a whole, with a smaller proportion of socioeconomically disadvantaged individuals.

Some health plans have a smaller fraction of the elderly than the general population, because individuals who are 65 years and older disproportionately receive their care through Medicare fee-for-service programs (see Chapter 9, "US government claims databases" section). Because membership is often associated with employment status, turnover of the population can occur when employers contract with different health plans or when individuals change jobs.

Some benefits, such as mental health services, may be "carved-out," i.e., contracted en bloc to another organization, and thus not captured in detail by HMOs' data systems. Some health plan benefit plans cap the amount of certain services, such as physical therapy, and would thus not necessarily capture services that the members pays for individually. Some individuals may have more than one source of health insurance, for instance if spouses each have separate family coverage. In this case, an HMO may not capture all care an eligible individual receives.

While the data are rich in elements related to health care, information on race/ethnicity, indicators of socioeconomic status, and health behaviors (e.g., smoking status, alcohol consumption) are not yet recorded for all members. However, data on some of these factors, such as race/ethnicity, body mass index, and smoking status, are increasingly available in EMRs.

Except for HMOs with EMRs where prescription orders are also available, drug information typically pertains to dispensed prescriptions. Prescription medications filled out-of-plan, nonprescription medications, and those dispensed in inpatient settings are not routinely captured in the health plan dispensing files, and inexpensive prescriptions relative to the cost of deductibles may not be completely captured. Some health plans have restrictive formularies. However, different HMOs often have formularies that include different drugs; thus multi-HMO projects often yield diverse drugs from a particular class. Newer agents may be somewhat slower to achieve widespread use than in the fee-for-service environment.

Particular applications

Examples below are drawn from the HMO Research Network (HMORN, http://www.hmoresearchnetwork.org/) and the Kaiser Permanente (KP) Center for Effectiveness and Safety Research (CESR) initiative, which are partially overlapping consortia of health plans that exemplify many characteristics of HMOs described above. The health plans that comprise these consortia (see Table 9.1) serve large, geographically and ethnically diverse defined populations, have varied health care delivery models and practice patterns, automated claims data, access to full text medical records, access to providers, and the ability to work with the health plans' members. The 19 member health plans of the HMORN (18 in the US and one in Israel) include approximately 16 million current enrollees, enough to address many questions that could not be addressed with any individual plan's population alone (see Table 9.2). A wide array of medical care delivery models is represented in the HMORN,

Table 9.1 Affiliated managed care organizations and research departments.

Managed care organization	Research department/institute	Acronym	Location	HMORN	CESR
Geisinger Health System	Geisinger Center for Health Research	GHS	Pennsylvania	√	
Group Health Cooperative	Group Health Research Institute	GHC	Washington State & Northern Idaho	√	
Harvard Pilgrim Health Care	Harvard Pilgrim Health Care Institute & Harvard Medical School: Department of Population Medicine	HPHC	Massachusetts, New Hampshire & Maine	√	
HealthPartners	HealthPartners Institute for Education and Research	HPIER	Minnesota	√	
Henry Ford Health System	Center for Health Services Research	HFHS	Michigan	√	
Kaiser Permanente Colorado	Institute for Health Research	KPCO	Colorado	√	√
Kaiser Permanente Georgia	Center for Health Research—Southeast	KPG	Georgia	√	√
Kaiser Permanente Hawaii	Center for Health Research—Hawaii	KPH	Hawaii	√	√
Kaiser Permanente Mid-Atlantic	Department of Research	KPMAS	Maryland & Virginia		√
Kaiser Permanente Northern California	Division of Research	KPNC	Northern California	√	√
Kaiser Permanente Northwest	Center for Health Research—Northwest	KPNW	Oregon & Washington	√	√
Kaiser Permanente Ohio	Division of Research	KPOH	Ohio		√
Kaiser Permanente Southern California	Department of Research and Evaluation	KPSC	Southern California	√	√
Lovelace Health System	Lovelace Clinic Foundation	LCF	New Mexico	√	
Maccabi Healthcare Services	Maccabi Institute for Health Services Research	MHS	Israel	√	
Marshfield Clinic/ Security Health Plan of Wisconsin	Marshfield Clinic Research Foundation	MCRF	Wisconsin	√	
Fallon Community Health Plan	Meyers Primary Care Institute	MPCI	Central Massachusetts	√	
Scott & White Health System	Scott & White Division of Research and Education	S&W	Texas	√	

Table 9.2 Demographic characteristics of HMO Research Network member health plans.

Health Plan	GHS	GHC	HPHC	HPIER	HFHS	KPCO	KPG	KPH	KPNC	KPNW	KPSC	LCF	MHS	MCRF	MPCI	S&W
Year established	1915	1947	1969	1957	1948	1969	1985	1958	1945	1942	1947	1973	1941	1916	1977	1982
Primary model	Mixed	HMO	Mixed	Mixed	Mixed	HMO	Mixed	HMO	HMO	HMO	HMO	HMO	HMO	Mixed	Mixed	HMO
Total enrolled, x1000	229	617	762	687	208	451	271	216	3,130	471	3,324	194	1,800	160	220	203
% with EMR data	36	69	35	83	60	83	100	98.5	100	98	100	100	100	100	60	75
Age																
% ≤ 17 yrs	19	20	24	35	18	22	24	22	22	23	25	39	41	24	19	30
% 18–44 yrs	29	33	39	28	29	34	39	35	35	34	36	25	32	33	33	24
% 45–64 yrs	28	33	33	30	35	30	31	30	29	31	28	20	19	26	29	28
% 65 +	24	13	4	4	18	14	7	13	13	13	11	15	5	17	19	9
Gender																
% female	52	53	52	52	55	53	53	50	52	52	52	55	52	52	52	53
Race[a]																
% White	96	82	75	81	54	74	63	25	51	84	38	55	95	97	87	84
% African American	<1	3	16	9	33	5	33	<1	8	3	8	1	0	<1	2	8
% Asian American	0	6	5	5	3	3	<1	63	17	5	10	1	0	<1	3	2
% American Indian	<1	1	<1	1	<1	1	<1	<1	<1	1	<1	2	0	<1	<1	1
% Hispanic	1.4	4	4	2	1	15	<1	3	19	6	41	38	0	<1	8	7
% Other	<1	3	0	2	8	2	4	17	5	1	<1	0	5	<1	0	7
Member Retention (% still enrolled at 1, 3, 5 yrs; 2003 – 2008)																
% enrolled at 1 year	82	84	78	73	99.5	83	87	85	87	82	87	78	99	92	95	81
% enrolled at 3 years	54	66	47	46	86.4	66	67	72	75	66	70	66	98	78	92	81
% enrolled at 5 years	41	55	35	38	62.6	56	54	63	66	57	59	57	98	68	92	62

[a] may be > 100% if multiple responses allowed at collection, "other" may include persons reporting multiple races.

including staff, group and network, as well as independent physicians associations (IPAs, organizations that contract with HMOs on behalf of physicians who are not employed by the HMO). The KP CESR initiative, established in 2009, is a culturally and geographically diverse, distributed research network spanning nine US states and the District of Columbia. It is comprised of all eight KP regions, six of which are also HMORN members.

Standard data layouts

The adoption of standard data layouts that use a common data model has facilitated multi-HMO research. The existence of data files that adhere to a common data model allows creation of libraries of reusable data management and analytic programs. These standard layout files also greatly facilitate multicenter research, as it is possible for a single program to be used in multiple sites with negligible modification. This practice improves the efficiency and consistency of multicenter research.

The core data resource for research in the HMORN is its virtual data warehouse (VDW). The VDW is "virtual" in the sense that it is a distributed research dataset, with the data transformed according to a common data model remaining at each site. Within each research center, data are extracted from the extensive, local health plan data systems into the site-specific VDWs and configured into 14 tables using standard variable names and values. The primary content areas of these data systems include enrollment, demographics, outpatient prescription drug dispensings, outpatient diagnoses and procedures, utilization of clinical services, hospitalizations, geocoding of member addresses, and tumor characteristics (for cancer patients). Other content areas include vital signs, laboratory results, and death.

For each content area, a data dictionary specifies the format for each element including variable name, variable label, extended definition, code values, and value labels. Local site programmers have mapped and transformed data elements from their local data systems into the standardized set of variable definitions, names, and codes.

Examples of current and past multisite, multiproject research programs within HMORN and KP CESR

The formal collaborations and research programs across the HMORN and KP CESR span multiple therapeutic topics that are funded by the US Food and Drug Administration (FDA), the US Centers for Disease Control and Prevention (CDC), the US Agency for Healthcare Research and Quality (AHRQ), the US National Institutes of Health (NIH), nonprofit foundations, and private organizations. Some current and past programs include:

- Cancer Research Network (CRN; supported by US National Cancer Institute, (NCI));
- Cardiovascular Research Network (CVRN; US National Heart, Lung, and Blood Institute, (NHLBI));
- Mental Health Research Network (MHRN; US National Institute of Mental Health (NIMH));
- The Vaccine Safety Datalink (VSD; CDC);
- Developing Evidence to Inform Decisions about Effectiveness (DEcIDE; AHRQ) center;
  - Diabetes Multi Center Research Consortium (DMCRC)
  - Distributed Research Network (DRN)
- Scalable PArtnering Network for Comparative Effectiveness Research (SPAN; AHRQ);
- Medication Exposure in Pregnancy Risk Evaluation Program (MEPREP; FDA);
- Mini-Sentinel program (FDA);
- contracts from the FDA's Center for Drug Evaluation and Research (CDER) and its Center for Biologics Evaluation and Research (CBER), and several other newly-emerging collaboratives;

Cancer Research Network (CRN)

The CRN (http://crn.cancer.gov/), originally funded by NCI in 1998, consists of the research programs, enrolled populations, and data systems of 14 HMORN sites nationwide. Its goal is to conduct research on cancer prevention, early detection, treatment, long-term care, surveillance, communication, and dissemination. The CRN is equipped to study cancer control at the patient, provider, and system levels, and has experience with a range of data collection strategies. CRN activities have generated more than 140 journal publications in a range of disciplines. Studies include evaluations of the patterns and trends in use of hormone therapy, tamoxifen, and other chemotherapy; assessments of the risk of cancer associated with exposure to statins and other cardiovascular medications; and an evaluation of the impact of a decision aid designed to educate women about their risk of breast cancer and the risks and benefits of tamoxifen.

Cardiovascular Research Network (CVRN)

The CVRN (http://www.cvrn.org/), funded by NHLBI since 2007, includes 15 HMORN sites. It has created a framework to address questions about contemporary cardiovascular epidemiology, optimal management, and associated clinical outcomes within large community-based populations where most clinical care is delivered. Examples of CVRN research projects include studies of (1) hypertension diagnosis, management and control; (2) quality of care and outcomes of warfarin therapy for atrial fibrillation and venous thromboembolism; and (3) the use and outcomes of implantable cardioverter defibrillators for prevention of sudden death. The network also established capacity to rapidly respond to emerging cardiovascular disease research questions and to facilitate external collaborations.

Mental Health Research Network (MHRN)

The MHRN was funded in 2010 by the NIMH. The 11 HMORN sites participating in MHRN cover a diverse population of over ten million members in 12 states. The goal of MHRN is to conduct research to answer questions about mental health care and financing that are important to health systems, policy-makers, and other stakeholders. Diversity of member demographics, insurance coverage, and organization of health services make this network an ideal environment for studying variation in care, comparing effectiveness and cost of treatments across practice environments, and studying dissemination and implementation of innovations. The initial 3-year funding supports the development of the core infrastructure for sharing data as well as four pilot research projects that leverage infrastructure in specific clinical areas: practice variation among

sites in high and low value care for mood disorders; behavioral activation therapy for perinatal depression; development of a registry for autism spectrum disorders; and the relation between boxed warnings of selective serotonin reuptake inhibitors (SSRIs) and suicidality in children.

Vaccine Safety Datalink (VSD)

The CDC-funded VSD (http://cdc.gov/vaccinesafety/ Activities/VSD.html; see also Chapter 22) is comprised of ten HMORN sites. The VSD was established in 1991 to monitor immunization safety and address the gaps in scientific knowledge about rare and serious events following immunization. Currently, VSD collects vaccination and comprehensive medical information on nearly ten million members from these HMOs annually (3% of the US population). While most of the VSD data sources are identical to the HMORN's VDW, the vaccine exposure data is obtained from the HMOs' EMRs. The VSD has developed a standardized approach for performing near-real time safety surveillance of new vaccines as these vaccines enter the US market. VSD Rapid Cycle Analysis (RCA) studies rely on data automatically updated weekly and sequential statistical analyses to compare the rate of occurrence of prespecified adverse events following receipt of a vaccine with expected rates among persons not exposed to the vaccine. An example of a VSD study is one by Lee and colleagues who used weekly sequential analyses and observed that H1N1 and seasonal influenza vaccines were not associated with greater risks of Guillain-Barré syndrome, other neurologic outcomes, and allergic and cardiac events in the 2009–10 season.

The Developing Evidence to Inform Decisions about Effectiveness (DEcIDE) Center, the Diabetes Multi Center Research Consortium (DMCRC), and the Distributed Research Network (DRN)

The DEcIDE network is part of AHRQ's Effective Health Care program, created in response to the Medicare Modernization Act of 2003. DEcIDE focuses primarily on comparative effectiveness of therapies, as assessed from observational studies and practical clinical trials in real-world populations. Examples of task orders awarded to the HMORN DEcIDE Center include: (1) observational studies of comparative effectiveness of β-blockers for heart failure on hospital readmission and mortality; (2) development of evidence and educational/system approaches to reduce prenatal exposure to medications with a potential for fetal harm; and (3) a cluster randomized trial in 45 hospitals of three different methods to reduce acquisition of methicillin-resistant Staphylococcus aureus (MRSA) in intensive care units.

The HMORN DEcIDE Center Diabetes Multi-Center Research Consortium (DMCRC) includes 12 HMORN health plans plus external partners. The DMCRC is developing a comprehensive comparative effectiveness research agenda, and a distributed research database of patients with diabetes. Examples of DMCRC studies include: (1) cohort studies comparing diabetes patients undergoing bariatric surgery with similar patients receiving usual clinical care, and (2) outcomes of further intensifying diabetes therapy in patients already on at least two oral medications or basal insulin to maintain "tight" glycemic control (glycosylated hemoglobin<7%). This study attempts to address the apparent lack of benefit on cardiovascular disease endpoints of tight glycemic control observed in recent trials.

AHRQ has also funded the HMORN DEcIDE Center to create new capabilities for distributed studies of the safety and effectiveness of treatments, including drugs, vaccines and medical devices. The program, PopMedNet (www.popmednet.org), allows data partners to create both large and small data networks, while retaining control over the uses and users of their data resources. PopMedNet is an efficient, reusable infrastructure through which routinely collected healthcare data and related information can be assembled and analyzed to support decision making by patients, providers, and policy-makers. Participating investigators can distribute queries through network software, execute queries against local data, and return aggregated results to the end-user. The software is capable of supporting a variety of study types, including observational studies, quasi-experimental studies, clinical trials, and registries.

Medication Exposure in Pregnancy Risk Evaluation Program (MEPREP)

The FDA-funded MEPREP includes ten HMORN sites plus Tennessee Medicaid (under the auspices of Vanderbilt University). Its purpose is to study the effects of prescription medications used during pregnancy. To overcome the challenges presented by the lack of clinical trial data about the use of medications during pregnancy, MEPREP links health care information for mothers and their babies. Collectively, the participating sites have health care information for about one million births from 2001 to 2008, and this number will grow by approximately 100 000 births with each subsequent study year. Examples of studies conducted in these environments include (1) assessment of medication use during pregnancy and birth outcomes, and (2) the effects of antidepressant medications and cardiovascular medications on birth defects and perinatal outcomes.

FDA Mini-Sentinel program

The FDA's Mini-Sentinel program (http://www.minisentinel.org) is a major component of the FDA's Sentinel Initiative (see also Chapter 22). The Mini-Sentinel program is creating a "laboratory" for developing and evaluating safety surveillance scientific methods and offers FDA the opportunity to evaluate medical product safety in existing automated healthcare data systems while learning about the barriers and challenges inherent in these activities. This consortium, led by the Harvard Pilgrim Health Care Institute, involves most HMORN sites, plus large national health plans, free standing registries, and hospitals.

FDA contracts: epidemiologic studies of adverse effects of marketed drugs

Nearly all HMORN sites participate in the FDA's Pharmacoepidemiologic Research Program, which assists FDA's Center for Drug Evaluation and Research (CDER) Office of Surveillance and Epidemiology. This program and its predecessors have evaluated both direct adverse effects of drugs, such as rhabdomyolysis associated with lipid lowering agents, and appropriateness of medication use. The latter study contributed to the withdrawal of cisapride.

Conclusion

HMO-based research is likely to evolve in several ways. These organizations are well suited to use cluster randomization, at the level of practices or health plans, to evaluate treatment strategies that cannot be evaluated through purely observational methods. As described above, the health plans' observational data makes such studies especially efficient and economical, while providing highly relevant real world data on comparative clinical effectiveness and safety. HMOs can also likely improve the efficiency of more conventional clinical trials, by using health plan data to obtain preliminary estimates of the number of potential eligible subjects and to support identification, recruitment, and follow-up of study participants.

HMOs are also early adopters of EMRs, and thus likely to be able to incorporate these data more quickly into pharmacoepidemiologic studies. The use of natural language processing methods to allow more effective use of EMRs' free text will also improve the depth and quality of data available. Additional initiatives that are likely to grow in importance include more linkage to external data sources, such as state birth certificate files, the National Death Index, and immunization registries. HMOs are well positioned to collect biological specimens, either for immediate use or to store in a specimen bank to support later research. HMOs are also well positioned to engage their members to obtain historical and behavioral information that is not routinely collected in health records.

Summary points for health maintenance organizations/health plans

• Routinely collected electronic data from US health plans, including both administrative claims and electronic medical record data, are used extensively to evaluate the benefits and risks of marketed medical products.

• Available data for health plans includes diagnoses and procedures resulting from care delivered in both ambulatory and inpatient settings, full text medical records, and outpatient pharmacy dispensing data from well-defined populations.

• Health plan-based research studies have the ability to readily work with providers and contact plan members.

• Researchers using this data resource must be cognizant of limitations, such as absence of complete information on race/ethnicity, other indicators of socioeconomic status or lifestyle factors; incomplete capture of nonprescription medications, medications filled out-of-plan, or inpatient drug use; and under-representation of uninsured population or, in some cases, of individuals aged 65 years or older.

Case Example 9.1: Health maintenance organizations/health plans

Background

• The use of second-generation antipsychotics (SGAs) has substantially increased in children and adolescents, although data on their comparative safety and effectiveness in this population are limited.
• Numerous case reports and studies suggest an association between SGAs and type 2 diabetes mellitus and impaired glucose tolerance in adult populations, although the evidence has often been inconsistent, particularly with regard to the differential effects of specific agents.
• Evidence to suggest an association between impaired glucose tolerance and antipsychotic use in children is limited.

Question

• Is use of SGAs associated with an increased risk of incident type 2 diabetes mellitus in children?

Approach

• A retrospective cohort study was conducted using the administrative databases of three health plans participating in the HMORN.
• The cohort included children ages 5 to 18 years who initiated SGA therapy from January 2001 to December 2008 and two comparison groups—nonusers of psychotropic drugs and users of antidepressant medications.
• Diagnoses from inpatient and outpatient records, pharmacy dispensings, and outpatient laboratory results were used to identify incident cases of type 2 diabetes mellitus.

Results

- The crude incidence rate of diabetes for the SGA exposed cohort was 3.23 per 1000 person years (95% confidence interval: 1.67, 5.65) compared to 0.76 per 1000 person years (0.49, 1.12) among nonusers of psychotropic medications, and 1.86 per 1000 person years (1.12, 2.90) among antidepressant users.
- The findings differed depending upon the comparison group and definition of the outcome of interest (i.e., if abnormal laboratory test results were considered in addition to diagnosis codes and pharmacy dispensings).

Strengths

- This cohort study utilized a large, diverse cohort of pediatric patients from three geographically distributed health plans.
- The study was able to follow patients for longitudinal exposures and clinical outcomes, including glucose laboratory values.

Limitations

- The small number of cases precluded detailed evaluation of the associations between individual agents and the risk of diabetes.
- Only diagnosed cases of diabetes were identified, some cases might go undetected.
- Residual confounding was possible, since potential confounders such as baseline body mass index (not available in the VDW of the three participating health plans), diet, exercise, race/ethnicity, or severity of underlying mental health conditions were not evaluated.

Key Points

- The study found a potential 4-fold increased rate of diabetes among children exposed to SGAs. However, the findings varied with the comparison group and definition of the outcome.
- Additional research is needed to better define the nature and magnitude of diabetes risk associated with SGA use in children.

US government claims databases

Introduction

The United States (US) government funds health care services for certain segments of the population via a number of programs. Data from three of these programs have been used extensively for pharmacoepidemiologic research, and are the focus of this chapter. These three programs are Medicaid, Medicare, and the Department of Veterans Affairs (VA) Heath Care System. These programs and their resulting data differ substantially with regard to populations covered, benefits provided, and data available.

Description

Medicaid

Description of the Medicaid program

Medicaid was established in 1965, and is administered separately by each state or territory that offers Medicaid coverage, with federal oversight from the Centers for Medicare & Medicaid Services (CMS). These programs are funded jointly by the federal government and individual state governments. Medicaid functions as a payer rather than a provider of health services. Each state establishes its own eligibility rules within general federal mandates.

Medicaid is currently the largest US government-funded healthcare program, providing coverage to 58 million US citizens and lawfully admitted immigrants, of whom approximately 75% are either low income pregnant women or members of low income families with children, with the remaining 25% consisting of chronically disabled or low-income elderly persons, including some who also receive Medicare benefits. Medicaid does not currently provide coverage for even the poorest individuals unless they belong to one of these specifically designated groups.

The services covered by Medicaid vary by state, within federal mandates. Certain services are mandatory, including inpatient and outpatient hospital services, and physician services. Although outpatient prescription drug coverage is not mandatory, all Medicaid programs provide such coverage for at least some enrollment categories. With certain exceptions (e.g., drugs for anorexia, weight gain, fertility, etc.), Medicaid programs are required to cover all drugs manufactured by companies that have entered into a federal rebate agreement, which includes all or nearly all manufacturers. However, programs can require prescribers to obtain prior authorization before the prescription will be covered. With the enactment of the Medicare drug benefit in 2006, outpatient prescription drugs for Medicaid-Medicare dual enrollees are now covered by Medicare rather than Medicaid. Most states pay the cost of drugs covered by the Medicaid program but not Medicare. Medicaid covers a large proportion of all nursing home care in the US, with over 40% of long-term care costs billed to the program.

Most Medicaid programs include beneficiaries who receive services on a fee-for-service basis as well as those enrolled in capitated plans. In fee-for-service plans, health care providers bill Medicaid for specific goods and services provided, such as visits, hospitalizations, and prescription drugs. In capitated managed care plans, an insurance company is paid a certain amount per person per time period (e.g., month) to cover all or specific aspects of that enrollee's health care. Importantly for researchers, the degree of completeness of encounter information for patients in capitated plans is believed to vary among plans, although this has not been formally studied.

Characteristics of Medicaid recipients

In 2008, 58.2 million persons, or 19% of the US population, received health care services covered by Medicaid. Baseline characteristics of the Medicaid population can be seen in Table 9.3. Children, females, and nonwhites are over-represented in Medicaid.

Sources of Medicaid data for research

CMS is the major source of Medicaid data for researchers. It receives data from individual state Medicaid programs, and performs extensive editing, range checks, and comparisons with previous data from that state when preparing research files, known as Medicaid Analytic Extract (MAX) files. Anomalies in the data are either reconciled with the state or published in an anomaly report, which is available to researchers. Crude data provided by states through the Medicaid Statistical Information System (MSIS) are also available, but do not undergo the same quality assurance checks as the MAX data. There is currently a lag of approximately three to four years between the end of a calendar year and when MAX data from that year become available.

The CMS' Research Data Assistance Center (ResDAC), operated through a contract with the University of Minnesota School of Public Health, provides free assistance to academic, government, and nonprofit researchers in obtaining and using Medicaid and Medicare data. ResDAC maintains a website of information on Medicaid and Medicare data (http://www.resdac.umn.edu/), conducts workshops and seminars, and provides individual technical assistance to researchers, including obtaining prices for data from CMS, assisting in preparation of data requests, and providing technical assistance in the use of the data.

Pharmacoepidemiologic research has also been conducted since the early 1980, using data obtained directly from individual states, including California, Florida, Iowa, Missouri, New Jersey, New York, Oregon, and Tennessee. Several commercial entities also make Medicaid data available.

Data structure of Medicaid databases

MAX files contain information on beneficiaries' demographics, enrollment, inpatient hospitalizations, outpatient physician visits, outpatient prescription drugs, outpatient laboratory and radiology studies, and stays in long term care facilities (i.e., nursing homes, mental health hospitals). All records except for demographic and enrollment data originate from healthcare providers seeking reimbursement for goods and services. Such records are called claims. Hospitalization claims exclude many details of the hospital stay, including drugs administered. Outpatient laboratory and radiology claims report the type of test performed, but not results. Diagnoses are coded in the

Table 9.3 Demographic characteristics of the Medicaid, Medicare, and Veterans Health Administration populations.

	Medicaid (2008)[+]		All Medicare[++]			Part D Enrolled[+++]			Veterans Health Administration (2009)[++++]	
	#	% US*	#	% US*		#	% Medicare		#	% US**
	#	%	#	%		#	%		#	%
Total enrollment	58,238,773	19.1	46,520,716	15.2		27,972,316	60.1		5,744,000	1.9
Gender										
Female	31,512,082	54.1	25,742,676	55.3	Female	16,517,856	59.1	Female	459,520	8
Male	21,824,014	37.5	20,778,040	44.7	Male	11,454,460	40.9	Male	5,280,800	93
Unknown	4,902,677	8.4	–	–	–	–	–	–	–	–
Age										
<1	2,006,749	3.4	–	–	–	–	–	–	–	–
1–5	9,670,094	16.6	–	–	–	–	–	–	–	–
6–12	9,516,371	16.3	–	–	–	–	–	–	–	–
13–14	2,334,030	4.0	–	–	–	–	–	–	–	–
15–18	4,837,569	8.3	2,658	0.0	<19	–	–	–	–	–
19–20	1,956,043	3.4	676,386	1.5	19–34	5,550,293	19.8	<65	3,452,144	60.1
21–44	12,637,182	21.7	3,574,913	7.7	35–54	6,272,615	22.4	65–69	–	–
45–64	5,639,547	9.7	3,501,360	7.5	55–64	5,355,331	19.1	70–74	2,291,856	39.9
65–74	2,011,317	3.5	20,606,076	44.3	65–74	4,205,434	15.03	75–79	≥65	
75–84	1,631,909	2.8	12,714,058	27.3	75–84	3,307,856	11.8	80–84	–	–
85+	1,103,551	1.9	5,445,265	11.7	85+	3,280,787	11.7	85+	–	–
Age group missing	4,894,411	8.4	–	–	–	–	–	–	–	–

(continued)

Table 9.3 (*Continued*)

Race/ethnicity	Medicaid (2008)[+]			Medicare (2009)					Veterans Health Administration (2009)[++++]	
				All Medicare[++]		Part D Enrolled[+++]				
	#	% US*		#	% US*	#	% Medicare		#	% US**
Non-hispanic white	22,135,196	38.0	White	38,589,288	83.0	22,438,315	80.2	Non-Hispanic White	4,554,992	79.3
Black/African American	12,403,508	21.3	Black	4,727,383	10.2	3,164,002	11.3	African American	649,072	11.3
Hispanic or Latino	10,820,941	18.6	Hispanic	1,168,699	2.5	928,411	3.3	Hispanic or Latino	333,152	5.8
Asian	1,446,157	2.5	Asian	898,809	1.9	686,657	2.5	Asian	86,160	1.5
American Indian/Alaska Native	730,574	1.3	N. American Native	201,887	0.4	122,557	0.4	American Indian/Alaska Native	45,952	0.8
Native Hawaiian/Pacific Islander	465,114	0.8	Other	853,488	1.8	570,323	2.0	Pacific Islander	–	–
Hispanic/Latino and one or more race	1,878,622	3.2	Unknown	81,162	0.2	62,051	0.2	Other	74,672	1.3
More than one race	147,061	0.3	–	–	–	–	–	–	–	–
Not identified	8,211,600	14.1	–	–	–	–	–	–	–	–

*US Population estimates from (http://www.census.gov/popest/states/NST-ann-est.html) N = 304,374,846 as of July 1, 2008.

**US Population estimates from (http://www.census.gov/popest/states/NST-ann-est.html) N= 307,006,550 as of July 1, 2009.

[+]FY 2008 Medicaid Beneficiaries by Gender (MSIS 2008 Table 13), Age (MSIS 2008 Table 12), Race/Ethnicity (MSIS 2008 Table 14).

[++]Medicare Enrollment: Hospital Insurance and/or Supplementary Medical Insurance Enrollees, by Demographic Characteristics, as of July 1, 2009 (Table 2.3).

[+++]Medicare Part D: Type of Coverage Category for Part D Enrollees, by Demographic Characteristics, as of December 2009 (Table 14.4).

[++++]FY 2009 National Center for Veterans Analysis and Statistics, VA Benefits and Health Care Utilization. Veteran Population as of Sept 30, 2009. http://www.va.gov/VETDATA/Pocket-Card/4X6_.pdf

International Classification of Diseases, 9th Edition, Clinical Modification (ICD9-CM). Inpatient and outpatient procedures are coded in ICD-9-CM Procedure Codes, Common Procedure Terminology (CPT), Healthcare Common Procedure Coding (HCPCS), or sometimes state-specific codes, depending on the state and file. ICD-10 will replace ICD-9 in the US on October 1, 2013. Drugs are coded according to the National Drug Code (NDC).

Medicaid data can be linked to Medicare to increase capture of care for dual enrollees. Such a link can be very important, since Medicaid utilization records can fail to document a considerable proportion of care provided to dual enrollees.

Medicare

Description of the Medicare program

Like Medicaid, Medicare was established in 1965. Medicare is funded by the US federal government without state funds, and administered directly by CMS. Medicare provides health care coverage for nearly all legal residents of the US age 65 and above, some disabled people younger than 65, and people with end-stage renal disease or amyotrophic lateral sclerosis.

Medicare functions as a payer rather than as a direct provider of health care, and is made up of four separate parts: A, B, C, and D. All parts of Medicare coverage require beneficiaries to pay deductibles; some stipulate cost sharing, where the beneficiary pays a percentage of costs, and premiums. Part A generally covers inpatient, short-term skilled nursing care, home health, and hospice care, and all Medicare beneficiaries are enrolled. Part B covers outpatient treatment and procedures, in addition to some drug therapies given in a physician's office or clinic, and is supplemental to Part A, with beneficiaries paying a monthly premium for coverage. Part C, also known as Medicare Advantage, is the Medicare managed care benefit. Part C enrollees typically should not be included in pharmacoepidemiologic studies because claims for Part C enrollees are unavailable from CMS.

Part D is the outpatient prescription drug coverage component of Medicare, which was instituted in 2006. It is administered by hundreds of private stand-alone prescription drug plans (PDPs), which supplement traditional fee-for-service Medicare (Parts A and B), as well as Medicare Advantage prescription drug (MA-PD) plans, which combine Parts A, B, and D in a managed care plan. PDP availability varies by state, and in 2010, a minimum of 41 stand-alone PDPs were available to beneficiaries in all states, with over 1,500 total available in the US, in addition to various MA-PDs. Each PDP has its own formulary, with certain classes of drugs (e.g., benzodiazepines, barbiturates) excluded by law from all plans.

Characteristics of Medicare recipients

In 2010, Medicare covered 47 million Americans, with permanently disabled adults younger than 65 consisting of 8 million, or 17%, of Medicare recipients. Baseline characteristics of the Medicare population are presented in Table 9.3. Females, whites, and the elderly are over-represented. Traditional fee-for-service (FFS) Medicare plans have a higher percentage of disabled beneficiaries under the age of 65.

Sources of Medicare data for research

CMS is the major source of Medicare data for researchers. ResDAC provides assistance to academic, government, and nonprofit researchers in obtaining and using Medicare data.

Data structure of Medicare databases

Medicare data are available in numerous file types that are linkable to each other, as well as to Medicaid data for dually enrolled beneficiaries. Some of these files contain information about enrollees, including date of birth, sex, address of residence, race, and, for decedents, death date. About half of the available files are claims-level standard analytic files (SAFs), which contain data based on claims submitted by providers. Institutional file types include: inpatient, outpatient, skilled nursing facility, hospice, and home health agency SAFs. Noninstitutional data on physicians/suppliers (Carrier file), as well as durable medical equipment (DME), provide useful claims to researchers. Also available is the Medicare Provider and Analysis Review File (MedPAR), which includes inpatient and skilled nursing facility (SNF) final action claims. Unlike the SAFs that are structured as one record per claim, the MedPAR file groups all claims for each inpatient or SNF stay into one line item. This makes it much easier to look at an entire hospitalization.

Of great interest to those interested in pharmacoepidemiologic research is the prescription drug file. Prescription drug information in Medicare is available in the Part D Drug Event (PDE) file, which contains one record per dispensed prescription. Supplementary files are also available that provide information on Part D plans, pharmacies, drugs, prescribers. Demographic information on Part D enrollees can be seen in Table 9.3.

The coding in Medicare files is similar to Medicaid. Diagnoses are coded in ICD-9-CM; while inpatient and outpatient procedures are coded in a combination of ICD-9-CM Procedure Codes, CPT and HCPCS codes, depending on the specific file. For example, MedPAR uses ICD-9-CM Procedures Codes only. Part D PDE files use NDCs to code individual drugs.

Department of Veterans Affairs health care

Description of the Veterans Affairs

The Department of Veterans Affairs (VA) was established in 1930 as the Veterans Administration, when Congress authorized President Hoover to "consolidate and coordinate Government activities affecting war veterans." The Department of Veterans Affairs' Veterans Health Administration (VHA) is one of the largest integrated health care systems in the United States, providing medical, surgical, and rehabilitative care to a diverse group of military Veterans who are mostly older, relatively sick, and often have multiple chronic medical and/or psychiatric conditions. In 2009, the VA health care system included 153 hospitals/medical centers, over 1000 ambulatory care, mobile, independent and community-based outpatient clinics, and 135 nursing homes. The VA health care system consists of 21 regional integrated networks (Veteran Integrated Service Networks or VISNs).

The VA health care system is primarily a direct provider of health care services, funded by the US government. Veterans who served in the military, as well as active duty Reservists and National Guard, are potentially eligible for VA health care. Veteran eligibility requirements are variable and depend on length of military service, type of discharge, and time of service. There are eight priority groupings used to rank eligibility status of veterans. The priority groups are defined by many factors, some of which include: various service-connected disabilities, theaters of war, and socioeconomic status. While veterans receiving health care are not required to pay premiums for coverage, some are charged co-payments for certain medical services and outpatient prescriptions, depending on their priority group. With minor exceptions, only prescriptions written by VA prescribers and filled in a VA pharmacy are covered by the VA's comprehensive medical care plan.

Characteristics of Veterans Affairs population

In 2009, approximately 5.7 million veterans were treated in the VA Health Care system, with over 4.5 million receiving prescriptions. Table 9.3 presents demographic characteristics of VA patients, which differ from those of the general adult population in terms of age and gender. Almost 40% of veterans were >65 years of age in 2009, and 92% of Veteran beneficiaries are male.

Sources of Veterans Affairs data for research

Access to VA data is limited to researchers employed by the VA and their collaborators.

Data structure of VA databases

Pharmacy data systems record drugs dispensed to inpatients in VA hospitals as well as outpatient prescriptions dispensed by its outpatient pharmacies, 80% of which are dispensed through the mail via VA's Consolidated Mail-order Pharmacies (CMOPs). Drugs are recorded and classified according to the VA Drug Classification System (http://www.pbm.va.gov/NationalFormulary.aspx), which is similar to the American Hospital Formulary Service categorization of pharmaceutical products. Clinical databases contain data on inpatient and outpatient encounters, including admissions, discharges, transfers, clinic visits, prescription orders, laboratory, radiology, surgery, and administrative services. Diagnoses are recorded in ICD-9, while ICD-10 will be used beginning in 2013. Death data are obtained from various sources, with cross-checks with the Social Security Administration Death Master File. In addition to the VA administrative databases, the VA has several disease-specific registries that are used for patient care and research. Examples of conditions with existing registries include cancer, diabetes, HIV, and hepatitis C. The VHA also maintains its own adverse drug event reporting system (see also Chapter 7), which currently contains over 200,000 reports related to drugs or vaccines.

Strengths

Population size and length of follow-up

An important strength of these databases is their large size: 58.2 million people in Medicaid, 46.5 million in Medicare, and 5.7 million in the VA. Because Medicaid and Medicare files are linkable to each other, beneficiaries can be followed across years, even if Medicaid enrollees join Medicare. With Medicare and the VA, patients who enter the system often remain for many years, permitting long-term follow-up.

Accuracy of pharmacy claims

Another notable strength of these data is that pharmacy claims record what was dispensed by the pharmacy, which is one step closer to ingestion than what was prescribed, which is recorded in medical record databases (see Chapter 9, 'Medical record databases" section). Further, outpatient prescription claims accurately record the date, drug, and quantity dispensed by the pharmacy. Traditionally, because of low co-payments, patients have had a strong financial incentive to use these programs to purchase their drugs instead of paying for them out-of-pocket. This served to increase the completeness of pharmacy claims data. However, with the recent offering of low priced (e.g., $4) generic prescriptions by many retail pharmacies, patients and pharmacists

may have little financial incentive to report low-cost prescriptions to the patient's drug benefit plan, and thus some prescriptions may not be recorded in US claims databases. Further, patients may not take all of the medicine dispensed as directed. However, for chronically administered drugs, dispensing records have been found to accurately reflect cumulative exposure and gaps in medication supply when compared with electronic medication containers that record when the bottle was opened (28), which are currently considered the best available means of measuring medication ingestion in community-dwelling patients (see Chapter 20).

In the VA, the outpatient database tracks prescription medications and nonprescription medications obtained through the VA, as well as certain medical supplies. As is the case with medications obtained through Medicaid services, the low co-payment, and in some instances no co-payment, associated with VA prescriptions has resulted in a strong financial incentive for Veterans to obtain their outpatient prescriptions through the VA. An additional advantage of the VA data is the recording of drugs dispensed by the pharmacy to patients hospitalized in VA hospitals. However, certain medications (e.g., those obtained from floor stock and medications administered acutely in acute care areas), though recorded in the electronic medical records, are not accessible in the prescription databases.

Validity of procedure claims

For Medicare and Medicaid, claims with codes for clinical procedures determine the amount of money paid to the health care provider. Therefore, procedure records are audited to detect fraud, and would thus be expected to be highly accurate with regard to performance of that procedure. Wysowski *et al.* performed medical record validation in a Medicaid study that used presence of a surgical procedure code as part of an algorithm to identify cases of hip fracture. They found that while all of the procedures billed for were actually performed, some of the procedures were used to correct orthopedic conditions other than hip fracture.

Over-representation of underserved populations

Another potential strength of Medicaid is over-representation of traditionally under-represented groups. Medicaid has substantially greater numbers of pregnant women, young children, and African Americans than other data sets. Seniors, who bear the greatest burden of medication-related adverse events, make up 86% of the Medicare population, 40% of the VA population, and 8% of Medicaid. This is particularly important given that seniors are underrepresented in US commercial insurance databases.

Ability to validate outcomes

Examining the validity of diagnosis codes frequently requires review of clinical records. Fortunately, a mechanism exists to obtain inpatient hospital and emergency department records corresponding to Medicare and Medicaid claims. Using this mechanism, researchers have been able to obtain approximately 70–75% of inpatient hospital and emergency department records. The cost of obtaining medical records, however, is not inexpensive (approximately $150/record in 2010). To our knowledge, this mechanism has not been tried for obtaining outpatient medical or dental records.

One of the strengths of the VA data is the mechanism for obtaining primary inpatient and outpatient medical records to validate outcomes. Records can be obtained electronically from the local health care system, where the medical care information is current and complete.

Ability to link to external data

In addition to the capability to link to each other, Medicaid and Medicare data have also been linked to sources of mortality data such as the Social Security Administration Death Master File, National Death Index, and state vital statistics registries. VA data can also be linked to Medicaid and Medicare and National Death Index data. Medicare data have also been linked to data from state pharmaceutical assistance programs for the elderly to identify outcomes in enrollees of the state programs. Linkage to birth certificate data has been performed for studies of the effects of fetal exposure to medications and for evaluations of the effects on newborns of policies that affect prenatal care. Drivers' license data and police reports of injurious crashes have also been linked to Medicaid data. Studies using registries have linked to Medicare, Medicaid, and VA data to identify outcomes. Medicare data can be linked to the Medicare Current Beneficiary Survey (MCBS) to obtain additional information about the subgroup of subjects who participated in the MCBS. Data from Medicaid and Medicare enrollees admitted to a nursing home can be linked to the nursing home Minimum Data Set to obtain additional information, including measures of physical, psychological, and psychosocial functioning in these enrollees. External data obtained on a subset of such linkages can be used to adjust for factors not recorded in the parent database (see also Chapter 21).

Weaknesses

Nonrepresentativeness

Each of the programs described in this chapter is unrepresentative of the general population in a different way. Nonrepresentativeness may be an important limitation for descriptive studies seeking to describe the overall population and its health care utilization. For example, newborn deliveries account for 40% of hospital admissions within Medicaid beneficiaries, but only 16% of admissions in the non-Medicaid US population. However, for etiologic studies, generalizability is compromised only for biologic relationships that vary by factors that differ between the studied and general populations. For example, Medicaid studies evaluating the gastrointestinal side effects of nonsteroidal anti-inflammatory drugs have produced similar results to those performed in other populations. On the other hand, studying groups with a high degree of comorbidity (e.g., Medicaid and VA beneficiaries) may be advantageous in some circumstances, such as when drug effects are more readily discernable in high-risk groups.

Unavailable information

Administrative and clinical data like those described here often lack information on many potentially important confounding factors, such as smoking, exercise, diet, environmental exposures, etc. Some of these factors can be obtained in a subset of patients by reviewing primary medical records to the degree that these factors are recorded in medical records. Linkages with external data sources, such as those described above, can also provide additional information on all or a subset of subjects.

Limitations in prescription coverage

Only drugs covered by the plan can be studied. A number of drug categories are generally not covered by the Medicare and Medicaid prescription drug benefits, such as agents for fertility, weight loss, hair growth, cosmetic effect, and over-the-counter smoking cessation. Coverage of nonprescription drugs varies by state in Medicaid, and is not included in Medicare Part D.

In Medicare, the Part D program is carried out by over a thousand private pharmacy benefit plans, each offering a selection of formularies and cost-sharing options. This leads to inconsistencies in drug availability across plans, which may limit which products beneficiaries can access.

In Medicaid, the coverage of injectable drugs and adult vaccines varies by state, although coverage for many childhood vaccines is required by federal law. Whether injectable drugs are recorded as prescription encounters or other types of encounters also varies by state. Medicare covers the cost of certain adult vaccinations and their administration (e.g., influenza, pneumococcal pneumonia, hepatitis B).

All prescriptions written by VA prescribers and filled in a VA pharmacy are covered by the VA's comprehensive medical care plan. The VA National Formulary lists all products (drugs and supplies) covered under the VA medical care plan. Any agent not on the Formulary and approved through a nonformulary mechanism is also covered. Only drugs dispensed and released by VA can be studied.

Eligibility and data limitations

An important potential challenge for all US claims databases is the availability of low cost prescriptions, which may reduce or eliminate incentives to submit prescription claims for payment.

When using Medicaid data, researchers may also experience gaps in beneficiary records due to periods of ineligibility. Since Medicaid is known to have frequent turnover in their beneficiaries, researchers must develop strategies to deal with this limitation. One approach to this is to use the Medicaid eligibility files. However, these files may not be completely accurate. Another approach to reducing this potential problem is to restrict consideration to time periods in which Medicaid encounters are present within some specified period (e.g., six months) both before and after the person-time under study, or there is evidence of death.

In Medicare and the VA, in contrast, turnover is low, as beneficiaries of both programs often remain enrolled once they are deemed eligible to receive benefits.

Data validity/access to medical records

The validity of data on exposures, outcomes, and covariates is a major consideration. It is important to keep in mind that these data were generated as a by-product of providing health care or administering health care benefits rather than for research purposes. This is true for all administrative and medical record databases. As a result, researchers need to consider whether a given research question can be addressed using preexisting data.

Our experience suggests that in each study, with few exceptions, investigators should obtain medical records in at least a sample of outcomes to confirm the validity of the encounter diagnoses, characterize the severity of the disease, and obtain information on potential confounding variables not found in the encounter data. One potential exception is studies of outcomes for which encounter diagnoses have previously been found to be sufficiently valid. Another potential exception is studies using a procedure or a prescription for a drug as the outcome of interest.

Out of plan care

The lack of completeness of VA data with regard to health care obtained outside the VHA is an important issue. Veteran patients can voluntarily go to any hospital for care. Moreover, for emergency and urgent conditions, Veteran patients are taken to the nearest hospital for care. Because of this, many acute conditions such as myocardial infarction, stroke, and severe hypoglycemic events are not captured as inpatient events and these important outcomes can be missed. For patients under the age of 65 these missing events must be taken into consideration for any study. For studies of VA enrollees aged 65 and above, out-of-plan medical care can often be identified by linking VA data to Medicare data. Because Medicaid and Medicare reimburse health care providers in the private sector, out-of-plan care is less likely to be an issue in those plans than in the VA.

Particular applications

Many methodological and applied studies have been performed using data from the Medicaid, Medicare, and VA systems. A few illustrative examples are presented here.

Methodological studies

Stürmer and colleagues used Medicaid data from New Jersey to compare three approaches to adjusting for measured confounding variables: conventional adjustment using the observed variables, adjustment using propensity scores (see Chapter 21), and adjustment using disease risk scores (see Chapter 21). They found that the three methods all produced similar results.

McKenzie and colleagues examined the validity of Medicaid pharmacy encounter records to estimate drug use in elderly nursing home residents. They found good agreement between Medicaid encounter records and nursing home records for presence or absence of drug ingestion (positive and negative predictive values > 85%), and that doses recorded using the two databases correlated well (correlation coefficients from 0.66 to 0.97).

Schneeweiss and colleagues used Medicare data linked to a state pharmaceutical assistance program for the elderly to assess high-dimensional propensity scores (see Chapter 21) as an approach to controlling for measured confounding factors. They found that high-dimensional propensity scores resulted in effect estimates closer to those produced by randomized trials than did conventional adjustment by predefined covariates.

Several studies have been conducted with VA data to assess the validity of ICD-9 codes to identify specific conditions. For example, Petersen *et al.* assessed the predictive value of myocardial infarction (MI), coronary bypass graft surgery, cardiac catheterization, and angioplasty. The positive predictive values of claims ranged from 90–100%.

Applied pharmacoepidemiologic studies

Roumie *et al.* used Tennessee Medicaid data to examine the association between different nonsteroidal anti-inflammatory drugs and stroke, myocardial infarction, and cardiovascular death. They found that current use of rofecoxib, valdecoxib, and indomethacin was associated with an increased risk of cardiovascular events in those without preexisting cardiovascular disease.

Ray and colleagues used Tennessee Medicaid data to examine the association between antipsychotic drugs and risk of sudden cardiac death. They found that at doses of greater than 100 mg/d of chlorpromazine equivalents, the rate ratio for use of any antipsychotic drug was 2.39 (95% confidence interval (CI), 1.77 to 3.22). Hennessy and colleagues used Medicaid data from three states to study the risk of a composite outcome of sudden death or ventricular arrhythmia in persons with schizophrenia who received antipsychotics. The primary comparison was thioridazine versus haloperidol. They found no overall difference in the rate of the composite outcome, although thioridazine had a higher risk of the composite outcome at doses of 600 mg/d or greater in chlorpromazine equivalents (rate ratio 2.6, 95% CI 1.0 to 6.6). A dose–response relationship was evident for thioridazine but not for haloperidol.

Patrick *et al.* used data from Medicare and the Pennsylvania state pharmaceutical assistance plan to examine the relationship between adherence to bisphosphonates and fracture risk. They found that good adherence (defined as 80–100% of days covered not clear what covered means in this context, see Chapter 20) was associated with a 22% reduction in overall fracture rate compared to worse adherence.

Lambert *et al.* evaluated the risk of new onset diabetes in Veterans exposed to specific antipsychotic agents. They found that the second-generation antipsychotic agents studied were associated with a higher risk of diabetes than first generation agents.

Conclusion

Because Medicaid has covered drugs and medical care for decades, its data have a long history of use in pharmacoepidemiology. Since Medicaid data have become available from CMS with assistance provided by ResDAC, use of Medicaid data for research has increased even more, and will probably continue to do so. With the anticipated expansion of Medicaid, the size of the population available should increase further, making these data even more valuable.

The Medicare drug benefit should be an enormously valuable resource for pharmacoepidemiology, and this is beginning to occur. We are hopeful that CMS will continue to permit researchers to obtain medical records to validate outcomes identified in Medicaid and Medicare data. In the future, perhaps it will be possible to access Medicare patients directly, obtaining supplemental historical and even biological information.

VA databases have existed for well over a decade but continue to evolve to include more detailed clinical information. In the future, more real-time databases will be available, as will newer VA databases, many of which are now in the pilot phase. These newer databases should allow for more timely evaluation and the ability to better evaluate population trends at the time of care. Some of the projects that are currently in an early or pilot phase are newer methods for creating common prevalent cohorts available for medical chart validations, automated text-based validation tools, and increased use of VA databases for comparative effectiveness research (see Chapter 22).

Also, databases that are currently being compiled by the Department of Defense (DoD) could prove very helpful in the examination of vaccines, as well as other medications. These DoD databases hold great potential for pharmacoepidemiologic research studies.

Finally, the potential use of US government health care data as part of FDA's sentinel initiative for active surveillance (see Chapter 22) holds great promise.

Summary points for Medicaid databases

- The US Medicaid program provides medical coverage for certain categories of disadvantaged individuals.
- Data on prescription drugs are audited to detect fraud, and have been found to be accurate.
- The accuracy of diagnostic codes depends on the specific condition. With few exceptions, researchers using Medicaid data should verify diagnoses using primary medical records.

Case Example 9.2: Medicaid databases

Background

- Based on spontaneous reports and effects on blood pressure and heart rate, there was concern that medications used to treat attention deficit hyperactivity disorder (ADHD) might increase the risk of certain cardiovascular events including myocardial infarction, stroke, and sudden cardiac death.

Questions

- Are ADHD medications associated with an increased risk of serious cardiovascular events in children and adults?

Approach

- Series of cohort studies using data from health plans and Medicaid, supplemented with Medicare claims in persons enrolled in both Medicaid and Medicare.
- The rate of serious cardiovascular events was measured in persons receiving ADHD medications and unexposed comparison groups.
- Confounding factors present in claims data were measured and controlled for.

Results

- None of the studies found consistently elevated risks of cardiovascular events associated with use of ADHD medications.

- The conduct of multiple studies in multiple populations by multiple research groups provided additional assurance that the results were valid.

Strengths

- The study was large, allowing meaningful comparisons of very rare events.
- In adults, the outcomes were either validated by record review or were based on well-validated outcomes.

Limitations

- Claims diagnoses of serious cardiovascular outcomes had poor positive value in children, possibly because of the low frequency of events in children.

Key Points

- Large sample sizes are needed to study rare outcomes.
- Studies in multiple populations by multiple research groups can permit assessment of the consistency of results.

Canadian provincial databases

Introduction

Canada, with its population of approximately 34 million, has a universal health care program which, under the federal Canada Health Act of 1984, requires provinces to provide hospitalization and physician services without payment by the patient at the time of service. The administration of the program is under the responsibility of each of its ten provinces and three territories. From east to west the provinces, where the vast majority of residents are located, consist of: Newfoundland/Labrador (NFLD), Prince Edward Island (PEI), Nova Scotia (NS), New Brunswick (NB), Quebec (QC), Ontario (ON), Manitoba (MB), Saskatchewan (SK), Alberta (AB), and British Columbia (BC). Drug regulation is centrally conducted through Health Canada, an organization under the jurisdiction of the federal health ministry, but the administration of the drug coverage programs is conducted by the provinces and territories. Since public drug programs are not included in the Canada Health Act, the characteristics of drug coverage differ greatly across provinces. These in turn determine the nature of the study populations and the

specific drugs that can be considered for pharmacoepidemiologic studies.

The health services program covers physician visits, diagnostic tests, procedures, and hospitalizations, and covers all residents regardless of age or income. Physicians are paid on a fee-for-service basis, and databases have been created in each province for the administration of the program. A small number of physicians may have all or a portion of their activities covered by salary, and hence the services they provide may not be included in the medical services databases.

Prescription drug programs have been available for varying lengths of time in different provinces. Unlike coverage for physician visits, diagnostic tests, procedures, and hospitalizations, drug coverage differs across provinces, ranging from the entire population (e.g., universal in Saskatchewan and Manitoba) to specific segments of the population (e.g., elderly and welfare recipients in Ontario). In some provinces, the program has distinctive coverage features, described below.

Within each province, three health databases are available: (1) medical services, (2) hospitalizations, and (3) prescription drugs. These databases are linkable through a unique patient identifier that remains unchanged over time. In addition, it is possible to link this information to the demographic characteristics of the patients and to a variety of prescriber characteristics. Additional linkage capacities are available through province-specific databases, such as registries (e.g., cancer or cardiac registries), or through research initiatives.

The Canadian government is currently reforming its drug regulation by the implementation of progressive licensing. Under this framework, the current point-in-time licensing system will be replaced by a cyclical progressive licensing model. This will be achieved through "the collection, analysis, and communication of knowledge and experience about a drug throughout its life cycle," including the post-approval setting. This change in landscape has led to the creation of the Drug Safety and Effectiveness Network (DSEN) of the Canadian Institute for Health Research (CIHR), which is the Government of Canada's agency responsible for funding health research. The objectives of DSEN are "to increase the available evidence on drug safety and effectiveness available to regulators, policy-makers, health care providers and patients; and, to increase capacity within Canada to undertake high-quality postmarket research in this area." In this context, an increase in the number of post-approval studies is forecasted.

Description

Prescription drug databases

Eligibility criteria for prescription drug programs vary greatly across provinces. For example, in Ontario, the drug program is universal for all elderly residents over the age of 65 as well as for welfare recipients. In Quebec the program also includes the vast majority of elderly (97%) and all welfare recipients. In addition, given that drug coverage is mandatory in Quebec since 2001, all residents and their dependents that do not have access to private insurance plans through their employers are covered by the public drug program. The public drug program imposes a deductible and co-payment, the amount of which depends on family income. In Alberta, the program also covers adults and children who are severely handicapped as well as those receiving palliative care. In British Columbia, the public drug program was expanded in 2003 to cover patients with AIDS and cystic fibrosis as well as prescriptions dispensed in mental health services centers. In Newfoundland/Labrador, patients with growth hormone deficiency are covered by the public drug program. Nova Scotia also offers coverage for seniors, welfare, and patients with cancer. In some provinces (e.g., British Columbia, Alberta, and Newfoundland/Labrador), expensive drugs may be covered by the public drug program but the level of co-payment depends on income, and may reach as much as 10% of a person's annual net income. In Manitoba, access to the public drug program depends on family income relative to the cost of drugs, and does not exceed 3.5% of a family's gross income. Saskatchewan offers a drug plan to all residents, and co-payment also depends on annual income.

Depending on the province, prescription data for sub-groups of the population who are neither elderly nor welfare recipients may therefore appear either in public drug program databases or in private insurance databases. Such coverage features may affect the generalizability of findings obtained in studies conducted in adults between the ages of 18 and 65. The availability of longitudinal data may also be compromised by residents who migrate between the public and private insurance programs. However, dates of membership are available and continuous membership in the public drug program may be used as a study eligibility criterion. Two exceptions are British Columbia and Manitoba. In British Columbia, a collaborative program has been implemented (BC PharmaNet) under the auspices of the Ministry of Health, which combines data on all prescriptions dispensed through the public drug program, private insurers, and out-of-pocket. Essentially, all prescriptions dispensed in community pharmacies regardless of coverage are centrally recorded in BC PharmaNet. In Manitoba, prescriptions are also combined although not segmented by private or out-of-pocket; those not covered by the province are designated as "nonadjudicated." This represents a major advantage over most of the other provinces where there is no universal drug program. However, this advantage is offset by restricted access policies, described below.

In summary, the majority of the Canadian population resides in provinces where the public drug program is restricted to specific segments of the population (e.g., elderly, welfare). Coverage features for the remainder may affect the generalizability of findings obtained in pharmacoepidemiologic studies, and this issue should be addressed in studies on a case by case basis. The population covered by a provincial prescription drug plan is therefore a major criterion in the selection of a Canadian database to conduct pharmacoepidemiologic research.

Prescription drug databases records all prescription drug dispensings received in an outpatient setting. Drugs obtained over-the-counter, in-hospital, or long-term care units are not usually included in the database. Drugs dispensed to nursing home residents are also included if the pharmacy where they acquire their prescriptions is considered to be community-based as opposed to institution-based. Claims databases require that the drug be approved in the formulary before they can be included in the database. Reimbursement is under the jurisdiction of each province. Consequently, the date of inclusion of the drugs in the formulary, and the type of listing (general or restricted), differs from the date of drug approval by Health Canada, and may vary across provinces. This is another important criterion in the selection of a Canadian database.

The main data elements found in the prescription drug databases are listed in Table 9.4. Apart from a few exceptions, data and coding systems are very similar across provinces. With the exception of the Saskatchewan database, prescribed daily dose may be derived directly from the quantity dispensed, prescribed duration, and dose per unit (strength). The prescribed duration may, however, be inaccurate for drugs taken as needed (PRN).

Therapeutic indication for a drug prescription is not recorded in any of the databases. For each patient, the year of entry and exit from the drug program are available in the patient information database. This is important information for studies that include segments of the population whose membership in the drug program may be transitory, such as membership based on income or access to private insurance programs.

For each province, the nature and size of the population covered by the public drug program, the database custodians, as well as their year of availability are summarized in Table 9.5. Year of availability refers to the earliest date when data became available through the database custodians, which may not correspond to the year of implementation of the public drug program. Furthermore, depending on the structure of the repository and archive processes, data availability for earlier years may be restricted. Overall, databases may be available for pharmacoepidemiologic research in seven provinces. The three remaining provinces, all located in the east, account for the smallest segments of the Canadian population.

In addition to the drug databases, custodians also act as a repository for other provincial databases and are responsible for their linkage.

Table 9.4 Information recorded in the prescription drug databases.

Common to all provincial databases	Specific to individual databases
Patient information	
Encrypted patient identifier	Category of membership (e.g., welfare recipient, elderly, level of deductible as a proxy for income)
Gender	
	Age: date of birth, birth year, age, or age group depending on database and confidentiality procedures
Drug information	
Date of dispensing	
Drug class (AHF[a] classification)	
Drug Information Number (DIN)[b]	
Generic name	
Brand name	
Strength	
Form of administration	
Quantity dispensed	
Prescribed duration[c]	
Prescriber information	
Encrypted prescriber information	
Cost information	
Unit cost	
Patient contribution	
Drug plan contribution	
Total cost, including dispensing fee	

[a]American Hospital Formulary.
[b]Assigned by Health Canada.
[c]Not available in Saskatchewan.

Table 9.5 Characteristics of the population covered in the public drug database, by province.

Province	Total population	Custodian	Population covered	Segments covered			Year of availability
				Welfare	Elderly	Other	
Prince Edward Island	135,000						N/A
New Brunswick	750,000						N/A
Newfoundland/ Labrador	100,000	DHCS[a]	N/A	√	√	Partial	2007
Nova Scotia	1 million	PHRU[b]	150,000	√	√	Partial	
Quebec	7.5 million	RAMQ[c]	3.5 million	√	√	Partial	2001
Ontario	13 million	ICES[d]	1.5 million	√	√	None	1990
Manitoba	800,000	MCHP[e]	800,000	√	√	√	2005
Saskatchewan	1 million	SK Health[f]	910,000	√	√	√	1976
Alberta	3.5 million	AHW[g]	374,000	√	√	√	Restricted
British Columbia	4 million	PopDataBC[h]		√	√	√	1985
		PharmaNet[i]				√	(expanded 2003)

[a]DHCS: Department of Health and Community Services (Government)
[b]PHRU: Population Health Research Unit (University)
[c]RAMQ: Régie de l'assurance-maladie du Québec (Government)
[d]ICES: Institute for Clinical Evaluative Sciences (Non-profit)
[e]MCHP: Manitoba Centre for Health Policy (University)
[f]SK Health: Saskatchewan Health (Government)
[g]AHW: Alberta Health and Wellness (Government)
[h]Population Data BC (University) (formerly available through the British Columbia Linked Health Database (BCLHD).
[i]BC Ministry of Health (Government)

Medical services databases

The health care system of Canada covers medical care (although not necessarily prescription drug coverage) for all residents regardless of age and income. For the administration of the program, each province has created a database which includes all claims submitted by the physicians who are paid fee-for-service. All patient encounters that are individually billed are recorded in the database regardless of setting (inpatient, outpatient, emergency department). Data elements that are included in each claim and which are relevant for pharmacoepidemiologic research are summarized in Table 9.6.

The nature of the information in the various medical services databases is similar. Practice region is either recorded in the database as a data element, such as in Saskatchewan, or may be derived indirectly from the main practice setting and region identified in a random sample of medical visits for a given physician.

Diagnostic coding depends on the province, following either the International Classification of Diseases, tenth edition (ICD-10) since 2006 or the ICD-9-CM for those provinces that have not yet implemented ICD-10 (e.g., Quebec). Diagnosis is the only field that is not mandatory for payment, which may pose a threat in the validity of study findings. Procedures are coded according to the Canadian Classification of Diagnostic, Therapeutic, and Surgical Procedures. Laboratory tests

Table 9.6 Information available in the medical services databases.

Common to all provincial databases	Specific to individual databases
Patient information	
Encrypted patient identifier	
Gender	
	Age: Date of birth, birth year, age, or age group depending on database
Service information	
Date of encounter	
Service rendered	Coding systems differ across provinces
Location of service (Hospital, community clinic, emergency department, long-term care unit, etc.)	Coding systems differ across provinces
Diagnosis	ICD-9 or ICD-10 depending on provinces
Physician information	
Encrypted physician information	
Practice region (urban, rural)	Category and source of information differs according to province
Year of graduation	Categories differ according to province

Table 9.7 Information available in the hospital discharge databases.

Patient information
Encrypted identifier
Gender
Age
Hospital admission information
Main diagnosis
Secondary diagnoses
Accident code
Admission date
Discharge date
Length of stay
Hospital identification
Patient destination (community, other hospital, long-term care unit, death)

performed at the hospital that are not individually billed will not be in the database. The vast majority of claims are submitted electronically, and the resulting medical services claims databases are populated in real-time. In a few provinces, such as Nova Scotia, Manitoba, and British Columbia, mental health services, including psychotherapy, are also recorded in a distinct database.

Hospitalization databases

Unlike the medical services databases, hospitalization databases were created for health statistics rather than reimbursement. The databases contain clinical data related to hospital discharges and day surgeries. With the exception of Quebec, all provinces contribute to the Discharge Abstract Database (DAD) maintained by the Canadian Institute for Health Information (CIHI). The information is therefore homogeneous across provinces. In Quebec, the hospital discharge database is called MED ECHO. The information included in the hospitalization databases is summarized in Table 9.7.

In the hospitalization databases, diagnosis was coded with ICD-9-CM until March 31st, 2006 and with ICD-10 since. In the DAD database, information on mental health resources, cancer staging and reproductive history have been added in 2009–10. Unlike claims databases, the hospitalization databases are mainly populated once a year and the fiscal year runs from April 1st to March 31st. Databases are typically available six months after the end of the fiscal year, at the earliest. In studies where such delay is unacceptable, it is possible to identify hospitalizations through the location of service in the medical services database (physician billings). However, since diagnoses in the hospital discharge database (one principal diagnosis and up to ten secondary diagnoses) are abstracted from hospital charts by medical archivists, they are believed to be more reliable than the single diagnosis recorded by physicians on their billings.

Linkage capacities

The medical services, hospitalization, and prescription drug databases may be linked through a unique identifier, which remains unchanged over time. Linkage provides a longitudinal accumulation of population-based information on all health care services received by residents of each province. Availability of prescription data may, however, be interrupted by out-of-province residency, admission to acute or long-term care units, or periods of non-eligibility in the public prescription drug programs due to access to private insurance programs, for example.

These databases may be linked to other data sources, such as registries or surveys. Technically, linkage with multiple data sources is feasible provided that the health insurance number has been collected. Cancer or infectious disease registries are available in each province, but many database custodians have not yet developed the linkage capacities with these other sources. An exception is Saskatchewan, where many studies involving linkage between the cancer registry and claims databases have been conducted. Some provincial database custodians, such as those of Ontario, Nova Scotia, and Manitoba, also act as a warehouse for other databases. Consequently, the linkage processes are already in place in those provinces.

Linkage capacities include linkage with other statistics or health databases, registries (e.g., cancer registries, vital statistics), national health surveys, or with database/registries created for research or clinical purposes (e.g., Dalhousie Multiple Sclerosis Research Unit database, Canadian Cardiac Network in Ontario). Although many databases have been identified across Canada, many have not yet been linked to health care databases for pharmacoepidemiologic research.

Database access and confidentiality

Access policies are a very important consideration in the selection of a database. As described below, some are available to academic researchers only, while others may also be accessible by employees of private or commercial organizations. Access may be sought directly from government agencies in Saskatchewan, Quebec. For the other provinces, access is sought through a repository, which may be an academic center (e.g., Nova Scotia, Ontario, British Columbia) or through a regional health board (e.g., Manitoba). For seven provinces (SK, QC, ON, BC, MB, NS, AB), health databases have been widely used for pharmacoepidemiologic research. For the remaining provinces, access is restricted because of absence of a common database custodian and/or absence of access procedures. Furthermore, databases from British Columbia, Manitoba, Newfoundland/Labrador, and Ontario are not accessible by the pharmaceutical industry. In Ontario and Manitoba, access is restricted to designated researchers only. The databases from Saskatchewan and Quebec are accessible to all researchers, regardless of sector.

Regardless of the province, a database request must be submitted to the custodians for review. Review consists of ethics approval and, for university-based custodians, a scientific review as well.

The data sets available to researchers vary greatly across provinces. In Saskatchewan, Quebec, and Nova Scotia, raw anonymized datasets are sent directly to the researchers. In Ontario, data must be analyzed in-house by a member or affiliate of the Institute for Clinical Evaluative Sciences (ICES). To maintain confidentiality of the data, no patient, health care professional (including pharmacist), or institution identifiers are transmitted to researchers. All identifiers are encrypted. Furthermore, in Quebec, to reduce the possibility of identifying a particular patient, only a random sample of approximately 75% of the population eligible for a given study may be obtained, and no birthdates are transmitted. Patient age is categorized in five-year intervals and year but exact date of death is not provided. More detailed information may be sought, but a special request must be submitted to the provincial Information Privacy Commissioner. In Saskatchewan, all drugs that are part of the data elements required for a given study must be identified *a priori*. Data extraction does not offer the possibility to obtain all drugs acquired by a given patient.

Linkage with medical charts or complementary sources of information

The variable validity of diagnostic codes recorded in health care databases is a well-known threat to pharmacoepidemiologic studies. In many instances, it may be desirable to access source information, such as hospital or outpatient charts, in order to obtain clinical characteristics and validate the diagnosis of cases ascertained in the databases. To obtain claims data on patients identified in a clinical or hospital setting is feasible, mainly through informed consent. However, one major barrier for the conduct of validation studies is the feasibility to link the information that appears in the claims databases back to the individual patient charts. Because of data protection rules and regulations, this process requires approval by the Access to Information and Privacy Commission and, in some provinces, it may not be acceptable.

Yet, some validation studies have been conducted, but validation data are far from comprehensive. According to a recent review, at least 18 validation studies of Canadian databases have been published in the literature, the majority of which having been conducted to validate the diagnostic codes present in the medical services databases.

Another methodological issue that would warrant access to patients or their health records is the collection of data that are not present in the databases. Indication, smoking, alcohol use, body mass index, over-the-counter drug use are examples of such variables. Two-stage sampling is a method that may be used to address unmeasured confounders through the collection of supplementary data in a subset of individuals. This requires identifying patients in the claims database and using nominal information to access medical charts. To our knowledge, this has been done only through the Saskatchewan and Quebec databases.

Strengths

Canadian databases have been widely used for pharmacoepidemiologic research. Although most studies found in the literature involve a limited number of databases, such as those from Saskatchewan, Ontario, Quebec, British Columbia, and Manitoba, as research capacity within Canada is expanding, one can foresee greater use of the other databases as well. Among the unique features of the Canadian databases are the availability of longitudinal population-based data on prescription drugs and health care use, and most importantly linkage capacities with other sources of data, such as registries or surveys.

Weaknesses

The technical advantages of the Canadian databases are somewhat offset by decentralization and the access restrictions described above. Although efforts to pool databases are currently ongoing in a number of countries, few attempts have been made in Canada to date. The difficulty in accessing patient health records through nominal information, for diagnostic validation or to control for unmeasured confounders, is a threat to the validity of studies that aim at assessing the safety or effectiveness of a drug.

Particular applications

Below are a few examples of studies conducted through linkage with various databases. Examples illustrate drug utilization studies, risk evaluation studies, and comparative effectiveness research.

Drug and health care utilization

Dalhousie Multiple Sclerosis Research Unit (DMSRU) database. The DMSRU database includes 25 years of clinical data and may be linked to Nova Scotia's provincial data. In a study conducted by Sketris *et al.*, drug use and costs by seniors with multiple sclerosis was compared to that of all senior residents of the province.

Through the *National Rehabilitation Reporting System* of Ontario, a study was conducted on health care utilization in nontraumatic and traumatic spinal cord injury patients using linkage with the *Ontario Health Insurance Plan* for physicians' fee-for-service claims and the *National Ambulatory Care Resource System* for all visits to emergency departments.

Another study compared health care use before and after a workplace injury using linkage between the *Workers' Compensation Board (WCB)* of British Columbia and the *British Columbia Linked Health Databaset*. All these databases may be accessible through PopulationData BC. Medical services and hospitalizations were obtained for five years before and five years after the injury. Use was also compared to injured workers who did not file a claim.

Comparative effectiveness research

A nonrandomized comparative effectiveness study on drug-eluting stents impregnated with paclitaxel versus sirolimus in diabetic and nondiabetic patients has also been conducted through linkage between patients identified in the *Cardiac Care Network of Ontario percutaneous coronary intervention registry* and linked to the administrative health databases of Ontario. Study outcomes consisted of target-vessel revascularization, myocardial infarction and death.

Risk evaluation studies

In Manitoba, there is a universal *Manitoba Bone Density Program*, which is accessible to all residents of the province provided that they meet the criteria for testing consistent with published guidelines. The program has managed all clinical bone density scanning of the province since 1997, and the database has been shown to be over 99% complete and accurate. A study assessed the association between weight and body mass index, and low bone mineral density and fractures in women age 40 and 59 years.

A study on the association between benzodiazepines and motor vehicle accidents also involved a specific linkage between the Quebec driver's license files, police reports of injurious crashes, and health care databases.

Canada-wide linkage has rarely been done, and never with prescription drug databases since they are province-specific. However, the *Canadian Organ Replacement Register (CORR)* is a national organ failure registry in Canada and is maintained by the Canadian Institute for Health Information (CIHI). This database was linked with the CIHI hospital discharge database which is also centralized. Such a linkage allowed researchers to create the Canadian Pediatric End-Stage Renal Disease database, a tool to perform longitudinal studies in this patient population. This database includes all provinces except Quebec, which has separate privacy legislation.

Other linkage capacities include health care databases with population health surveys, Provincial Vital Statistics databases (birth, death, and cause of death), Canadian Reduction of Atherothrombosis for Continued Health (REACH) Registry, Nova Scotia, Saskatchewan, British Columbia

Cancer Registry (available through database custodians), and Ontario diabetes database. There are many such clinical databases in Canada and they will be increasingly linked, but so far it has been uncommon.

Conclusion

Medical services, hospitalizations, and prescription drug databases are widely available in Canada. At present, their potential for use in pharmacoepidemiologic research is somewhat hampered by access restriction and/or delays. Great potential exists for linkage with complementary sources of information such as registries. However, such registries are often local initiatives, with no information centralized in a common repository. Greater linkage capacities between databases and other complementary data sources would be valuable to augment the data sources in Canada, such as for example, laboratory test results. At the present time, the Manitoba bone mass registry is the only provincial source of data on diagnostic test results.

The fragmentation of databases across provinces and heterogeneity in custodians leads to a taxonomy of databases that is very complex. In the future, database access and linkage capacities will need to be better communicated in order to implement collaborative projects across provinces.

Summary points for Canadian provincial databases

• Each of the 10 Canadian provinces maintains a prescription, medical services, and hospital admissions database.

• In all provinces except British Columbia and Manitoba, only drugs covered by public drug programs are recorded in the prescription database.

• Medical services and hospital admissions databases are universal, i.e., they cover all residents regardless of age or income.

• Population included in the prescription databases depends on the public drug coverage program, which varies from province to province (e.g., universal in Saskatchewan, restricted to elderly and welfare recipients in Ontario).

• Subjects are identified by a unique health insurance number that is used in each of the health care services databases (e.g., prescription drug data, hospitalizations, physician services) and can be used to link records across the databases and longitudinally.

• Linkage between health care databases and other sources of information, such as registries, is feasible and is subject to approval by the provincial Access to Information and Privacy Commission.

• Several Canadian databases have been widely used for drug safety and effectiveness research. However, restrictions on access as well as delay of data extraction in most provinces are important limitations.

Medical record databases

Introduction

Medical record databases are longitudinal patient record databases that are used by health care providers in caring for their patients, and anonymized for the purpose of research. They often record information unavailable in administrative databases. Such information may include smoking status, alcohol use, and body mass index. Further, diagnosis codes entered for administrative rather than clinical purposes may not reflect the clinician's view of the

---

Case Example 9.3: Administrative claims databases in Canada Pariente *et al.* (2012)

Background

• Antipsychotic agents are frequently prescribed to elderly patients with dementia, despite numerous regulatory safety warnings for this population.
• Studies published in the literature have shown that antipsychotics increase the risk of stroke among demented elderly.
• The impact of antipsychotics on the risk of cardiovascular events, such as myocardial infarction (MI), remain poorly examined.

Issue

• Using the Quebec administrative claims databases, a population-based study was conducted to evaluate the association between antipsychotics and MI in a community-dwelling elderly population with dementia.

Approach

• A historical cohort design.
• Cohort of elderly with dementia was assembled, using dispensing of cholinesterase inhibitors (ChIs) as a proxy for dementia.
• Subcohort of new antipsychotic users and antipsychotic non-users were created.
• Subjects were followed to the study end date defined as the earliest of the following: date of MI, date of death, date of institutionalization, end of follow-up (1 year after index date), or end of the study period.
• The effects of age, gender, cardiovascular comorbidity or history (previous MI, stroke, diabetes, hypertension or heart failure), use of statins, sedatives, antidepressants, anxiolytic agents, acetylsalicylic acid, or NSAIDs, were considered. Propensity scores were also used in a secondary analysis. Effects of potential confounders not measured in administrative claims databases were considered, using a self-controlled case series analysis.

Results

• 10 969 antipsychotic users and 10 969 non-exposed subjects were identified.
• During the year following initiation of antipsychotic treatment, the risk of MI was 1.3% compared to 1.2% in the unexposed cohort.
• Adjusting for covariates, the hazard ratio for the risk of MI after initiation of AP treatment was 2.19 (95% CI: 1.11–4.32).
• Self-controlled case series analysis yielded incidence rate ratios of 1.78 (95% CI: 1.26–2.52) for 1–30 day period after AP initiation.

Strengths

• Population-based data enabled identification of a large number of elderly patients with dementia who were using antipsychotics.
• Multiple methods to control for measured or unmeasured confounders (covariates, propensity scores, self-controlled case-series analysis) were used.
• Dementia diagnosis is largely under-reported in administrative claims database; hence dispensing of ChI was used as a proxy.

Limitations

- The number of cases was not sufficiently large to examine risk of MI for each of the antipsychotic drugs individually.
- Limited statistical power to study effect modification by the presence of a cardiovascular history.
- Administrative databases lack information on indication for antipsychotic use in this population, such as agitation, aggressiveness, or motor behaviors associated with delusion. If such factors are also associated with an increased risk of MI, then it could lead to a bias.

Key Points

- Due to the prevalence of use of antipsychotics among elderly patients with dementia treated with cholinesterase inhibitors, adverse events induced by these medications have an important public health impact.
- Effect of antipsychotics on the risk of MI appears to be time-limited, which highlights the need for close monitoring of patients in the early phase of treatment.
- Due to the limitations of claims databases, it is important to use advanced analytical strategies for the control of measured and unmeasured confounding.

true clinical state of the patient. In contrast, information from medical record databases may be more likely to reflect the patient's true clinical state, because the data are collected for patient care.

The completeness of primary care medical record databases in recording outside care should be evaluated rather than assumed. Further, data from medical record databases still require careful study to assess the validity of the exposure and diagnosis data. In addition, there may be a high proportion of missing or absent data for some variables of interest, such as smoking, alcohol use, and occupation. In this section, we focus on primary care medical record databases, electronic patient records taken from interactions with primary care givers, and in some cases specialists based in the outpatient setting, which include information on past and current medical problems and therapies including prescriptions and other modalities.

The medical record databases highlighted in this section include the Clinical Practice Research Datalink (CPRD) (formerly known as the General Practice Research Database or GPRD), The Health Improvement Network (THIN), and the Intercontinental Marketing Services (IMS) Disease Analyzer (previously known as Mediplus). Other more localized electronic medical record databases exist but are less likely to be useful by themselves in pharmacoepidemiologic research, either because of incomplete data collection, small populations, or other reasons. CPRD GP OnLine Data (GOLD) and THIN are derived from the medical records of

patients within the United Kingdom (UK), whereas Disease Analyzer contains records from France, Germany, and UK. These databases have been widely used by pharmacoepidemiologists. While there are many similarities among the databases, there are also important differences (see Table 9.8).

The UK has advantages for obtaining electronic medical records data as a "gatekeeper" system exists in which all patients must be registered with general practitioners (GP) to get "free at the point of care" National Health Service (NHS) treatment. Almost the entire population in the UK is registered with a GP and most GPs have computerized medical records. GPs are informed of all medical care including hospitalizations. The UK was the setting of the first of these databases, now called CPRD GOLD, established in 1987 as a tool for conducting public health research. Since then, several more medical record databases have been developed for research purposes. The IMS Disease-Analyzer, while including patients from the UK, also includes patients from Germany and France. Both Germany and France have universal health care, but patients frequently have additional private insurance. Unlike the UK, medical care in Germany and France is not necessarily driven by the primary care physicians, as patients may see a specialist without first visiting a GP depending on their insurance coverage.

The CPRD datalink system includes the CPRD GOLD, which was initially called Value Added Medical Products (VAMP) Research Databank. This

Table 9.8 Overview of CPRD, THIN, and IMS Disease-Analyzer.

	CPRD	THIN	IMS Disease-Analyzer
Year data collection initiated	1987 In 2012 CPRD became the English NHS 52 million data system	2002	1992
Number of patients Included	5+ million active patients in CPRD GOLD. 12.93 million total patients. In all, CPRD has as many 52 million individuals with varying types of data.	3.6 million "active" patients who can be followed prospectively; 10.0 million total patients contributing over 57.1 million patient years.	UK: 4.2 million total patients with 17.9 million patient years Germany: 29.9 million (incl. 17.2 million German Specialty patients) with 54.5 million patient yrs France: 5.2 million patients with 6.0 million patient years.
Number of Physician Practices Included	629 in CPRD GOLD	498	UK: 218; Germany: 2357 (plus 2010 specialty practices); France: 2091
Coding Used	READ, Multilex	READ, Multilex	ICD10, READ, ATC Codes
Software Used	Vision	Vision	Various
Regular quality checks performed	Permanent ongoing data checks on all practices: Data quality assurance processes are undertaken as part of data processing. Patients are flagged as "acceptable" for use in research by a process that identifies and excludes patients with non-contiguous follow up or patients with poor data recording that raises suspicion as to the validity of that patient's record. Up to standard dates (described in text)	For the first 100 practices, preliminary audits of consultations and prescriptions as compared to national levels were performed. Ongoing, all data collected undergo consistency and integrity checks. Feedback is provided to practices regarding UK quality metrics performances, medical history recording, and comparison of prevalence of disease with national levels where available. Acceptable mortality recording (described in text).	All data checked to meet quality standards and for plausibility. Feedback reports are given to each physician monthly, showing the physician's prescription patterns and those of colleagues within the IMS panel and within their specialty group.

provided GPs with software that enabled them to contribute anonymized patient information to a central database. In order to participate, GPs agreed to undergo training in data entry and provide a copy of the entire anonymous medical record to VAMP including photocopied (but de-identified) letters from specialists and hospitals. Since inception, there have been many changes in management of the database.

The Health Improvement Network began collecting data in 2002. CPRD GOLD and THIN collect similar information from representative sample populations within the UK (e.g. individual practices). Some practices participate in both THIN and CPRD. It is important to recognize that pooling results from both databases would need to account for this overlap. The IMS Disease Analyzer differs from CPRD and THIN in that data are collected from three countries with most of the patient records obtained from Germany and the UK and a smaller number from France. IMS Disease Analyzer also directly includes data from some specialist groups in Germany: cardiologists, diabetologists, dermatologists, gynecologists, otolaryngology, neurologists, psychiatrists, pediatricians, urologists, and some surgeons, including orthopedists.

Description

Data collection and structure

Each year, practitioners record information on 3–5 million patients for each of these databases, accounting for nearly 5–7% of the population within the UK in each of the databases (and 5–7% within Germany in Disease-Analyzer). Practitioners use the electronic medical record to document information about their patients. Data are extracted electronically from the medical record, examined for completeness and accuracy by the database administrators, and then uploaded into the database in an anonymous form. Data are collected initially and then updated over differing intervals, adding information on new patients entering the system and updating the longitudinal profiles of existing patients. All three databases abstract this data specifically for research purposes. Table 9.9 shows the data collected in each database.

CPRD-GOLD, THIN, and the IMS Disease-Analyzer are representative of their respective populations in terms of age, sex, most diseases, and prescriptions written, so that the prevalence of these will be similar to the general population. Complete CPRD datasets encompass all of England. In general, most regions of the represented countries are included, though the density of patients within each region in the database may not represent the exact proportion of people living in the region. However, the reported frequency of some diseases and characteristics are not representative of the population. For example, there is variability in the recording of musculoskeletal diseases. Similarly, the spectrum of socioeconomic status found in the databases may not reflect the true distribution in the country.

Researchers utilizing the databases have access to anonymized patient medical history including comorbidities. Diagnoses and symptoms are entered using diagnostic codes, described below. Additional information can sometimes be elicited by reading through anonymized free text entries. Most free text entries are available to researchers, and additional records can be requested for an associated cost for anonymizing data. Some practitioners may still keep paper record files, which may include precomputerization records, hospital discharge paperwork, or consultant letters. Both CPRD and THIN have additional data services that will obtain these data, for a fee, from the GP.

Laboratory tests, blood pressure, height, and weight are available in all three databases to varying degrees. For example, in both CPRD GOLD and THIN laboratory data from recent years is nearly complete but some older lab tests may not be available electronically if they were received by the GP in hard copy. In IMS, hemoglobin A1C for diabetic patients is nearly complete but many other laboratory values are not recorded. Prescriptions issued by the general practitioner are well captured in these databases, though not all prescriptions are linked to a diagnosis code.

Hospitalizations, referrals and the resulting consultation letters are recorded to varying degrees among the databases. In CPRD, complete hospitalization data (including hospital specialist

Table 9.9 Selected variables available for epidemiologic research.

	CPRD	THIN	IMS Disease-Analyzer
Health care professional demographics	Can determine if nurse or doctor entering data	Can determine if nurse or doctor entering data	Age, sex and years in practice of physician.
Types of physicians	General practitioners and in other CPRD datasets, all parts of NHS	General practitioners	Mainly general practitioners, but in Germany also specialists, e.g., cardiology, gastroenterology, dermatology.
Practice and patient demographics	*Practice* Region, Practice size, Practice-level socioeconomic status (index multiple deprivation), Up-to-standard date, date of last registration, status of practice (what is status?) *Patient* Year of birth, sex, ethnicity (currently about 25% recorded, but also available via census data), socioeconomic class and other census data to small area level, hospital and disease registry data. Additionally, approximately 60% of patients have practice level Index of Multiple Deprivation and Townsend scores through linkage in addition to post code derived socioeconomic status (CPRD internal data).	*Practice* Computerization date, Vision date, patients per practice, region sometimes provided *Patient* Year of birth for adults, month and year for children. Patient-level socioeconomic status (Townsend deprivation scores), region, ethnicity (20%)	*Practice* Region, community size and patients per practice, number of doctors, number of employees, emphasis (e.g., GP vs. specialty) *Patient* Age, sex, health insurance status (e.g., private, statutory), medical insurance company, region, town size (>100,000 vs. <100,000).
Social history:	Smoking (83–93%), obesity (61–79%), alcohol (approx 80%)	Smoking (86–94%), obesity (73–83%), alcohol intake (75–85%)	Obesity (~40% had BMI), smoking and alcohol recording unknown
Referrals and results of investigations	Linkage to hospital data (England) shows the majority of records and provides greater detail. Most labs are electronic.	Available electronically where referral is made using Vision though some may be in paper files. Most labs are electronic.	HbA1C, blood sugar, cholesterol, LDL and HDL are available but others are variably available but can be requested. Test results can be requested from paper files.
Therapy	Drug name, route, dose, frequency, duration, Immunizations including batch. Cost of drug can be added.	Drug name, route, dose, frequency and duration. Cost of drugs is available in linked file.	Drug name, route, dose, frequency, duration, cost of therapy.

Health care Utilization	Visit frequency, hospitalizations, and consultant visits. Links to hospital episode statistics (HES) provides detailed ward level resource utilization in England only.	All GP visits recorded, hospitalizations are entered by GP, not directly from hospital. Sick leave recorded if GP issues a note.	Visit frequency, hospitalizations, sick leave included.
Identification of pregnancy and families	Pregnancy and pregnancy outcomes. Mother–baby link via a family/household algorithm/family identification number.	Pregnancy recorded. Families are identified by a number given to each household.	Pregnancy status. Family documentation incomplete
Identification of death and cause of death	Date of death and cause(s) available via CPRD data and from linkage to Office for National Statistics central mortality data (ONS).	Death date recorded. If the cause is not recorded, death certificates can be requested for a fee. Some cause of death information is also available as a linked file. Acceptable Mortality Reporting (AMR) is a quality indicator given for the year in which mortality records are deemed complete.	Seldom recorded.
Available additional data (e.g., consult records, labs, paper files)	Hospital discharge summaries, consultant letters. All free text available.	Hospital discharge summaries, consultant letters. Most free text available.	Available upon request.
Questionnaires	Prospective data collections possible from both healthcare professionals and from patients. Response rates from three recent studies were about 90% (and CPRD internal data).	Prospective data collections possible from both healthcare professionals and from patients. Response to paper questionnaires is about 90% (and THIN internal data).	Available upon request.

consultations) are automatically linked to the patient's record for practices in England. In THIN, hospitalization data often depend on the GP manually entering this information, and mainly includes discharge date and discharge diagnostic code but will soon include some linkages to hospitalization as well. Hospitalizations are not recorded in the Disease-Analyzer unless the patient was referred to the hospital by the GP. Consultant letters and referrals are also not available for the Disease-Analyzer database. Referrals are captured in both CPRD and THIN, although consultations may be obtained in the form of hard copy letters. Finally, components of social history such as occupation are not routinely recorded.

All three services allow for questionnaires directed toward practitioners or patients, to augment the data provided in the database. Fees are paid to the database for administration of the questionnaire and practitioners receive a fee for questionnaire completion.

In all three databases, most data are entered using codes rather than free-text entries. READ codes are a comprehensive clinical language developed in the UK utilizing standard alphanumeric codes to record patient diagnoses, symptoms, laboratory and radiographic tests, and processes of care (e.g., referrals). In the UK, Multilex codes encode drugs prescribed by the GP. The Disease Analyzer uses READ codes in the UK and International Classification of Disease 10th edition (ICD-10) codes in the other countries, and Anatomical Therapeutic Chemical classification (ATC) codes rather than Multilex codes for medications in Germany and France.

Data quality: accuracy and completeness

Data completeness varies among variables and databases. Pregnancy, family structure, mortality, and cause of death are variably recorded and can be difficult to ascertain or can require the use of complicated coding algorithms (particularly for family structure). Factors such as smoking and obesity may have gaps; before 2004 these data were often not recorded, though after the introduction of the UK national initiative of Quality and Outcomes Framework (QOF), there has been a substantial increase in the completeness of recording of these and other variables. For example, prior to 2004, smoking was recorded for around 75% of patients in CPRD GOLD, whereas in a 2007 study, it was found to be recorded in nearly 90%. Additionally, software improvements and quality improvement initiatives have increased overall data capture. However, some information may not be captured in these databases. For example, medications mainly given by specialists and over-the-counter medications may be missing. However, the long-term use of medications also available over-the-counter, such as aspirin and nonsteroidal anti-inflammatory drugs may be recorded. In patients over the age of 60, chronically used nonprescription medications seem likely to be captured given that the NHS provides free access to these medications when prescribed by the GP.

Data quality checks are performed by all three databases at regular intervals. In general, each record is examined for presence of birth date, registration date, sex, and continuity of data recording. If a particular provider or practice regularly provides data in which these elements are missing, they will receive feedback on their performance and may even be dropped from the database altogether. When data are uploaded or abstracted from the medical records, the database company performs additional quality checks to make sure the data have been correctly uploaded or extracted. Patients who have transferred out of the practice or who have died are censored at that time but not removed from the database; the date of entry into the practice and date the patient left the practice are available. Finally, subsequent updates to the databases are verified for accuracy. All three databases undergo routine updating of the software used to collect, check, transfer and present data.

Several quality measures encourage physician participation and accurate data collection. Contributing GPs receive monetary compensation and training in the use of their software, and regular evaluation of their prescribing behavior and data recording. Specific types of compensation differ depending on the database. Feedback reports are given to recording practitioners with tips on improving performance and in some cases, a summary of the practitioner's prescribing habits relative to similar practices or across the country. Other quality measures include audits of newly added practices and comparison of acquired data to national databases (e.g., mortality, hospitalizations, cancer, and cardiovascular registries).

The UK NHS also has made changes in recent years that have affected data quality. For example, pay for performance measures instituted in 2004 increased GP reliance on the electronic medical record, leading to more complete data recording, especially for specific medical conditions. Pay for performance was designed to increase performance using 146 quality indicators for ten chronic diseases: asthma, cancer, chronic obstructive pulmonary disease, coronary artery disease, diabetes, epilepsy, diabetes, hypertension, hypothyroidism, mental health, and stroke. Upon entering the medical record to begin an encounter, yellow quality indicator boxes appear for completion if a patient has one of these diseases. In 2004–05 under the new pay for performance program, 99% of patients with diabetes had a reported hemoglobin A1c value in the past 15 months, as compared to 87% in 1998. It is unclear whether reporting has also improved for diseases outside of the ten specified above. Other quality improvement strategies within the UK include national standards for treatment of diabetes (2003) and heart disease (1999), incentives for cervical cytology and immunizations (early 1990s), and widespread use of audit and feedback to the GPs by Primary Care Trusts (1990s).

Access to the databases

Access to the latest versions of the databases can be purchased through the following administrators: CPRD (www.cprd.com), THIN (www.epic-uk.org), and Disease-analyzer (www.ims.com).

Studies must be first reviewed by the home institution's institutional review board (IRB) and the ethics board of each database. Given researchers' inability to identify individual patients, such studies often meet the criteria for IRB exemption. However, ethics approval must still be sought through the databases (for CPRD, through the Independent Scientific Advisory Committee—ISAC; for THIN, through the Scientific Review Committee—SRC). The companies additionally require the completion of a data use agreement prior to initiation of the study.

Strengths

Population-based data and sample size

Population-based studies draw subjects from the greater population to arrive at a sample that is reflective of the source of individuals from which the sample was derived. All three medical record databases allow researchers to use population-based study designs, minimizing selection bias and improving validity and generalizability. In these databases, whole practices are enrolled rather than individual patients, although patients can opt out of having their information used. Very few patients opt out; although the number is not known, it is suspected to be <0.1%.

Population-based data sources are ideal for case-control studies in which cases (e.g., individuals with disease) are all or a representative sample of all cases in a precisely defined population and controls are sampled randomly from the source population from which the cases were derived. Similarly, population-based data allow for the design of cohort studies given the prospective data capture with long follow-up periods. As the data are largely representative of the general population, results are generalizable to the broader population.

Information about practices in which the patients are seen allows researchers to measure individual practice effects on health outcomes. Furthermore, the large number of patients with longitudinal follow up allows for sufficient statistical precision to study many rare outcomes.

Validity of information

The validity of the information in these databases has been extensively studied, with the highest number of validation studies in CPRD GOLD followed by THIN, and much a smaller number in Disease-Analyzer. This wealth of information provides a major advantage over other types of databases. Studies of agreement between recording in the electronic medical record and capture of data (e.g., prescription medications and specialist referrals) have been performed for some of the databases. Numerous studies have validated a variety of outcomes and diseases. If not previously performed, validation of the desired exposure and outcome to be studied should be performed prior to or as part of the study to ensure that a particular diagnostic code reflects the patient's true state.

Access to original medical records

Obtaining data from the medical record allows for a complete overview of the patient's history. Most, if not all, data about the patient are funneled through the GP and therefore accessible to the researcher. Laboratory and radiology data are mostly available and therapy data are complete except for medications administered in the hospital or by specialists (e.g., chemotherapy) and over-the-counter medications. Notably, via requests to the database administrators, anonymized copies of paper records, more detailed patient history and consultation letters are obtainable. Response rates for medical record requests have been greater than 80–90% in published studies in THIN and CPRD. An additional benefit in CPRD is the availability of original electronic medical records from hospitalizations, cancer registry data, cardiovascular registry data as well as links to many NHS audit datasets, and direct link to these data for each patient in specific geographical regions. The population for linked data is dependent upon a number of factors but can range from 2 million to 52 million. Data specific to cancer, myocardial infarction, and air pollution are currently available for 52 million people. In addition, all hospitalization data are thought to be captured for these individuals. Diagnostic codes are recorded by unit clerks coding from the medical charts and all labs and testing procedures are uploaded electronically. Additional datasets will be available over time.

Weaknesses

Completeness of data

As the data are derived from the patient's GP medical record, the investigator is relying on the GP's complete and accurate recording of the patient's history and events. Any information received by the GP from consultants, hospitalizations, or test results in hard copy would need to be manually entered into the electronic medical record, and thus may not be fully captured. Radiology and laboratory reports received in hard copy may not be entered in all cases (and may be more likely to be entered if abnormal).

In general, much of specialist care is missing from these databases, as they are designed to capture GP activity. Exceptions include IMS disease analyzer's capture of data from specialist offices in Germany, inpatient specialist information captured in the hospitalization data in CPRD, and the GP recording of consultation data in THIN and CPRD, although all consultations may not be recorded, particularly specialist information during hospitalization. In one GPRD study, 10% of data on specialist consultations were missing. These are old estimates, however.

Because codes for each chronic disease may not be repeated at each visit, episodes of care involving acute events may be better recorded than chronic diseases. Nonsignificant medical events or medical problems that are no longer clinically active may not be documented.

Limited information on patient-based socioeconomic status is included in CPRD GOLD and THIN, and these data are unavailable in Disease-Analyzer. Occupation and employment are rarely if ever recorded in any of the databases. THIN provides a patient-level measure of socioeconomic status derived from the patients' postal code of residence (around 95% of patients have this information), whereas CPRD provides a practice-level measure of socioeconomic status for nearly all practices and has recently added a patient-level measure for 60% of patients.

Data on variables such as smoking, alcohol use, body mass index, and height are not available for all patients (see Table 9.9 for data on percent recording). Data on medications given during hospitalization, those medications restricted to specialist care, and hospital discharge medications may be particularly problematic (though patients generally only receive up to two weeks of medications upon discharge). In addition, not all medications are linked to a particular diagnosis. Around 50% are linked to Disease Analyzer. While medications are not directly linked to a diagnosis in CPRD and THIN, one can use diagnoses recorded during the visit when the medication was prescribed. Medication adherence is often not recorded so notation of a prescription does not necessarily mean the medication was taken. Also, prescription records only capture prescriptions written but do not indicate which prescriptions were filled. However, in THIN and CPRD GOLD, refills or repeat prescriptions are recorded. New prescriptions are generated when the current refills have been used and a new record is created.

Finally, although these are longitudinal databases, patients may only be in the database for a few years if they transfer out of the practice or if the practice ceases to participate in the database. Thus, studies of incident exposure in which patients need to be followed for many years may suffer from loss to follow-up over time.

Particular applications

Numerous peer-reviewed manuscripts have been published, and many abstracts have been presented at international conferences using these three databases (greater than 700 from GPRD/CPRD alone, over 150 in Disease-Analyzer, and more than 200 in THIN).

Representative incidence and prevalence studies include shoulder complaints in UK primary care, newly diagnosed heart failure in primary care, bullous pemphigoid, and pemphigus vulgaris. Other epidemiologic studies include the natural history of disease (e.g., irritable bowel syndrome), the risk of a particular outcome occurring (e.g., lymphoma among inflammatory bowel disease patients, myocardial infarction in patients with psoriasis, and complications of diabetes), defining associated conditions (e.g., obesity and liver disease), and patterns of diseases or symptoms and the rate of referral (e.g., chronic pelvic pain).

Hundreds of pharmacoepidemiologic studies have been published. These include studies assessing risks and outcomes of medication (e.g., risk of myopathy and myalgias by statin class), safety and tolerability of medications, studies of medication exposure and pregnancy outcomes, reduction of morbidity or mortality by medications or interventions such as vaccinations, and trends in prescribing.

Finally, pharmacoeconomics and health services studies have used medical record databases for population-based studies. Cost-effectiveness of bisphosphonates in elderly women, comparison of cost between glaucoma therapies, cost-effectiveness of long-term hormonal contraception, and the cost-effectiveness of treatment of gastroesophageal reflux disease are a few examples. Health services researchers have examined health insurance-related barriers in obtaining new medicines and delay in access to new medical therapies, health care utilization in fibromyalgia and diabetes, prescribing trends and their budget impact, equivalent care of the elderly and non-elderly in terms of investigating a symptoms concerning for ovarian cancer, and vaccination uptake and distribution in the UK. As one can see, the diversity of studies and variety of disciplines utilizing these databases are immense.

Conclusion

It is important to recognize that changes in the national health systems may have an impact on data collection, quality, and variables included. For example, pay for performance increased the recording of data with regard to the diseases of interest, particularly diabetes. CPRD and THIN are working on data quality initiatives including practice level data quality indicators. CPRD has created linkage to death certificates, other healthcare databases, and national registry data (e.g., hospitalization, cancer, cardiovascular, and mortality registries) and will in future include many new linkages both within the NHS and to social care data; although published data have not yet resulted, studies are underway. THIN has also added such linkages which will be available to researchers by Fall 2012. THIN has recently added pop-up questionnaires that appear for completion while the GP is charting within the medical record. When an investigator is requesting additional information, this feature allows the GP to complete the investigator's questionnaire at the point of care. CPRD has added the ability to perform genetic studies allowing for collection of blood samples, and interventional studies in which patients are randomized at the point of care. CPRD is also developing a new data collection system for new to the market drugs.

This system already has permission to collect full prior and future electronic data on patients prescribed new to the market medications for over 15% of the UK population. IMS has developed several new information databases over the past few years including IMS Contract Monitor which contains information regarding the volume of drug delivery by public pharmacies, the health insurance plans, and the drug manufacturers. This information can then be merged with patient information from the Disease-Analyzer. More developments like those mentioned here can be expected in the future.

Summary points for medical record databases

• Medical records databases contain anonymized data on diagnoses, therapies, and health related behaviors recorded by general practitioners as part of the patients' electronic medical record.

• CPRD and THIN are broadly representative of the United Kingdom. Disease-analyzer contains data from the UK, Germany, and France. Each database has population-based data on several million patients with over 50+ million years of follow up time, allowing researchers to investigate rare outcomes.

• Medical record databases have been used to study a wide variety of medical conditions using numerous study designs. Validation of the key exposure and/or outcome improves study validity. Many such validation studies have already been conducted.

• Incomplete information on some data from specialists as well as health related behaviors can be problematic within medical record databases. Investigators may obtain additional information by sending questionnaires to GPs through third party vendors.

• The size and complexity of the medical record databases require that individuals or institutions working with them have adequate computer software and hardware, as well as experienced data managers.

Case Example 9.4: Medical record databases

Background

• Psoriasis is a common inflammatory disease which is associated with an increased risk of cardiovascular disease. Small studies have demonstrated an increased prevalence of metabolic syndrome among patients with psoriasis. Metabolic syndrome also shares similar pro-inflammatory pathways with psoriasis and could be an important mediator in the relationship between psoriasis and cardiovascular disease.
• It has been hypothesized that patients with psoriasis have elevated rates of metabolic syndrome when compared to the general population and that this association increases in strength as severity of psoriasis increases.

Question

• Is there an increased prevalence of metabolic syndrome among patients with confirmed psoriasis compared to those without psoriasis in the general population, and does prevalence vary by severity of psoriasis?

Approach

• A cross-sectional study was performed in THIN among patients with psoriasis (exposed) and matched patients without psoriasis (unexposed).
• Patients with psoriasis age 45–65 were randomly selected from patients with psoriasis in THIN who belonged to a practice participating in Additional Information Services (AIS). Questionnaires were sent the GPs of 4900 patients to query about the validity of the diagnosis of psoriasis and the extent of disease (in terms of body surface area covered by psoriasis).
• Up to 10 controls within the same age range (45–65) and practice were randomly selected for each psoriasis patient. All patients had to have at least one GP visit within two years at the time of sampling.
• The outcome of interest was metabolic syndrome defined by National Cholesterol Education Program ATP III diagnostic criteria: central obesity (determined by body mass index or BMI $\geq$ 30), hypertriglyceridemia, low high-density lipoprotein cholesterol, high blood pressure and high fasting glucose level. These values were obtained from the database by selecting the most recent BMI and the maximum laboratory value.
• Conditional logistic regression was used to determine the association between psoriasis (overall and stratified by severity as minimal, moderate, and severe) and metabolic syndrome. The results were adjusted for age, sex, and duration of observation within THIN. Potential confounders including smoking status and social class (by Townsend score) were also explored.

Results

- The response rate to the survey was 95%. Of those surveys returned, 90% had a confirmed diagnosis of psoriasis and of these 96% has useable data regarding body surface area of skin affected by psoriasis. Metabolic syndrome was identified in 34% of participants with psoriasis compared to 26% of controls (Odds Ratio (OR) 1.50, 95%CI: 1.40–1.61). The OR adjusted for age, sex, and duration of observation time was 1.41 (95%CI: 1.31–1.51). Adjusting for smoking and social class did not change the results and were not retained in the model.
- Psoriasis severity affected the degree of association. OR for mild (<=2% BSA), moderate (3–10% BSA, and severe psoriasis (>10% BSA) were 1.22 (95%CI: 1.11–1.35), 1.56 (95%CI: 1.38–1.76), and 1.98 (95%CI: 1.62–2.43), respectively.
- Obesity, hypertriglyceridemia, hypertension, and hyperglycemia were all more common in patients with psoriasis than control patients. In addition, hypertriglyceridemia, for example, had a dose–response relationship with psoriasis severity independent of other risk factors such as obesity.

Strengths

- This cross-sectional study utilized a well-defined source population which minimizes bias and enhances generalizability.
- The large sample size allowed for adjustment for many potential confounding variables.
- There was a high response rate to the survey, and severity of psoriasis was objectively measured based on GP categorization of body surface area affected.
- The findings were robust to sensitivity analyses (not described here).

Limitations

- When a laboratory value is not present, it is treated as if it were not performed. There is a possibility that the laboratory values are stored in paper charts by the GP. Similarly, weight and height values may be missing in the electronic medical record. In our study, 8% of patients were missing data on BMI.
- It is possible that patients with severe psoriasis are seen more frequently by the GP and are therefore more likely to have their dyslipidemia diagnosed (detection bias).

Key Points

- Psoriasis is associated with metabolic syndrome. Furthermore, a "dose–response" relationship was observed between psoriasis severity and metabolic syndrome.
- Obesity, hyperglycemia, and dyslipidemia are common among patients with psoriasis and patients with psoriasis should be screened for these disorders.
- Further studies are needed to understand the biological mechanism by which metabolic syndrome and psoriasis are related.

Pharmacy-based medical record linkage systems

Introduction

Pharmacy-based medical record linkage (PbMRL) systems have drug dispensing files as the primary exposure source. These are linked with different outcomes databases (e.g., hospitalization, mortality, clinical laboratory), and all are linked to a central patient router. The central patient router file includes unique, anonymized patient identification numbers, which are used to draw together patient exposure and outcome data stored in the different linked databases into a single new research database. PbMRLs are therefore best described as federated or virtual database networks which transparently integrate multiple autonomous databases into a single system. Since the constituent databases remain autonomous, these systems offer an alternative when stringent privacy and governance rules of the individual databases do not permit storage of data in a central repository. PbMRLs are dynamic systems in the sense that they can be linked to new databases, disease registries or patient-reported outcomes to add detail to data needed to answer pharmacoepidemiologic questions.

PbMRLs have been established in the Nordic countries (Denmark, Sweden, Norway, Finland, Greenland, and Iceland), Scotland, and the Netherlands. In these countries, prescriptions issued by both GPs and medical specialists are filled in community pharmacies. These systems are among the oldest systems for pharmacoepidemiologic research in Europe, created in the early 1990s. At that time, pharmacies were among the first organizations in health care that used computers that store coded files to administrate the dispensing process, amongst other to comply with complex reimbursement requirements. A major advantage of these systems is that they capture detailed information of dispensings resulting from prescriptions by general practitioners, medical specialists, and those with a license to prescribe.

The dynamic architecture of the PbMRL, having the capability to link multiple different files to a central patient repository, is a major advantage,. A drawback of these systems is that they cannot produce simple statistics of required data because access to some variables requires governance clearance of one or several of the linked databases. For governance clearance, a scientific protocol is needed. In most EU countries, many specific record linkage-based systems are available, ranging in size from several thousand up to millions of patients, but are limited to a particular disease and have limited use for PbMRL pharmacoepidemiologic research. In this chapter comparison of PbMRL systems have been limited to the Nordic countries and the Netherlands that are remarkably similar with respect to available exposure data (Table 9.10) and linked clinical outcome data (Table 9.11). As examples of pharmacy-based medical record linkage systems, we will discuss the Danish OPED (Odense University Pharmacoepidemiologic Database), the Danish AUHD (Aarhus University Prescription Database), and the Dutch PHARMO record linkage system.

Description

Pharmacy-based medical record linkage systems have at least three types of files in common: a patient router file containing the characteristics of patients in the catchment population; a pharmacy-based drug exposure registry; and one or more linked clinical registries obtained from other organizations or health professionals. The exposure and clinical registries are linked to the patient router file using a variety of record linkage methods. Below,

we first discuss the methods used to link the different databases, and then the linked outcomes databases.

Record linkage

A major challenge when constructing a network consisting of multiple databases is the method to be used to link records that comprise information on the same patient as recorded in different databases to a unique patient in the patient roster file. This process is simplified if unique patient identification numbers can be used. However, in some databases such identifiers are not recorded, or cannot be used because laws and regulations do not permit. At least three methods can be used to link different patient-based databases. The most straightforward is a *deterministic* linkage, based on unique personal identification numbers used across multiple systems. This is the main linkage method for the OPED and AUPD databases in Denmark and can also be used for the entire population of Denmark. Alternatively, in the absence of unique personal identification numbers, a sequence of patient characteristics can be used to construct a unique, semi-deterministic linkage key. The Medicine Monitoring Unit (MEMO) database in the Scotland Tayside region uses such a key. This is a ten-digit integer, in which the first six digits indicate the date of birth, digits seven and eight provide information on region of residence, the ninth digit indicates gender, and the tenth digit incorporates a checksum to ensure the number's validity. A third method, probabilistic record linkage, is used to link databases and registries in the PHARMO system. Several patient characteristics and complex relational variables are used to create identifiers. Records from two files to be linked are grouped into record pairs, based on initial agreement of date of birth and gender. Additional characteristics then are added to each side of the pair, such as first initial of surname, surname, postal code, name of general practitioner, name compression algorithms, and date of death. Bayesian likelihood estimations and learning-based rules are applied to estimate the likelihood that two records from two distinct files belong or do not belong to the same individual. Although the use of personal identification

Table 9.10 Data available in drug exposure files in Denmark, Northern countries and the Netherlands.

Record linkage system	OPED[a] (1990)	AUPD[b] (1989)	Other Northern countries	PHARMO[c] (1986)
Geographic area	Regional	Regional	National	Regional
Population	1.2 million	1.8 million	17 Million	3.2 million
Pharmacy				
Unique identifier	YES	YES	YES	YES
Location	YES	YES	YES	YES
Monthly updated	YES	YES	YES	YES
Dispensed drugs				
Unique identifier	YES	YES	YES	YES
ATC code	YES	YES	YES	YES
DDD number	YES	YES	MOST	YES
Amount dispensed	YES	YES	YES	YES
Prescribed dose	NO	NO	FREETEXT	YES
Reimbursed drugs	YES	YES	SOME	YES
Nonreimbursed drugs	NO	NO	MOST	YES
Duration of use	NO	NO	SOME	YES
Dispensing date	YES	YES	YES	YES
Indication for use	NO	NO	NO	NO
Prescriber				
Unique identifier	YES[d]	YES	SOME	YES
Profession[e]	YES	YES	YES	YES
Practice	YES	YES	SOME	YES
Date started practice	YES	YES	SOME	YES
Year of birth	YES	YES	YES	YES
Sex	YES	YES	YES	YES

[a]Odense University Pharmacoepidemiologic Database.
[b]Aarhus University Prescription Database, Denmark.
[c]PHARMO Record Linkage Network.
[d]PHARMO ID, after deduplication.
[e]physician, nurse, dentist, midwife.

numbers (deterministic or semi-deterministic) is often regarded the most accurate linkage strategy, such numbers may have been reused, have not yet been assigned, may change over time, may be recorded incorrectly, or may be missing. Deterministic, semi-deterministic, and probabilistic record linkage each have advantages and disadvantages that have to be balanced to construct sustainable

Table 9.11 Linked databases in the Danish network and the PHARMO record linkage system.

Database	Characteristics	
	Denmark	PHARMO
Clinical laboratories http://www.pharmo.nl/	Test name, IUPAC test code, local analysis number, result, measurement unit, date or ordering and carrying out the analysis Different Laboratories Information System Population Subset 1999–2009	Test name, WCIA-test code, local analysis number, result, measurement unit, date or ordering and carrying out the analysis PHARMO ClinLab Population Subset (1.2M) 1991–2010 (update 3Month)
Birth Registers	Multiplicity (singleton, twin etc), weight, length, fetal presentation, gestational age, Apgar scores, congenital disease, mode of delivery. Maternal status includes previous stillbirths, live birth (parity), age at delivery, smoking, location of birth. Mortality. Danish Medical Birth Register http://www.ssi.dk	Multiplicity (singleton, twin etc), weight, length, fetal presentation, gestational age, Apgar scores, congenital disease, mode of delivery. Maternal status includes previous stillbirths, live birth (parity), age at delivery, smoking, location of birth. Mortality Dutch Perinatal Registration http://www .perinatreg.nl
Hospitalizations	Admission/discharge date, diagnoses (ICD10), operations, surgeries (ICD10) and Selected In-Hospital treatments Danish National Registry of Patients http://www.ssi.dk	Admission/discharge date, diagnoses (ICD10), operations and surgeries (ICD10) IUPAC testcode, local analysis number, result, measurement unit, date or ordering and carrying out the analysis, ID hospital or GP ordering the test. Dutch Hospital Data http://www.dutchhospitaldata.nl/
Death Registry	Date of death, cause of death Danish Registry of Causes of Death http://www.ssi.dk	Date of death, demographic history National Centre Family history http://www.cbg.nl/
Cancer	Date of cancer diagnosis, method of verification, morphology, topography, initial treatment, surgery, radiotherapy, chemotherapy, hormonal and immunotherapy, comorbidity. Additional information for specific cancers. http://www.ssi.dk	Date of cancer diagnosis, method of verification, morphology, topography, initial treatment, surgery, radiotherapy, chemotherapy, hormonal and immunotherapy, comorbidity at diagnosis. Additional information for specific cancers. http://www.ikcnet.nl/
Pathology	Test date, pathological specimens, morphology, topography procedures, diagnoses National Pathology Registration http://www.ssi.dk	Test date, pathological specimens morphology, topography, procedures, diagnoses PALGA http://www.palga.nl

record linkage networks. Most networks use all these techniques and hence validation of the linkage quality against a gold standard is needed but not always possible.

Patient router files

A patient router file, in which all patients have a unique identification number, represents essentially all inhabitants of a population in a defined geographic area, such as a region or country. Patient router files typically include a constructed or given unique personal identifier, year of birth, gender, and place of residence, and serve as a router pointing to the files where exposure and clinical histories are stored. Patients may enter the population by birth or immigration, and may depart from the population through death or emigration. In Denmark, information regarding date of birth and date of death is available from the Civil Registration System (CRS). In the Netherlands this information is obtained through linkage to birth or death registries. The time periods between date of entry into and date of exit from the catchment area are defined as the "event eligible" periods for individual patients. Within these eligible periods, cohorts can be extracted based on defined events (e.g., exposure, outcomes) or particular patient characteristics (e.g., age). Follow-up almost always ends with death or end of the registration period, if not otherwise specified. Changes in health care in recent years have led patients to shop among community pharmacies, creating the need to identify duplicate patients and to define new unique patient numbers.

Exposure databases

Community pharmacies are the source of exposure information in pharmacy-based medical record linkage systems. In both Denmark and the Netherlands, for example, drugs prescribed by GPs, medical specialists, or others with a prescribing license have to be filled in community pharmacies. In response to financial and other incentives, most patients have designated a single pharmacy to fill all their prescriptions. The PHARMO pharmacy database holds dispensing information going back to 1986; OPED began collecting data in 1990 and AUPD in 1989. There are about 1,600 community pharmacies in the Netherlands and 300 in Denmark. Prescriptions originating from the primary health care sector account for approximately 96% of the total volume of medicinal product sales in Denmark. These databases typically use the Anatomical Therapeutic Chemical (ATC) coding system to code drugs.

Some important national and regional differences in systems should be noted. In the Danish Government Statistical Office, a nationwide prescription database has been available since the 2004, regardless of reimbursement status, but all analyses must be made on their server, with no access to the civil registration number. Registration in the regional Danish prescription databases depends on reimbursement status, and hence data on sedatives, hypnotics, oral contraceptives, and laxatives are incomplete. The Dutch PHARMO database is not restricted to reimbursed drugs, but also contains information on nonreimbursed drugs, homeopathic drugs, and herbal remedies, as well as some medical devices (e.g., blood glucose monitors), urinary incontinence pads, and other nonpharmaceutical products. The PHARMO database also includes dosage instructions as well as duration of use. The PHARMO Institute also holds a database of in-hospital drug exposures since 2000 from 12 out of 80 hospital pharmacies in the Netherlands, with a total catchment population of 2.5 million. The 12 hospitals record all medication orders for patients during their hospital stays. Data for approximately one million of these 2.5 million hospitalized patients are linked to the PHARMO patient router files.

Hospitalizations

Denmark has a registry containing information on hospitalized patients since 1977 and the Netherlands has had a similar registry since 1963. They completely cover the period for which drug exposure information is available, and include all clinical discharge diagnoses. In Denmark, diagnoses are coded using either the *International Classification of Diseases, 8th edition* (ICD-8) or 10th edition (ICD-10) systems. In the PHARMO region, discharge diagnoses are coded using the ICD-9–CM (clinical modification). Denmark's hospital registry also includes information on visits to emergency departments and outpatient hospital clinics since 1995. Both the Denmark and Dutch hospital databases include information on more than 10 discharge diagnoses and procedures per hospitalization, but are incomplete regarding noninvasive diagnostic procedures such as magnetic resonance imaging and computed tomography.

Clinical laboratory data

Both the PHARMO record linkage system and the Danish databases have been linked to laboratory test results. Data are collected from individual laboratories, including all clinical tests ordered by GPs and hospitals. Orders for tests and test results are communicated electronically between GPs and hospitals. Individual laboratories in Northern Denmark and in the PHARMO region use different software systems. The PHARMO database includes data on more than 500 different hematological and serological tests for more than 2.3 million patients, of whom 1.2 million overlap and are linked to the PHARMO roster files. Data are updated every three months. In Denmark, the population covered by the laboratory database is located in a well-defined geographical area representing approximately 30% of the population. These tests include lipid and glycosylated hemoglobin (HbA1c) levels in patients with diabetes. Nonlaboratory measurements include blood pressure, smoking status, body mass index, and results of fundoscopic examinations. At the PHARMO Institute, some test results are recorded in a function test database (e.g., blood pressure, electrocardiograms (ECGs), forced expiratory volume in one second, fundoscopic examinations, and microfilament assessments), and are available for research.

Pathological findings

In both countries, clinical pathology data are transferred by national organizations into a national pathology registry. In Denmark, pathology data have been used for research and measurement of quality in diagnostics and treatment since 1997. In the Netherlands, the Pathological Anatomy National Automated Archive (PALGA) register is a central depository of pathological findings used in routine daily practice. Excerpts of pathological findings are anonymized, and an excerpt of the complete data set is stored in a national research database, accessible to researchers upon request. The PALGA network includes data from all 64 histopathology and cytopathology laboratories in the Netherlands, with a continuously expanding automated archive of excerpts of pathology reports (currently about 42 million excerpts on nearly 10 million patients since 1991). In both Denmark and the Netherlands, the pathology databases are used to assess the quality of cancer registrations, and to identify and alert cancer registries about new cases. Pathology in Denmark is coded according to the Systemized Nomenclature of Medicine (SNOMED); a classification system comparable in scope to SNOMED is used in the Netherlands.

Cancer registries

Denmark and the Netherlands national organizations and governments have established cancer registries to collect data on incident cancers. In both countries, registries are based on notification forms completed in hospitals. In the Netherlands, trained staff members from one of the regional cancer centers visit hospitals to abstract information from medical records onto specific data forms. The PHARMO record linkage system is restricted to the Eindhoven Cancer Registry (IKZ), which covers a catchment area of approximately two million patients; to date one million patients are linked to the PHARMO roster files. By this linkage, incidence cases, staging, and other therapies are added to the PHARMO record linkage scheme. The data recorded in the Danish and Dutch national cancer registries are comparable, with diagnoses coded using ICD-10.

Birth registry, maternal linkage, and death

The National Perinatal Registration (PRN) program in the Netherlands (PHARMO) and the Medical Birth Registry in Denmark were established for surveillance of birth rates and other factors related to birth. Since 1973 the Danish Medical Birth Registry has stored prospectively collected information on all live births and stillbirths, including the personal identification numbers of both infant and mother. Other variables are maternal age, body mass index, maternal smoking status during pregnancy, pregnancy complications, and infant characteristics. Both the PRN database and the Danish Medical Birth Registry are used for research purposes. Linkage of these registries to the core pharmacy databases permits study of drug teratogenicity, delivery complications, and maternal diseases, as well as short-term and long-term consequences to children of in utero drug exposure. Mortality statistics are available and coded in the patient router files through linkage to national vital statistics databases in Denmark, and through linkage to the genealogy database in the Netherlands.

Other linkages

The Danish and PHARMO systems can also be linked to many other databases and cohorts, including GP records (PHARMO), the national registry of traffic accidents, the national registry of driver licenses, the national registry of kidney transplants, the Rotterdam study, local and regional laboratories with records of digital ECGs, and a database including food constituents. These food constituents are collected in an annual survey of a project that focus on cardiovascular disease (MORGEN). Both the Danish data network and the PHARMO network facilitate patient contact, to request their cooperation in providing patient-reported outcomes or DNA.

Strengths

Linkage possibilities in the Netherlands and Denmark, and also in Sweden, Iceland, and Norway, are great in number. In theory, the databases can be expanded to include the complete countries. They constitute powerful resources for collecting detailed information for pharmacoepidemiologic research. A major strength of the pharmacy-based medical record linkage systems is the quality of the drug exposure information. Misclassification is not introduced by failure to fill prescriptions, as these data indicate what drugs were actually dispensed. The PHARMO system has an additional advantage, in that information on completeness of exposure does not depend on reimbursement status. A second strength of the PbMRL systems discussed here is that, even in the absence of unique patient identifiers, databases can be linked with a high sensitivity and specificity using semi-deterministic or probabilistic record linkage methods. Linkage possibilities are not restricted to the healthcare domain, e.g., it is possible to link drug exposure files to food inventories or driver's license databases.

Another key asset of PbMRL systems is that exposure and outcomes are recorded separately, by the relevant health professionals, thereby minimizing the potential for ascertainment bias. Record linkage is also much less expensive than collecting data de novo.

Through contact with patients, biosamples and patient-reported outcomes can be obtained and linked to these databases. PbMRL systems also have the advantage of having well-defined denominators, including everyone in a given geographic area, regardless of whether information is recorded in hospitals, in the general practitioner's office, in clinical laboratories, or elsewhere. Researchers can focus on information in these databases that is most reliable and complete. Through linkage to nationwide registries and use of vital statistics, it is possible to assess the representativeness of findings for a complete nation.

Pharmacy files include prescriptions not only from GPs, but also from medical specialists, who are responsible for about a quarter of all prescriptions and more than half of all prescriptions given to patients with complicated diseases, although the percentage might differ slightly by country. Omitting these prescriptions could cause bias by overrepresentation of healthier patients. This does not occur in pharmacy-based systems.

Pharmacy-based systems also contain great detail regarding type of drug, dose, and duration, permitting assessment of adherence and compliance to different types of medications, in relation to dose or route of administration. They also provide precise and detailed product information— major assets for pharmacoepidemiologic studies.

Weaknesses

Inevitably, the weaknesses of medical record linkage systems are related to their strengths. The different organizations maintaining the patient-level databases must safeguard the integrity of the record linkage systems through rules of governance and access limitations. These organizations have to address many administrative issues, including confidentiality, conflicts of interest of health professionals and researchers, and procedures to ensure data quality. It is possible for individual organizations and data providers to prevent linkage for political and commercial reasons.

Constant political experimenting with health care systems is a major threat to the existence of medical record linkage systems. There is always a potential for a sudden, unexpected termination of registries or content of registries. For example, the Danish regional drug dispensing databases depend on the reimbursement status of drugs. As costs of sedatives, hypnotics, oral contraceptives, and laxatives are not reimbursed, these drugs cannot be studied. Although these data systems are not claims databases, they are used to claim reimbursement of dispensings to the different health insurance companies that require full identification of patients, their enrollees. If nonreimbursed drugs are dispensed without full patient identification, data may become incomplete. The possibility exists that in the near future many inexpensive generics will cease to be reimbursed, which might affect the completeness of dispensing in pharmacy-based medical record linkage databases. In the Netherlands, for instance, internet pharmacies and central distribution systems of biologicals can affect the completeness of data available to record linkage systems. Networks have to adapt and collaborate with these new drug sources to ensure data completeness.

Although the linkage domains seem unlimited, the complexity of PbMRL systems extends to the diverse governance structures responsible for protecting the privacy of patients and health care professionals and for addressing potential conflicts of interest between them. Linked study data sets need to comply with the governance schemes of different organizations. Privacy laws in the European Union are not clear about whether needed data transfer is allowed, even after anonymization. Therefore, most registries do not give permission to distribute individual, anonymized patient records, whether linked or unlinked.

The steady growth in computerization of health administration, and the high costs involved, as well as financial and other incentives, has led health care providers to increase requests for reimbursement to provide data. Such price increases will increase the costs of studies.

Record linkage systems potentially can cover 35 million European inhabitants in Northern Europe and the Netherlands, still far below the size of pharmacoepidemiologic databases in the US. Obviously, the primary advantage of the European systems is not size but detail.

Particular applications

Studies examining aspects of drug exposure

One study conducted in the PHARMO system showed an increased persistence rate (which might be expected to prolong treatment effect) for weekly versus daily alendronate (relative risk: 1.84, 95% CI: 1.65–2.20). Dose–response relationships can also be examined. For example, dose–response relationships have been studied for statins and oral antidiabetic drugs concerning goal attainment of low density lipoprotein cholesterol (LDL-c) and HbA1c levels, respectively. A study performed by Eussen *et al.* linked medication use to responses to a food questionnaire. They studied the relationship between the intake of phytosterol/-stanol-enriched margarines in relation to persistence with statins, and found that overall statin discontinuation rates were not significantly different between users and non-users of enriched margarine. However, in the subgroup of starters, combination users had a higher risk of discontinuing statin therapy than single-component product users within twelve months (adjusted hazard ratio (HR): 2.52, 95% CI: 1.06–6.00).

Studies using clinical laboratory files

Results obtained from GP PHARMO medical records showed that GPs tend to over-record abnormal values (as they obviously are of interest for further diagnostic and treatment decisions), compared to normal values. Average total cholesterol levels recorded in the GP files were 7.1 mmol/L, while the average total cholesterol values for the same patients in the clinical laboratory files were 5.6 mmol/L. Only 70% of the total cholesterol tests could be found in the GP files, measured against the clinical laboratory files. The differences were explained by tests ordered by medical specialists and by underreporting of tests for patients who had reached their treatment goal.

Linking clinical laboratory data to drug exposure data from community pharmacies permits detailed research into the effect of drugs on biochemical parameters. For example, a study of patients with type 2 diabetes starting insulin compared glycemic control between those initiated on insulin detemir and those initiated on insulin glargine. One year after start of insulin, there was no difference in mean HbA1c level or proportion of patients at goal (HbA1c < 7%) between users of the two preparations. Kornum *et al.* studied whether diabetes is a risk factor for hospitalization with pneumonia and assessed the impact of HgbA1C level on such risk. The adjusted relative risk for pneumonia-related hospitalization among patients with diabetes was 1.26 (95% CI: 1.21–1.31) compared with non-diabetic individuals. The adjusted relative risk was 4.43 (95% CI: 3.40–5.77) for patients with type 1 diabetes and 1.23 (95% CI: 1.19–1.28) for patients with type 2 diabetes. Compared with patients without diabetes, the adjusted relative risk was 1.22 (95% CI: 1.14–1.30) for diabetic patients whose HgbA1C level was < 7%, and 1.60 (95% CI: 1.44–1.76) for diabetic patients whose HbA1C level was greater than > 9%. They concluded that poor long-term glycemic control among patients with diabetes increases the risk of hospitalization with pneumonia. The impact of poor adherence on HgbA1c goal attainment was also studied using data from the PHARMO database. In patients starting oral glucose-lowering drugs (OGLD), the effect of nonpersistent OGLD use on HbA1c goal attainment (< 7%) was quantified, revealing that nonpersistent patients were about 20% less likely to attain the goal compared to persistent patients.

Pathology

The linkage of PHARMO and PALGA (the Dutch nationwide registry of histo- and cytopathology) and counterpart databases in Denmark allow the study of the relationship between drug exposure and morbidity, assessed by pathology specimens retrieved via biopsy or resection. For example, in a study investigating estrogen exposure (retrieved via the PHARMO database) and the outcome of melanoma (retrieved via the PALGA database), a relationship between risk of cutaneous melanoma and cumulative dose of estrogens was identified. In addition to the conclusion that exposure to certain drugs might increase the risk of cancer, drugs have also been found that prevent, reverse, suppress, or delay premalignant lesions. Recent studies have shown that both statins and nonsteroidal anti-inflammatory drugs (NSAIDs) are associated with reduced incidence and progression of melanoma.

Cancer

Relationships between drug use and cancer, either occurrence or treatment, also can be studied using linked data from hospitals, GP files, and clinical pathology laboratory findings. Several studies have examined the effectiveness of cytostatics and co-medication in cancer patients. The added value of linkage to the cancer registries, in addition to hospital registries, is that incident cases can be identified and extra information is available, such as cancer type, staging of the cancer, and nondrug treatment.

The possible relationship between the use of oral glucocorticoids and increased risk of basal cell carcinoma (BCC), squamous cell carcinoma (SCC), malignant melanoma (MM), and non-Hodgkin's lymphoma (NHL) was studied using the AUPD database. The results showed slightly elevated risk estimates for BCC: incidence rate ratio (IRR): 1.15 (95% CI: 1.07–1.25), SCC IRR: 1.14 (95% CI: 0.94–1.39), MM IRR: 1.15 (95% CI: 0.94–1.41), and NHL IRR: 1.11 (95% CI: 0.85–1.46). These results support an overall association between glucocorticoid use and the risk of BCC.

In-hospital drug use

In addition to cancer treatment, treatment of other morbidities during hospitalization can be studied through linkage of the hospital registry data to inpatient pharmacy data. For example, opioid use has been examined in patients admitted for genitourinary, digestive, or abdominal surgery. Use of (nico)morphine was associated with the risk for developing postoperative paralytic ileus (POI) (OR: 12.1, 95% CI: 5.4–27.1). The association between opioids and POI was most obvious in patients with abdominal surgery (OR: 33.8, 95% CI: 6.2–184.6) and patients without colon/colorectal/rectal tumors (OR: 13.2, 95% CI: 5.7–30.3). A clear association was found between the use of opioids and the risk for POI, as coded in the Dutch hospital registry. In another study, the relationship between initial antibiotic treatment of secondary intra-abdominal infections and related outcomes was assessed. It was found that inappropriate initial antibiotic treatment was associated with a 3.4-fold (95% CI: 1.3, 9.1) risk of clinical failure. The length of hospital stay and costs of hospitalization were significantly increased for patients with antibiotic failure.

Birth registries

The effect of drugs and adverse drug reactions in children and the effect of drugs during pregnancy are an important area of study, as these relationships can only be examined to a very limited extent, if at all, in clinical trials. Linkage to perinatal registries permits detailed research into drug exposures and comorbidities during pregnancy and short- and long-term health status of offspring, topics that are well established in the Northern countries. In their study of the safety of metoclopramide use during pregnancy, Sorensen *et al.* found no associations between metoclopramide and malformations, low birth weight, or preterm delivery.

Conclusion

The major future challenge of medical record linkage systems is to protect the structures that make possible linkage between different databases. The Northern countries and the Netherlands, together covering almost 35 million inhabitants, have the potential to build extremely detailed databases for use in pharmacoepidemiologic research. The databases described above already cooperate in several projects financed by the European Commission (FP7) (http://cordis.europa.eu/fp7/) and are part of the European Network for Centres of Pharmacoepidemiology and Pharmacovigilance (ENCePP) (www.encepp.eu). However, given the complexity of EU privacy protection laws, governance models are needed to safeguard access to medical record linkage systems. Data sharing and integration of different national resources will be a true challenge in coming years. Experience in the Northern countries and the Netherlands show that independent organizations with stringent control of access can help to safeguard medical record linkage systems.

Future goals are to add patient-reported outcomes and DNA to the pharmacy-based medical record linkage systems. Studies in the Netherlands have shown the feasibility of these linkages and their capacity to support pharmacogenetic research (see Chapter 14), outcomes research, research on quality of life (see Chapter 18), as well as research on adverse outcomes and risk factors that will contribute to a better understanding of the risk and effectiveness of drugs in daily life.

Summary points for pharmacy-based record linkage systems

- PbMRL systems combine information recorded in different databases and registries into a single network, respecting the governance rules for data access and data sharing of the contributing organizations.
- PbMRL are dispensing-based, record dosing schemes, and are the best representation of drugs prescribed by general practitioners and medical specialists in the Nordic countries and the Netherlands.
- Access to data is limited by scientific research protocols that need scientific and governance clearance. Therefore, PbMRL systems are best described as cohort servers to be constrcuted to anewer specific PE questions.
- PbMRL systems in the Netherlands and Nordic countries are comparable with respect to their capabilities although access to data might be different because of country-specific laws, regulations and governance issues.
- PbMRL systems require predefined governance clearance rules and expertise to expedite rapid access to data
- The complex nature of these multi-detailed data systems require advanced data analysis skills and close collaboration with data providers.

Case Example 9.5: Endocrine treatment discontinuation in patients with breast cancer
  Study by Van Herk-Sukel *et al.* (2010)

Background
- Adjuvant endocrine treatment in women with early stage breast cancer significantly prolongs disease-free and overall survival time.

- The guidelines recommend treatment of (at least) five years with tamoxifen only, five years of aromatase inhibitors (AIs; anastrozole, letrozole and exemestane) or sequential therapy of 2–3 years of tamoxifen followed by 2–3 years of AIs.

Question

- What is the rate of discontinuation of endocrine treatment in women with early stage breast cancer, and which factors are related to this discontinuation?

Approach

- Linkage of the Cancer Registry and the PHARMO Data Network to combine drug use as registered in community and hospital pharmacies with detailed information on all newly diagnosed cancer patients in the southeastern part of the Netherlands.
- Continuous use (allowing a 60-day gap between refills) of endocrine treatment (either tamoxifen or AIs) was determined after 5 years of follow-up.

Results

- Half of the breast cancer patients discontinued endocrine treatment before the end of the recommended treatment period of five years.
- Older age and more concomitant diseases independently increased the likelihood to discontinue endocrine therapy.

Strengths

- A population-based study showing true rates of discontinuation in daily clinical practice.
- Including both tamoxifen and aromatase inhibitors.
- Five years of follow-up.

Limitation

- The reason why patients discontinued their treatment was not collected.

Key Point

- Identification of patients at risk of discontinuation will assist in the development of interventions to improve cancer treatment continuation comparable to that of patients included in clinical trials.

Further reading

Health maintenance organizations/health plans

Andrade SE, *et al.* (2011) Antipsychotic medication use in children and risk of diabetes mellitus. *Pediatrics* **128** (6): 1135–41.

Andrade SE, *et al.* (2012) Medication Exposure in Pregnancy Risk Evaluation Program. *Matern Child Health J.* **16** (7): 1349–54.

Arterburn DE, *et al.* (2010) Body mass index measurement and obesity prevalence in ten US health plans. *Clin Med Res* **8** (3–4): 126–30.

Boudreau DM, *et al.* (2007) Statin use and breast cancer risk in a large population-based setting. *Cancer Epidemiol Biomarkers Prev* **16** (3): 416–21.

Brown JS, *et al.* (2007) Early detection of adverse drug events within population-based health networks: application of sequential testing methods. *Pharmacoepidemiol Drug Saf,* **16** (12): 1275–84.

Davis RL, *et al.* (2007) Risks of congenital malformations and perinatal events among infants exposed to antidepressant medications during pregnancy. *Pharmacoepidemiol Drug Saf* **16** (10): 1086–94.

Davis RL, *et al.* (2005) Active surveillance of vaccine safety data for early signal detection. *Epidemiology* **16** (3): 336–41.

Donahue JG, *et al.* (2002) Gastric and duodenal safety of daily alendronate. *Arch Intern Med* **162** (8): 936–42.

Finkelstein JA, *et al.* (2001) Reducing antibiotic use in children: a randomized trial in 12 practices. *Pediatrics* **108** (1): 1–7.

Go AS, *et al.* (2008) The Cardiovascular Research Network: a new paradigm for cardiovascular quality and outcomes research. *Circ Cardiovasc Qual Outcomes* **1** (2): 138–47.

Go AS, *et al.* (2008) Comparative effectiveness of different beta-adrenergic antagonists on mortality among adults with heart failure in clinical practice. *Arch Intern Med* **168** (22): 2415–21.

Graham DJ, *et al.* (2004) Incidence of hospitalized rhabdomyolysis in patients treated with lipid-lowering drugs. *JAMA* **292** (21): 2585–90.

Lafata JE, *et al.* (2007) Academic detailing to improve laboratory testing among outpatient medication users. *Med Care* **45** (10): 966–72.

Lee GM (2011) H1N1 and seasonal influenza vaccine safety in the Vaccine Safety Datalink project. *Am J Prev Med* **41** (2): 121–8.

Platt R, *et al.* (2001) Multicenter epidemiologic and health services research on therapeutics in the HMO Research Network Center for Education and Research on Therapeutics. *Pharmacoepidemiol Drug Saf* **10** (5): 373–7.

Platt R, *et al.* (2012) The US Food and Drug Administration's Mini-Sentinel program: status and direction. *Pharmacoepidemiol Drug Saf* **21** (S1): 1–8.

Raebel MA, *et al.* (2005) Laboratory monitoring of drugs at initiation of therapy in ambulatory care. *J Gen Intern Med* **20** (12): 1120–6.

Selby JV, *et al.* (2010) Trends in time to confirmation and recognition of new-onset hypertension, 2002–2006. *Hypertension* **56** (4): 605–11.

Toh S, *et al.* (2011) Comparative-effectiveness research in distributed health data networks. *Clin Pharmacol Ther* **90** (12): 883–7.

Wagner EH, *et al.* (2005) Building a research consortium of large health systems: the Cancer Research Network. *J Natl Cancer Inst Monogr* **35**: 3–11.

US government claims databases

Choudhry NK, Shrank WH (2010) Four-dollar generics–increased accessibility, impaired quality assurance. *N Engl J Med Nov 11;* **363** (20): 1885–7.

Cooper WO, Habel LA, Sox CM, Chan KA, Arbogast PG, Cheetham TC, Murray KT, Quinn VP, Stein CM, Callahan ST, Fireman BH, Fish FA, Kirshner HS, O'Duffy A, Connell FA, Ray WA (2011) ADHD drugs and serious cardiovascular events in children and young adults. *New England Journal of Medicine* **365**: 1896–1904.

Faught R, Weiner J, Guerin A, Cunnington M, Duh M (2009) Impact of nonadherence to antiepileptic drugs on health care utilization and costs: Findings from the RANSOM study. *Epilepsia* **50** (3): 501–9.

Habel LA, Cooper WO, Sox CM, Chan KA, Fireman BH, Arbogast PG, Cheetham TC, Quinn VP, Dublin S, Boudreau DM, Andrade SE, Pawloski PA, Raebel MA, Smith DH, Achacoso N, Uratsu C, Go AS, Sidney S, Nguyen-Huynh MN, Ray WA, Selby JV (2011) ADHD medications and risk of serious cardiovascular events in young and middle-aged adults. *JAMA* **306**: 2673–83.

Hennessy S, Bilker WB, Weber A, Strom BL (2003) Descriptive analyses of the integrity of a US Medicaid claims database. *Pharmacoepidemiology and Drug Safety* **12**: 103–11.

Hennessy S, Leonard CE, Bilker WB (2007) Researchers and HIPAA. *Epidemiology* **18**: 518.

Morrato E, Nicol G, Maahs D, Druss B, Hartung D, Valuck R, *et al.* (2010) Metabolic screening in children receiving antipsychotic drug treatment. *Arch Pediatr Adolesc Med* **164** (4): 344–51.

Ray WA, Meredith S, Thapa PB, Hall K, Murray KT (2004) Cyclic antidepressants and the risk of sudden cardiac death. *Clin Pharmacol Ther Mar;* **75** (3): 234–41.

Ray WA, Meredith S, Thapa PB, Meador KG, Hall K, Murray KT (2001) Antipsychotics and the risk of sudden cardiac death. *Arch Gen Psychiatry Dec;* **58** (12): 1161–7.

Schelleman H, Bilker WB, Kimmel SE, Daniew GW, Newcomb C, Guevara JP, Cziraky MJ, Strom BL, Hennessy S (2012) Methylphenidate and risk of serious cardiovascular events in adults. *Am J Psychiatry* **169**: 178–85.

Schelleman H, Bilker WB, Strom BL, Kimmel SE, Newcomb C, Guevara JP, Daniel GW, Cziraky MJ, Hennessy S (2011) Cardiovascular events and death in children exposed and unexposed to ADHD medications. *Pediatrics* **127**: 1102–10.

Schneeweiss S, Rassen JA, Glynn RJ, Avorn J, Mogun H, Brookhart MA (2009) High-dimensional propensity score adjustment in studies of treatment effects using health care claims data. *Epidemiology Jul;* **20** (4): 512–22.

Sohn M, Arnold N, Maynard C, Hynes D (2006) Accuracy and completeness of mortality data in the Department of Veterans Affairs. *Population Health Metrics* **4**: 2–8.

Shrank WH, Choudhry NK (2011) Time to fill the doughnuts—health care reform and Medicare Part D. *N Engl J Med Feb 17;* **364** (7): 598–601.

Canadian provincial databases

BC Ministry of Health. http://www.health.gov.bc.ca/pharmacare/(accessed June 18, 2012).

BC PharmaNet. http://www.health.gov.bc.ca/pharmacare/pharmanet/netindex.html (accessed June 18, 2012).

Canadian Cardiac Network of Ontario. http://www.ccn.on.ca (accessed June 18, 2012).

Canadian Institute for Health Information. http://www.cihi.ca (accessed June 18, 2012).

Downey W, *et al.* (2000) *Health databases in Saskatchewan. In: Pharmacoepidemiology*, 3rd Edition. Ed Strom BL. John Wiley & Sons Ltd.

Government of Alberta. Health and Wellness http://www .health.alberta.ca (accessed June 18, 2012).

Hemmelgarn B, *et al.* (1997) Benzodiazepine use and the risk of motor vehicle crash in the elderly. *JAMA* **278**: 27–31.

Jacobs P, Yim R (2009) *Using Canadian Administrative Databases to Derive Economic Data for Health Technology Assessments.* Ottawa ON: Canadian Agency for Drugs and Technologies in Health.

Leslie WE, *et al.* (2005) Construction and validation of a population-based bone densitometry database. *J. Clin. Densitom* **8**: 25–30.

Manitoba Health. http://www.gov.mb.ca/health/ pharmacare/(accessed June 18, 2012).

Moride Y, *et al.* (2002) Suboptimal duration of antidepressant treatments in the older ambulatory population of Quebec: association with selected physician characteristics. *J Am Geriatr Soc* **50** (8): 1365–71.

Moride Y, Metge C (2010) Data sources to support research on real world drug safety and effectiveness in Canada: An environmental scan and evaluation of existing data elements http://www.pharmacoepi.ca (accessed June 18, 2012).

Nova Scotia Ministry of Health. http://www.gov.ns.ca/ health/pharmacare/(accessed June 18, 2012).

Ontario Drug Benefit. Ontario Ministry of Health and Long-term Care. http://www.health.gov.on.ca (accessed June 18, 2012).

Pariente A, *et al.* (2012) Antipsychotic use and myocardial infarction in older patients with treated dementia. *Arch Intern Med* **172**: 648–53.

Population Data BC. http://www.popdata.bc.ca/data/ internal/health/mentalhealth (accessed June 18, 2012).

Rawson N (2009) Access to linked administrative healthcare utilization data for pharmacoepidemiology and pharmacoeconomics research in Canada: anti-viral drugs as an example. *Pharmacoepidemiol. & Drug Safety* **18**: 1072–9.

Régie de l'assurance-maladie du Québec http://www .ramq.gouv.qc.ca/fr/statistiques/banques/vuedensemble.shtml (Accessed 18 June 2012)

Sketris IS, *et al.* (1996) Drug therapy in multiple sclerosis: a study of Nova Scotia senior citizens. *Clin. Ther.* **18**: 303–18.

Smith PM, *et al.* (2010) Research opportunities using administrative databases and existing surveys for new knowledge in occupational health and safety in Canada, Quebec, Ontario and British Columbia. *Can. J. Public Health* **101**Suppl 1: S46–52.

Medical record databases

CPRD website. http://www.cprd.com/intro.asp2012.

THIN website. http://csdmruk.cegedim.com/(accessed Apr. 2012).

IMS health website. www.imshealth.com (accessed Apr. 2012).

Becher H, Kostev K, Schroder-Bernhardi D (2009) Validity and representativeness of the disease analyzer patient database for use in pharmacoepidemiological and pharmacoeconomic studies. *Int J Clin Pract* **47** (10): 617–26.

Dave S, Peterson I (2009) Creating medical and drug code lists to identify cases in primary care databases. *Pharmacoepidemiol Drug Saf* **18**: 704–7.

Dietlein G, Schroder-Bernhardi D (2002) Use of the mediplus patient database in healthcare research. *Int J Clin Pract* **40** (3): 130–3.

Ehrenstein V, Antonsen S, Pedersen L (2010) Existing data sources for clinical epidemiology: Aarhus University Prescription Database. *Clin Epidemiol* **2**: 273–9.

Hall GC, Sauer B, Bourke A, Brown JS, Reynolds MW, Casale RL (2012) Guidelines for good database selection and use in pharmacoepidemiology research. *Pharmacoepidemiol Drug Saf* **21** (1): 1–10.

Hall G (2009) Validation of death and suicide recording on the THIN UK primary care database. *Pharmacoepidemiol Drug Saf* **18**: 120–31.

Hardy J, Holford T, Hall G, Bracken M (2004) Strategies for identifying pregnancies in the automated medical records of general practice research database. *Pharmacoepidemiol Drug Saf* **13**: 749–59.

Haynes K, Bilker WB, Tenhave TR, Strom BL, Lewis JD (2011) Temporal and within practice variability in the health improvement network. *Pharmacoepidemiol Drug Saf* **20** (9): 948–55.

Herrett E, Thomas S, Schoonen S, Smeeth L, Hall A (2010) Validation and validity of diagnoses in the general practice research database: A systematic review. *Br J Clin Pharmacol* **69** (1): 4–14.

Jick S, Kaye J, Vasilakis-Scaramozza C, *et al.* (2003) Validity of the general practice research database. *Pharmacotherapy* **23** (5): 686–9.

Khan N, Harrison S, Rose P (2010) Validity of diagnostic coding within the general practice research database: A systemic review. *Br J General Practice* **60** (572): e128–e136.

Khan N, Perera R, Harper S, Rose P (2010) Adaptation and validation of the charlson index for Read/OXMIS coded databases. *BMC Family Prac* **5** (11): 1.

Lester H (2008) The UK quality and outcomes framework. *BMJ* **337**: a2095.

Lewis JD, Schinnar R, Bilker WB, Wang X, Strom BL (2007) Validation studies of the health improvement network (THIN) database for pharmacoepidemiology research. *Pharmacoepidemiol Drug Saf (THIN)* **16**: 393–401.

Lewis J, Bilker W, Weinstein R, Strom B (2005) The relationship between time since registration and measured incidence rates in the general practice research database. *Pharmacoepidemiol Drug Saf* **14**: 443–51.

Lewis J, Brensinger C (2004) Agreement between GPRD smoking data: A survey of general practitioners and a population-based survey. *Pharmacoepidemiol Drug Saf* **13**: 437–41.

Maguire A, Blak B, Thompson M (2009) The importance of defining periods of complete mortality reporting for research using automated data from primary care. *Pharmacoepidemiol Drug Saf.* **18**: 76–83.

Langan SM, Seminara NM, Shin DB, Troxel AB, Kimmel SE, Mehta NN, Margolis DJ, Gelfand JM (2012) Prevalence of metabolic syndrome in patients with psoriasis: a population-based study in the United Kingdom. *J Invest Derm* **132**: 556–62.

Pharmacy-based medical record linkage systems

Dezentje VO, van Blijderveen NJ, Gelderblom H, Putter H, van Herk-Sukel MP, Casparie MK, *et al.* (2010) Effect of concomitant CYP2D6 inhibitor use and tamoxifen adherence on breast cancer recurrence in early-stage breast cancer. *J Clin Oncol.* **28** (14): 2423–9.

Furu K, Wettermark B, Andersen M, Martikainen JE, Almarsdottir AB, Sørensen HT (2010) The Nordic countries as a cohort for pharmacoepidemiological research. *Basic Clin Pharmacol Toxicol* **106** (2): 86–94.

Hallas J (2001) Conducting pharmacoepidemiologic research in Denmark. *Pharmacoepidemiol Drug Saf* **10** (7): 619–23.

Heintjes EM, Hirsch MW, Van der Linden MW, O'Donnell JC, Stalenhoef AF, Herings RMC (2008) LDL-c reductions and goal attainment among naive statin users in the Netherlands: real life results. *Curr Med Res Opin* **24** (8): 2241–50.

Johnsen SP, Larsson H, Tarone RE, *et al.* (2005) Risk of hospitalization for myocardial infarction among users of rofecoxib, celecoxib, and other NSAIDs: a population-based case-control study. *Arch Intern Med* **165** (9): 978–84.

Koomen ER, Joosse A, Herings RM, Casparie MK, Guchelaar HJ, Nijsten T (2009) Estrogens, oral contraceptives and hormonal replacement therapy increase the incidence of cutaneous melanoma: a population-based case-control study. *Ann Oncol* **20** (2): 358–64.

Lash TL, Pedersen L, Cronin-Fenton D, *et al.* (2008) Tamoxifen's protection against breast cancer recurrence is not reduced by concurrent use of the SSRI citalopram. *Br J Cancer* **99** (4): 616–21.

Nielsen GL, Sørensen HT, Larsen H, Pedersen L (2001) Risk of adverse birth outcome and miscarriage in pregnant users of non-steroidal anti-inflammatory drugs: population based observational study and case-control study. *BMJ* **322** (7281): 266–70.

Nielsen GL, Sørensen HT, Zhou W (1997) The Pharmacoepidemiologic Prescription Database of North Jutland—a valid tool in pharmacoepidemiological research. *Int J Risk Safety Med* **10**: 203–5.

Pedersen CB, Gotzsche H, Moller JO, Mortensen PB (2006) The Danish Civil Registration System. *A cohort of eight million persons. Dan Med Bull* **53** (4): 441–9.

Penning-van Beest F, van Herk-Sukel M, Gale R, Lammers JW, Herings R (2011) Three-year dispensing patterns with long-acting inhaled drugs in COPD: a database analysis. *Respir Med* **105** (2): 259–65.

Penning-van Beest FJ, Termorshuizen F, Goettsch WG, Klungel OH, Kastelein JJ, Herings RM (2007) Adherence to evidence-based statin guidelines reduces the risk of hospitalizations for acute myocardial infarction by 40%: a cohort study. *Eur Heart J* **28** (2): 154–9.

Peters BJ, Rodin AS, Klungel OH, Stricker BH, de Boer A, Maitland-van der Zee AH (2010) Variants of ADAMTS1 modify the effectiveness of statins in reducing the risk of myocardial infarction. *Pharmacogenet Genomics* **20** (12): 766–74.

Ruiter R, Visser LE, van Herk-Sukel MP, Coebergh JW, Haak HR, Geelhoed-Duijvestijn PH, *et al.* (2012) Lower risk of cancer in patients on metformin in comparison with those on sulfonylurea derivatives: results from a large population-based follow-up study. *Diabetes Care* **35** (1): 119–24.

Sorensen HT, Pedersen L, Skriver MV, Norgaard M, Norgard B, Hatch EE (2005) Use of clomifene during early pregnancy and risk of hypospadias: population based case-control study. *BMJ* **330** (7483): 126–7.

Thomsen RW, Johnsen SP, Olesen AV, *et al.* (2005) Socioeconomic gradient in use of statins among Danish patients: population-based cross-sectional study. *Br J Clin Pharmacol.* **60** (5): 534–42.

van der Linden MW, van der Bij S, Welsing P, Kuipers EJ, Herings RM (2009) The balance between severe cardiovascular and gastrointestinal events among users of selective and non-selective non-steroidal anti-inflammatory drugs. *Ann Rheum Dis* **68** (5): 668–73.

van Herk-Sukel MP, Lemmens VE, Poll-Franse LV, Herings RMC, Coebergh JW (2012) Record linkage for pharmacoepidemiological studies in cancer patients. *Pharmacoepidemiol Drug Saf* **21** (1): 94–103.

van Herk-Sukel MP, van de Poll-Franse LV, Lemmens VE, Vreugdenhil G, Pruijt JF, Coebergh JW, Herings RMCl (2010) New opportunities for drug outcomes research in cancer patients: the linkage of the Eindhoven Cancer Registry and the PHARMO Record Linkage System. *Eur J Cancer* **46** (2): 395–404.

CHAPTER 10
Field Studies

David W. Kaufman

Slone Epidemiology Center at Boston University and Boston University School of Public Health, Boston, MA, USA

Epidemiologic studies in which data are collected in the field are known as "field" or "ad hoc" studies. These are contrasted with studies that use preexisting data, principally from healthcare databases. While studies using existing data have advantages of time-efficiency, cost, and some validity benefits, there are potential drawbacks in terms of subject definitions and data availability, and there may not be appropriate data available to address particular questions. With the ability to tailor subject enrollment and data collection to a specific research question, field studies continue to play an important role in pharmacoepidemiology.

All types of epidemiologic research designs, including cohort, case-control, and cross-sectional designs can be conducted as field studies, as long as subject enrollment and data collection are part of the process. Field studies are by their nature more expensive and slower than studies using existing data, but there are situations where a field study is the only way to recruit the subjects and/or obtain the information needed to answer specific research questions.

Strengths

The strengths and weaknesses of field studies are generally complementary to those of database studies. On the strength side, it is often possible to more rigorously define outcomes, it may be more feasible to enroll subjects with very rare conditions, and it is especially more feasible to obtain the information needed to study questions for which administrative data are inadequate.

Outcome definition

A general problem with health care databases is that outcomes are generally defined by diagnosis codes, which are frequently insufficient for confirming the validity of diagnoses. An example is Stevens-Johnson syndrome, where a detailed review of clinical information that ideally extends to evaluating photographs of patients' lesions is necessary to ensure outcome validity. In database studies, the choice is to create an algorithm based on diagnosis codes and perhaps some treatment information, or better, to obtain access to patient records for the needed information, which can be a difficult process unless electronic medical records are available. Even if a validated algorithm is used, it is generally advisable to conduct a validation study based on medical records in a sample of patients. In contrast, collection of the needed information can be built into the protocol of a field study.

Studying extremely rare diseases

While databases cover large numbers of subjects, some diseases are so rare that until recently even the largest databases were insufficient to identify a sufficient number of cases. In these situations, it has been necessary to set up large population-based case finding networks. Examples are agranulocytosis, aplastic anemia, and Stevens-Johnson syndrome/toxic epidermal necrolysis (SJS/TEN), conditions that are of frequent

Textbook of Pharmacoepidemiology, Second Edition. Edited by Brian L. Strom, Stephen E. Kimmel, and Sean Hennessy.

interest because they are often induced by drugs and disproportionately result in regulatory action. The International Agranulocytosis and Aplastic Anemia Study (IAAAS), conducted in Israel and Europe in the 1980s, covered a population of 23 million persons over a period of six years to prospectively enroll 270 cases of agranulocytosis and 154 of aplastic anemia. It would have been difficult to provide such a large population experience in any other way, although with the use of large government databases, especially the availability of Medicare data (see Chapter 9), and the linking of multiple databases, that is becoming feasible.

Exposure and covariate information tailored to the research question

Setting up a data collection system specifically to study a particular question has the major advantage of allowing the collection of precisely the information needed. While databases have the advantage of prescription records that are independent of any research agenda, drugs are not always taken as prescribed, and prescription drugs can be obtained from other sources, such as friends and relatives. Use of nonprescription (OTC) drugs can usually only be ascertained directly from the subjects. The same is true of herbals and other dietary supplements. Habits such as alcohol and tobacco consumption, and patient-reported outcomes such as quality of life (see also Chapter 18), generally require access to the subjects themselves. Other sources of information, such as medical records and medical care providers, can also be accessed in a field study, for example to ascertain specifics of oncology treatment regimens beyond the simple fact of prescriptions. Obtaining detailed information from records and providers for the rigorous definition of diseases under study and collecting appropriate and specifically relevant exposure and covariate information are two of the principal advantages of field studies.

Weaknesses

Time, cost, and logistics

Because of the need to set up and maintain data collection networks, enroll subjects, and obtain data, field studies are time consuming and expensive. A prospective follow-up study, in particular, usually requires actually following the individual subjects for a period of years, depending on the latency period of the events of interest. While ad hoc case-control studies are generally faster than cohort studies, with exposures of interest occurring prior to enrollment, the prospective enrollment of incident cases as they occur can also take years. Many questions in pharmacoepidemiology are urgent in nature, especially if driven by regulatory concerns; thus, the time required to conduct a field study can be a real barrier that must be balanced against the requirement for information that cannot be obtained by other approaches.

The corollary to the time requirements of field studies is that a substantial staff is usually needed to manage the logistics of the enrollment network and data collection, which are not issues with database studies. Personnel costs are always by far the largest component of a field study budget, which can frequently run to millions of dollars.

Issues of study validity

Avoidance of selection bias

Although more precise inclusion criteria are usually possible compared to database studies, it is still necessary to identify and enroll most subjects who meet the criteria to avoid selection bias, and this can present a substantial challenge. An effective general strategy to maximizing subject identification is to avoid more passive approaches such as voluntary referrals from clinicians or self-selection by subjects. Further, when eligible subjects are identified, assiduous efforts must be made to recruit them to ensure a reasonable participation rate. Recruitment rates and the potential for nonresponse bias must always be considered in judging the validity of field studies.

Avoidance of information bias

The other major validity concern that is more particularly a problem for field studies is information bias. This can apply either to the identification of outcomes in a cohort study, or the ascertainment of exposure in case-control studies. A particularly important source of information bias is differential recall of information by study subjects according to their exposure or disease status (i.e., recall bias). In ad hoc case-control studies, where information about drug exposures and potential confounding factors is often obtained by interview, the general concern is that cases may remember and report their histories more completely than controls, who are often relatively healthy and lacking a reason to search their memory for events that explain an illness.

However it arises, information bias can lead either to over- or under-estimation of epidemiologic measures of association. While information bias can never be ruled out, it can be minimized by good practices, including rigorous training of data collection staff, careful design of questionnaires to maximize recall, and procedures that ensure consistent data collection. Sometimes it is possible to assess the validity of exposure information in a subset of subjects, for example by comparison to pre-existing records.

Other methodological issues

Other potential problems, such as confounding, affect all pharmacoepidemiologic studies and cannot be considered particular weaknesses of field studies. Indeed, such studies often have the ability to obtain more appropriate and detailed information on potential confounding factors.

Particular applications

This section describes some of the practical aspects of field studies in the areas of design, setup, conduct, and analysis.

Design

What kind of study and data are needed?

The first design consideration is a careful understanding of the study question, which in turn informs the most appropriate approach to providing a valid answer. Relevant issues that determine design choices include:

• *Incidence of the outcome of interest*—rare outcomes, such as acute hematological or cutaneous reactions with an annual incidence of a few cases per million, generally require a case-control approach to enroll a sufficient number of cases, whereas more common outcomes, such as myocardial infarction, with an incidence measured in cases per thousand, can be studied by either a case-control or follow-up (cohort) approach (see Chapters 2 and 3).

• *Frequency of exposure to the relevant drug*—uncommonly used drugs generally must often be studied with a follow-up approach in which the primary criterion for enrollment focuses on users and non-users. It is obvious that at some point, the combination of a rare outcome with a rare exposure reaches the level where it becomes infeasible for reasons of logistics or cost to conduct an informative field study (see Chapter 3).

• *Nature of the putative association*—is it large in relative terms? This influences the sample size requirements (see Chapter 3). Is it an acute effect that occurs soon after exposure, or are latent intervals possible? Does it occur early in treatment with the drug or is a substantial length of exposure required? These latter questions indicate the relevant time window for identifying exposure and outcome, and also determine the level of detail that must be obtained. A study of acute effects may also require considerable detail about the clinical onset of the outcome, in order to properly discern the temporal sequence between exposure and outcome.

• *Where the study should be conducted*—political/regulatory considerations may dictate the need for data from specific countries. Obviously the study must be conducted in regions where both the exposure and outcome of interest occur.

• *Sources of information needed to rigorously define the outcome of interest*—is a diagnostic label sufficient? Can patient reports be relied upon? Are medical records or provider reports needed? Is the diagnosis sufficiently inconsistent that a separate review process should be established to ensure uniformity?

• *Sources of information needed to characterize exposure*—patient reports, medical records, healthcare providers? The sources will help to determine the nature of the data collection process, including such issues as self-administered questionnaires vs. personal interviews, having nonstudy medical staff

complete abstraction forms to provide relevant data from records vs. interviewing physicians vs. requesting the records for abstraction by study staff.
• *Likely confounding that will need to be addressed*—understanding this issue will help determine the information needed on potential confounding factors and other relevant covariates, and the analytic strategy. In turn, the information requirements will determine the sources that need to be tapped to obtain covariate details. Frequently the best source will be the study subjects themselves.

Protocol development

Once the basic design questions have been answered, the detailed study protocol can be developed. The first key point in this process is to determine what is required to enroll subjects who meet the inclusion criteria, both in terms of the specific infrastructure and the size of the data collection network needed to meet the sample size goals. Then the actual data collection procedures can be specified, a process in which practical considerations play a crucial role, since the protocol has to be not only rigorous, but also feasible. For example, it may be desirable to obtain blood samples for the extraction of DNA among nonhospitalized subjects, but this requires them to come to a site where blood can be drawn, or a home visit by a trained phlebotomist. An alternative that does not yield as much DNA, but is sufficient for many purposes, is the use of buccal swabs or saliva samples, which can be collected by the subjects themselves at home and shipped in prepaid mailers to the study office or laboratory. If data are to be obtained directly from study subjects, a key question is whether this should be done by interview (in-person or via telephone) or self-administered questionnaire (e.g., completing a mailed or online form). In general, interviews allow for more control over the consistency of the data collection process, since it is guided by the interviewer, who can be trained and supervised. Self-administered questionnaires are less expensive since an interviewing staff is not required, but they rely on individual interpretation of the questions by subjects. The anonymity of filling out a questionnaire in private can be an advantage for sensitive topics, although

it can be argued that the rapport developed by an experienced interviewer is also beneficial in this regard. Practical considerations of cost and feasibility generally dictate the approach chosen.

Data collection instruments

Because a study is only as informative as the data that are recorded, developing instruments that allow for the collection of the needed items is critical. Depending on the details and source of the data to be collected, the instruments may include case report and record abstraction forms, self-administered questionnaires, and interview questionnaires.

Case report forms (CRFs) to be filled out by health care personnel should be avoided or minimized. Indeed, a major principle in the conduct of field studies is to minimize the work needed from cooperating clinical sites, since their continuing willingness to support the project is essential to its success. If CRFs are required, they should be as simple as possible, both to reduce errors and the level of effort required to complete them. An alternative is for study staff to directly abstract information from medical records, either on-site or at the study office. However, this a labor-intensive process, particularly when the records are on paper rather than electronic. The format of paper medical records is not standardized, and the quality and completeness of the information varies greatly. If the abstraction is to be done at the study headquarters instead of the clinical sites, copies of the medical records must be requested. The balance between this additional step and the logistical complications and expense of travelling to the individual sites varies depending on the number and location of the sites.

Self-administered questionnaires are commonly used in large field studies. Because there is no interviewer to control and standardize the process of filling out a questionnaire, it must be designed to lead the subject very clearly through the steps. Numerical answers or check boxes are preferred over free text, which is not readily amenable to quantitative analysis. If the questionnaire is being completed online, it can incorporate branching that leads the respondent through the questions and sections in logical order contingent on their responses at each point, as well as error checks that direct the respondent to fill in missed questions or that flag out-of-range answers. Frequently, standardized validated instruments are incorporated into study questionnaires to obtain information on psychosocial factors, dietary history, physical activity, etc. It is always good practice to take advantage of previously developed (and if possible, validated) instruments when these are available, since they have been shown to work in the field and produce results that can be more readily compared with other research. Specifically with regard to medication histories, standardized instruments are rare and the questions will likely have to be tailored to the specific needs of the project. It is important to keep questionnaires as brief as possible.

The principles guiding the design of interview questionnaires (see Chapter 12) are similar to those covering self-administered questionnaires, but there are also differences. A major difference is that a well-trained interviewer can be relied upon to lead the subject through the questions, which can allow for a less rigid structure that permits probing for additional information. A highly scripted interview that is simply administered verbatim is very standardized, which is desirable, and also minimizes the training and educational requirements for interviewers (and hence staff costs). However, it is more difficult to establish rapport with the subject and tight scripting does not easily accommodate probing, which may be essential to obtaining certain types of information. The other end of the spectrum is a very open-ended approach, which has the important drawback of reducing consistency, and is more often used in qualitative research. Perhaps most effective is a middle ground that retains structure and scripts for at least some of the questions and statements while still allowing interviewers latitude to probe and develop a style that is successful for them.

Medication histories in case-control studies are frequently obtained by interview (see Chapter 12), and the development of appropriate questionnaires to elicit this information is of particular importance in pharmacoepidemiology. Questions on medication use can range from open-ended–"did you take any drugs in the last month?"–to asking about the use of specific medications of interest by name, and even showing cards with drug names. An approach that has been proven to be effective in many studies is to ask systematically about drug use for specific indications–"did you take anything for pain in the last month?" A methodological study that evaluated these different approaches sequentially found that 0–45% of the use of a number of drugs was identified by an open ended question, with a structured list of reasons adding 35–81%, and finally a specific question by name adding 19–39%. From this it can be inferred that asking about use by indication would cover 61–81% of the total. If only a few drugs are of particular interest, it is desirable to ask about them by name. Requesting subjects to refer to medication packages, or using product photographs during in-person interviews, have also been shown to be helpful. Another memory aid which is sometimes used is a diary of life events.

Obtaining the names of medications taken is only half the battle, since details of use also need to be recorded. The level of detail is determined by the research question, but also by practical considerations of what a subject can be expected to report with reasonable accuracy. Precise information on timing and amount of use is generally relevant only for the evaluation of acute effects, where a recent exposure period is of primary interest, for example, use of an antibiotic on days X, Y, and Z in the previous two weeks in relation to the development of agranulocytosis. Studies of long-term effects generally require information on substantial use with less fine detail, which is likely to be well-remembered even if in the more distant past, for example use of an antihypertensive agent for at least one year in relation to lung cancer.

Setup

Three key aspects of the setup of a field study involve the data collection network, the study staff, and the computing infrastructure (including the main database).

Data collection network

The particulars of the network are determined by the study population, sample size, and any specific considerations that require data from particular countries. In some instances it may be possible to conduct a field study in a single center, but in practice the sample size requirements usually call for data collection in multiple centers. Any multicenter study will need a coordinating center to maintain the overall operation and ensure consistency of data collection. If the study will be conducted in multiple countries, it will be necessary to have at least one co-investigator in each country who has knowledge of local conditions and connections with the appropriate institutions, and who can be responsible for setting up and running the project there. A key factor in the success or failure of a large multicenter study is the level of engagement of the co-investigators. Thus, building a good collaboration is an essential step in getting the study off the ground.

In case-control studies in particular, cases are generally identified through the health care system, most often relevant hospital departments, but occasionally doctors' offices. Recruiting the institutions is likely to be a large challenge, especially with modern privacy regulations and other human subjects considerations. Large multicenter studies require applications to many institutional review boards (IRBs), which can take months to complete. These applications require a local investigator in each institution. The participation of local co-investigators requires their commitment to the topic and minimization of their effort in the setup and operation of the study. Often the setup is a larger burden than the actual ongoing operation of the network when the study is up and running.

Study staff

As with other clinical studies that involve data collection, an experienced staff is an important component of success. One of the key positions is the study coordinator, who is responsible for the day-to-day running of the data collection network. Typical responsibilities for the coordinator include training and supervising field and office staff, monitoring the progress of subject enrollment and data collection, monitoring or performing quality control of the data, communication with co-investigators in multicenter studies, assisting with IRB applications, and providing information for data analyses. It is advisable and sometimes a requirement because of privacy or other institutional regulations for data collection personnel in specific hospitals to be employees of those institutions. Other central staff may include research assistants, coders, and research pharmacists. Another key position, although not unique to field studies, is that of data analyst. Studies that involve data collection frequently require the input of experienced clinicians to ensure that subjects meet inclusion criteria. In such situations it is often appropriate to engage the appropriate clinicians as consultants to the study team.

Computing infrastructure

In modern field studies, the importance of the computer infrastructure can scarcely be overstated. It behooves any group that is continually engaged in the conduct of these studies to build a good programming and computer operations department. There are three main components to the infrastructure: (1) logs to track subject enrollment and data collection; (2) software for data collection and management, which may include among other modules, data entry software for computerized interviews, online questionnaires, scanning software for paper forms, quality control and coding software, and a system for producing automated letters to subjects and providers; and (3) the study database itself.

Pilot phase

During the set-up phase, it is generally advisable to test the methods by initiating data collection in a few sites. Such a pilot period allows adjustment of study procedures before full scale operations begin. For example, it may be that the initial inclusion criteria do not yield the expected number of subjects, and need to be relaxed (after determination that this will not jeopardize validity). The originally planned subject identification and enrollment procedures in the study sites may prove to be infeasible or overly inefficient, with pilot experience suggesting modifications that improve the process. Experience with the data collection instruments may point the way to improvements that increase the likelihood that the desired information will be obtained.

Conduct of the study

Most pharmacoepidemiologic field studies are multicenter, giving rise to some general operational principles that underlie their conduct:

• *Communication*—the imperative of maintaining good communication between the coordinating center and field operations and among co-investigators cannot be stressed too highly. Communication is necessary to understand what is happening at the study sites, to maintain consistency in the conduct of the study throughout the network, and to keep a geographically separated team of investigators fully informed of problems and involved in the solutions.

• *The study team should actively conduct the study*— particularly in subject enrollment, but also in data collection, a passive approach that relies on the good will and efforts of individuals who are not part of the study team is likely to lead to recruitment difficulties and substandard data. The primary commitment of clinicians and their staffs is to provide clinical care, and as much as possible, a study should rely on their granting access to patients and information and nothing more. Voluntary referrals of subjects are likely to be biased and in low numbers. Expectations that clinical personnel will actively assist with data collection, whether through filling out case report forms or interacting with subjects, are generally unrealistic. A highly active approach to the conduct of field studies is more expensive, but it is essential to producing valid, informative results in a timely manner.

• *Do not cut corners to save costs or time*—there may be pressure from sponsors to accelerate the timetable and cut costs. Field studies are usually commissioned only when studies of existing data, which can be conducted rapidly and at relatively modest cost, are infeasible. Thus, sponsors need to be aware of the different realities that apply to field study operations. A substandard study conducted rapidly without sufficient financial resources serves no one's interests.

Subject enrollment

There are two key goals in the enrollment phase of all field studies: to reach the targeted number of subjects meeting the inclusion criteria so as to meet the sample size requirements, and to maximize the participation rate in order to reduce the possibility of selection bias. There are numerous approaches to achieving these goals. Follow-up studies, which tend to be very large, may enroll subjects through the use of magazine subscriber lists, registries of professionals, and advertisements. The numbers of subjects in case-control studies are usually much smaller, a few hundred or at most, a few thousand cases and controls, but the enrollment of cases of rare conditions that are often of interest in pharmacoepidemiology (e.g., blood dyscrasias) may require large and even international networks to obtain the needed numbers.

Cases are most often identified through contact with the health care system, and the principle of active ascertainment, which involves members of the study staff taking the initiative to identify cases, is the most important defense against selection bias during the enrollment process. Specific approaches include regular telephone contact with the relevant sites, or visits by study staff to identify subjects and approach them for participation. The rapid turnaround and reliability of email has opened up further possibilities for efficiently communicating with sites. A complicating factor is privacy regulations, which in the US now prohibit outside personnel from examining medical records and approaching patients without prior permission or a waiver of authorization. On the other hand, medical personnel can examine records with a Health Insurance Portability and Accountability Act (HIPAA) preparatory to research waiver, and health care providers can then invite potentially eligible subjects to participate, either in person or by letter. The latter process can be simplified for the sites by developing a computerized system to generate letters of invitation. Patients approached in this way can either indicate their agreement to have contact information forwarded to the study staff (opt-in) or indicate by mail or phone that they do not wish to participate, in which case the information is not forwarded (opt-out). With the opt-out approach, the contact information is forwarded to the study staff if the subject has not opted out within a specified time period. In either instance, once the contact information has been sent to the study office, actual enrollment, including informed consent, is controlled by study personnel and not reliant on individual sites.

The different recruitment mechanisms require IRB approval for the individual study sites. For reasons related to study validity and practicality, opt-out is greatly to be preferred to opt-in, because it usually results in higher participation rates of eligible subjects. However, many IRBs will only approve an opt-in approach, which can sometimes make a study infeasible. Variations on the opt-out approach exist, for example, recruiting Medicare recipients in the US through the Centers for Medicare and Medicaid Services (CMS). This has the further advantage of initially identifying subjects from a comprehensive list, which is less subject to bias. Other list-based recruitment approaches, such as identifying potential subjects through cancer registries, may occasionally be feasible, and preferable to working with clinical sites because they do not require the step of medical personnel identifying subjects to approach.

More problematic enrollment approaches include those that have clinical personnel recruit and consent subjects, or some form of advertising, e.g., by internet, flyers, newspapers, or through patient organizations. The former is logistically cumbersome, requires an impractical level of effort from the sites, and is likely to lead to low and biased recruitment

The optimal enrollment situation is one that is controlled by study staff as early in the process as possible. Once a potentially eligible subject is identified, assiduous efforts must be made to contact her or him, determine final eligibility through a screening process (e.g., a brief screening interview or questionnaire), and obtain consent to participate. Depending on the nature of the data collection, this can be done by phone, in person, by mail, or via the internet. Meeting the general goal of enrolling as many identified eligible subjects as possible often requires multiple contacts by telephone, email, or regular mail.

In certain instances a more elaborate process for determining the eligibility of cases is required. This is particularly important in studies of rare conditions for which the diagnoses are not straightforward and subjects are enrolled from multiple countries where health care practices may differ. For example, in two multicenter studies of Stevens-Johnson syndrome and toxic epidermal necrolysis, it was deemed necessary to have a committee of dermatologists review photographs as well as relevant clinical and pathological information to confirm the diagnoses. The review committees met twice a year during the course of the studies. A similar approach was taken for agranulocytosis and aplastic anemia in the IAAAS, where actual bone marrow biopsy specimens were obtained for review for more than 95% of the cases. This general approach assures the most consistent case definitions, but requires considerable resources to assemble all of the relevant materials and cover the costs of the review sessions.

The enrollment of controls in case-control studies may be done through health care providers (e.g., other hospitalized patients), which generally requires permission from providers to approach potential subjects for enrollment. This, of course, risks selection bias if the illnesses which result in the medical attention that qualifies the controls are related to the exposure of interest, and also from incomplete enrollment. Appropriate specification of diagnoses for hospital controls is a key design issue that requires considerable attention in developing protocols for hospital-based case-control studies. "Population" or "community" controls can be identified by means of random digit dialing, lists of licensed drivers, Medicare rolls, or municipal census lists. With the latter approaches, identified potential controls can then be approached for participation directly by study staff, except in the instance of Medicare, where subjects are first approached by CMS, with their contact information given to investigators after an opt-out period has expired. Another possibility is nominations by cases (e.g., relatives, friends), but this has considerable potential for bias. Maximum effort by study personnel to contact and enroll targeted hospital or community controls is crucial for validity as well as efficiency.

Data collection

Once subjects are enrolled, the primary goal of the data collection phase of a field study is to obtain the specified data with as much completeness and consistency as possible. With self-administered data collection procedures, including mailed or internet questionnaires, study staff needs to follow up with subjects who do not complete them in a timely manner. The follow-up process can involve repeat mailings and telephone or email contact as appropriate. To ensure maximum participation in this phase of a study, it may be advisable to offer the option of an interview for subjects who will not complete the questionnaires on their own.

Interviews (see Chapter 12) are often the primary source of data in pharmacoepidemiologic field studies, and have the advantage over self-administered questionnaires of being a more consistent and controlled process, albeit more costly. Interviews can either be conducted in person (in the hospital, at a subject's home, or at some other site) or by telephone. It is important for comparability that the interview setting be as similar as possible for cases and controls.

Regardless of the type of interview, modern field studies generally involve the use of computerized data entry systems; this technology is referred to as computer-assisted telephone interview (CATI) and computer-assisted personal interview (CAPI). CATI is used when interviews are conducted by telephone from a call center, research office, or even the interviewer's home. CAPI involves the use of laptop computers to conduct interviews in person. In either instance, the software operates similarly, providing the questions for the interviewer to ask and checkboxes or entry fields to record the answers. In CAPI, where the laptop is not connected to a central server, all the necessary software is resident on the computer and the data are saved locally and uploaded later. Because computerized interviews save a separate data entry step that would be needed with paper questionnaires, they are cost-effective and reduce entry errors. Sophisticated branching of questions can be readily accommodated, leading the interviewer and subject through what may be a complex set of questions. Another advantage of computerized interviews is that automatic coding during the interview, e.g., for drug product names, can be built into the software, increasing accuracy and again saving a data processing step.

If data are obtained from medical records, these must be requested (with a signed release from the subject) and abstracted by study staff, often a labor-intensive process that may require repeat requests to providers for the information. In some instances with relatively small data collection networks, it is feasible for study staff to actually visit the sites and abstract the information there, although this has become uncommon because of privacy regulations.

Some field studies require the collection of biological samples, e.g., blood, urine, or tissue (such as biopsy material). With today's focus on genetics, DNA samples are increasingly sought. DNA can be obtained either from blood samples or from cheek cells collected through buccal swabs or saliva samples, which can be done by subjects at home. A drawback to cheek cell samples is the restricted amount and reduced quality of DNA compared to that obtained from whole blood, but it is sufficient for many purposes. If blood samples are needed, these must be drawn by a professional, either at the subject's home or at some sort of collection site, which complicates logistics and adds to costs. In addition to procedures related to the sample collection itself, freezers and other storage facilities must be maintained, and relationships with appropriate laboratories developed for conducting the relevant tests.

Data management

An important aspect of the data management process is coding and quality control (QC). Many data items, including drug product names, medical conditions, procedures, occupation, and so on, may be collected as text that must be numerically coded for analysis. Interview software can provide a head start on this process by linking with computerized dictionaries that will automatically code data entries that match up with dictionary entries, but there is always a need for at least some coding after data collection because of misspelled entries or those that require some interpretation. In some studies, all coding is done after the data have been collected.

Appropriate coding can make a major contribution to efficient analyses. Diagnoses are frequently coded with International Classification of Diseases (ICD) codes. For drug names, there are various dictionaries available, including among others, the

WHO Drug Dictionary (WHO-DD), Iowa Drug Information Service (IDIS) Drug Vocabulary and Thesaurus, and the Slone Drug Dictionary. The WHO dictionary includes drug names linked to the Anatomical Therapeutic Chemical (ATC) Classification System while the IDIS and Slone dictionaries utilize a modified version of the American Hospital Formulary Service (AHFS) Pharmacologic Therapeutic Classification. These classification systems facilitate the identification and grouping of agents with similar pharmacologic properties and therapeutic uses. These dictionaries have been used in various pharmacoepidemiologic studies and have varied content. While no single dictionary is comprehensive for all prescription and nonprescription medications, each of them is well suited for the coding of most drug names that have been encountered in Europe and the United States.

The QC process is an important step in ensuring that the data are consistent and as free from errors as possible. The first line of defense with computerized interviews or online self-administered questionnaires is built-in checks in the software to not accept entry of inappropriate answers, e.g., out of range ages, impossible height and weight values. Another common feature that maximizes completeness of the information is to require that certain questions be answered before the interview can proceed. Good practice for interviewers is to review the questionnaires (whether computerized or on paper) immediately after completion to clean up inconsistencies in filling them out. At the central office there are usually two levels of QC. Another series of automatic checks built into the software for uploading interview and self-administered data to the main database flags inappropriate entries for correction. There should also be some level of manual QC of the data, which can range from a complete review of all items for each subject in small studies to review of key items such as medication histories or random spot checking the data for individual subjects in very high volume studies where individual checking of all data is not feasible. Errors and inconsistencies identified at this stage can be corrected by contacting the interviewer and sometimes even the subject if necessary. After all QC checks have been completed, the data can be released for use in analyses.

The process of uploading data to central databases is usually fairly automated in modern field studies. Computerized interviews and online self-administered questionnaires can be transferred directly, with some built-in QC checks as described above. Paper questionnaires are designed to be scanned whenever possible, although text fields may require manual entry. Abstraction of medical records is ideally accomplished with a computerized form that again allows direct uploading to a central database. When computer-assisted data collection processes such as interviews and abstraction are done locally rather than from a central office, automated uploading is still possible via secure internet connection. Entry of laboratory test results and other similar data items may require a manual process, which can be greatly facilitated by appropriately designed software.

Analysis

Most analytical issues are not unique to field studies, and will not be covered here. A sometimes underappreciated step that is worth mentioning involves the creation from the raw data of analytical files that contain the variables on exposures, outcomes, and covariates needed for a particular analysis. The goal in the data collection phase of a study is to obtain information on all items that may be needed to address all the research questions. The format of the data should be designed to facilitate accurate and complete collection, and may not be appropriate for analysis without some transformation. For example, complex medication histories may need to be simplified into analytical variables by combining information from the use of several products, calculating total dosage ingested over a specified time period, and defining the temporal sequence of drug use and clinical events. The latter process may require comparing information on the timing of drug use and the clinical course of a medical condition that has been obtained using a common reference point that is consistent for all subjects (e.g., the day of hospital admission). This "pre-analysis" creation of analytical files requires first a conceptual process to define the variables needed for the analysis. The actual preparation of a file can involve substantial computing from the raw data. Whether in a field study or a database study, once an analytical file is prepared, the epidemiologic analyses, while defined by the data items and specific questions addressed, are similar.

Conclusions

As databases and other ongoing resources such as registries become more computerized and better adapted for research, there will be less call for field studies. However, it is not envisioned that the day will come where all pharmacoepidemiologic research questions can be answered with already-collected data. There will always be situations that require more detailed information about the disease under study than is available from preexisting data, information about OTC medication use, details of habits that are not routinely recorded, or information on factors that can only be provided by subjects, such as quality of life. In these instances, field studies will be needed. It is to be hoped that investigators and organizations with the capacity to mount such studies continue to be available, so

that the conduct of field studies does not become a lost art in the practice of pharmacoepidemiology.

Key points

- "Field" or "ad hoc" studies involve data collection in the field to answer specified research questions, to be distinguished from studies that use preexisting data.
- Field studies are needed when there is no existing database that can adequately answer the questions posed.
- The outcome(s) can be defined rigorously because information needed for this purpose can be specified and obtained.
- Exposure and covariate information can be tailored specifically to the research question.
- An important limitation is that field studies generally take years to complete. They are also more expensive than studies utilizing existing data, with often-complicated logistics.
- Care must be taken to avoid biases in enrollment of subjects and collection of information, which can be less of a concern with preexisting data collected for another purpose.

Case Example 10.1: International study of severe cutaneous adverse reactions (Roujeau JC *et al.*, 1995)

Background

- Stevens-Johnson syndrome and toxic epidermal necrolysis (SJS/TEN) are extremely rare but life-threatening dermatological conditions that are associated with the use of numerous medications, and are frequently cited in regulatory action to remove drugs from the market. Until the present study was conducted, much of the information linking specific drugs with the risk of SJS/TEN was derived from case reports.

Question

- The study goal was to quantify the risk of SJS/TEN among users of specific drugs in absolute as well as relative terms.

Approach

- Case-control study conducted in France, Germany, Italy, and Portugal. For the initial report, 245 cases of SJS/TEN were identified through active ascertainment in hospital networks covering all of Germany and substantial portions of the other three countries.
- All relevant clinical and laboratory information, including photographs, was reviewed by a committee of dermatologists to confirm that potential cases met study criteria as SJS/TEN. An index day corresponding to the clinical onset of the condition was specified for each case.

(*continued*)

- 1147 controls were other hospital patients with specified diagnoses judged unrelated to the prior use of medications.

- Medication histories were obtained by interview of the patients or family members.

- Standard case-control analytic methods were used to estimate odds ratios (ORs), controlling for confounding. Absolute (excess) risks were also estimated.

Results

- Overall ORs for associated drugs were high, ranging from 5.5 to infinity. These included previously suspected drugs such as sulfonamides, other anti-infectives, anticonvulsants, and certain NSAIDs.

- In general, the risk was highest early in the course of therapy.

- Excess risks were low, ranging from 0.2 to 4.5 per million users in one week.

Strengths

- Very rigorous definition of cases. The study contributed to standardizing the classification of SJS/TEN.

- Provided quantitative risk estimation with control for confounding, especially important with multiple associated drugs with overlapping use.

- Covered a sufficiently large population to enroll several hundred cases of a disease spectrum with an incidence of the order of a few cases per million per year.

Limitations

- Potential information bias due to interview-based drug histories.

- Potential underascertainment of cases in the very large base population.

Key points

- For the first time, quantified risk of SJS/TEN for many previously implicated drugs.

- Demonstrated the importance of determining absolute as well as relative measures of risk when studying very rare diseases.

Further Reading

Abenhaim L, Moride Y, Brenot F, *et al.* (1996) Appetite-suppressant drugs and the risk of primary pulmonary hypertension. International Primary Pulmonary Hypertension Study Group. *N Engl J Med* **335**: 609–16.

Bastuji-Garin S, Rzany B, Stern RS, *et al.* (2004) Clinical classification of cases of toxic epidermal necrolysis, Stevens-Johnson syndrome, and erythema multiforme. *Arch Dermatol* **129**: 92–6.

Cozier YC, Palmer JR, Rosenberg L (2004) Comparison of methods for collection of DNA samples by mail in the Black Women's Health Study. *Ann Epidemiol* **14**: 117–22.

Kaufman DW, Kelly JP, for the International Collaborative Study of Severe Anaphylaxis (2003) Risk of anaphylaxis in a hospital population in relation to the use of various drugs: an international study. *Pharmacoepidemiol Drug Safety* **12**: 195–202.

Kaufman DW, Kelly JP, Levy M, Shapiro S (1991) *The Drug Etiology of Agranulocytosis and Aplastic Anemia: The International Agranulocytosis and Aplastic Anemia Study.* New York: Oxford University Press.

Kazis LE, Miller DR, Skinner KM, *et al.* (2004) Patient-reported measures of health: The Veterans Health Study. *J Ambul Care Manage* **7**: 70–83.

Louik C, Lin AE, Werler MM, *et al.* (2007) First-trimester use of selective serotonin-reuptake inhibitors and the risk of birth defects. *N Engl J Med* **356**: 2675–83.

Mitchell AA, Cottler LB, Shapiro S (1986) Effect of questionnaire design on recall of drug exposure in pregnancy. *Am J Epidemiol* **123**: 670–6.

Roujeau JC, Kelly JP, Naldi L, *et al.* (1995) Medication use and the risk of Stevens-Johnson syndrome or toxic epidermal necrolysis. *N Engl J Med* **333**: 1600–7.

Sakamoto C, Sugano K, Ota S, *et al.* (2006) Case-control study on the association of upper gastrointestinal bleeding and nonsteroidal anti-inflammatory drugs in Japan. *Eur J Clin Pharmacol* **62**: 765–72.

Strom BL (2001) Data validity issues in using claims data. *Pharmacoepidemiol Drug Saf* **10**: 389–92.

Willett WC, Sampson L, Stampfer MJ, *et al.* (1985) Reproducibility and validity of a semiquantitative food frequency questionnaire. *Am J Epidemiol* **122**: 51–65.

CHAPTER 11

How Should One Perform Pharmacoepidemiologic Studies? Choosing Among the Available Alternatives

Brian L. Strom
Perelman School of Medicine at the University of Pennsylvania, Philadelphia, PA, USA

Introduction

As discussed in the previous chapters, pharmacoepidemiologic studies apply the techniques of epidemiology to the content area of clinical pharmacology. Between 500 and 3000 individuals are usually studied prior to drug marketing. Most postmarketing pharmacoepidemiologic studies need to include at least 10 000 subjects, or draw from an equivalent population for a case-control study, in order to contribute sufficient new information to be worth their cost and effort. This large sample size raises logistical challenges. Chapters 7 through 10 presented many of the different data collection approaches and data resources that have been developed to perform pharmacoepidemiologic studies efficiently, meeting the need for these very large sample sizes. This chapter synthesizes this material, to assist the reader in choosing among the available approaches.

Choosing among the available approaches to pharmacoepidemiologic studies

Once one has decided to perform a pharmacoepidemiologic study, one needs to decide which of the data collection approaches or data resources described in earlier chapters of this book should be used. Although, to some degree, the choice may be based upon a researcher's familiarity with given data resources and/or the investigators who have been using them, it is very important to tailor the choice of pharmacoepidemiologic resource to the question to be addressed. One may want to use more than one data collection strategy or resource, in parallel or in combination. If no single resource is optimal for addressing a question, it can be useful to use a number of approaches that complement each other. Indeed, this is probably the preferable approach for addressing important questions. Regardless, investigators are often left with a difficult and complex choice.

In order to explain how to choose among the available pharmacoepidemiologic data resources, it is useful to synthesize the information from the previous chapters on the relative strengths and weaknesses of each of the available pharmacoepidemiologic approaches, examining the comparative characteristics of each (see Table 11.1). One can then examine the characteristics of the research question at hand, in order to choose the pharmacoepidemiologic approach best suited to addressing that question (see Table 11.2). The

Textbook of Pharmacoepidemiology, Second Edition. Edited by Brian L. Strom, Stephen E. Kimmel, and Sean Hennessy.
© 2013 John Wiley & Sons, Ltd. Published 2013 by John Wiley & Sons, Ltd.

assessment and weights provided in this discussion and in the accompanying tables are arbitrary. They are not being represented as a consensus of the pharmacoepidemiologic community, but represent the judgment of this author alone, based on the material presented in earlier chapters of this book. Nevertheless, most would agree with the general principles presented, and even many of the relative ratings. My hope is that this synthesis of information, despite some of the arbitrary ratings inherent in it, will make it easier for the reader to integrate the large amount of information presented in the prior chapters.

Note that there are other data sources not discussed here, some of which have been, or in the future may be of importance to pharmacoepidemiologic research. Examples include the old Boston Collaborative Drug Surveillance data, MEMO, Pharmetrics, Aetna, Humana, and many others. Given the proliferation of pharmacoepidemiologic data resources, we make no attempt to include them all. Instead, we will discuss them in categories of type of data, as we did in the chapters themselves.

Table 11.1 Comparative characteristics of pharmacoepidemiologic data resources[a].

Pharmacoepidemiologic approach	Relative size	Relative cost	Relative speed	Representativeness	Population-based	Cohort studies possible	Case-control studies possible
Spontaneous reporting	++++	+	++++	++	—	—	+ (with external controls)
Health maintenance organizations/health plans	++	+++	+++	+++	++	++++	++++
Commercial insurance databases	++	+++	+++	+++	++	++++	++++
US Government claims databases	+++	++	++	variable	++++	++++	++++
UK medical record databases	++	++	+++	+++	+++	++++	++++
In-hospital databases	+	++	+++	++	—	++	++
Canadian provincial databases	++	++	+++	++++	++++	++++	++++
Pharmacy-based medical record linkage systems	++	++	+++	++++	++++	++++	++++
Ad hoc studies							
Case-control surveillance	variable	+++	+	variable	—	—	++++
Prescription-event monitoring	+++	+++	+	+++	++	++++	+ (nested)
Registries	variable	+++	+	variable	variable	+++	+++
Field studies							
Ad hoc case-control studies	as feasible	+++	+	as desired	as desired	—	++++
Ad hoc cohort studies	as feasible	++++	—	as desired	as desired	++++	++ (nested)
Randomized trials	as feasible	++++	—	—	—	++++	++ (nested)

(continued)

Table 11.1 *(Continued)*

Pharmacoepidemiologic approach	Validity of exposure data	Validity of outcome data	Control of confounding	Inpatient drug exposure data	Outpatient diagnosis data	Loss to follow-up
Spontaneous reporting	+++	++	—	+++	+++	N/A
Health maintenance organizations/health plans	++++	+++	++	—	++	3–15%/yr
Commercial insurance databases	++++	+++	++	—	++	about 25%/yr
US Government claims databases	++++	+++	++	—	++	variable
UK medical record databases	+++	++++	++	—	++	Nil
In-hospital databases	++++	+++	++	++++	—	Nil
Canadian provincial databases	++++	+++	++	—	++	Nil
Pharmacy-based medical record linkage systems	++++	+	+	—	—	Nil
Ad hoc studies						
Case-control surveillance	++	++++	+++	—	+	N/A
Prescription-event monitoring	+++	+++	++	—	+++	variable
Registries	+++	+++	++	+	Variable	N/A
Field studies						
Ad hoc case-control studies	++	++++	+++	++	+	N/A
Ad hoc cohort studies	+++	+++	+++	++	++++	Variable
Randomized trials	++++	+++	++++	++	++++	N/A

[a]See the text of this chapter for descriptions of the column headings, and previous chapters for descriptions of the data resources.

Comparative characteristics of pharmacoepidemiologic data resources

Table 11.1 lists each of the different pharmacoepidemiologic data resources that were described in earlier chapters, along with some of their characteristics.

The *relative size* of the database refers to the population it covers. Only spontaneous reporting systems, US Medicare, some of the pharmacy-based medical record linkage systems, and Prescription Event Monitoring in the UK cover entire countries or large fractions thereof. Of course, population databases differ considerably in size, based on the size of their underlying populations. Medicaid databases are next largest, with the commercial databases approaching that. The UK electronic medical record databases would be next in size, as would the health maintenance organizations, depending on how many are included. The Canadian provincial databases again could be equivalently large, depending on part on how many are included in a study. The other data resources are generally smaller. Case-control surveillance, as conducted by the Slone Epidemiology Unit, can cover a variable population, depending on the number of hospitals and metropolitan areas they include in their network for a given study. The population base of registry-based case-control studies depends on the registries used for case finding. Ad hoc studies can be whatever size the researcher desires and can find resources for.

As to *relative cost*, studies that collect new data are most expensive, especially randomized trials and cohort studies, for which sample sizes generally need to be large and follow-up may need to be prolonged. In the case of randomized trials, there are additional logistical complexities. Studies that use existing data are least expensive, although their cost increases when they gather primary medical records for validation. Studies that use existing data resources to identify subjects but then collect new data about those subjects are intermediate in cost.

As regards *relative speed* to completion of the study, studies that collect new data take longer, especially randomized trials and cohort studies. Studies that use existing data are able to answer a question most quickly, although considerable additional time may be needed to obtain primary medical records for validation. Studies that use existing data resources to identify subjects but then collect new data about those subjects are intermediate in speed.

Representativeness refers to how well the subjects in the data resource represent the population at large. US Medicare, Prescription Event Monitoring in the UK, the provincial health databases in Canada, and the pharmacy-based medical record linkage systems each include entire countries, provinces, or states and, so, are typical populations. Spontaneous reporting systems are drawn from entire populations, but of course the selective nature of their reporting could lead to less certain representativeness. Medicaid programs are limited to the disadvantaged, and so include a population that is least representative of a general population. Randomized trials include populations limited by the various selection criteria plus their willingness to volunteer for the study. The GPRD and THIN use a nonrandom large subset of the total UK population, and so may be representative. Health maintenance organizations (HMOs) and commercial databases are

closer to representative populations than a Medicaid population would be, although they include a largely working population and, so, include few patients of low socioeconomic status and fewer than usual elderly. Some of the remaining data collection approaches or resources are characterized in Table 11.1 as "variable," meaning their representativeness depends on which hospitals are recruited into the study. Ad hoc studies are listed in Table 11.1 "as desired," because they can be designed to be representative or not, as the investigator wishes.

Whether a database is *population-based* refers to whether there is an identifiable population (which is not necessarily based in geography), all of whose medical care would be included in that database, regardless of the provider. This allows one to measure incidence rates of diseases, as well as being more certain that one knows of all medical care that any given patient receives. As an example, assuming little or no out-of-plan care, the Kaiser programs are population-based. One can use Kaiser data, therefore, to study medical care received in and out of the hospital, as well as diseases which may result in repeat hospitalizations. For example, one could study the impact of the treatment initially received for venous thromboembolism on the risk of subsequent disease recurrence. In contrast, hospital-based case-control studies are not population-based: they include only the specific hospitals that belong to the system. Thus, a patient diagnosed with and treated for venous thromboembolism in a participating hospital could be readmitted to a different, nonparticipating, hospital if the disease recurred. This recurrence would not be detected in a study using such a system. The data resources that are population-based are those which use data from organized health care delivery or payment systems. Registry-based and ad hoc case-control studies can occasionally be conducted as population-based studies, if all cases in a defined geographic area are recruited into the study, but this is unusual (see also Chapter 2).

Whether cohort studies are possible within a particular data resource would depend on whether individuals can be identified by whether or not they were exposed to a drug of interest. This would be true in any of the population-based systems, as well as any of the systems designed to perform cohort studies.

Whether case-control studies are possible within a given data resource depends on whether patients can be identified by whether or not they suffered from a disease of interest. This would be true in any of the population-based systems. Data from spontaneous reporting systems can be used for case finding for case-control studies, although this has been done infrequently.

The *validity of the exposure data* is most certain in hospital-based settings, where one can be reasonably certain of both the identity of a drug and that the patient actually ingested it. Exposure data in spontaneous reporting systems come mostly from health care providers and, so, are probably valid. However, one cannot be certain of patient adherence in spontaneous reporting data. Exposure data from claims data and from pharmacy-based medical record linkage systems are unbiased data recorded by pharmacies, often for billing purposes, a process that is closely audited as it impacts on reimbursement. These data are likely to be accurate, therefore, although again one cannot assure adherence. Refill adherence though has been found to correlate closely with adherence measured using microchips embedded in medication bottles (see Chapter 20). In addition, there are drugs that may fall beneath a patient's deductibles or co-payments, or not be on formularies. Also, since drug benefits vary depending on the plan, pharmacy files may not capture all prescribed drugs if beneficiaries reach the drug benefit limit. In the UK medical record systems, drugs prescribed by physicians other than the general practitioner could be missed, although continuing prescribing by the general practitioner would be detected. Ad-hoc case-control studies generally rely on patient histories for exposure data. These may be very inaccurate, as patients often do not recall correctly the medications they are taking. However, this would be expected to vary, depending on the condition studied, type of drug taken, the questioning technique used, etc. (see Chapter 12).

The *validity of the outcome data* is also most certain in hospital-based settings, in which the patient is subjected to intensive medical surveillance. It is least certain in outpatient data from organized systems of medical care. There are, however, methods of improving the accuracy of these data, such as using drugs and procedures as markers of the disease and obtaining primary medical records. The outcome data from automated databases are listed as variable, therefore, depending on exactly which data are being used, and how. The UK medical record systems analyze the actual medical records, rather than claims, and can access additional questionnaire data from the general practitioners, as well. Thus, their outcome data are probably more accurate.

Control of confounding refers to the ability to control for confounding variables. The most powerful approach to controlling for confounding is randomization. As discussed in Chapter 2, randomization is the most convincing way of controlling for unknown, unmeasured, or unmeasurable confounding variables. Approaches that collect sufficient information to control for known and measurable variables are next most effective. These include HMOs, the UK medical record systems, case-control surveillance, ad hoc case-control studies, and ad hoc cohort studies. Users of health databases in Canada, commercial databases, and Medicaid (sometimes) can obtain primary medical records, but not all information necessary is always available in those records. They generally are unable to contact patients directly to obtain supplementary information that might not be in a medical record. Finally, spontaneous reporting systems do not provide for control of confounding.

Relatively few of the data systems have data on *inpatient drug use*. The exceptions include spontaneous reporting systems, the in-hospital databases, and some ad hoc studies if designed to collect such.

Only a few of the data resources have sufficient *data on outpatient diagnoses* available without special effort, to be able to study them as outcome variables. Ad hoc studies can be designed to be able to collect such information. In the case of ad hoc randomized clinical trials, this data collection effort could even include tailored laboratory and physical examination measurements. In some of the resources, the outpatient outcome data are collected observationally, but directly via the physician, and so are more likely to be accurate. Included are spontaneous reporting systems, the UK medical record systems, HMOs, Prescription Event Monitoring, and some ad hoc cohort studies. Other outpatient data come via physician claims for medical care, including Medicaid databases, commercial databases, and the provincial health databases in Canada. Finally, other data resources can access outpatient diagnoses only via the patient, and so they are less likely to be complete; although the diagnosis can often be validated using medical records, it generally needs to be identified by the patient. These include most ad hoc case-control studies.

The degree of *loss to follow-up* differs substantially among the different resources. They are specified in Table 11.1.

Characteristics of research questions and their impact on the choice of pharmacoepidemiologic data resources

Once one is familiar with the characteristics of the pharmacoepidemiologic resources available, one must then examine more closely the research question, to determine which resources can best be used to answer it (see Table 11.2).

Table 11.2 Characteristics of research questions and their impact on the choice of pharmacoepidemiologic data resources[a].

Pharmacoepidemiologic approach	Hypothesis generating[b]	Hypothesis strengthening[c]	Hypothesis testing[d]	Study of benefits (versus risk)	Incidence rates desired	Low incidence outcome	Low prevalence exposure
Spontaneous reporting	++++	+	—	—	—	++++	++++
Health maintenance organizations/health plans	++	++++	+++	++	+++	+++	+++
Commercial insurance databases	++	++++	+++	++	+++	+++	+++
US Government claims databases	++	++++	+++	++	+++	++++	++++
UK medical record databases	++	++++	+++	++	++++	+++	+++
In-hospital databases	+	++++	+++	++	+++	+	+
Canadian provincial databases	++	++++	+++	++	+++	+++	+++
Pharmacy-based medical record linkage systems	+	++	++	++	+++	+++	+++
Ad hoc Studies							
Case-control surveillance	+++	+++	+++	+++	—	++++	+
Prescription-event monitoring	++	++	+++	+++	+++	+++	+++
Registries	+	+++	+++	+++	+++	+++	+++
Field Studies							
Ad hoc case-control studies	+	++	+++	+++	+	++++	+
Ad hoc cohort studies	+	++	+++	+++	++++	++	+++
Randomized trials	+	+	++++	++++	++++	+	++++

(continued)

Table 11.2 (*Continued*)

Pharmacoepidemiologic approach	Important confounders	Drug use inpatient (versus outpatient)	Outcome does not result in hospitalization	Outcome does not result in medical attention	Outcome a delayed effect	Exposure a new drug	Urgent question
Spontaneous reporting	—	+++	++++	+	+	++++	++++
Health maintenance organizations/health plans	+++	—	+++	—	+	++	+++
Commercial insurance databases	++	—	+++	—	+	+++	+++
US Government claims databases	++	—	+++	—	+ to +++	++	++
UK medical record databases	+++	—	+++	—	+++	+++	+++
In-hospital databases	++	++++	—	—	—	+++	+++
Canadian provincial databases	++	—	+++	—	+++	++	+++
Pharmacy-based medical record linkage systems	+	—	—	—	++	+++	+++
Ad hoc studies							
Case-control surveillance	+++	+	—	—	++	+	+
Prescription-event monitoring	++	+	++++	+	+	++++	+
Registries	++	++	+	++	++	+++	+
Field studies							
Ad hoc case-control studies	+++	++++	++	—	++	+	+
Ad hoc cohort studies	+++	+++	++++	+++	+	++++	+
Randomized trials	++++	+++	++++	++++	+	++++	+

[a]See the text of this chapter for descriptions of the column headings, and previous chapters for descriptions of the data resources.

[b]Hypothesis-generating studies are studies designed to raise new questions about possible unexpected drug effects, whether adverse or beneficial.

[c]Hypothesis-strengthening studies are studies designed to provide support for, although not definitive evidence for, existing hypotheses.

[d]Hypothesis-testing studies are studies designed to evaluate in detail hypotheses raised elsewhere.

Pharmacoepidemiologic studies can be undertaken to generate hypotheses about drug effects, to strengthen hypotheses, and/or to test *a priori* hypotheses about drug effects. *Hypothesis-generating studies* are studies designed to raise new questions about possible unexpected drug effects, whether adverse or beneficial. Virtually all studies can and do raise such questions, through incidental findings in studies performed for other reasons. In addition, virtually any case-control study could be used, in principle, to screen for possible drug causes of a disease under study, and virtually any cohort study could be used to screen for unexpected outcomes from a drug exposure under study. In practice, however, the only settings in which this has been attempted systematically have been HMOs/health plans, case-control surveillance, Prescription Event Monitoring, and Medicaid databases. To date, the most productive source of new hypotheses about drug effects has been spontaneous reporting. However, this is the goal of Sentinel, a Congressionally-mandated data system of over 100 million US lives, being built primarily for hypothesis generation (see "FDA's Sentinel Initiative" in Chapter 22). In the future, new approaches using the internet (e.g., health websites with consumer posting boards) could potentially be used for hypothesis generation of events, including those not coming to medical attention.

Hypothesis-strengthening studies are studies designed to provide support for, although not definitive evidence for, existing hypotheses. The objective of these studies is to provide sufficient support for, or evidence against, a hypothesis to permit a decision about whether a subsequent, more definitive, study should be undertaken. As such, hypothesis-strengthening studies need to be conducted rapidly and inexpensively. Hypothesis-strengthening studies can include crude analyses conducted using almost any dataset, evaluating a hypothesis which arose elsewhere. Because not all potentially confounding variables would be controlled, the findings could not be considered definitive. Alternatively, hypothesis-strengthening studies can be more detailed studies, controlling for confounding, conducted using the same data resource that raised the hypothesis. In this case, because the study is not specifically

undertaken to test an *a priori* hypothesis, the hypothesis-testing type of study can only serve to strengthen, not test, the hypothesis. Spontaneous reporting systems are useful for raising hypotheses, but are not very useful for providing additional support for those hypotheses. Conversely, randomized trials can certainly strengthen hypotheses, but are generally too costly and logistically too complex to be used for this purpose. (Post-hoc analyses of randomized trials can obviously be re-analyzed, for the purposes of generating or strengthening hypotheses, but then they are really being analyzed as cohort studies.) Of the remaining approaches, those that can quickly access, in computerized form, both exposure data and outcome data are most useful. Those that can rapidly access only one of these data types, only exposure or only outcome data, are next most useful, while those that need to gather both data types are least useful, because of the time and expense that would be entailed.

Hypothesis-testing studies are studies designed to evaluate in detail hypotheses raised elsewhere. Such studies must be able to have simultaneous comparison groups and must be able to control for most known potential confounding variables. For these reasons, spontaneous reporting systems cannot be used for this purpose, as they cannot be used to conduct studies with simultaneous controls (with rare exception). The most powerful approach, of course, is a randomized clinical trial, as it is the only way to control for unknown or unmeasurable confounding variables. (On the other hand, studies of dose–response, duration–response, drug–drug interactions, determinants of response, etc. are more readily done in nonrandomized than randomized studies.) Techniques which allow access to patients and their medical records are the next most powerful, as one can gather information on potential confounders that might only be reliably obtained from one of those sources or the other. Techniques which allow access to primary records but not the patient are next most useful.

The research implications of questions about the *beneficial effects* of drugs are different, depending upon whether the beneficial effects of interest are expected or unexpected effects. Studies of *unexpected beneficial effects* are exactly analogous to studies of unexpected adverse effects, in terms of their implications to one's choice of an approach; in both situations one is studying side effects. Studies of *expected beneficial effects*, or drug efficacy, raise the special methodological problem of confounding by the indication: patients who receive a drug are different from those who do not in a way which usually is related to the outcome under investigation in the study. It *is* sometimes possible to address these questions using nonexperimental study designs. Generally, however, the randomized clinical trial is far preferable, when feasible.

In order to address questions about the *incidence of a disease* in those exposed to a drug, one must be able to quantify how many people received the drug. This information can be obtained using any resource that can perform a cohort study. Techniques that need to gather the outcome data *de novo* may miss some of the outcomes if there is incomplete participation and/or reporting of outcomes, such as with Prescription Event Monitoring, ad hoc cohort studies, and outpatient pharmacy-based cohort studies. On the other hand, ad hoc data collection is the only way of systematically collecting information about outcomes that need not come to medical attention (see below). The only approaches that are free from either of these problems are the hospital-based approaches. Registry-based case-control studies and ad hoc case-control studies can occasionally be used to estimate incidence rates, if one obtains a complete collection of cases from a defined geographic area. The other approaches listed cannot be used to calculate incidence rates.

To address a question about a *low incidence outcome*, one needs to study a large population (see Chapter 3). This can best be done using spontaneous reporting, US Medicare, Prescription Event Monitoring, or the pharmacy-based medical record linkage systems, which can or do cover entire countries. Alternatively, one could use commercial databases, HMOs/health plans, or Medicaid databases, which cover a large proportion of the United States, or the medical record systems in the UK. Canadian provincial can also be fairly large, and one can perform a study in multiple such databases. Ad hoc cohort

studies could potentially be expanded to cover equivalent populations. Case-control studies, either ad hoc studies, studies using registries, or studies using case-control surveillance, can also be expanded to cover large populations, although not as large as the previously-mentioned approaches. Because case-control studies recruit study subjects on the basis of the patients suffering from a disease, they are more efficient than attempting to perform such studies using analogous cohort studies. Finally, randomized trials could, in principle, be expanded to achieve very large sample sizes, especially large simple trials (see Chapter 16), but this can be very difficult and costly.

To address a question about a *low prevalence exposure*, one also needs to study a large population (see Chapter 3). Again, this can best be done using spontaneous reporting, US Medicare, the pharmacy-based medical record linkage systems, or Prescription Event Monitoring, which cover entire countries. Alternatively, one could use commercial databases, large HMOs, or Medicaid databases, which cover a large proportion of the United States, or the medical record databases in the UK. Ad hoc cohort studies could also be used to recruit exposed patients from a large population. Analogously, randomized trials, which specify exposure, could assure an adequate number of exposed individuals. Case-control studies, either ad hoc studies, studies using registries, or studies using case-control surveillance, could theoretically be expanded to cover a large enough population, but this would be difficult and expensive.

When there are *important confounders* that need to be taken into account in order to answer the question at hand, then one needs to be certain that sufficient and accurate information is available on those confounders. Spontaneous reporting systems cannot be used for this purpose. The most powerful approach is a randomized trial, as it is the most convincing way to control for unknown or unmeasurable confounding variables. Techniques which allow access to patients and their medical records are the next most powerful, as one can gather information on potential confounders that might only be reliably obtained from one of those sources or the other. Techniques which allow access to primary records but not the patients are the next most useful.

If the research question involves *inpatient* drug use, then the data resource must obviously be capable of collecting data on inpatient drug exposures. The number of approaches that have this capability are limited, and include: spontaneous reporting systems and inpatient database systems. Ad hoc studies could also, of course, be designed to collect such information in the hospital.

When the *outcome under study does not result in hospitalization, but does result in medical attention*, the best approaches are randomized trials and ad hoc studies which can be specifically designed to be sure this information can be collected. Prescription Event Monitoring and the UK medical record systems, which collect their data from general practitioners, are excellent sources of data for this type of question. Reports of such outcomes are likely to come to spontaneous reporting systems, as well. Medicaid databases and commercial databases can also be used, as they include outpatient data, although one must be cautious about the validity of the diagnosis information in outpatient claims. Canadian provincial databases are similar, as are HMOs. Finally, registry-based case-control studies could theoretically be performed, if they included outpatient cases of the disease under study.

When the *outcome under study does not result in medical attention at all*, the approaches available are much more limited. Only randomized trials can be specifically designed to be certain this information is collected. Ad hoc studies can be designed to try to collect such information from patients. Finally, occasionally one could collect information on such an outcome in a spontaneous reporting system, if the report came from a patient or if the report came from a health care provider who became aware of the problem while the patient was visiting for medical care for some other problem. In the future, as noted above, new approaches using the internet (e.g., health websites with consumer posting boards) could potentially be used for hypothesis generation of events not coming to medical attention.

When the *outcome under study is a delayed drug effect*, then one obviously needs approaches capable of tracking individuals over a long period of time. The best approach for this are some of the provincial health databases in Canada. Drug data are available in some for more than 25 years, and there is little turnover in the population covered. Thus, this is an ideal system within which to perform such long-term studies. Some HMOs have even longer follow-up time available. However, as HMOs' they suffer from substantial turnover, albeit more modest after the first few years of enrollment. Commercial databases are similar. Any of the methods of conducting case-control studies can address such questions, although one would have to be especially careful about the validity of the exposure information collected many years after the exposure. Medicaid databases have been available since 1973. However, the large turnover in Medicaid programs, due to changes in eligibility with changes in family and employment status, makes studies of long-term drug effects problematic. Similarly, one could conceivably perform studies of long-term drug effects using Prescription Event Monitoring, the pharmacy-based medical record linkage systems, ad hoc cohort studies, or randomized clinical trials, but these approaches are not as well-suited to this type of question as the previously discussed techniques. Theoretically, one also could identify long-term drug effects in a spontaneous reporting system. This is unlikely, however, as a physician is unlikely to link a current medical event with a drug exposure long ago.

When *the exposure under study is a new drug*, then one is, of course, limited to data sources that collect data on recent exposures, and preferably those that can collect a significant number of such exposures quickly. Ad hoc cohort studies or a randomized clinical trial are ideal for this, as they recruit patients into the study on the basis of their exposure. Spontaneous reporting is similarly a good approach for this, as new drugs are automatically and immediately covered, and in fact reports are much more common in the first three years after a drug is marketed. The major databases are next most useful, especially the commercial databases, as their large population base will allow one to accumulate a sufficient number of exposed individuals rapidly, so one can perform a study sooner. In some cases, there is a delay until the drug is available on the plan's formulary, however; that especially can be an issue with HMOs. The US government claims databases (Medicare and especially Medicaid) have a delay in processing of their data, which makes them less useful for the newest drugs. Ad hoc case-control studies, by whatever approach, must wait until sufficient drug exposure has occurred that it can affect the outcome variable being studied.

Finally, if *one needs an answer to a question urgently*, potentially the fastest approach, if the needed data are included, is a spontaneous reporting system; drugs are included in these systems immediately, and an extremely large population base is covered. Of course, one cannot rely on any adverse reaction being detected in a spontaneous reporting system. The computerized databases are also useful for these purposes, depending on the speed with which the exposures accumulate in that database; of course, if the drug in question is not on the formulary in question, it cannot be studied. The remaining approaches are of limited use, as they take too long to address a question. One exception to this is Prescription Event Monitoring, if the drug in question happens to have been a subject of one of its studies. The other, and more likely, exception is case-control surveillance, if the disease under study is available in adequate numbers in its database, either because it was the topic of a prior study or because there were a sufficient number of individuals with the disease collected to be included in control groups for prior studies.

Examples

As an example, one might want to explore whether nonsteroidal anti-inflammatory drugs (NSAIDs) cause upper gastrointestinal bleeding and, if so, how often. One could examine the manufacturer's premarketing data from clinical trials, but the number of patients included is not likely to be large enough to study clinical bleeding, and the setting is very artificial. Alternatively, one could examine

premarketing studies using more sensitive outcome measures, such as endoscopy. However, these are even more artificial. Instead, one could use any of the databases to address the question quickly, as they have data on drug exposures that preceded the hospital admission. Some databases could only be used to investigate gastrointestinal bleeding resulting in hospitalization (e.g., Kaiser Permanente, except via chart review). Others could be used to explore inpatient or outpatient bleeding (e.g., Medicaid, Canadian provincial databases). Because of confounding by cigarette smoking, alcohol, etc., which would not be well measured in these databases, one also might want to address this question using case-control or cohort studies, whether conducted ad hoc or using any of the special approaches available, for example case-control surveillance or Prescription Event Monitoring. If one wanted to be able to calculate incidence rates, one would need to restrict these studies to cohort studies, rather than case-control studies. One would be unlikely to be able to use registries, as there are no registries, known to this author at least, which record patients with upper gastrointestinal bleeding. One would not be able to perform analyses of secular trends, as upper gastrointestinal bleeding would not appear in vital statistics data, except as a cause of hospitalization or death. Studying death from upper gastrointestinal bleeding is problematic, as it is a disease from which patients usually do not die. Rather than studying determinants of upper gastrointestinal bleeding, one would really be studying determinants of complications from upper gastrointestinal bleeding, diseases for which upper gastrointestinal bleeding is a complication, or determinants of physicians' decisions to withhold supportive transfusion therapy from patients with upper gastrointestinal bleeding, for example age, terminal illnesses, etc.

Alternatively, one might want to address a similar question about nausea and vomiting caused by NSAIDs. Although this question is very similar, one's options in addressing it would be much more limited, as nausea and vomiting often do not come to medical attention. Other than a randomized clinical trial, for a drug that is largely used on an outpatient basis one is limited to systems which request information from patients, or ad hoc cohort studies.

As another example, one might want to follow-up on a signal generated by the spontaneous reporting system, designing a study to investigate whether a drug which has been on the market for, say, five years is a cause of a relatively rare condition, such as allergic hypersensitivity reactions. Because of the infrequency of the disease, one would need to draw on a very large population. The best alternatives would be Medicare or Medicaid databases, HMOs, commercial databases, case-control studies, or Prescription Event Monitoring. To expedite this hypothesis-testing study and limit costs, it would be desirable if it could be performed using existing data. Prescription Event Monitoring and case-control surveillance would be excellent ways of addressing this, but only if the drug or disease in question, respectively, had been the subject of a prior study. Other methods of conducting case-control studies require gathering exposure data *de novo*.

As a last example, one might want to follow-up on a signal generated by a spontaneous reporting system, designing a study to investigate whether a drug which has been on the market for, say, three years is a cause of an extremely rare but serious illness, such as aplastic anemia. One's considerations would be similar to those above, but even Medicare or Medicaid databases would not be sufficiently large to include enough cases, given the delay in the availability of their data. One would have to gather data *de novo*. Assuming the drug in question is used mostly by outpatients, one could consider using Prescription Event Monitoring or a case-control study.

Conclusion

Once one has decided to perform a pharmacoepidemiologic study, one needs to decide which of the resources described in the earlier chapters of this book should be used. By considering the characteristics of the pharmacoepidemiologic resources available as well as the characteristics of the question to be addressed, one should be able to choose

those resources that are best suited to addressing the question at hand.

Key points

• There are many different approaches to performing pharmacoepidemiologic studies, each of which has its advantages and disadvantages.
• The choice of pharmacoepidemiologic resource must be tailored to the question to be addressed.
• One may want to use more than one data collection strategy or resource, in parallel or in combination.
• By considering the characteristics of the pharmacoepidemiologic resources available and the characteristics of the question to be addressed, one should be able to choose those resources that are best suited to address the question at hand.

Further reading

Anonymous (1986) Risks of agranulocytosis and aplastic anemia. A first report of their relation to drug use with special reference to analgesics. The International Agranulocytosis and Aplastic Anemia Study. *JAMA* **256**: 1749–57.

Klemetti A, Saxen L (1967) Prospective versus retrospective approach in the search for environmental causes of malformations. *Am J Public Health* **57**: 2071–5.

Coulter A, Vessey M, McPherson K. The ability of women to recall their oral contraceptive histories. *Contraception* 1986; **33**: 127–39.

Glass R, Johnson B, Vessey M. (1974) Accuracy of recall of histories of oral contraceptive use. *Br J Prev Soc Med* **28**: 273–5.

Mitchell AA, Cottler LB, Shapiro S. (1986) Effect of questionnaire design on recall of drug exposure in pregnancy. *Am J Epidemiol* **123**: 670–6.

Paganini-Hill A, Ross RK. Reliability of recall of drug usage and other health-related information. *Am J Epidemiol* 1982; **116**: 114–22.

Persson I, Bergkvist L, Adami HO. (1987) Reliability of women's histories of climacteric oestrogen treatment assessed by prescription forms. *Int J Epidemiol* **16**: 222–8.

Rosenberg MJ, Layde PM, Ory HW, Strauss LT, Rooks JB, Rubin GL. (1983) Agreement between women's histories of oral contraceptive use and physician records. *Int J Epidemiol* **12**: 84–7.

Schwarz A, Faber U, Borner K, Keller F, Offermann G, Molzahn M. (1984) Reliability of drug history in analgesic users. *Lancet* **2**: 1163–4.

Stolley PD, Tonascia JA, Sartwell PE, Tockman MS, Tonascia S, Rutledge A. *et al.* (1978) Agreement rates between oral contraceptive users and prescribers in relation to drug use histories. *Am J Epidemiol* **107**: 226–35.

Strom BL, West SL, Sim E, Carson JL. (1989) Epidemiology of the acute flank pain syndrome from suprofen. *Clin Pharmacol Ther* **46**: 693–9.

PART III
Special Issues in Pharmacoepidemiology Methodology

CHAPTER 12

Validity of Pharmacoepidemiologic Drug and Diagnosis Data

Suzanne L. West[1,3], Mary Elizabeth Ritchey[2], and Charles Poole[3]

[1]*RTI International, Research Triangle Park, NC, USA*
[2]*Food and Drug Administration, Center for Devices and Radiological Health, Silver Spring, MD, USA*
[3]*Gillings School of Global Public Health, University of North Carolina, Chapel Hill, NC, USA*

The opinions expressed in this chapter by Mary Elizabeth Ritchey are those of the author and do not necessarily represent the official policies of the US Food and Drug Administration.

Introduction

Whether to have confidence in the results of a pharmacoepidemiology study depends on proper study design, appropriate statistical analysis, and robust data. We begin this chapter by discussing the validity of the drug and diagnostic information used by clinicians in patients' care. Next, we discuss measurement error, describing the different types of error and error detection methods, exploring how errors may affect the point estimate, and describing current techniques for mitigation. In the remainder of the chapter we illustrate validity concerns when data from administrative claims, electronic health records, or questionnaire responses are used, using as examples studies of the associations between nonsteroidal anti-inflammatory drugs (NSAIDs) and myocardial infarction (MI), and between NSAIDs and gastrointestinal (GI) bleeding.

Clinical problems to be addressed by pharmacoepidemiologic research

Physicians rely on patient-supplied information on past drug use and illness to assist with the diagnosis of current disease. Proper diagnosis and treatment of current illnesses may be compromised by poor recall of past illnesses and drugs. Patients' recall abilities compromise a physician's ability to diagnose and/or prescribe successfully and may play a role in the success of drug therapy. The patient needs to recall the physician's instructions for most effective drug use and research shows many do not recall their therapeutic regimens immediately after seeing their physician. Patient recall may be even poorer for illnesses and medication use that occurred many years previously.

Of particular concern to the subject of this book is the validity of data on drug exposure and disease occurrence, because the typical focus of pharmacoepidemiologic research is often the association between a medication and an adverse drug event. Further, many potential confounders of importance in pharmacoepidemiologic research (although certainly not all) are either drugs or diseases. As noted,

Textbook of Pharmacoepidemiology, Second Edition. Edited by Brian L. Strom, Stephen E. Kimmel, and Sean Hennessy.
© 2013 John Wiley & Sons, Ltd. Published 2013 by John Wiley & Sons, Ltd.

clinicians recognize that patients very often do not know the names of the drugs they are taking currently. Thus, it is a given that patients have difficulty recalling past drug use accurately, at least absent any aids to this recall. Superficially at least, patients cannot be considered reliable sources of diagnosis information either; in some instances they may not even have been told the correct diagnosis, let alone recall it. Yet, these data elements are crucial to pharmacoepidemiology studies that ascertain data using questionnaires. Special approaches have been developed by pharmacoepidemiologists to obtain such data more accurately, from patients and other sources, but the success of these approaches needs to be considered in detail.

Methodological problems to be solved by pharmacoepidemiologic research

Indices of measurement error relevant to pharmacoepidemiologic research

Two main comparisons may be drawn between two (or more) methods of data collection or two (or more) sources of information on exposure or outcome: *validity* and *reliability*. Many different terms have been used to describe each, resulting in some confusion. Although the literature uses the term *validation* or *verification* to describe the agreement between two sources of information, *concordance* or *agreement* may more appropriately indicate comparison of data sources. Used properly, the term *validation* requires that one of the methods or sources be clearly superior to the other, a "gold standard." In recognition that a method or source can be superior to another method or source without being perfect, the term "alloyed gold standard" has been used.

Quantitative measurement of validity

For a binary exposure or outcome measure, such as "ever" versus "never" using a particular drug, two measures of validity, whose synonym is *accuracy,* are used. *Sensitivity,* also called *completeness,* measures the degree to which the inferior source or method correctly identifies individuals who,

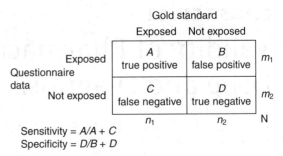

$$\text{Sensitivity} = A/A + C$$
$$\text{Specificity} = D/B + D$$

Figure 12.1 Formulas for calculating sensitivity and specificity.

according to the superior method or source, possess the characteristic of interest (i.e., ever used the drug). *Specificity* measures the degree to which the inferior source or method correctly identifies individuals who, according to the superior method or source, lack the characteristic of interest (i.e., never used the drug). Figure 12.1 illustrates the calculation of sensitivity and specificity.

Sensitivity and specificity are the two sides of the validity "coin" for a dichotomous exposure or outcome variable. In general, sources or methods with high sensitivity tend to have low specificity, and methods with high specificity tend to have low sensitivity. In these very common situations, neither of the two sources or methods compared can be said to have superior overall validity. Depending on the study setting, either sensitivity or specificity may be the more important validity measure. Moreover, absolute values of these measures can be deceiving. For example, if the true prevalence of ever using a drug is 5%, then an exposure classification method or information source with 95% specificity (and perfect sensitivity) will double the measured prevalence to 10%. The ultimate criterion of importance of a given combination of sensitivity and specificity is the degree of bias exerted on a measure of effect, such as an estimated relative risk due to misclassification.

Because the degree of bias depends on such study-specific conditions as the true prevalence of exposure, no general guidelines can be given. Each study situation must be evaluated on its own merits. For example, suppose in a case–control study that the true odds ratio (OR) is 3.0, that the sensitivity of an exposure measure is higher among cases (90%) than among controls (80%), that the specificity is lower among cases (95%) than among controls (99%), and, for simplification, that the outcome is measured perfectly and no control-selection bias exists. The exposure misclassification will bias the expected effect estimate upward to OR = 3.6 if the true exposure prevalence in the source population is 10%, will bias it downward to OR = 2.6 if the true exposure prevalence is 90%, and will leave it unbiased at OR = 3.0 if the true exposure prevalence is 70%.

As measures of validity, sensitivity and specificity have "truth" (i.e., the classification according to a gold standard or an alloyed gold standard) in their denominators. Investigators should take care not to confuse these measures with positive and negative predictive values, which include the inferior measure in their denominators. We distinguish here between the persons who *actually* do or do not have an exposure or outcome, and those who are *classified* as having it or not having it. The *positive predictive value* is the proportion of persons classified as having the exposure or outcome who are correctly classified. The *negative predictive value* is the proportion of persons classified as lacking the exposure or outcome who are correctly classified. Predictive values are measures of performance of a classification method or information source, not measures of validity. Predictive values depend not only on the sensitivity and specificity (i.e., on validity), but also on the true prevalence of the exposure or outcome. Thus, if a method or information source for classifying persons with respect to outcome or exposure has the same validity (i.e., the same sensitivity and specificity) in two populations, but those populations differ in their outcome or exposure prevalence, the source or method will have different predictive values in the two populations.

In many validation studies, the confirmation or verification rates are not measures of validity, but merely measures of agreement. In other such investigations, one method or source may be used as a gold standard or as an alloyed gold standard to assess another method or source with respect to only one side of the validity "coin." Studies that focus on the completeness of one source, such as studies in which interview responses are compared with prescription dispensing records to identify drug exposures forgotten or otherwise unreported

by the respondents, may measure (more or less accurately) the sensitivity of the interview data. However, such studies are silent on the specificity unless strong assumptions are made (e.g., that the respondent could not have obtained the drug in a way that would not be recorded in the prescription dispensing records). Similarly, validation of cases in a case-control study using self-report or administrative data often provides only the positive predictive value that the cases are true cases and does not evaluate the negative predictive value that the controls are truly controls. Ideally, one would design a validation study to calculate sensitivity and specificity, as well as positive and negative predictive values and the key patient characteristics and other variables on which they depend. It is important to note that positive and negative predictive values are useful only for internal validation studies.

In general, studies that measure mere agreement are all too commonly interpreted as though they measured validity or accuracy. The term *reliability* tends to be used far too broadly to refer not only to reliability but also to agreement or validity. For a drug exposure, a true gold standard is a list of all drugs the study participant has taken, including dose, duration, and dates of exposure. This drug list may be a prescription diary that the study participants kept or a computerized database of filled prescriptions. Neither of these data sources is a genuine gold standard, however. Prescription diaries cannot be assumed to be kept with perfect accuracy. For example, participants may record drug use as more regular and complete than it actually was, or as more closely adhering to the typically prescribed regimen. Similarly, substantial gaps may exist between the time that a prescription is filled and the time that it is ingested, if it is ingested at all. (See Chapter 20 for discussion of adherence.)

Two methods are used to quantify the validity of continuously distributed variables, such as duration of drug usage. The mean and standard error of the differences between the data in question and the valid reference measurement are typically used when the measurement error is constant across the range of true values (i.e., when measurement error is independent of where an individual's true exposure falls on the exposure distribution in the study

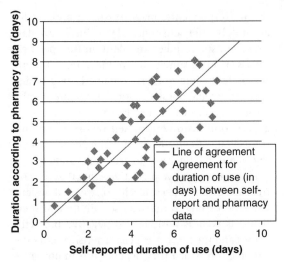

Figure 12.2 Line of agreement for continuous variables.

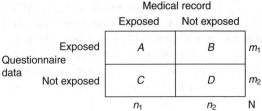

Accuracy = $A + D/N$

Chance agreement (expected) = $((n_1 \times m_1) + (n_2 \times m_2))/N^2$

$$\kappa = \frac{\text{accuracy} - \text{chance agreement}}{1 - \text{chance agreement}}$$

Figure 12.3 Formulas for calculating the percent agreement and κ.

population). With the caveat that it is generalizable only to populations with similar exposure distributions, the product–moment correlation coefficient may also be used.

High correlation between two measures does not necessarily mean high agreement. The correlation coefficient could be very high (i.e., close to 1), for example, even though one of the variables systematically overestimates or underestimates values of the other variable. The high correlation means that the over- or underestimation is systematic and very consistent. When the two measures being compared are plotted against each other and they have the same scale, full agreement occurs only when the points fall on the line of equality, which is 45° from either axis (Figure 12.2). However, perfect correlation occurs when the points lie along any straight line parallel to the line of equality. It is difficult to tell from the value of a correlation coefficient how much bias will be produced by using an inaccurate measure of disease exposure.

Quantitative measurement of reliability

To evaluate reliability or agreement for categorical variables, the percentage agreement between two or more sources and the related kappa (κ) coefficient are used. They are used only when two imperfect classification schemes are being compared, not when one classification method may be considered,

a priori, superior to the other. The κ statistic is the percentage agreement corrected for chance. Agreement is conventionally considered poor for a κ statistic less than zero, slight for κ between zero and 0.20, fair for a κ of 0.21–0.40, moderate for a κ of 0.41–0.60, substantial for a κ of 0.61–0.80, and almost perfect for a κ of 0.81–1.00. Figure 12.3 illustrates the percentage agreement and κ calculations for a reliability assessment between questionnaire data and medical record information.

The intraclass correlation coefficient is used to evaluate the reliability of continuous variables. It reflects both the average differences in mean values and the correlation between measurements. The intraclass correlation coefficient indicates how much of the total measurement variation is due to the differences between the subjects being evaluated and how much is due to differences in measurement for one individual. When the data from two sets of measurements are identical, the intraclass correlation coefficient equals 1.0. Under certain conditions, the intraclass correlation coefficient is exactly equivalent to Cohen's weighted κ.

It is impossible to translate values of measures of agreement, such as κ, into expected degrees of bias in exposure or disease associations.

Measurement error in pharmacoepidemiologic research

Epidemiologic assessments of the effects of a drug on disease incidence depend on an accurate assessment of both drug exposure and disease occurrence.

Measurement error for either factor may identify a risk factor in the study that does not exist in the population or, conversely, may fail to detect a risk factor when one truly exists.

In an epidemiologic study, the measure of association is often based on the number of subjects categorized by the cross-classification of presence or absence of disease and exposure. If one were to use questionnaire data to study the association between drug A and disease B, and if some study participants forgot their past exposure to drug A, they would be incorrectly classified as nonexposed. This misclassification is a measurement error. Although the measurement process often involves some error, if this measurement error is of sufficient magnitude, the validity of the study's findings is diminished.

Two types of measurement error or misclassification may occur: nondifferential and differential. The difference between these errors relates to the variables under study. In particular, differential misclassification occurs when the misclassification of one variable (e.g., drug usage) varies according to the level of another variable (e.g., disease status), so that the direction of the bias is toward or away from the null. For example, in a case–control study of NSAIDs and MI, patients with an MI may recall past NSAID use differently from those who had not had a recent MI. MI cases may ponder the origins of their illness and recall and report NSAID use they otherwise would have forgotten or failed to report (Figure 12.4). Alternatively, patients may be distracted by their illness during the interview and forget their past NSAID use, fail to report it to end the interview more quickly, or fail to report it because of psychological denial of it as an explanation for their disease (Figure 12.4).

Case-Control Study of NSAIDs and Myocardial Infarction (MI)

No exposure misclassification
MI cases recall exposure just as well as those without MI

	NSAID use	No NSAIDs	
MI	200	200	OR = 2.5
No MI	240	600	

MI cases recall exposure better than those without an MI

MI	Sens=	0.95
	Spec=	0.9
No MI	Sens=	0.8
	Spec=	0.7

	NSAID use	No NSAIDs	
MI	210	190	OR = 1.4
No MI	372	468	

MI cases do not recall exposure as well as those who did not have an MI

MI	Sens=	0.8
	Spec=	0.9
No MI	Sens=	0.9
	Spec=	0.7

	NSAID use	No NSAIDs	
MI	180	220	OR = 0.9
No MI	396	444	

Figure 12.4 Example of differential misclassification of exposure.

Thus, the respondent's state of mind, and possibly the interviewer's, at the time of the interviews affects the overall accuracy of the interview or questionnaire information and the degree to which the accuracy may differ by respondent characteristics (e.g., case or control status). Patients who learn that they have serious diseases, and parents who learn that their children do, often experience stages in questioning how these illnesses arose. In earlier stages, patients often blame themselves. Over time, they frequently seek external explanations. The time course of the psychological state of seriously ill patients and their close family members varies highly but may be critical to the validity of their interview and questionnaire data. The traditional assumptions that cases remember true exposures better than noncases (i.e., that exposure classification has higher sensitivity among cases than among noncases) and that cases intentionally or unintentionally report more false-positive exposures than noncases (i.e., that exposure classification has lower specificity among cases than among noncases) are undoubtedly too simplistic for general reliance.

A difference in the accuracy of recall between cases and noncases could influence the determination of NSAID exposure and the resulting measure of association. In case-control studies, differential misclassification of exposure can result from recall bias. A common belief is that the potential for recall bias can be minimized if the study is designed to obtain complete exposure data (i.e., information on the names and usage dates for every drug used in the time period of interest).

Nondifferential misclassification of exposure occurs when the misclassification of one variable does not vary by the level of another variable and may occur if both cases and controls simply forget their exposures to the same degree. The measure of association is affected by nondifferential misclassification of exposure as well; it is usually biased toward the null. Exceptions can occur when classification errors are not independent of each other, as when participants who are particularly reluctant to report health outcomes that they have experienced are especially unwilling to report medications that they have taken as well. Other exceptions to the rule about bias toward the null from nondifferential misclassification can occur with more than two categories of exposure. A simple hypothetical example using a case-control study to illustrate the potential for bias away from the null from independent, nondifferential misclassification of an exposure with more than two categories of exposure (low, medium, and high) is provided in Figure 12.5. If 40% of the cases and controls in the high-exposure group are misclassified into the medium-exposure group, then

No Exposure Misclassification

	Exposure				
	Low	Medium	High		
Cases	100	200	600	Medium vs Low	OR = 2
Controls	100	100	100	High vs Low	OR = 6

40% of cases and controls in the high exposure group
are misclassified as medium exposure

	Exposure				
	Low	Medium	High		
Cases	100	440	360	Medium vs Low	OR = 3.1
Controls	100	140	60	High vs Low	OR = 6

Figure 12.5 Example of nondifferential misclassification of exposure when exposure is polychotomous.

the OR for medium exposure is relatively unbiased, but the OR for high exposure is biased upward to 2.6.

Under some circumstances, no bias occurs from independent, nondifferential misclassification of a binary outcome measure. For example, if no false-positive cases exist, then the expected risk ratio will be the risk ratio, given correct disease classification, multiplied by the ratio of the sensitivity in the exposed group to the sensitivity in the unexposed group. If the sensitivity is independent and nondifferential, this ratio equals unity and the risk ratio is unbiased.

Effects of measurement error on the point estimate of association

Copeland *et al.* evaluated misclassification in epidemiologic studies, using a series of computer-generated graphs. They showed that the bias—discrepancy between the point estimate and the true value of the measure of association—was a function of the disease frequency, exposure frequency, sensitivity, and specificity of the classification. Notably, Copeland *et al.* were not able to describe bias as a function of the product-moment correlation coefficient, the intraclass correlation coefficient, percentage agreement, or κ. Thus, higher or lower values of these measures, even when one of the measurement methods is a gold standard, should not be interpreted as evidence of greater or lesser degrees of bias. When nondifferential misclassification occurred, the point estimate was biased toward the null. Their results for nondifferential misclassification of disease also indicated that the rarer the disease, the more the potential for bias in cohort studies. Likewise, the less prevalent the exposure, the more the potential for bias in case–control studies. For differential misclassification, the point estimate could be biased toward or away from the null. Differential misclassification is problematic for ad hoc case–control studies in which recall bias is always a concern.

All Copeland *et al.*'s simulations were done on binary disease and exposure variables. For a continuous variable, nondifferential misclassification may not produce a bias toward the null if a perfect correlation exists between the variable as measured and the true value. For example, if both cases and controls in a case-control study underestimate duration of drug use by an equal percentage, a bias toward the null will not occur.

Correcting measures of association for measurement error

Estimates of sensitivity and specificity are required to correct effect estimates for measurement error. These estimates can be derived from previous research or from a subsample within the study analyzed. However, estimates of sensitivity and specificity of exposure classification from previous research are rarely available. When these estimates are available, they may not be useful, because the classification methods have to be similar in both the correctly classified and misclassified data. The classification probabilities will vary according to the questionnaire design, study population, and time period of administration. In addition, the correction methods most familiar to epidemiologists are appropriate for bivariate, not multivariate, data.

For differential misclassification of exposure by disease status (e.g., recall bias), the researcher is responsible for either presenting a strong case that recall bias did not threaten the study's validity, or controlling for it statistically. One approach to estimate the effects of bias is to conduct a sensitivity analysis. Sensitivity analysis is the last line of defense against biases after every effort has been made to eliminate, reduce, or control them in study design, data collection, and data analysis. As used in this context, the meaning of the term *sensitivity* differs from its other epidemiologic meaning as the counterpart to specificity as a measure of classification validity. In a sensitivity analysis, one alters key assumptions or methods reasonably to see how sensitive the results of a study are to those variations. One key assumption, usually implicit, is that the exposure and the outcome in a study have been measured accurately. With estimates from previous research, or "guesstimates" from expert experience and judgment, one can modify this assumption and use a variety of analytic methods to "back calculate" what the results might have looked like if more accurate methods had been used to classify participants with respect to outcome, exposure, or both. Sometimes wildly implausible degrees of inaccuracy would have to have been present to produce observed associations. Other times, the overall study results may seem sufficiently close to being nondifferential if viewed in isolation and out of the context of the particulars of the study; but they may be viewed as appreciably biased by knowledgeable researchers.

For many years, this kind of assessment has been conducted informally and qualitatively. However, the net result is controversy, with investigators judging the bias small and critics judging it large. Furthermore, intuitive judgments, even those of the most highly trained and widely experienced investigators, can be poorly calibrated in such matters. Formal sensitivity analysis makes the assessment of residual bias transparent and quantitative, and forces the investigator (and other critics) to defend criticisms that in earlier times would have remained qualitative and unsubstantiated. An important and well-known historical example is the bias from nondifferential misclassification of disease proposed by Horwitz and Feinstein to explain associations between early exogenous estrogen preparations and endometrial cancer. When proper sensitivity analyses were conducted, only a negligible proportion of these associations were explained by bias.

Epidemiologic applications of quantitative methods with long histories in the decision sciences can now probabilistically quantify uncertainties about multiple sources of systematic error. These methods permit incorporation of available validation data, expert judgment about measurement error, uncontrolled confounding, and selection bias, together with conventional sampling error and prior probability distributions for effect measures themselves, to form uncertainty distributions. These approaches have been used in pharmacoepidemiology in assessing:

- selection bias in a study of topical coal tar therapy and skin cancer among severe-psoriasis patients;
- exposure misclassification and selection bias in a study of phenylpropanolamine use and stroke;
- selection bias, confounder misclassification, unmeasured confounding in a study of less than definitive therapy and breast cancer mortality; and
- other clinical and nonclinical applications.

Sometimes biases can be shown to be of more concern and sometimes of less concern than intuition or simple sensitivity analysis may suggest. Almost always the probabilistic uncertainty about these sources of systematic error dwarfs the uncertainty reflected by conventional confidence intervals. With the use of these methods, the assessment of systematic error can move from a qualitative discussion of "study limitations," beyond sensitivity analyses of one scenario at a time for one source of error at a time, to a comprehensive analysis of all sources of error simultaneously. The resulting uncertainty distributions not only supplement, but also can supplant, conventional likelihood and p-value functions, which reflect only random sampling error. Consequently, much more realistic, probabilistic assessments of total uncertainty attending effect measure estimates are possible.

Methodological problems in pharmacoepidemiologic research

Self-reported drug and diagnostic data are often found to be inaccurate when compared with medical records or other data sources, but these data inaccuracies may be due to the consistency of documentation and the terminology used—from the medical records, to what the health care provider communicated to the patient, to what appears on the questionnaire. Case example 12.1 summarizes the published literature on studies that have validated drug exposure information (NSAIDs) or health outcomes (MI and GI bleeding) and that collected data via self-report.

Self-reported drug data from ad hoc survey studies: recall accuracy

The methodological literature on recall accuracy indicates that study participants have difficulty remembering drug use from the distant past, which contributes to misclassification of exposure in ad hoc case–control studies. The literature to date suggests that recall accuracy of self-reported medication exposures is sometimes, but not always, influenced by type of medication, drug use patterns, design of the data collection materials, and

Case Example 12.1

Background

- Much of the pharmacoepidemiologic research to assess the relation between medication exposures and clinical outcomes in the past 10 to 15 years has used administrative claims databases.

- Before a researcher embarks on a study using administrative claims or electronic health records, it is useful to conduct a literature search to determine whether validated algorithms for identifying exposures or outcomes exist.

- Validated medication and outcome algorithms that are consistent across multiple databases may obviate the need for *de novo* algorithm development. However, when the literature contains multiple algorithms, inconsistently validated algorithms, or algorithms that lack reliability, *de novo* algorithm development may be necessary.

Question

- Are there validated algorithms in the published literature for identifying nonsteroidal anti-inflammatory drug (NSAID) exposure and gastrointestinal (GI) bleeding as an outcome?

Approach

- Using PubMed, we conducted a literature search to identify publications that used validated algorithms for identifying NSAID exposure and GI bleeding outcomes for use in claims or electronic health care record studies. In addition, we queried researchers who use specific health care databases for their research, in order to identify additional validation studies.

- Articles had to include the data sources, NSAID use, and GI bleeding outcome.

- Abstracts and full texts were read to determine whether reliability or validation of NSAID use, GI bleeding, or both was conducted or referenced.

- Results of reliability and validation measures from each study were abstracted into evidence tables (final tables available in *Pharmacoepidemiology*, 5th edition).

Results

- We identified several algorithms using different combinations of ICD-9-CM and CPT codes to measure GI bleeding; results varied across studies.

- In Veteran's Affairs (VA) administrative data, sensitivity and specificity of GI bleeding were higher when only ICD-9 or CPT codes were used, but the positive predictive value (PPV) for determining a GI event increased with combined assessment of ICD-9 and CPT codes or limitation to patients with NSAIDs.

- PPV in claims and health care records outside the VA system ranged from 56% to 90% when ICD-9 algorithms were compared with chart review. The reported PPV was lowest in the HealthCore Integrated Research Database, but increased marginally when we assessed severe bleeding among only patients taking NSAIDs. PPV of the Read codes in the United Kingdom General Practice Research Database was 99.0% when compared with ICD-10.

- The reliability of classifying GI bleeding was considerably lower in claims compared with health care records (e.g., 23–28% in HMO Research Network), independent of NSAID use. However, algorithms developed with the use of other data systems fared better (e.g., 76.8% confirmation of GI bleeding at autopsy in Saskatchewan Health data and 68% sensitivity for acute GI bleeding in Tayside Medical Monitoring Unit data).

Strengths

- This literature scan involved searching a major database (PubMed) and soliciting input from experts in the field.

- We were able to evaluate the reliability and validity of multiple algorithms for GI bleeding and multiple databases as they were used in the peer-reviewed, published studies.

Limitations

- Our literature scan was not systematic or all-inclusive, and it used only the PubMed database. It did not include nonpublished reliability or validation studies, nor were study authors contacted to determine whether unreported values were available (i.e., sensitivity and specificity often not reported).

Key points

- Reliability and validity of an outcome may differ by database, algorithm, and patient population. In this literature scan, we noted different study results across the databases, depending on which algorithm (e.g. ICD-9/10 or CPT) was used, and whether patients using NSAIDs were included as the sample of interest.

(*continued*)

- Validation of a specific algorithm, using original documents such as medical records, is a necessary step to enhance the quality and credibility of the research findings; this necessity is especially true for new algorithms with which no previous validation study has been performed.

- Although other studies may have reviewed original documents to validate a particular algorithm, varying findings across studies using the same algorithm suggest a need for validation in new databases or for any changes to the algorithm.

- As medical practice changes, further validation of previously validated claims is also warranted.

respondent characteristics. Given the current state of the literature, epidemiologists who plan to use questionnaire data to investigate drug–disease associations will need to consider which factors may influence recall accuracy in the design of their research protocols.

The influence of medication class

Several studies have compared self-reported recall accuracy for current or past medication use with prospectively collected cohort data or pharmacy, hospital, and outpatient medical record documentation. Overall, published studies indicate that people accurately remember ever having used a medication and when they first began using it, for some medications, although they do not remember brand names and duration of use as well. In general, inaccuracies correlated with more time elapsed between occurrence of exposure and its subsequent reporting. Accuracy of self-reporting varies by medication, with:

- regularly used medications (especially those with more refills) being recalled more often than short-term medications;
- first and most recent brands in a class being recalled more frequently than other medications in the class;
- multiple medications in one class being recalled more frequently than single medication exposure; and
- salient medications (those that prompted study initiation) being more accurately recalled than common and less disconcerting medications.

For prescription drugs, self-reported use from recall, as compared with medical records, was found to be moderately accurate; however, for over-the-counter medications and vitamin supplements, recall was poor. Discrepancies were due to both underreporting (e.g., respondent forgot that the medication was taken) and overreporting (e.g., physician was unaware of medication use or failed to record patient's use in chart) and differed by therapeutic class. When self-reported data were compared with multiple sources, such as medical records and pharmacy dispensing, instead of with a single source, better verification of self-reported use occurred.

The influence of questionnaire design

As reported in a recent systematic review, several factors affect the accuracy of medication exposure reported via questionnaire. The type of question asked influences how well respondents answer medication questions, as is illustrated by a study seeking use of analgesics in the week before questionnaire administration. Design also influences the completeness of self-reported psychoactive medication use. Medication-specific or indication-specific questions were found to identify most medications in current use, but a general medication question, "Have you taken any other medications?" failed to identify all of the medications respondents were currently taking. Similarly, open-ended questions such as "Have you ever used any medications?" yielded less than half of the affirmative responses for actual use of three different medications. The addition of indication-specific questions to open-ended questions also adds incremental affirmative responses concerning exposures. Finally, 20–35% of respondents reported drug exposure only when asked medication-name-specific questions. Similar findings were reported for self-reported medication use in a university population.

Response order may affect recall, as noted with malaria medications when respondents had more than one episode of malaria. Medications listed earlier tended to be selected more frequently than those listed later—a finding that may be related to "satisficing," which occurs when respondents expend the least psychological and emotional effort possible to provide an acceptable answer to a survey question rather than an optimal answer.

A comparison of self-report for current and recent medication use (within the past 2 years) with pharmacy records of dispensed prescriptions for multiple drug classes found that the number of drug dispensings recalled was highest for cardiovascular medications (66%) and poorest for alimentary tract medications (48%). Recall was influenced by the number of regularly used medications: 71% for one drug, 64% for two drugs, and 59% for three or more drugs, although duration of use was not related to recall. However, the questionnaire did not allow sufficient space to record all medications used in the time period for this study. Thus, if respondents were unable to record all medications because of space limitations, then a misleading finding may have resulted: namely, that respondents were unable to recall all their medications.

Another methodological study evaluated whether question structure influenced the recall of currently used medications in 372 subjects with hypertension who had at least 90 days of dispensings in the PHARMO database. The questionnaire asked indication-specific questions first (e.g., medications used for hypertension, medications used for diabetes), followed by an open-ended question that asked whether the participants used any *other* medications not already mentioned. For hypertension, the sensitivity was 91% for indication-specific questions and 16.7% for open-ended questions. About 20% of participants listed medications on the questionnaire that were not in the database; a similar proportion failed to list medications on the questionnaire that were in use according to the pharmacy database. According to these results on sensitivity of recall, indication-specific questions invoke better recall accuracy. However, to adequately assess question structure, the questionnaire should have been designed to query medications with an open-ended question before querying with indication-specific questions. This sequencing would have allowed a comparison

of the number of medications recalled by each question structure.

The influence of patient population

With regard to predictors of recall accuracy, factors such as questionnaire design, use of memory aids, recall period, extent of past drug use, age, and education sometimes influence how well respondents remember past drug use, the effect often seeming to vary by therapeutic class. Behavioral characteristics such as smoking and alcohol use have rarely been evaluated as predictors of accuracy, and inconsistent findings were noted. Because of the paucity of information on predictors of recall, further research in this area is warranted.

Few studies have evaluated whether demographic and behavioral characteristics influence the recall of past medication use. No differences in recall accuracy have been noted by gender. With ever having used an antidepressant, inconsistent results were noted for evaluation of age, household income, and education as predictors of recall accuracy. Racial and socioeconomic differences in reporting were noted with oral contraceptive use, with white participants having better agreement than participants of other races, and with privately paying users having better agreement than those receiving public health care funds. For any past estrogen use, small variations in recall accuracy were noted by ethnicity and education, with more college-educated women having poorer recall than women without a college education.

A study of medication use during pregnancy reported better recall in mothers with higher educational attainment and poorer pregnancy outcome (low birth weight, gestational age, or Apgar score) whereas other authors found that factors such as maternal age, marital and employment status, and pregnancy outcome did not influence the reporting of pregnancy medication exposures.

Medication-specific questions substantially increased reporting accuracy for certain subgroups, including 25- to 44-year-olds, males, African-Americans, and those who completed the eighth grade. Age affected recall accuracy for hormone shots, NSAIDs, and other medications, with younger respondents having better recall accuracy.

However, this finding did not hold true for oral estrogen or oral contraceptive use. Study design may explain the different results noted; the two studies that reported an age effect were methodological studies evaluating recall accuracy, whereas the two that reported no age effects were etiologic studies that reported verification of drug use as a measure of exposure misclassification for the association under study.

Self-reported diagnosis and hospitalization data from ad hoc studies: recall accuracy

Just as recall accuracy of past medication use varies by drug class, the recall accuracy of disease conditions varies by disease. Several factors influence reporting of a medical condition during an interview, including the type of condition and the interviewee's understanding of the problem. Reporting also depends on the respondent's willingness to divulge the information. Conditions such as sexually transmitted diseases and mental disorders may not be reported because the respondent is embarrassed to discuss them with the interviewer or worries about the confidentiality of self-administered questionnaires. As a result, conditions considered sensitive are likely to be underreported when ascertained by self-report.

In studies comparing self-reports to clinical evaluation, depending on the type of condition, both under- and overreporting have been found. Studies using medical records to assess recall accuracy for common ailments typically found poor agreement, with patients' underreporting often being the major cause of the disagreement. Overreporting occurred, as well, especially for conditions for which the diagnostic criteria are relatively nonspecific. Comparing self-reported symptom and quality of life information at two different time periods also showed both over- and underestimation.

The influences of medical condition type

Comparing patient self-report with data from a provider questionnaire (gold standard) on previous history of cardiovascular disease or GI events, researchers found better agreement for previous acute myocardial infarction than for upper GI bleeding (see Case example 12.2).

Case Example 12.2: (Fourrier-Reglat, 2010)

Background

- Researchers may have to query the subject to assess medication exposure and outcome diagnoses. Accuracy of ad hoc questionnaire studies has been determined via comparison with pharmacy, practitioner, and hospital records.

- In some cases, pharmacy or medical records may not be available or there may be reason to question both the patient and practitioner rather than conducting medical record review. In addition, questionnaires can provide concurrence regarding patient history and indication for use, which are not available from claims data or easily found in many medical records.

Question

- When questionnaires are self-administrated, is there concordance of patient-derived and physician-derived data on medical information such as previous medical history and initial indication for nonsteroidal anti-inflammatory drug (NSAID) prescriptions?

Approach

- The Kappa statistic (κ) was used to measure concordance in self-administered questionnaires completed by 18,530 pairs of NSAID patients and their prescribers for the French national cohort study of NSAID and Cox-2 inhibitor users.

- Both patients and prescribers were asked about patients' previous history of cardiovascular events, including myocardial infarction (MI), and gastrointestinal events, including upper digestive hemorrhage. Patients and prescribers were asked to identify which of the following was the initial indication for NSAID use: rheumatoid arthritis, psoriatic rheumatism, spondylarthritis, osteoarthritis, back pain, muscle pain/sprain/tendonitis, migraine/headache, flulike symptoms, dysmenorrhea, or other indication.

Results

- Agreement between patients and prescribers was substantial for MI ($\kappa = 0.75$, 95% CI: 0.71–0.80), and minimal for upper GI bleeding ($\kappa = 0.16$, 95% CI: 0.11–0.22).
- With prescriber data as the gold standard, patient reports of MI provided moderately complete data (sensitivity: 77.7%; specificity: 99.6%, PPV: 74.1%, NPV: 99.6%), but reports of upper GI bleeding by patients were less well documented in the prescriber reports (sensitivity: 44.6%; specificity: 98.5%, PPV: 10.4%, NPV: 99.8%).
- For the index NSAID indication, the proportion of agreement ranged from 84.3% to 99.4%, and concordance was almost perfect (k = 0.81–1.00).

Strengths

- Concurrent evaluation of patients and prescribers allows corroboration of patient history and indication for medication usage, which are difficult to assess in claims and electronic health care records.
- Self-administered questionnaires provide data on a list of potential confounders that are often missing from electronic records.

Limitations

- Study was carried out in an established cohort in a single country. Results may not be generalizable to other data in other locations.
- Neither the patient nor the prescriber reports "truth"; accuracy of recall was not assessed in this study.

Key points

- Prior history and indication for prescriptions are often missing from claims and electronic health care record databases. Questionnaires from both patients and prescribers may collect data on these potential confounders, as well as determine the reliability of the collected variables.
- Patients and prescribers may have differing recall of patient history, especially as related to nonspecific diagnoses.
- Relying on patient-reported data may be necessary but inaccurate, especially for over-the-counter medication use. However, corroboration with another information source, such as data from the prescriber, may provide an estimate of the reliability of patient-reported data.

The best reporting has been noted with conditions that are specific and familiar, such as diabetes mellitus, hypertension, asthma, and cancers such as breast, lung, large bowel, and prostate. However, assessing reporting accuracy is more difficult for common, symptom-based conditions such as sinusitis, arthritis, low back pain, and migraine headaches, which many people may have, or believe they have, without having been diagnosed by a clinician.

Poor agreement with cardiovascular conditions likely stems from both over- and underreporting, depending on the data source used for comparison. In most instances of recall error, persons who had incorrectly reported MIs and stroke had other conditions that they may have mistakenly understood, during communications from their physician, as coronary heart disease, MI, or stroke. Underreporting is the primary reason for poor agreement comparing interview data to clinical evaluation, although it is unclear whether this is due to the respondent's unwillingness to admit to mental illness or underdiagnosis of the conditions.

The influences of timing of diagnosis and its emotional effects on the patient

Factors influencing accuracy of past diagnoses and hospitalizations also include the number of physician services for that condition and the recency of services. For reporting of diagnoses, the longer the interval between the date of the last medical visit for the condition and the date of interview, the poorer the recall. These differences in recall may be explained in part by recall interval, patient age, a cohort (generational) effect, or some intertwining of all three factors. Diagnoses considered sensitive by one generation may not be considered sensitive by subsequent generations. Furthermore, terminology changes over time, with prior generations using different nomenclature than recent generations.

Conditions with substantial impact on a person's life are better reported than those with little or no impact on lifestyle. More patients with current restrictions on food or beverage due to medical problems reported chronic conditions that were confirmed in medical records than those without these restrictions. Similarly, those who had restrictions on work or housework reported their chronic conditions more often than those who did not have these restrictions. The major determinant of recall for spontaneous abortions was the length of the pregnancy at the time the event occurred; nearly all respondents who experienced spontaneous abortions occurring more than 13 weeks into the pregnancy remembered them, compared with just over half of those occurring in the first 6 weeks of pregnancy.

Perhaps because of attending emotional stress, lifestyle changes, and potential financial strain, hospitalizations tend to be reported accurately. Only a 9% underreporting of hospitalizations occurred when surgery was performed, compared with 16% when surgery was not performed. Underreporting in those with only a 1-day hospital stay was 28%, compared with 11% for 2–4 day stays, and approximately 6% for stays lasting 5 or more days.

Researchers also agree that respondents remember the type of surgery accurately. Recall accuracy was very good for hysterectomy and appendectomy, most likely because these surgeries are both salient and familiar to respondents. For induced abortions, marginal agreement occurred, as noted by records from a managed care organization: 19% of women underreported their abortion history, 35% overreported abortions, and 46% reported accurately, according to their medical records. Cholecystectomy and oophorectomy were not as well recalled and were subject to some overreporting. However, apparent overreporting may have been due to possible incompleteness of the medical records used for comparison.

The influence of patient population

The influence of demographic characteristics on reporting of disease has been thoroughly evaluated, although the results are conflicting. The most consistent finding is that recall accuracy decreases with age, although this may be confounded by recall interval, or cohort (generational) effects. Whether gender influences recall accuracy is uncertain. Men have been found to report better than women, independent of age, whereas conflicting evidence found that women reported better than men, especially in older age groups. Further studies indicate that gender and age differences depended on the disease under investigation, with women overreporting malignancies and men overreporting stroke. No differences were found by age or gender for reporting of hospitalizations.

Reporting of illnesses, procedures, and hospitalizations was more accurate among white patients than among patients of other races, but the number of study participants who were not white was relatively small. Reporting by educational level was equivocal and was more complete for self-respondents than for proxy respondents. For self-respondents, those with a poor or fair current health status reported conditions more completely than those with good to excellent health status.

The influence of questionnaire design

Questionnaire design also influences the validity of disease and hospitalization data obtained by self-report. Providing respondents with a checklist of reasons for visiting the doctor improves recall of all medical visits. Simpler questions yield better responses than more complex questions, presumably because complex questions require the respondent to first comprehend what is being asked and then provide an answer. Redundancy that often occurs in longer questions and greater time allowances to develop an answer may increase recall; however, longer questions may tire the respondents, leading to satisficing, as well as increase the cost of the research.

Currently available solutions

Following best practices for questionnaire design

Designing a questionnaire to collect epidemiologic data requires careful planning and pretesting. The data analysis phase requires validation of response to ensure that the data collected yield measurements responsive to the study question and hypothesis. The following steps should be considered during the design and analysis stages:

1. Use validated instruments or validated questions whenever possible, realizing that the fact that a validation study has been done does not, by itself, render a question or questionnaire "validated."

2. Strive for a fifth-grade literacy level if you must develop new survey questions to be used for a general population. Use cognitive testing to assess respondent comprehension of new questions.

3. Evaluate the accuracy of respondents' answers by comparing them to a truly accurate comparison source (i.e., gold standard) whenever possible so that sensitivity and specificity can be calculated for use in bias analyses.

4. Compute the percent agreement and κ to test the reliability of self-report. For example, when evaluating medication use, compare with pill counts, chemical markers inserted into the pills, electronic monitoring caps, or pharmacy dispensing databases. Note, however, that percent agreement and κ do not provide information on bias and, in fact, may be misleading with regard to bias. A measure with a percent agreement that seems high or a κ that falls into conventional categories of "good" or "excellent" agreement can nonetheless produce substantial bias.

5. Assess validity and reliability on a subset of the respondent population. Internal validation studies (sample size notwithstanding) offer special opportunities that external validation studies do not, notably the ability to use positive and negative predictive value, not just sensitivity and specificity.

6. Use validation studies to assess differential and possibly even dependent measurement error: for instance, validation studies of exposure metrics in cases and controls.

As with history taking during a clinical visit, epidemiologic research using questionnaires often asks respondents to recall past events or exposures, with recall intervals spanning days to several years. Researchers can facilitate recall and reporting of medication use in particular by using indication-specific questions, a drug photo prompt, a list of drug names, or a calendar for recording life events.

To appreciate the accuracy of data derived by recollection, one must understand the response process in general and the organization of memory, a key element of the response process. The adequacy of the response process depends on four key respondent tasks:

• question comprehension and interpretation;
• search for and retrieval of information to construct an answer to the question;
• judgment to discern the completeness and relevance of memory for formulating a response; and
• development of the response based on retrieved memories.

If survey instrument developers attend too little to the first two key tasks, then questions may be too vague or complex for respondents to marshal retrieval processes appropriate to them. (For discussion of the theory of survey response and the cognitive process underlying retrieval, see Tourangeau *et al.*, 2000.)

Most pharmacoepidemiologic research requires assessment of the time between exposure occurrence and observation of outcome, which may range from several hours to many years. Thus, questionnaires used in pharmacoepidemiology typically include one or more different types of temporal questions:

• time of occurrence, to provide an event date, such as date of diagnosis;
• duration, such as length of time a drug was taken;
• elapsed time, to determine time passed since an event occurred, such as time since a drug was last taken; and
• frequency, determine the number of events that occurred over a specific time period, such as the number of visits to a primary care provider over a 6-month period.

An example best illustrates the theory of Tourangeau and colleagues on how respondents use a cyclic process of recalling details about a particular event: As new information is recalled, it helps shape the memory and adds details to describe the event in question. For this example, the question may be asked, "When was your major depression first diagnosed?" The respondent uses the following process to provide the correct date of January 2008: The respondent begins by being uncertain whether the depression was diagnosed in 2007 or 2008. To work toward identifying the correct year, the respondent recalls that the depression was the result of his losing his job. The job loss was particularly traumatic because he and his wife had just purchased their first home a few months previously and, with the loss of his income, were at risk of losing the house. The home purchase is a landmark event for this respondent, and he remembers that it occurred in mid-2007, just as their children finished the school year. So, in 2007 he lost his job, near the end of the year, because the holiday season was particularly grim. He remembers that his depression was diagnosed after the holidays, but was it January or February of 2008? It was January 2008 because he was already taking antidepressants by Valentine's Day, when he went out to dinner with his wife and he could not drink wine with his meal (Figure 12.6).

As illustrated in Figure 12.6, landmark events probably serve as the primary organizational units of autobiographical knowledge and anchor information retrieval. In particular, the example shows how the respondent used landmark and other notable events, relationships among datable events, and general knowledge (holiday period and children finishing the school year) to reconstruct when his major depression was first diagnosed. An important caveat is that this respondent was willing to expend considerable effort searching his memory to determine when his depression was diagnosed, which may not be true for all respondents.

In contrast, to minimize satisficing, questionnaire developers should consider the length of the instrument and the number of response categories. When faced with a long list of choices, respondents more frequently choose answers at the top of the list rather than those at the bottom, to minimize effort. Respondents with lower cognitive skills and less education, where discerning the best possible response poses a challenge, are more apt to settle for a satisfactory rather than an optimal response. Because accuracy of response is critical for pharmacoepidemiologic research, questionnaire developers must consider methods to minimize response burden that leads to satisficing.

In addition to survey design and respondent motivation, measurement error can be attributed to improper training of interviewers and poor data entry. Understanding the measurement error associated with key variables is critical to the analysis. Measurement error can be assessed with the use of several different modeling approaches (for details, see Biemer, 2009).

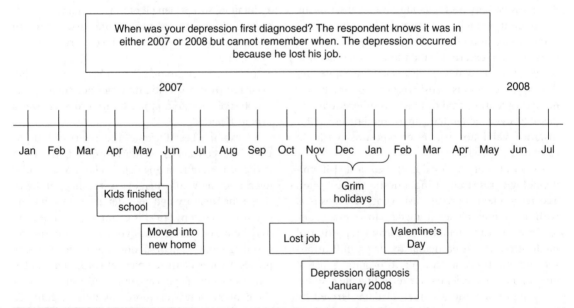

Figure 12.6 Recall schematic for showing how date of depression diagnosis was determined.

Conducting validation studies to assess self-reported data

Exposure confirmation performed as part of etiologic studies is often only partial verification, for two reasons. First, the comparison data source may be an alloyed gold standard, which means the rate calculated is a measure of agreement, not a measure of validity. Second, and more commonly, verification studies using a gold or an alloyed gold standard can assess only one of the two validity measures, either sensitivity or specificity.

Methodological studies that use alternative data sources such as prospectively collected data or databases of dispensed drugs can measure both sensitivity and specificity, if one assumes that the prescription database is a gold standard. Lower sensitivity is often more of a concern than lower specificity, depending on the data source used. Drug exposures or diseases underreported on questionnaires or missing due to incomplete claims processing in a record-linked database—that is, data sources with low sensitivity—cannot be rigorously evaluated as risk factors for the association under investigation. Alternatively, low specificity is often less of a problem in pharmacoepidemiology unless the characteristic with low specificity also has very low prevalence in the population being studied. For example, because the incidence of Stevens–Johnson syndrome is low, a small degree of misclassification will occur when the case definition in administrative claims data uses the ICD-9-CM code 695.1; included in the class will be several skin problems other than Stevens–Johnson (i.e., the false-positive rate will be high).

While data for each individual must be complete, data for all persons who are covered by the health plan also must appear in the database. Systematic omissions of specific population groups, such as specific ethnic or racial groups, diminish the quality of the database.

Considering the influence of comparator selection on validation studies

The medical record cannot be relied on to document all medications prescribed for individuals. Because people see a variety of health care providers, retrieval of medical records depends not only on the patient's ability to remember and report who prescribed a drug or diagnosed a condition, but also on the health care provider's attention to recording the information and on the availability of the medical record for review. Even if the outpatient or inpatient medical record is available, it may be incomplete for medications prescribed. Completeness may depend on the type of medication, as well: psychotropic medications, such as benzodiazepines, tend to be omitted more frequently than nonpsychotropic medications.

Medical records are often used to validate self-reported information about diagnoses, but the diagnosis documentation in the medical record may be incomplete. With conversion from paper to electronic medical records (EMRs), more studies are evaluating the completeness of the EMRs than are evaluating the completeness of paper medical records. This trend will likely continue as the use of this newer technology increases and as the documentation of clinical performance and quality of care is increasingly acknowledged as a critical factor in health care delivery.

Validation of pharmacoepidemiologic drug and diagnosis data from electronic encounter databases

In addition to ad hoc studies to evaluate drug–disease associations (see Chapter 10), various computerized, administrative databases may be used for pharmacoepidemiologic research—the structure, strengths, and limitations of which were reviewed in Chapters 8 and 9. The discussion below is specific to claims or encounter databases, rather than medical record databases.

The drawbacks and limitations of these data systems are important. Their most critical limitation for pharmacoepidemiologic research is the way health insurance is currently covered in the United States, typically through the place of employment. If the employer changes plans, which may be done annually, or the employee changes among the plans offered by the employer, or the employee changes jobs, then the plan no longer covers that employee or his or her family. Thus, the continual enrollment and disenrollment of plan members hinders the opportunity for longitudinal analyses. Unclear is whether and how enrollment and longitudinal follow-up capabilities will change because of the 2010 Patient Protection and Affordable Care Act.

Completeness and validity of data are the most critical elements in the selection of a database for research. *Completeness* is defined as the proportion of all exposures or, all events of interest that occurred in the population covered by the database that appear in the computerized data. Missing subjects, exposures, or events can introduce bias in the study results. For example, completeness of the drug data may vary by income level if persons with higher incomes and drug copayments choose to obtain their medications at pharmacies not participating in a prescription plan, which is the means of pharmacy data collection. Similarly, a bias may be introduced in the association between a drug and a serious adverse drug reaction if hospitalizations for that adverse reaction are missing from the database.

Special considerations with drug data

In 1984 Lessler and colleagues reported that drug dispensing data in Medicaid files are typically valid but that the same is not true for diagnosis data. Likely because of this research, drug data in administrative databases are often not validated. However, assumptions that claims for a drug are accurate and reflect complete representations of exposures may be incorrect and should be tested when the drug exposure or database is new. Other caveats for use of drug dispensing data are that they cannot address actual medication adherence or ingestion and that over-the-counter medication data are typically unavailable.

When using drug data from administrative databases for pharmacoepidemiologic studies, researchers may want to consider an incident ("new user") study design when appropriate. This design, in which the risk period begins when drug use is initiated, minimizes prevalent user bias. This bias may occur, for instance, if risk varies with exposure time and if early use affects, or is affected by, determinants of outcome. The new user design allows control of confounding variables at the point of drug initiation (i.e., before drug exposure may alter their measurement).

Special considerations with diagnosis and hospitalization data

Unlike the drug data in administrative databases, inpatient and outpatient diagnoses in these databases raise considerable concern for investigators. The accuracy of outpatient diagnoses is less certain than that of inpatient diagnoses for several reasons: hospitals employ experienced persons to code diagnoses for reimbursement, but individual physicians' offices may not. Moreover, hospital personnel scrutinize inpatient diagnoses for errors, which is unusual in the outpatient setting.

Systematic errors because of diagnostic coding may influence the validity of both inpatient and outpatient diagnostic data. For example, diseases listed in record-linked databases are often coded according to the International Classification of Disease (ICD). Poorly defined diseases are difficult to code under the ICD system; no way exists to indicate that an ICD code is the result of "ruling out" other codes. How health care plans address "rule-out" diagnoses is unclear: Are they included or excluded from the diagnoses in the physician claims files? In a study of transdermal scopolamine and seizure occurrence, many patients with ICD codes indicating seizures received this diagnosis code as a "rule-out" code, according to the actual diagnoses in their medical records. This result suggests that "rule-out" codes do become part of administrative claims data. In addition, reimbursement standards and patient insurance coverage limitations may influence the selection of ICD codes for billing. The potential for abuse of diagnostic codes, especially outpatient codes, may arise when physicians apply to either an insurance carrier or the government for reimbursement; the abuse would be less likely to occur in staff/group model health maintenance organizations, such as Group Health Cooperative or Kaiser Permanente. Lastly, ICD version changes may produce systematic errors.

Continuing with the NSAID example, we conducted another literature scan of published studies validating, in administrative databases, MI or GI bleeding outcomes following the use of NSAIDs. Validation studies often compare administrative data with medical records without calculating sensitivity and specificity. Most of these studies provide only positive predictive values, which indicate whether the coding scheme is accurately classifying observed measures as compared with another source. Case

Example 12.3 summarizes the findings from a study using the data from the Veteran's Administration to identify upper GI events with an algorithm consisting of ICD-9 and Current Procedural Terminology (CPT) codes. The measurement characteristics of the diagnosis codes selected for the algorithm depended on which codes were used.

Case example 12.3: (Abraham, 2006)

Background

- A variety of electronic administrative databases are available for pharmacoepidemiologic research. One major advantage of using such databases for pharmacoepidemiologic research is the comparative validity of the drug data in lieu of questionnaire data, for which recall bias is always a concern. However, databases differ in terms of demographic, clinical, diagnosis, and procedure data capture.

- New algorithms for identifying an outcome may have different reliability and validity than previously used algorithms, even in the same database. It is important to validate claims within each new database and to validate new algorithms upon development.

Question

- Within the Veteran's Affairs (VA) administrative data, what is the reliability and validity of various measures of diagnosis for nonsteroidal anti-inflammatory drug (NSAID)–related upper gastrointestinal events (UGIE)?

Approach

- A retrospective cohort database and medical record abstraction study was conducted of 906 veterans to determine the reliability and validity of ICD-9 and CPT codes to determine UGIE and to develop an algorithm to predict events among NSAID users.

- The ICD-9 codes used for UGIE were 531.x-534.x and 578.x. CPT procedural codes were 432xx, 443xx, 435xx, 436xx, 440xx, 446xx, 44120, 78278, 7424x, 7425x, and 74260.

- Multivariable logistic regression analysis was used to derive a predictive algorithm using ICD-9 codes, CPT codes, source of code (outpatient/inpatient), and patient age. The algorithm was developed and tested in separate cohorts from VA data.

Results

- Table 12.1 presents the sensitivity, specificity, positive predictive value (PPV), and negative predictive value (NPV) for the three claims-based diagnoses of UGIE evaluated and the algorithm PPV among NSAID users. The sensitivity dropped as diagnosis included broader parameters, while the PPV increased. Using both ICD-9 and CPT codes led to the highest specificity and NPV.

Table 12.1 Sensitivity, specificity, PPV and NPV for claims-based diagnoses of UGIE. Adapted from Abraham (2006) with permission from John Wiley and Sons.

Claims-based diagnosis of UGIE	Sensitivity (%)	Specificity (%)	Positive predictive value (%)	Negative predictive value (%)
Only ICD-9 codes for UGIE	100	96	27	100
ICD-9 and CPT codes for UGIE	82	100	51	99
ICD-9 and CPT algorithm for UGIE	66	88	67	88
Algorithm in only NSAID users	NA	NA	80	NA

NA = not applicable. UGIE = upper gastrointestinal events.

(*continued*)

Strengths

- Evaluation of sensitivity, specificity, PPV, and NPV provides the full picture of reliability and validity of claims for both patients diagnosed with UGIE and those without the diagnosis.
- Multiple diagnoses codes and a predictive algorithm were assessed, providing a robust evaluation for this data set, one that is suitable for future study and clinical decision-making.
- Data were from routine clinical and billing processes, so no additional burden of data collection for research purposes was necessary.

Limitations

- The study was conducted in one database (VA) only; validation results for the algorithm may not be applicable to different databases or patient populations.
- Multivariable logistic regression did not include multiple demographic or clinical factors that may affect occurrence of outcome. Additional factors may improve the reliability and validity of algorithm.

Key points

- Within the same database, different algorithms or codes used to assess a diagnosis may substantially affect the number of diagnoses captured. For instance, use of both ICD-9 and CPT codes for UGIE substantially decreased the sensitivity and increased the PPV for UGIE within claims data. Thus, validation of the specific codes or algorithm used to assess a diagnosis is key to understanding the findings from pharmacoepidemiologic research.
- Inclusion of a broader base of diagnoses, procedures, or other factors forming an algorithm to provide a diagnosis may increase specificity, but it does so at the expense of sensitivity. Sensitivity, specificity, PPV, and NPV are *all* necessary to provide a complete picture of the agreement between claims data and medical records.

Best practices

For the data in an administrative database to be considered valid, subjects who appear in the computerized files as having a drug exposure or disease should truly have that attribute, and those without the exposure or disease should truly not have the attribute. Validating the case definition for observational studies by comparing administrative databases with original documents, such as inpatient or outpatient medical records, is necessary to enhance research quality and credibility. Although many studies have reviewed original documents to validate the diagnoses under study, or have referenced validation studies, a need still exists for validation of drug exposures and disease diagnoses in other administrative databases or when no previous validation has been performed. As medical practice changes, further validation of previously validated claims will be warranted.

Evaluating the completeness of the databases is much more difficult because it requires an external data source known to be complete. Researchers determine validity and completeness by comparing the database information with other data sources,

such as medical records, administrative or billing records, pharmacy dispensings, or procedure logs. Choice of an appropriate comparator varies by study question, information used from the database and comparator, and availability of other data sources. Completeness is typically assessed for a particular component of a study, such as the effect of drug copayments on pharmacy claims, or the availability of discharge letters in the General Practice Research Database. The study by Lessler published almost 30 years ago indicated that pharmacy data from administrative databases were of high quality; because claims are used for reimbursing pharmacy dispensings, this finding should hold true today. However, adherence is an issue (see Chapter 20), and not every dispensing indicates exposure; the extent of unclaimed prescriptions and whether they affect research is unknown.

The investigator must be aware of the limitations of both the administrative database and the chosen comparison data set. For example, over-the-counter medications are unlikely to be available for study in either administrative claims or pharmacy dispensing records. The chosen comparator should provide sufficient data to validate both the exposure and outcome algorithms used for the study and to evaluate the completeness and accuracy of the chosen cohort. A variable that provides exact linkage between the data sets, such as a medical record number, should be available so that exact algorithms can be evaluated for accuracy within a subset of known study patients. For example, if a single claim contains six diagnosis codes and 6 months of claims were used to determine outcomes in patients, then all six diagnosis codes for all claims across the 6-month study time must be available in a comparison data set to establish the validity of the algorithm used for the outcome. A validation assessment should include evaluation of patients with and without the exposure or outcome: combined, positive predictive value, negative predictive value, sensitivity, and specificity provide a complete understanding of the agreement between the two data sets.

A validation study should include the following steps:

1. Choose a meaningful number of patients for validation. This sample size should be statistically grounded; however, considerations of data availability, cost, and labor are understandable.

2. Abstract variables required to determine cohort selection, exposure, outcome, and other variables for validation. Calculate measures of agreement between the two data sets.

3. Consider strengths and limitations of the two data sets to ascertain validity and completeness of the administrative database to answer the study question.

Analyses conducted to evaluate the usefulness of administrative databases for observational studies include assessment of:

- consistency among data files in the same system,
- surrogate markers of disease, and
- time-sequenced relationships, such as diagnostic procedures preceding surgery.

The future

This chapter reflects published methodological data-quality work as applied to the conduct of

pharmacoepidemiology studies, whether the medication and diagnostic data arise from questionnaires, administrative claims, or EMRs. It has discussed ways to minimize measurement error in epidemiologic studies, to validate important study variables in order to assess whether measurement errors have occurred, and to evaluate the impact of these errors on the direction and magnitude of effect.

Methods for conducting pharmacoepidemiology studies have shifted over the past 25–30 years from reliance on studies requiring *de novo* data collection from individuals, to extensive use of electronic data from either administrative health claims or EMRs. This evolution will increasingly incorporate studies using distributed data networks (see "FDA's Sentinel Initiative" in Chapter 22) and data from health information exchanges. Nevertheless, *de novo* data collection must still ascertain information on quality of life, patient-reported outcomes, and medications either not included in pharmacy dispensing files or not reliably entered into EMRs.

The improved computer technology that has resulted in faster processor speeds and increased storage capacity has facilitated the storage of health care data in an electronic format and has allowed development of distributed data networks, which use data from multiple health plans. The availability of these data for research has improved researchers' ability to conduct studies that require knowledge not only about whether a procedure or laboratory test was done, but also about the results of these clinical events. The advantage of access to electronic clinical data is lessened reliance on paper medical records to confirm diagnoses, which is especially important when little or no paper copy is available for review.

Although clinical practice in the United States has been moving toward EMRs slowly, the Health Information Technology for Economic and Clinical Health (HITECH) provisions of the 2009 American Recovery and Reinvestment Act established financial incentives for US providers to begin using EMRs in 2011. The increasing uptake of EMRs will lead to increased availability of more granular clinical data for pharmacoepidemiologic research. However, as with the validation process for research using administrative claims, data from EMRs will have to undergo scrutiny. Initial evaluation of EMR data suggests great promise, but data mapping and standardization of terminology and codes will be required to make these data, which are collected for clinical care, useful for research.

As part of the standardization process, data holders will have to document that their data are valid for conducting research and surveillance activities. This documentation will require investigators to apply their knowledge and practices from use of administrative claims data to EMR data and to data from health information exchanges, as both claims and EMR data are linked. The concern that Lessler and colleagues resolved about the validity of medication data for administrative claims is now being raised for prescribing data from EMRs—it is clear when the patient starts a medication, but the duration of use may not be adequately documented. Diagnosis data from EMRs do not carry the same level of concern for validity as claims data, because they are initially used for patient care, not for reimbursement; however, confirmation of the accuracy assumption still is needed. In the future, because EMR data will increasingly be used for research, we hope and expect to see studies validating EMR data.

Key points

• The validity of self-reported diagnosis and drug use data is a function of two properties: how accurately persons who have medical conditions or use drugs of interest are ascertained (sensitivity), and the accuracy with which those who do not have the conditions or do not use the drugs are identified (specificity).
• Misclassification of drug and diagnosis information obtained from study participants by questionnaires or interviews can be differential or nondifferential and depends on factors such as the training and experience of interviewers, the elapsed time since the events of interest took place, and characteristics of the participants, such as their medical status and age.
• If drug and diagnosis misclassification is nondifferential, or essentially random, associations

between drugs and diagnoses will usually be underestimated (i.e., biased toward the null). If the misclassification is systematic, or differential, associations that do not truly exist can appear to be present, or true associations can be overestimated or underestimated.
• Misclassification of drug and diagnosis information obtained from administrative databases is more likely to be nondifferential than differential, but the accuracy of diagnoses is of greater concern than the accuracy of drug information.
• The medical record is typically used as the gold standard for verifying drug and diagnosis information, but it may be incomplete and, with the increasing focus on privacy, such as the US Health Insurance Portability and Accountability Act, may be difficult to obtain.

Further reading

Abraham NS, Cohen DC, Rivers B, Richardson P (2006) Validation of administrative data used for the diagnosis of upper gastrointestinal events following nonsteroidal anti-inflammatory drug prescription. *Aliment Pharmacol Ther* **24** (2): 299–306.

Biemer P. Measurement errors in sample surveys. In: Pfeffermann D, Rao CR (eds.), *Handbook of Statistics—Sample Surveys: Design, Methods and Applications*. The Netherlands: North-Holland, pp. 281–316.

Bland JM, Altman DG (1986) Statistical methods for assessing agreement between two methods of clinical measurement. *Lancet* **1** (8476): 307–10.

Copeland KT, Checkoway H, McMichael AJ, Holbrook RH (1977) Bias due to misclassification in the estimation of relative risk. *Am J Epidemiol* **105** (5): 488–95.

Dosemeci M, Wacholder S, Lubin JH (1990) Does nondifferential misclassification of exposure always bias a true effect toward the null value? *Am J Epidemiol* **132** (4): 746–8.

Fourrier-Reglat A, Cuong HM, Lassalle R, Depont F, Robinson P, Droz-Perroteau C, *et al.* (2010) Concordance between prescriber- and patient-reported previous medical history and NSAID indication in the CADEUS cohort. *Pharmacoepidemiol Drug Saf* **19** (5): 474–81.

Gama H, Correia S, Lunet N (2009) Questionnaire design and the recall of pharmacological treatments: a systematic review. *Pharmacoepidemiol Drug Saf* **18** (3): 175–87.

Lash TL, Fox MP, Fink AK (2009) *Applying Quantitative Bias Analysis to Epidemiologic Data*. New York: Springer.

Lessler JT, Harris BSH (1984) *Medicaid Data as a Source for Postmarketing Surveillance Information*. Research Triangle Park, NC: Research Triangle Institute.

Maclure M, Willett WC (1987) Misinterpretation and misuse of the kappa statistic. *Am J Epidemiol* **126** (2): 161–9.

Mitchell AA, Cottler LB, Shapiro S (1986) Effect of questionnaire design on recall of drug exposure in pregnancy. *Am J Epidemiol* **123** (4): 670–6.

Poole C (1985) Exceptions to the rule about nondifferential misclassification. *Am J Epidemiol* **122**: 508.

Ray W (2003) Evaluating medication effects outside of clinical trials: New-user designs. *AJE* **158**: 915–20.

Rodgers A, MacMahon S (1995) Systematic underestimation of treatment effects as a result of diagnostic test inaccuracy: implications for the interpretation and design of thromboprophylaxis trials. *Thromb Haemost* **73** (2): 167–71.

Rothman KJ, Greenland S (2008) Precision and validity in epidemiologic studies. In: *Modern epidemiology*. 3rd ed. Philadelphia, PA: Lippincott, Williams & Wilkins.

Tourangeau R, Rips LJ, Rasinski K (2000) *The Psychology of Survey Response*. Cambridge, MA: Cambridge University Press.

Wacholder S, Armstrong B, Hartge P (1993) Validation studies using an alloyed gold standard. *Am J Epidemiol* **137** (11): 1251–8.

West SL, Ritchey ME, Poole C (2012) Validity of pharmacoepidemiology drug and diagnosis data. In: BL Strom, S Hennessy, SE Kimmel (eds.), *Pharmacoepidemiology* (5th ed.), Sussex: John Wiley & Sons, Ltd, pp. 757–94.

West SL, Savitz DA, Koch G, Strom BL, Guess HA, Hartzema A (1995) Recall accuracy for prescription medications: self-report compared with database information. *Am J Epidemiol* **142** (10): 1103–12.

CHAPTER 13

Assessing Causality of Case Reports of Suspected Adverse Events

Judith K. Jones

The Degge Group Ltd, Arlington, VA and Georgetown University, Washington, DC, USA

Introduction

An important component in evaluating suspected adverse drug reaction reports in clinical and/or clinical trial settings is the assessment about the degree to which any reported event is causally associated with the suspected drug. In reality, a particular event is either caused or not caused by a particular drug, but current assessment tools almost never permit a definitive determination. Several approaches to assessing the probability of a causal connection have evolved. This chapter will review current approaches and place them into their regulatory context and application.

Clinical problems to be addressed by pharmacoepidemiologic research

The basic clinical problem with applying causality assessment is that clinical events may be associated with multiple possible causal factors. The task is to conduct a differential diagnosis and evaluate the degree to which the occurrence of an event is linked to one particular suspected causal agent: a drug or other medicinal agent.

Evaluating causality in epidemiologic studies of chronic diseases differs from causality assessment in individual case reports. In epidemiologic studies, causality determination relates to events in one or more defined population studies. In contrast, in case reports of suspected adverse reactions to a medicinal product (typically submitted to the manufacturer, regulatory agency, or the literature), data are often incomplete and causal assessment is challenging. Reports often represent a clinician's suspicion of a causal association, thus the reporter and the evaluator often make an implicit judgment of causality. Single reports often have several attributes that represent obstacles to causality assessments, specifically:

1. The reporter usually *suspects* that the clinical event is associated with the exposure. This suspicion can often bias the collection of data required to evaluate other possible causes.
2. The data on exposure to suspect and concomitant drugs are often incomplete, usually missing information on duration, actual dose, and past history.
3. Available data on the adverse event, including onset, characteristics, and time course are typically incomplete, partly because the suspicion is usually retrospective and desired data (e.g., baseline laboratory data) are often not available at initial report.
4. Complete data on patient history of concomitant diseases, diet, lifestyle, and other confounders are typically not available, often because reports are based upon suspicion of a product, rather than on a differential diagnosis.

Textbook of Pharmacoepidemiology, Second Edition. Edited by Brian L. Strom, Stephen E. Kimmel, and Sean Hennessy.
© 2013 John Wiley & Sons, Ltd. Published 2013 by John Wiley & Sons, Ltd.

Adverse reactions to drugs can be acute, sub-acute, or chronic, can be reversible or not (e.g., birth defects and death), can be rare or common. They can be pathologically unique or identical to known diseases. Thus, defining general data elements and criteria for assessing causality that will apply to most types of suspected adverse reactions is challenging. For example, for irreversible events (birth defects or death), data on drug dechallenge (discontinuation) and rechallenge (reintroduction) are inapplicable. Furthermore, the reporter's motivation and the impact of a causal inference on his/her actions is a factor in the assessment's rigor; if the assessment will have little impact on future patients (in a clinical setting) or to product labeling (in the regulatory environment), the assessment might be less rigorous. Conversely, if, for example, continuation of a clinical trial or development program depends upon the assessment, the rigor of the method of assessment becomes more critical.

Historical perspectives: development of concepts

Thinking about the causality of adverse reactions evolved at approximately the same time in two disciplines: (1) in epidemiology, and (2) in the evaluation of individual case reports of suspected adverse reactions.

In 1959, Yerushalmy and Palmer drew upon the Koch–Henle postulates for establishing causation for infectious diseases and proposed analogous criteria for the causal nature of an association in epidemiologic studies. In 1965, Bradford-Hill expanded these concepts further when he proposed nine criteria – *strength, consistency, specificity, temporality, biological gradient, plausibility, coherence, experiment,* and *analogy* – to further guide assessment of causality in epidemiologic studies. These criteria continue to be generally used in chronic disease epidemiology.

However, in assessment of adverse drug reactions, prior to the development of specific criteria for these reports, as described below, the typical approach to case reports was to consider the events

as possibly associated with the drug simply if there were a number of similar reports. Considerations of pharmacologic plausibility, dose-response, and timing factors were sometimes implicit, but seldom explicit. This unstructured approach, called "global introspection," is still used. In a *qualitative* probability scale, judgments are expressed as "definite," "probable," "possible," "doubtful" or "unrelated."

The subjective nature of global introspection led Nelson Irey, a pathologist at the US Armed Forces Institute of Pathology, and two clinical pharmacologists, Karch and Lasagna, to simultaneously develop approaches for a more standardized assessment: They used very similar basic data elements:

1. Timing relative to drug exposure;
2. Presence/absence of other potential causal factors;
3. Dechallenge;
4. Rechallenge;
5. Other supportive data, *e.g.,* previous cases.
   See Case Example 13.1.

The objective was to evaluate causality from either a single case or a group of cases from an ill-defined exposed population. Without all nine Bradford-Hill criteria, there would be no way to evaluate the consistency, strength, or specificity of the association (with some exceptions). The temporal relationship does apply in both Irey and Karch and Lasagna and in some cases biological plausibility has been included in the criteria for single cases with a specific pharmacologic mechanism or dose response.

Following the introduction of these methods for the assessment of suspected adverse drug reactions, a large number of other approaches were developed in the form of algorithms, decision tables, and in one case, as a diagrammatic method. Most share basic elements and an example of a widely used scoring method is presented in Figure 13.1.

To address the inherent limitations, a more advanced approach to causality assessment, based on the Bayes probability theorem, emerged. This approach considered the probability of an event occurring in the presence of a drug relative to its probability of occurring in the absence of the drug, considering all known background information and all details of the case. The different types of

Case Example 13.1: General approach to causality assessment of a suspected adverse drug reaction

Background

- Application of a structured causality assessment can serve as a template for standardized assessment of the different elements of a case report of an adverse event that is suspected to be caused a drug.

- A formal approach helps avoids "global introspection," which is naturally biased by an assessor's own knowledge and preconceived notions.

Issue

- A 68-year-old Caucasian female with a history of severe osteoarthritis and occasional angina pectoris is given a prescription for a moderately potent nonsteroidal anti-inflammatory drug (NSAID) to be used at the lowest dose. Five days after starting therapy, she experiences two episodes of angina on exertion in the same day. Upon contacting her physician, she is instructed to discontinue the NSAID. She experiences no further anginal attacks, but is also distressed at the return of her painful arthritis. On her own, she restarts the NSAID. Within three days, she experiences four episodes of angina on exertion and notifies her physician who instructs her to stop the NSAID and come in the next day for an office examination. She has no further episodes of angina after discontinuing the drug.

Approach

- Identify key components that may help assess causality and a differential diagnosis: (1) timing (in both cycles); (2) other causes of the event and prior history of the event; (3) dechallenge (improvement upon discontinuing suspected drug); (4) rechallenge (return of event on reintroduction of drug); and (5) prior history of the drug–event association (not always used if event is the first observed).

Results

- Timing is consistent in both cycles with initiation of drug intake, but also with the ability to increase exercise level (see other factors, below).

- Other factors that may explain the event include prior history of angina, an intermittent condition, and increased exercise with relief of the arthritis.

- Dechallenge is positive both times.

- Rechallenge is positive.

- There are no data on dose or blood levels (biological plausibility).

- Global introspection on this case might reflect assessor's information biases. One oriented to NSAID GI effects might consider this a masked GI event. Another might consider the improved exercise tolerance as a cause, while another might suspect a direct vasoconstrictor effect of the NSAID. Despite the presence of positive dechallenges and a rechallenge, if the algorithm used gives "other factors" higher weight to offset the score or weight of dechallenge/rechallenge, then many methods would find this event "possibly related" to the NSAID.

- Confounding by the increased exercise tolerance and the intrinsic intermittency of the angina would make a stronger association less likely in the absence of further data.

- A Bayesian approach would try to identify, from clinical trials or observational data on the pattern of angina pectoris, the prior odds of the pattern of the two separate intermittent episodes of angina episodes occurring in (1) the absence and (2) the presence of the NSAID. Then the actual case is analyzed by evaluating the likelihood (if drug caused or not) of *each* of the following components: history of angina (e.g., the ratio of the probability of the pattern of angina given NSAID causation / the probability of the angina pattern given non-NSAID causation), timing of the episodes relative to drug start; dechallenge and its timing in both episodes; and rechallenge and its timing.

Strengths

- Use of specific categories of data to understand the dynamics of the event and the dosing and possible pharmacologic properties of the drug directs the deliberation to consider more possibilities to explain the pathophysiology and ultimately the probability of drug causation of the event.

- The Bayesian approach is more structured and intensive.

(*continued*)

Limitations

- Methods that are verbal or have numerical scores that do not always relate to actual pathophysiology may lead to misleading conclusions.
- Methods that require more data are often frustrated by the simple lack of data needed, and, when applying the Bayesian method specifically, the lack of baseline data in the population to make prior probability or likelihood judgments.

Key points

- Applications of a structured causality method can standardize and help reduce biases in assessing the possible cause-effect relationship of an event to a particular drug exposure.
- The components of causality assessment methods can help structure data collection on individual and groups of cases; ultimately, these aggregate data can improve the description of the event of interest, and possibly its relationship to a drug, or the disease of indication.
- The detailed probabilistic and explicit approach in the Bayesian method can, if data are available, provide a basis for developing more precise statements of the hypothesis that is posed in a spontaneous report of a suspected adverse drug reaction.

methods are described more fully and compared in the "Current tools" section below.

Uses of causality assessment

Pharmaceutical manufacturers

Pharmaceutical sponsors must apply causality assessment for events associated with their drugs for regulatory compliance in different countries and for product liability. In the US, FDA's regulations contain an implicit requirement for causality assessment. Sponsors must report serious unexpected events in clinical trials where there is a "reasonable possibility" that the events may have been caused by the drug (21 CFR § 312.32). However, a report *is not* an admission of causation. These regulations do not provide criteria or a

CAUSALITY ASSESSMENT
NARANJO SCORED ALGORITHM

QUESTION	ANSWER			SCORE
	Yes	No	Unk	
Previous reports?	+1	0	0	_____
Event after drug?	+2	−1	0	_____
Event abate on drug removal?	+1	0	0	_____
+ Rechallenge?	+2	−1	0	_____
Alternative causes?	−1	+2	0	_____
Reaction with placebo?	−1	+1	0	_____
Drug blood level toxic?	+1	0	0	_____
Reaction dose-related?	+1	0	0	_____
Past history of similar event?	+1	0	0	_____
ADR confirmed objectively?	+1	0	0	_____
Total Score				_____

Figure 13.1 A critical scored algorithm illustrated by the method of Naranjo *et al.* in wide use. This particular method uses some of the basic data elements as well as more details of the history and characteristics of the case, and a score is designated for the response to each question.

suggested method. Postmarketing regulations in the US also require reporting of all events associated with the drug "whether or not thought to be associated with the drug" (21 CFR §314.80). These reports are commonly referred to as "spontaneous reports."

Internationally, many regulatory agencies have suggested method(s) to minimize the number of nonspecific events reported, described below.

Drug regulators

Many countries have some method of approaching causality and the tools they use vary widely. In Europe, assessment methods were formally considered, and a European Medicines Agency's CPMP Working Party on Pharmacovigilance reached consensus on causality terms to be used that became a European Community Directive (*EC Document III/3445/91* -EN, July 1991). In 1994, Health Canada instituted a formal method of causality assessment for reports of vaccine-associated adverse events. France has required a formal imputability method for more than two decades.

Reports of adverse reactions to journals

Medical journals containing case reports of suspected adverse reactions largely avoid assessing causality. The majority of single case reports, letters to the editor, or short publications do not provide an explicit judgment using any of the published algorithms. Further, many reports do not provide information on confounding therapies or medical conditions–data elements considered essential for considering causality. However, the *Annals of Pharmacotherapy* requires that the Naranjo method (see Figure 13.1) be applied and reported in all case reports published.

Lack of a structured approach to publication of case reports was recognized in the early 1980s, and publications from a consensus conference proposed that publication of case reports require at minimum the five elements of the criteria for causality – timing, nature of the reaction, dechallange, rechallenge, and alternate causes based on prior history. Harumbaru and colleagues compared 500 published reports with 500 spontaneous reports to determine whether they contained the information

needed in most standard causality assessments. They found that although the published reports contained significantly more information, data were sparse on alternate causes / other diseases and other drugs in both types of reports. In an effort to address this problem of incomplete published reports, augmented publication guidelines with illustrative examples were published in two drug safety journals in 2006 by a task force of the International Society of Pharmacoepidemiology.

Other applications

There are other settings where standard assessments of causality of serious events could be useful: in clinical trials; formal consensus evaluations of new serious postmarketing spontaneous reports by sponsors and regulators; in the clinical setting as part of the differential diagnosis; and possibly in the courtroom or the newsroom.

Methodological problems to be addressed by pharmacoepidemiologic research

Drug-associated adverse events vary in frequency, manifestations, timing relative to exposure, and mechanisms; they mimic almost the entire range of human pathology, and have added unique new pathologies (e.g., kidney stones consisting of drug crystals, and the oculomucocutaneous syndrome caused by practolol). Symptom variations compound the causality assessment due to inadequate case definitions. Additionally, drug-associated events are often accompanied by other pathologies associated with the original illness. But unknown or unexpected events are not consistently recognized and/or described; therefore baseline and other detailed measurements are often not recorded.

Two divergent philosophies have developed. Some discount the value of causality assessment of individual reactions, deferring judgment to the results of formal epidemiologic studies or clinical trials. In contrast, Naranjo and others contend that the information in single reports can be evaluated to determine some degree of association, and that this can be useful–sometimes critical–when considering discontinuation of a clinical trial or development or market withdrawal of a drug. This latter view has spurred the evolution of causal assessment from expert consensual opinion (global introspection) to structured algorithms and elaborate Bayesian probabilistic approaches.

Current tools

Illustrative examples of four basic types of assessments that have been widely described in publications are described below.

Unstructured clinical judgment/global introspection

The most common approach is probably unstructured clinical judgment/global introspection. One or more experts review available clinical information and judge the likelihood that the adverse event resulted from drug exposure. However, it has been amply demonstrated that global introspection does not work well.

First, cognitive psychologists have shown that the ability of the human brain to make unaided assessments of uncertainty in complicated situations is poor, especially when assessing the probability of a cause and effect, precisely the task of causality assessment. This limitation has been repeatedly demonstrated in studies examining the evaluation of suspected adverse reactions. Several studies have used "expert" clinical pharmacologists to review suspected reactions and compared individual evaluations. They documented considerable disagreement and illustrated, thereby, how unreliable global introspection is as a causality assessment method.

Second, global introspection is uncalibrated. One assessor's "possible" might be another's "probable." This discrepancy was well demonstrated in Venulet's study of one pharmaceutical company's spontaneous report reviewers (who used both verbal and numerical scales).

Despite these concerns, global introspection continues to be used. For example, the WHO

International Centre for Drug Monitoring in Uppsala, Sweden, collects the spontaneous reports from national centres worldwide. It has published causality criteria ranging from "certain" to "unassessable/unclassifiable" that essentially represent six levels of global introspection, though they also generally incorporate consideration of the more standard criteria for causality.

Algorithm/criterial method with verbal judgments

These methods range from simple (10 or fewer questions) to lengthy (up to 84 questions) questionnaires. They share a basic structure based on the five criteria: timing, dechallenge, rechallenge, confounding, and prior history of the event. Information relevant to each element is elicited by a series of questions; the answers are restricted to "yes/no" (and for some methods "don't know"). These approaches are used by some drug regulatory agencies, including Australia's, and was used previously in an FDA algorithm.

Combining global introspection with an algorithm improved the consistency of ratings among reviewers. Since consideration of each case is segmented into components (e.g., timing, confounding diseases, etc.), this approach can highlight areas of disagreement. However, considerable global introspection is required to make judgments on the separate elements. These judgments require, in some cases, "yes" or "no" answers where a more quantitative estimate of uncertainty would be more appropriate. For example, the reviewer might have to consider whether the appearance of jaundice within one week represented a sufficient duration of drug exposure to be consistent with a drug–event association.

Algorithms requiring scoring of individual judgments

Several algorithms permit quantitative judgments by requiring the scoring of their criteria. The answers to questions are converted into a score for each factor, the scores summed, and this overall score converted into a value on a quantitative probability scale. These quantitative methods are used in a number of settings, from evaluations of suspected adverse reactions by hospital committees to applications by French and other regulators. Some pharmaceutical manufacturers also use them, although generally in a research context. A more practical example, Naranjo's, discussed previously, is shown in Figure 13.1.

In the 1990s, the Roussel Uclaf Causality Assessment Method (RUCAM) was developed by Bénichou and Danan. It has six criteria, with three or four levels of scoring for each, to derive an overall score. This method was recently applied in evaluation of adverse events in HIV clinical trials and was cited in a recent review of methods of assessment of hepatic injury. However, other critics stated that RUCAM's reliability is mediocre and that other methods may be more appropriate.

Probabilistic methods

The Bayesian method assesses the probability of an event occurring in the presence of a drug, relative to the probability of that event occurring in its absence (see Figure 13.2). Estimation of this overall probability, the "posterior probability," is based on two components:

1. What is known prior to the event (the "prior probability"), based on clinical trial and epidemiologic data; and
2. The likelihood for drug causation of *each* of the components of the specific case, including history, timing, characteristics, dechallenge and its timing components, rechallenge, and any other factors, such as multiple rechallenges.

Full application of this method requires detailed knowledge of the clinical event, its epidemiology, and relatively specific information about the event. Examples have been published for several types of events, including Stevens-Johnson syndrome, renal toxicity, lithium dermatitis, ampicillin-associated colitis, agranulocytosis, and Guillain-Barré syndrome. It appears useful for analyzing perplexing first events in new drug clinical trials, serious spontaneous adverse reaction reports, and possibly rare events discovered in cohort studies, when standard methods of statistical analysis do not provide sufficient clues as to causality because of inadequate sample size.

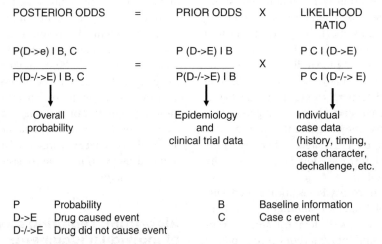

Figure 13.2 The basic equations for the Bayesian analysis of suspected drug-associated events. These provide a structured, yet flexible and explicit approach to estimating the probability that an event is associated with one or more, drugs, as described in the text and extensive literature dating from Auriche (1985), Lane (1990), and others. Since the prior probability estimate is dependent on explicit data from clinical trials and epidemiologic studies, this approach can provide a framework for specific event-related questions in these studies.

As disease natural histories and drug-induced diseases are now being described in large population databases, it will be essential to apply these analyses to population data. An excellent example of the application of this Bayesian method, with an additional complimentary method developed by Begaud and colleagues using the Poisson method for estimating the probability of rare events in populations was published recently by Zapater and colleagues. They have demonstrated the feasibility of utilizing clinical trial *and* population data to estimate the posterior probabilities of association in complex cases of ticlopidine-associated hepatitis.

Comparison among the different methods

Several efforts have been made to evaluate and compare these methods. Pere published an elegant and detailed evaluation of six representative algorithmic methods, identified standard evaluation criteria, and evaluated 1134 adverse reactions using various methods. Significantly, he found only moderate agreement between all pairs, and considerable disagreements on weightings of three of the major criteria–timing, dechallenge, and alternate etiologies–which underscores the lack of considerable information on the events and their characteristics.

Even today there is no consensus. In 2008, Agbabiaka and colleagues assessed 34 different methods and determined that there is still no universally accepted method. These findings were similar to those of Macedo's group in 2006. Others have stated that experts, working independently without a framework, frequently disagree on causality assessments because they are subjective, which leads to poor reproducibility and to disagreements. This lack of consensus by experts exists regardless of the adverse event type examined (e.g., vaccines, hypersensitivity reactions, hepatotoxicity).

Given the current state of affairs, where a number of published methods exist, the choice of a method for use in evaluating individual adverse effects will likely be determined by a number of practical factors. These include:

1. *How the evaluation will be used.* This refers to both short-term use (e.g., a rating suggesting more-than-possible association may be needed to result in a "signal") and long-term use (e.g., will a single "highly probable" case in a file, not otherwise acted upon, be a source of liability for the evaluator?).

2. *The importance of the accuracy of the judgment.* If this evaluation will determine either a specific clinical outcome, the continuation of a clinical trial, or the continued marketing of a drug, the accuracy of the judgment may be critical, then use of quantitative or the Bayesian method would be more appropriate. Conversely, if little hinges upon the judgment, unrefined estimates and methods may suffice.

3. *The number of causality evaluations to be made.* These considerations must also be weighed against the time required to make judgments on large numbers of reports, a dilemma for regulatory agencies and sponsors. Here the need for accurate judgments is pitted against the volume of evaluations to be considered. FDA's approach is to identify high priority problems according to their newness and seriousness.

4. *The accrued value of thorough evaluations.* In some circumstances, careful, rigorous evaluation of certain categories of drug-associated events facilitates more accurate evaluation of subsequent, related events. For example, consider a case where a drug under development is anticipated to cause hepatic events. Detailed evaluations of hepatic events induced by *older* drugs may allow more satisfactory causality evaluation of reports received on the new drug. Sometimes, this results from data collection being focused to a much greater degree on disease-specific criteria for events. France is even developing special disease-specific reporting forms.

5. *Who will be performing the evaluation?* Although no specific studies have been carried out to evaluate the differences among differently trained professionals, it is likely that knowledge held by each reviewer will have considerable impact on any method used, including the Bayesian method.

The future

The field of adverse reaction causality assessment has many unresolved issues, both methodological and practical. Originally there was hope a consensus method would be found, but the current state of the field would suggest that this is unlikely for several reasons.

First, some individuals and institutions have adopted one or a few methods and have committed to their use, often through their choice of data collecting systems or software. Second, practical aspects in using them appear to play a very real role. Although discussed with excitement as the possible "gold standard" for adverse reaction causality, the Bayesian method has not been widely embraced, partly because it is difficult to use without automation. With the lifting of that barrier, and with further practical applications, its potential may be realized. Third, the misuse of judgment terms or scores within the legal arena has generated concern, particularly given the fact that there is no reliable standard terminology.

All of these factors suggest the need for considerable further work in several areas:

1. Determining the *applications* of causality assessment, that is, the "output" of the process, so as to better define the desired rigor, accuracy, and usability of the methods. It would appear that there will probably always be needs for simpler and rougher methods, as well as more complete and rigorous methods, when the determination has considerable impact.

2. Further defining of the *critical elements needed* for evaluation of causality for different types of adverse reactions (e.g., hepatic, hematological, skin, etc.) so that this information may be collected at the time of reporting or publishing a spontaneous event. Such improvements can have a major impact on:

    a. collection of better information on the different drug-associated events, using data collection instruments tailored to the event of interest; and

    b. better definition of the dynamics and, ultimately, the pathophysiology and mechanisms of certain types of drug-induced conditions, which

is actively underway for some events such as liver toxicity.

3. Gathering of data on *critical elements* of the specific adverse events in the course of both clinical trials and epidemiologic studies. Risk factor, history, timing, characteristics, and resolution patterns of adverse events should be described in these studies and incorporated into general data resources on the characteristics of medical events and diseases.

4. Further work on *automation* of the causality evaluation process. Global introspection is still widely used because of the cumbersome nature of many of the more complete methods. Fortunately, some methods are now being automated, including the French method. Convenient access to the proper questions, arrayed in logical order, as well as background data meeting quality criteria on the state of information to date, has potential for considerably improving the state of adverse reaction causality evaluation.

5. Consideration of *new and different* methods. Although it is likely that further work will use one or more of the many available methods, it is interesting that other approaches have emerged. For example, as part of work on patient safety in the US, "root cause analysis" is used to identify important contributors to adverse events in clinical settings. This approach creates functional maps of possible contributing factors to not only identify a cause but also preventative measures. Another approach is the *N*-of-1 trial, which can evaluate the causality of adverse events in individuals, particularly those who have experienced multiple reactions to drugs.

In conclusion, the topic of assessing causality of adverse reactions continues to represent a challenge. With increased awareness of the need to consider causality as part of the regulatory process, the need for consensus, possibly on more than one method depending on use, continues. One major result of the application of detailed causality assessment, particularly when viewed prospectively with collection of data in both pharmacovigilance centres and clinical studies, is that these data can ultimately contribute to the overall understanding of the many drug-associated diseases.

Key points

• Applications of a structured causality method can standardize and help reduce biases in assessing the possible cause-effect relationship of an event to a drug exposure.

• The use of a clinical nonstructured approach ("global introspection") to assess adverse events believed to be associated with a drug has been shown to yield inconsistent results between raters; its lack of structure does not further the development of the hypothesis raised in the report of the event.

• The choice of a method is based upon the use of the judgment; if pivotal to continued development of a drug, the most rigorous methods such as the Bayesian approach may help; if used to sort out well-documented cases that may probably be associated with a drug, then simple algorithms or scoring algorithms usually suffice.

• The components of causality assessment methods can help structure data collection on individual and groups of cases; ultimately, these aggregate data can improve the description of the event of interest, and possibly its relationship to a drug, or the disease of indication.

• The detailed probabilistic and explicit approach in the Bayesian method can, if data are available, provide a basis for developing more precise statements of the hypothesis that is posed in a spontaneous report of a suspected adverse drug reaction.

Further reading

Agbabiaka TB, Savović J, Ernst E (2008) Methods for causality assessment of adverse drug reactions: a systematic review. *Drug Saf* **31** (1): 21–37.

Arimone Y, Miremont-Salamé G, Haramburu F, Molimard M, Moore N, Fourrier-Réglat A, Bégaud B (2007) Inter-expert agreement of seven criteria in causality assessment of adverse drug reactions, *Br J Clin Pharmacol* **64** (4): 482–8.

Arimone Y, Bégaud B, Miremont-Salamé G, Fourrier-Réglat A, Molimard M, Moore N, Haramburu F (2006) A new method for assessing drug causation provided agreement with experts' judgment. *J Clin Epidemiol* **59** (3): 308–14.

Benahmed S, Picot MC, Hillaire-Buys D, Blayac JP, Dujols P, Demoly P (2005) Comparison of pharmacovigilance algorithms in drug hypersensitivity reactions. *Eur J Clin Pharmacol* **61** (7): 537–41.

Bénichou C, Danan G (1994) A new method for drug causality assessment: RUCAM. In: *Adverse Drug Reactions. A Practical Guide To Diagnosis and Management*. New York: John Wiley & Sons Ltd, pp. 277–84.

Collet J-P, MacDonald N, Cashman N, Pless R (2000) The Advisory Committee on Causality Assessment. Monitoring signals for vaccine safety: the assessment of individual adverse event reports by an expert advisory committee. *Bull World Health Organ* **78**: 178–85.

Drug Information Association (1986) Proceedings of the Drug Information Association Workshop, Arlington, Virginia, February 1986, *Drug Inf J* **20**: 383–533.

García-Cortés M, Lucena MI, Pachkoria K, Borraz Y, Hidalgo R, Andrade RJ (2008) Spanish Group for the Study of Drug-induced Liver Disease (grupo de Estudio para las Hepatopatías Asociadas a Medicamentos, Geham). Evaluation of Naranjo adverse drug reactions probability scale in causality assessment of drug-induced liver injury. *Aliment Pharmacol Ther* **27** (9): 780–9.

Haramburu F, Begaud B, Pere JC (1990) Comparison of 500 spontaneous and 500 published reports of adverse drug reactions. *Eur J Clin Pharmacol* **39**: 287–8.

Irey NS (1976) Adverse drug reactions and death: a review of 827 cases. *JAMA* **236**: 575–8.

Jones JK (2012) Assessing causality of case reports of suspected adverse events. In: Strom BL, Kimmel SE, Hennessy S, eds., *Pharmacoepidemilogy*. 5th edn, John Wiley & Sons, Ltd, pp. 583–600.

Karch FE, Lasagna L (1977) Toward the operational identification of adverse drug reactions. *Clin Pharmacol Ther* **21**: 247–54.

Kelly WN, Arellano FM, Barnes J, Bergman U, Edwards IR, Fernandez AM, Freedman SB, Goldsmith DI, Huang K, Jones JK, McLeay R, Moore N, Stather RH, Trenque T, Troutman WG, Van Puijenbroek E, Williams, Wise RP (2007) Guidelines for submitting adverse event reports for publication. *Pharmacoepidemiol Drug Safety* **16**: 581–7.

Lane D (1990) Causality assessment for adverse drug reactions: a probabilistic approach. In Berry D, ed., *Statistical Methodology in the Pharmaceutical Sciences*. New York: Marcel Dekker, pp. 475–507.

Macedo AF, Marques FB, Ribeiro CF (2006) Can decisional algorithms replace global introspection in the individual causality assessment of spontaneously reported ADRs? **29** (8): 697–702.

Pere JC, Begaud B, Harambaru F, Albin H (1986) Computerized comparison of six adverse drug reaction assessment procedures. *Clin Pharmacol Ther* **40**: 451–61.

Rochon J, Protiva P, Seeff LB, Fontana RJ, Liangpunsakul S, Watkins PB, Davern, T, McHutchison JG; Drug-Induced Liver Injury Network (DILIN) (2008) Reliability of the *Drug Saf* Roussel Uclaf Causality Assessment Method for assessing causality in drug-induced liver injury, *Hepatology* **48** (4): 1175–83.

Rockey DC, Seeff LB, Rochon J, Freston J, Chalasani N, Bonacini M, Fontana RJ, Hayashi PH, US Drug-Induced Liver Injury Network (2010) Causality assessment in drug-induced liver injury using a structured expert opinion process: comparison to the Roussel-Uclaf causality assessment method, *Hepatology* **51** (6): 2117–26.

Sabaté M, Ibáñez L, Pérez E, Vidal X, Buti M, Xiol X, Mas A, Guarner C, Forné M, Solà R, Castellote J, Rigau J, Laporte JR (2011) Paracetamol in therapeutic dosages and acute liver injury: causality assessment in a prospective case series. *BMC Gastroenterol* **15** (11): 80.

Yerushalmy J, Palmer CE (1959) On the methodology of investigations of etiologic factors in chronic diseases. *J Chronic Dis* **10** (1): 27–40.

Zapater P, Such J, Perez-Mateo M, Horga JF (2002) A new Poisson and Bayesian -based method to assign risk and causality in patients with suspected hepatic adverse drug reactions. *Drug Safety* **25**: 735–50.

CHAPTER 14

Molecular Pharmacoepidemiology

Stephen E. Kimmel[1], Hubert G. Leufkens[2], and Timothy R. Rebbeck[1]

[1]*Perelman School of Medicine at the University of Pennsylvania, Philadelphia, PA, USA*
[2]*Utrecht Institute for Pharmaceutical Sciences, Utrecht University, Utrecht, The Netherlands*

Introduction

One of the most challenging areas in clinical pharmacology and pharmacoepidemiology is to understand why individuals and groups of individuals respond differently to a specific drug therapy, both in terms of beneficial and adverse effects. Reidenberg observed that, while the prescriber has basically two decisions to make while treating patients (i.e., choosing the right drug and choosing the right dose), interpreting the inter-individual variability in outcomes of drug therapy includes a wider spectrum of variables, including the patient's health profile, prognosis, disease severity, quality of drug prescribing and dispensing, adherence with prescribed drug regimen (see Chapter 20), and last, but not least, the genetic profile of the patient.

Molecular pharmacoepidemiology is the study of the manner in which molecular biomarkers alter the clinical effects of medications in populations. Just as the basic science of pharmacoepidemiology is epidemiology, applied to the content area of clinical pharmacology, the basic science of molecular pharmacoepidemiology is epidemiology in general and molecular epidemiology specifically, also applied to the content area of clinical pharmacology. Thus, many of the methods and techniques of epidemiology apply to molecular pharmacoepidemiologic studies. However, there are features of molecular pharmacoepidemiology that are unique to the field, as discussed later in this chapter. Most of the discussion will focus on studies related to genes, but the methodological considerations apply equally to studies of proteins and other biomarkers.

On average for each medication, it has been estimated that about one out of three treated patients experience beneficial effects, one out of three do not show the intended beneficial effects, 10% experience only side effects, and the rest of the patient population is nonadherent so that the response to the drug is difficult to assess. This highlights the challenge of individualizing therapy to produce a maximal beneficial response and minimize adverse effects. Although many factors can influence medication efficacy and adverse effects, including age, drug interactions, and medication adherence (see Chapter 20), genetics is an important contributor in the response of an individual to a medication. Genetic variability can account for a large proportion (e.g., some estimates range from 20% to 95%) of variability in drug disposition and medication effects.

In addition to altering dosing requirements, genetics can influence response to therapy by altering drug targets or the pathophysiology of the disease states that drugs are used to treat.

Definitions and concepts

Genetic variability

Building on the success of the various human genome initiatives, it is now estimated that there are approximately 25 000 regions of the human genome that are recognized as genes because they

Textbook of Pharmacoepidemiology, Second Edition. Edited by Brian L. Strom, Stephen E. Kimmel, and Sean Hennessy.
© 2013 John Wiley & Sons, Ltd. Published 2013 by John Wiley & Sons, Ltd.

contain *deoxyribonucleic acid (DNA)* sequence elements including exons (sequences that encode proteins), introns (sequences between exons that do not directly encode amino acids), and regulatory regions (sequences that determine gene expression by regulating the transcription of DNA to RNA, and then the translation of RNA to protein). Some of these sequences have the ability to encode *RNA* (*ribonucleic acid*, the encoded messenger of a DNA sequence that mediates protein translation) and proteins (the amino acid sequence produced by the translation of RNA). In addition, we are learning a great deal about genomic regions that do not encode RNA or protein, but play important roles in gene expression and regulation.

Thanks to numerous human genome initiatives, we also have substantial information about inter-individual variability in the human genome. The most common form of genomic variability is a *single nucleotide polymorphism (SNP)*, which represents a substitution of one nucleotide (i.e., the basic building block of DNA, also referred to as a "base") for another, which is present in at least 1% of the population. Each person has inherited two copies of each allele (one from the paternal chromosome and one from the maternal chromosome). The term allele refers to the specific nucleotide sequence at one point in the genome inherited either from the father or mother, and the combination of alleles in an individual is denoted a *genotype*. When the two alleles are identical (i.e., the same nucleotide sequence on both chromosomes), the genotype is referred to as "homozygous;" when the two alleles are different (i.e., different nucleotide sequences on each chromosome), the genotype is referred to as "heterozygous." Approximately 10 million SNPs are thought to exist in the human genome, with an estimated 2 common missense (i.e., amino acid changing) variants per gene. It is likely that only a subset (perhaps 50 000–250 000) of the total number of SNPs in the human genome will actually confer small to moderate effects on *phenotypes* (the biochemical or physiological manifestation of gene expression) that are causally related to disease risk.

However, SNPs are not the only form of genetic variation that may be relevant to human traits and diseases. For example, copy number variants (CNV) have also been recently identified as another common form of genomic variation that may have a role in disease etiology.

Finally, we also recognize that the genome is not simply a linear nucleotide sequence, but that population genomic structure exists in which regions as large as 100 kilobases (a kilobase being a thousand nucleotides, or bases) in length define units that remain intact over evolutionary time. These regions define genomic block structure that may define *haplotypes*, which are sets of genetic variants that are transmitted as a unit across generations.

Thus, the complexity of genome structure and genetic variability that influences response to medications provides unique challenges to molecular pharmacoepidemiology.

Pharmacogenetics and pharmacogenomics

While the term *pharmacogenetics* is predominantly applied to the study of how genetic variability is responsible for differences in patients' responses to drug exposure, the term *pharmacogenomics*, also encompasses approaches simultaneously considering data about thousands of genotypes, as well as responses in gene expression to existing medications. Although the term "pharmacogenetics" is sometimes used synonymously with pharmacogenomics, the former usually refers to a candidate-gene approach as opposed to a genome-wide approach in pharmacogenomics (both discussed later in this chapter).

The interface of pharmacogenetics and pharmacogenomics with molecular pharmacoepidemiology

Pharmacogenetic and pharmacogenomic studies usually are designed to examine intermediate endpoints between drugs and outcomes (such as drug levels, pharmacodynamic properties, or surrogate markers of drug effects) and often rely on detailed measurements of these surrogates in small groups of patients in highly controlled settings. Molecular pharmacoepidemiology focuses on the effects of genetics on clinical outcomes and uses larger observational and experimental methods to evaluate the effectiveness and safety of drug treatment in the population. Molecular pharmacoepidemiology uses similar methods as pharmacoepidemiology to answer questions related to the effects of genes on drug response. Thus, molecular pharmacoepidemiology answers questions related to:

1. the population prevalence of SNPs and other genetic variants;
2. evaluating how these genetic variants alter disease outcomes;
3. assessing the impact of gene–drug and gene–gene interactions on drug response and disease risk; and
4. evaluating the usefulness and impact of genetic tests in populations exposed, or to be exposed, to drugs.

There are, however, some aspects of molecular pharmacoepidemiology that differ from the rest of pharmacoepidemiology. These include the need to understand the complex relationship between medication response and the vast number of potential molecular and genetic influences on this response; a focus on interactions among these factors and interactions between genes and environment (including other medications) that raise issues of sample size and has led to interest in novel designs; and the need to parse out the most likely associations between genes and drug response from among the massive number of potentially important genes identified through bioinformatics (the science of developing and utilizing computer databases and algorithms to accelerate and enhance biological research). As stated previously, the basic science of epidemiology underlies molecular pharmacoepidemiology just as it underlies all pharmacoepidemiology. What is different is the need for approaches that can deal with the vast number of potential genetic influences on outcomes; the possibility that "putative" genes associated with drug response may not be the actual causal genes, but rather a gene near or otherwise associated with the causal gene on the

chromosome in the population studied (and that may not be similarly linked in other populations); the potential that multiple genes, each with a relatively small effect, work together to alter drug response; and the focus on complex interactions between and among genes, drugs, and environment. By discussing the potential approaches to these challenges in this chapter, it is hoped that both the similarities and differences between pharmacoepidemiology and molecular pharmacoepidemiology will be made clear.

Clinical problems to be addressed by pharmacoepidemiologic research

It is useful to conceptualize clinical problems in molecular pharmacoepidemiology by thinking about the mechanism by which genes can affect drug response.

Three ways that genes can affect drug response

The effect that a medication has on an individual can be affected at many points along the pathway of drug distribution and action. This includes absorption and distribution of medications to the site of action, interaction of the medication with its targets, metabolism of the drug, and drug excretion (see Chapter 4). These mechanisms can be categorized into three general routes by which genes can affect a drug response: pharmacokinetic, pharmacodynamic, and gene–drug interactions in the causal pathway of disease. These will be discussed in turn below.

Pharmacokinetic gene–drug interactions
Genes may influence the pharmacokinetics of a drug by altering its metabolism, absorption, or distribution. Metabolism of medications can either inactivate their effect or convert an inactive prodrug into a therapeutically active compound. The genes that are responsible for variable metabolism

of medications are those that code for various enzyme systems, especially the cytochrome P450 enzymes.

The gene encoding CYP2D6 represents a good example of the various ways in which polymorphisms can alter drug response. Some of the genetic variants lead to low or no activity of the CYP2D6 enzyme whereas some individuals have multiple copies of the gene, leading to increased metabolism of drugs. Thus, patients using the CYP2D6-dependent antipsychotic drugs (e.g., haloperidol) who are poor metabolizers (low CYP2D6 activity) are more than four times more likely to need antiparkinsonian medication to treat side effects of the antipsychotic drugs than high metabolizers. The decreased metabolic activity of CYP2D6 may also lead to lower drug efficacy, as illustrated for codeine, which is a prodrug that is metabolized to the active metabolite, morphine, by CYP2D6. It has been estimated that approximately 6–10% of Caucasians have variants that result in CYP2D6 genotypes that encode dysfunctional or inactive CYP2D6 enzyme, in whom codeine is an ineffective analgesic.

Although many drug-CYP2D6 genetic variant interactions have been reported based on experimental or epidemiologic associations, predicting clinical outcomes in daily practice based on such CYP2D6 genetic data in a valid fashion remains complex. Drug–gene associations shown in one study cannot always be replicated in another one. Obviously, variance in drug response has many determinants and singling out only one genetic factor fails to account for the cooccurrence, interplay, and interactions of several other factors (e.g., disease severity, exposure variability over time, physiological feedback mechanisms, testing bias), all also important for molecular pharmacoepidemiology.

In addition to metabolism, genes that alter the absorption and distribution of medications may also alter drug levels at tissue targets. These include, for example, genes that code for transporter proteins such as the ATP-binding cassette transporter proteins (ABCB, also known as the multidrug-resistance (MDR)-1 gene), which has polymorphisms that have been associated with, for example, resistance to antiepileptic drugs. Patients with drug-resistant epilepsy (approximately one of three patients with epilepsy is a nonresponder) are more likely to have the CC polymorphism of ABCB1, which is associated with increased expression of this transporter drug-efflux protein. Of note, the ABCB1 polymorphism falls within an extensive block of linkage disequilibrium (LD). LD is defined by a region in which multiple genetic variants (e.g., SNPs) are correlated with one another due to population and evolutionary genetic history. As a result, a SNP may be statistically associated with disease risk, but is also in LD with the true causative SNP. Therefore, the SNP under study may not itself be causal but simply linked to a true causal variant. One of the major challenges in genetics research at this time is developing methods that can identify the true causal variant(s) that may reside in an LD block.

Pharmacodynamic gene–drug interactions

Once a drug is absorbed and transported to its target site, its effect may be altered by differences in the response of drug targets. Therefore, polymorphisms in genes that code for drug targets may alter the response of an individual to a medication.

This is well illustrated by the polymorphisms of the $\beta(2)$-adrenergic receptor ($\beta(2)$-AR), known for their role in affecting response to β-agonists (e.g., albuterol) in asthma patients. In particular, the coding variants at position 16 within the $\beta(2)$-AR gene ($\beta(2)$-AR-16) have been shown to be important in determining patient response to albuterol treatment (see Case example 14.1).

Pharmacodynamic gene–drug interactions may also affect the risk of adverse reactions. One example is a polymorphism in the gene coding for the bradykinin B2 receptor that has been associated with an increased risk of angiotensin converting enzyme (ACE) inhibitor-induced cough. Cough is one of the most frequently seen adverse drug reactions (ADRs) in ACE therapy and very often a reason for discontinuation of therapy. The TT genotype and T allele of the human bradykinin B(2) receptor gene are found to be significantly higher in patients with cough.

Case Example 14.1

Background

- *Regular use* of inhaled B-agonists for asthma may produce adverse effects and be no more effective than *as-needed* use of these drugs.

Question

- Can genetic polymorphisms in the B2-agonist receptor alter responsiveness to inhaled B-agonists?

Approach

- Perform genetic analysis within a randomized clinical trial of regular versus as-needed use of inhaled B-agonists, and
- Compare the effects of multiple genetic polymorphisms on drug-response.

Results

- Regular use of inhaled B-agonist is associated with decline in efficacy among those with B(2)-AR-16 variants but not among those with other variants tested.
- No effect of genotype in those using inhaled B-agonists in an as-needed manner.

Strengths

- Randomized trial design eliminates confounding by indication for frequency of medication use.
- Candidate genes enhances biological plausibility.

Limitations

- Multiple polymorphisms tested on multiple outcomes leads to concern of false positives.
- Linkage disequilibrium: polymorphisms identified could be "innocent bystanders" by being linked to the true causative mutations.

Key points

- Genetic polymorphisms of drug targets may alter drug response.
- Because of the concern of false positives and/or linkage disequilibrium, replication studies and mechanistic studies remain critical to identifying true putative mutations that alter drug response.
- Effects of a gene may vary by the pattern of drug use, making it important to consider all aspects of drug use (dose, duration, frequency, regularity, etc.) in molecular pharmacoepidemiology studies.

Gene–drug interactions and the causal pathway of disease

Along with altering the pharmacokinetic and pharmacodynamic properties of medications, genetic polymorphisms may also alter the disease state that is the target of drug therapy. For example, antihypertensive medications that work by a particular mechanism, such as the increasing sodium excretion of some antihypertensive medications, may have different effects depending on the susceptibility of the patient to the effects of the drug. Patients with a polymorphism in the α-adducin gene have greater sensitivity to changes in sodium balance. A case-control study has suggested that those with the α-adducin polymorphism may be more likely to benefit from diuretic treatment than those without the polymorphism.

Genetic variability in disease states also can be critical for tailoring drug therapy to patients with a specific genotype related both to the disease and drug response. One example is the humanized monoclonal antibody trastuzumab (Herceptin®), which is used for the treatment of metastatic breast cancer patients with overexpression of the HER2 oncogene. The HER2 protein is thought to be a unique target for trastuzumab therapy in patients with this genetically associated overexpression, occurring in 10–34% of females with breast cancer. The case of trastuzumab, together with another anti-cancer drug, imatinib, which is especially effective in patients with Philadelphia chromosome-positive leukemias, has pioneered successful genetically targeted therapy.

Genetic polymorphisms that alter disease states can also play a role in drug safety. For example, factor V Leiden mutation, present in about one out of twenty Caucasians, is considered an important genetic risk factor for deep vein thrombosis and embolism. A relative risk of about 30 in factor V carriers and users of oral contraceptives compared to noncarriers and non-oral-contraceptive users has been reported. This gene–drug interaction has also been linked to the differential thrombotic risk associated with third-generation oral contraceptives compared with second-generation oral contraceptives. Despite this strong association, Vandenbroucke *et al.* have calculated that mass screening for factor V would result in denial of oral contraceptives for about 20 000 women positive for this mutation in order to prevent 1 death.

Table 14.1 Hypothetical response to medications by genetic variants in metabolism and receptor genes.

	Drug response		
Gene affecting metabolism*	Gene affecting receptor response*	Efficacy	Toxicity
Wild-type	Wild-type	70%	2%
Variant	Wild-type	85%	20%
Wild-type	Variant	20%	2%
Variant	Variant	35%	20%

Data from Evans and McLeod (2003).
*Wild-type associated with normal metabolism or receptor response and variants associated with reduced metabolism or receptor response.

Therefore, these authors concluded that reviewing personal and family thrombosis history, and only if suitable, factor V testing before prescribing oral contraceptives, is the recommended approach to avoid this adverse gene–drug interaction. This highlights another important role of molecular pharmacoepidemiology: determining the utility and cost-effectiveness (see also Chapter 17) of genetic screening to guide drug therapy.

The interplay of various mechanisms

It is useful to conceptualize how the effects of genetic polymorphisms at different stages of drug disposition and response might influence an individual's response to a medication. As an example, an individual may have a genotype that alters the metabolism of the drug, the receptor for the drug, or both. Depending on the combination of these genotypes, the individual might have a different response in terms of both efficacy and toxicity (see Table 14.1). In the simplified example in Table 14.1, there is one genetic variant that alters drug metabolism and one genetic variant that alters receptor response to a medication of interest. In this example, among those who are homozygous for the alleles that encode normal drug metabolism and normal receptor response, there is relatively high efficacy and low toxicity. However, among those who have a variant that reduces drug metabolism, efficacy at a standard dose could actually be greater (assuming a linear dose–response relationship within the possible drug levels of the medication) but toxicity could be increased (if dose-related). Among those who have a variant that reduces receptor response, drug efficacy will be reduced while toxicity may not be different from those who carry genotypes that are not associated with impaired receptor response (assuming that toxicity is not related to the receptor responsible for efficacy). Among those who have variants for both genes, efficacy could be reduced because of the receptor variant (perhaps not as substantially as those with an isolated variant of the receptor gene because of the higher effective dose resulting from the metabolism gene variant), while toxicity could be increased because of the metabolism variant.

The progression and application of molecular pharmacoepidemiologic research

Medications with a narrow therapeutic index are good targets for the use of molecular pharmacoepidemiology to improve the use and application of medications. One example is warfarin. This example illustrates both the logical progression of pharmacogenetics through molecular pharmacoepidemiology and the complexity of moving pharmacogenetic data into practice. The enzyme primarily responsible for the metabolism of warfarin to its inactive form is the cytochrome P450 2C9 variant (CYP2C9). Case example 14.2 illustrates both the logical progression of pharmacogenetics through molecular pharmacoepidemiology and the complexity of moving pharmacogenetic data into practice.

Methodological problems to be addressed by pharmacoepidemiologic research

The same methodological problems of pharmacoepidemiology must be addressed in molecular pharmacoepidemiology. These problems include those

---

Case Example 14.2: The complexity of the progression and application of molecular pharmacoepidemiology research

Background

- Warfarin is a narrow therapeutic index drug. Underdosing or overdosing, even to a minimal degree, can lead to significant morbidity (bleeding and/or thromboembolism).

Question

- Can genetic variants be identified and used to alter the dosing of warfarin and thus improve safety and effectiveness?

Approach and results

- Multiple study designs have been used to address this question.
- First, pharmacogenetic studies identified the effect of CYP2C9 polymorphisms on warfarin metabolism.
- Second, a case-control study comparing warfarin patients requiring low doses versus patients not requiring low doses found that CYP2C9 polymorphisms were associated with lower dose. By design, this study selected subjects based on warfarin dose requirements, not genotype, and could only determine that lower doses of warfarin were more common among those with CYP2C9 variants. The other associations noted were between lower dose requirements and bleeding, not between genotype and bleeding.
- Third, in order to address the clinically relevant question of bleeding, a retrospective cohort study was performed that demonstrated an increased risk of bleeding among patients with at least one CYP2C9 variant. The retrospective nature of the study left unanswered the question of whether knowing that a patient carries a variant can alter therapy in a way that can reduce risk.
- The recent development of algorithms to predict a maintenance warfarin dose that combines clinical and genetic data suggests that improvements may be made by incorporating genetic data into dosing algorithms. However, small clinical trials have not demonstrated the utility of genotyping. Large-scale trials are underway.

Strengths

- A logical series of studies, each with its own strengths and limitations, has improved our understanding of genetic variability in response to warfarin.

Limitations

- No randomized trials have yet shown that one can reduce adverse events and enhance effectiveness of warfarin by knowing a patient's genetic make-up.
- Only about 50% of variability in warfarin response can be explained by existing algorithms–other polymorphisms or clinical factors (e.g., adherence) may be important.

Key points

- The process of fully understanding the effects of polymorphisms on drug response requires multiple studies and often substantial resources.
- Our understanding of genetic variants has progressed so rapidly that new questions are often raised that have implications for clinical practice even as old ones are answered.
- Before using genetic data to alter drug prescribing, prospective evaluation is needed.

of chance and statistical power, confounding, bias, and generalizability (see Chapters 2, 3 and 21).

However, the complex relationship between medication response and molecular and genetic factors generates some unique challenges in molecular pharmacoepidemiology. These challenges derive from the large number of potential genetic variants that can modify the response to a single drug, the possibility that there is a small individual effect of any one of these genes, the low prevalence of many genetic variants, and the possibility that a presumptive gene–drug response relationship may be confounded by the racial and ethnic mixture of the population studied. Thus, the methodological challenges of molecular pharmacoepidemiology are closely related to issues of statistical interactions, type I and type II errors, and confounding. First and foremost, however, molecular pharmacoepidemiologic studies rely on proper identification of putative genes. In addition, in all research of this type, use of appropriate laboratory methods, such as high-throughput genotyping technologies, is necessary. Similarly, appropriate quality control procedures must be considered to obtain meaningful data for research and clinical applications. This section will begin by highlighting the nature of gene discovery and then focus on the methodological challenges of studying interactions, minimizing type I and type II errors, and accounting for confounding, particularly by population admixture (defined below).

Approaches to gene discovery: genome-wide versus candidate gene approaches

Two schools of thought have emerged about the genetic architecture of pharmacogenetics: the common disease-common allele hypothesis and the common disease-rare variant hypothesis. The common disease-common allele hypothesis, which postulates that commonly occurring inherited variants confer small effects on drug response. These so-called "low penetrance" alleles have been hypothesized to explain a large proportion of drug response because the attributable risk associated with these variants could be large if the alleles are carried by a large proportion of the population. Accompanying

this hypothesis is the notion that the overall disposition of drugs, and the attendant pharmacologic consequences and treatment effects observed in an individual, may result from numerous allelic variants of this type. These variants are typically identified via case-control association studies, including genome-wide association studies (GWAS). Genome wide association studies are studies in which randomly selected DNA sequences (selected across the genome to try to identify as much of the variability in DNA as possible) are examined for associations with outcomes, initially irrespective of biological plausibility (discussed in further detail under "Currently available solutions").

While there are examples of such pharmacogenetic association studies, including GWAS, that have revealed validated associations, there has been limited success in translating these findings into clinical practice. One reason for this limited success can be found from the experience of translating commonly occurring, low penetrance alleles to risk prediction in disease etiology studies. Despite the success in defining many such risk alleles in a wide variety of diseases, few of these have been translated into clinical practice as tools to refine risk assessment, screening, treatment, or other clinically relevant activities. In part, this is due to the small effect sizes of each single risk allele, and because combinations of these alleles, if they can be found, confer only clinically relevant effect sizes for extremely rare combinations of alleles having an effect on very limited subsets of the populations.

An additional concern of the identification of low penetrance alleles is that they have not yet been able to explain the majority of the estimated genetic contribution to disease etiology. Based on studies of families or phenotypic variability, most loci have been found to explain less than half (and at times as little as 1%) of the predicted heritability of many common traits. This "missing heritability" of complex disease suggests that other classes of genetic variation may explain the genetic contribution to common disease.

This "missing heritability" in common disease etiology may be explained by a large number of rare variants, each of which may confer very small effects To date, there has been little success in confirming the hypothesis that rare variants explain common disease or drug responses. The limited data are due both to the high cost of methods that may allow the detection of these rare variants, as well as statistical methods that allow researchers to identify associations in this setting. The former limitation is being resolved as technology for genetic sequencing becomes cheaper and more available. Methods for identifying associations remain limited, but include employing linkage disequilibrium in regions of interest to identify collections of rare variants; combining common and rare variants to provide joint information about the effect of variation in a region; studying individuals with extreme phenotypes to target deep sequencing activities; making use of admixture (defined below) and ancestry genomic differences to identify rare variants (discussed further below); using well-annotated families to study inheritance; studying structural variants including deletions and duplications; novel case-control matching strategies that consider not only epidemiologic matching or adjustment algorithms but also matching to specific genomic regions; using pooling strategies to study rare variants; and employing copy number variation (DNA segments that are 1 kilobase or larger and present at variable copy number in comparison with a reference genome).

Despite the debate about whether common low penetrance variants or rare variants explain disease and pharmacogenetic effects, it seems likely that both classes of these variants, as well as rare variants with large effects, are likely to be responsible for the phenotypic effects of interest. Therefore, hybrid strategies that consider all of these classes of genetic variants must be developed to explain the genetic architecture of common disease and pharmacogenetic response.

Interactions

Along with examining the direct effect of genes and other biomarkers on outcomes, molecular pharmacoepidemiologic studies must often be designed to examine effect modification between medication use and the genes or biomarkers of interest. That is, the primary measure of interest is often the role of biomarker information on the effect of a medication. For purposes of simplicity, this discussion will use genetic variability as the measure of interest.

Effect modification is present if there is a difference in the effect of the medication depending on the presence or absence of the genetic variant. This difference can be either on the multiplicative or additive scale. On the multiplicative scale, interaction is present if the effect of the combination of the genotype and medication exposure relative to neither is greater than the product of the measure of effect of each (genotype alone or medication alone) relative to neither. On the additive scale, interaction is present if the effect of the combination of the genotype and medication exposure is greater than the sum of the measures of effect of each alone, again all relative to neither.

For studies examining a dichotomous medication exposure (e.g., medication use versus nonuse), a dichotomous genetic exposure (e.g., presence versus absence of a genetic variant), and a dichotomous outcome (e.g., myocardial infarction occurrence versus none), there are two ways to consider presenting and analyzing interactions. The first is as a stratified analysis, comparing the effect of medication exposure versus non-exposure on the outcome in two strata: those with the genetic variant and those without (e.g., see Table 14.2). The second is to present a 2×4 table (also shown in Table 14.2). In the first example (stratified analysis), one compares the effect of the medication among those with the genetic variant to the effect of the medication among those without the genetic variant. In the second example (the 2×4 table), the effect of each combination of exposure (i.e., with both genetic variant and medication; with genetic variant but without medication; with medication but without genetic variant) is determined relative to the lack of exposure to either. The advantage of the 2×4 table is that it presents separately the effect of the drug, the gene, and both relative to those without the genetic variant and without medication exposure. In addition, presentation of the data as a 2×4 table allows one to directly compute both multiplicative and additive interactions. In the example given in Table 14.2, multiplicative interaction would be assessed by comparing the odds ratio

Table 14.2 Two ways to present effect modification in molecular pharmacoepidemiologic studies using case-control study as a model.

			Stratified analysis		
Genotype	Medication	Cases	Controls	Odds ratio	Information provided
+	+	a	b	ad/bc	Effect of medication vs. no medication among those with the genotype
	−	c	d		
−	+	e	f	eh/fg	Effect of medication vs. no medication among those without the genotype
	−	g	h		

			2 × 4 Table		
Genotype	Medication	Cases	Controls	Odds ratio	Information provided
+	+	a	b	ah/bg = A	Joint genotype and medication vs. neither
+	−	c	d	ch/dg = B	Genotype alone vs. neither
−	+	e	f	eh/fg = C	Medication alone vs. neither
−	−	g	h	Reference	Reference Group

Data from Botto and Khoury 2004.

for the combination of genotype and medication exposure to the product of the odds ratios for medication alone and genotype alone. Multiplicative interaction would be considered present if the odds ratios for the combination of medication and genotype (A in Table 14.2) was greater than the product of the odds ratios for either alone (B × C). Additive interaction would be considered present if the odds ratio for the combination of genotype and medication use (A) was greater than the sum of the odds ratios for medication use alone and genotype alone (B + C). The 2 × 4 table also allows the direct assessment of the number of subjects in each group along with the respective confidence interval for the measured effect in each of the groups, making it possible to directly observe the precision of the estimates in each of the groups and therefore better understand the power of the study. Furthermore, attributable fractions can be computed separately for each of the exposures alone and for the combination of exposures. In general, presenting the data in both manners is optimal because it allows the reader to understand the effect of each of the exposures (2 × 4 table) as well as the

effect of the medication in the presence or absence of the genotypic variant (stratified table).

Type I error

The chance of type I error (concluding there is an association when in fact one does not exist) increases with the number of statistical tests performed on any one data set (see also Chapter 3). It is easy to appreciate the potential for type I error in a molecular pharmacoepidemiologic study that examines, simultaneously, the effects of multiple genetic factors, the effects of multiple nongenetic factors, and the interaction between and among these factors. One of the reasons cited for nonreplication of study findings in molecular pharmacoepidemiology is type I error. Limiting the number of associations examined to those of specific candidate genetic variants that are suspected of being associated with the outcome is one method to limit type I error in pharmacoepidemiology. However, with increasing emphasis in molecular pharmacoepidemiologic studies on identifying all variants within a gene (and all variants within the genome) and examining multiple interactions, this method of limiting type I error is often not tenable. Some other currently available solutions are discussed in the next section.

Type II error

Because it has been hypothesized that much of the genetic variability leading to phenotypic expression of complex diseases results from the relatively small effects of many relatively low prevalence genetic variants, the ability to detect a gene–response relationship is likely to require relatively large sample sizes to avoid type II error (concluding there is no association when in fact one does exist). The sample size requirements for studies that examine the direct effect of genes on medication response will be the same as the requirements for examining direct effects of individual risk factors on outcomes. With relatively low prevalences of polymorphisms and often low incidence of outcomes (particularly in studies of adverse drug reactions), large sample sizes are typically required to detect even modest associations. For such studies, the case–control (see Chapter 2) design has become a particularly favored approach for molecular pharmacoepidemiologic studies because of its ability to select participants based on the outcome of interest (and its ability to study the effects of multiple potential genotypes in the same study).

Studies that are designed to examine the interaction between a genetic polymorphism and a medication will require even larger sample sizes. This is because such studies need to be powered to compare those with both the genetic polymorphism and the medication exposure with those who have neither. As an example, the previously mentioned case–control study of the α-adducin gene and diuretic therapy in patients with treated hypertension examined the effects of the genetic polymorphism, the diuretic therapy, and both in combination. There were 1038 participants in the study. When comparing the effect of diuretic use with no use and comparing the effect of the genetic variant with the nonvariant allele, all 1038 participants were available for comparison (Table 14.3). However, when examining the effect of diuretic therapy versus nonuse among those with the

Table 14.3 Gene-exposure interaction analysis in a case-control study.

Diuretic Use	Adducin Variant	Cases	Controls	Odds Ratio (OR) for Stroke Myocardial Infarction
0	0	A_{00}	B_{00}	1.0
		103	248	
0	1	A_{01}	B_{01}	1.56
		85	131	
1	0	A_{10}	B_{10}	1.09
		94	208	
1	1	A_{11}	B_{11}	0.77
		41	128	

Case control OR in variant carriers: $OR_{variant} = A_{11}B_{01}/A_{01}B_{11} = 41 \times 131/85 \times 128 = 0.49$
Case control OR in wild-type carriers: $OR_{wild-type} = A_{10}B_{00}/A_{00}B_{10} = 94 \times 248/103 \times 208 = 1.09$
Synergy index $= OR_{variant}/OR_{wild-type} = 0.45$
Case-only OR $= A_{11}A_{00}/A_{10}A_{01} = 41 \times 103/94 \times 85 = 0.53$
Data from Psaty et al., 2002.

genetic variant, only 385 participants contributed to the analyses. Of note, this study presented the data for interaction in the two ways presented in Table 14.3.

In order to minimize false negative findings, further efforts must be made to ensure adequate sample sizes for molecular pharmacoepidemiologic studies. Because of the complex nature of medication response, and the likelihood that at least several genes are responsible for the variability in drug response, studies designed to test for multiple gene–gene and gene–environment interactions (including other medications, environmental factors, adherence to medications, and clinical factors) will, similarly, require large sample sizes.

Confounding by population admixture

When there is evidence that baseline disease risks and genotype frequencies differ among ethnicities, the conditions for population stratification (i.e., population admixture or confounding by ethnicity) may be met. Population admixture is simply a manifestation of confounding by ethnicity, which can occur if both baseline disease risks and genotype frequency vary across ethnicity. For example, the African-American population represent admixture of at least three major continental ancestries (African, European, and Native American). The larger the number of ethnicities involved in an admixed population, the less likely that population stratification can be the explanation for biased associations. Empirical data show that carefully matched, moderate-sized case–control samples in African-American populations are unlikely to contain levels of population admixture that would result in significantly inflated numbers of false-positive associations. There is the potential for population structure to exist in African-American populations, but this structure can be eliminated by removing recent African or Caribbean immigrants, and limiting study samples to resident African-Americans. Based on the literature that has evaluated the effects of confounding by ethnicity overall, and specifically in African-Americans, there is little empirical evidence that population stratification is a likely explanation for bias in point estimates or incorrect inferences. Nonetheless, population admixture must be considered in designing and analyzing molecular pharmacoepidemiologic studies to ensure that adequate adjustment can be made for this potential confounder. It is important to note that poor study design may be more important than population stratification in conferring bias to association studies.

Currently available solutions

Gene discovery: genome-wide versus candidate gene approaches

As discussed in the "Methodological problem" section, there are two primary approaches for gene discovery: candidate gene association studies and genome-wide screens (GWAS). In the former, genes are selected for study on the basis of their plausible biological relevance to drug response. In the latter, randomly selected DNA sequences are examined for associations with outcomes, initially

irrespective of biological plausibility. GWAS rely on linkage disequilibrium (LD), defined above as the correlation between alleles at two loci. The GWAS approach uses DNA sequence variation (e.g., SNPs) found throughout the genome, and does not rely on a priori functional knowledge of gene function. A number of factors influence the success of these studies. Appropriate epidemiologic study designs and adequate statistical power remain essential. Thorough characterization of LD is essential for replication of genome-wide association studies: the haplotype mapping (HapMap) consortium and other groups have shown that the extent of LD varies by ethnicity, which may affect the ability to replicate findings in subsequent studies. Particularly informative SNPs that best characterize a genomic region can be used to limit the amount of laboratory and analytical work in haplotype-based studies. It has been hypothesized that studies that consider LD involving multiple SNPs in a genomic region (i.e., a haplotype) can increase power to detect associations by 15–50% compared with analyses involving only individual SNPs. Finally, even if genome-wide scans may identify markers associated with the trait of interest, a challenge will be to identify the causative SNPs.

Clearly, candidate gene and genome-wide approaches are not mutually exclusive. It has been suggested that gene discovery can focus on SNPs or haplotypes based on: (i) strong, prior information about biological pathways or linkage data; (ii) information about the functional significance of an SNP or haplotype; and/or (iii) studies that start with a "simple" haplotype involving a small number of SNPs that can be expanded to increase the number of SNPs that constitute haplotypes in a specific region of the genome.

Interactions

Along with traditional case–control and cohort studies, the case-only study can be used for molecular pharmacoepidemiologic studies designed to examine interactions between genes and medications. In this design, cases, representing those with the outcome or phenotype of interest, are selected for study, and the association between genetic variants and medication use is determined among these cases. Assuming that the use of the medication is unrelated to the genotype, the case-only study provides a valid measure of the interaction of the genotype and the medication on the risk of the outcome.

One strength of the case-only study design is that it eliminates the need to identify controls, often a major methodological and logistical challenge in case–control studies. One limitation of the case-only design is that it relies on the assumption of independence between exposure (medication use) and genotype. Although this assumption may be valid (in the absence of knowing genotype clinically, it may be reasonable to assume that the use of the medication is not related to patients' genotypes), it is certainly possible that the genotype, by altering response to medications targeted at a specific disease, could affect the medications being prescribed to patients.

Case Example 14.3

Background

- Identifying the effect of interactions between genes and medications on outcomes often requires large sample sizes. In addition, proper selection of a control group in case-control studies can be challenging.

Question

- Can a case-only study be used to more efficiently identify interactions between medications and genes?

Approach

- Select cases with the outcome of interest.
- Measure the association between genetic variants and the medication of interest among the cases.

Results

- Under the assumption that there is no association between the gene and medication exposure among those without the disease (i.e., controls), the odds ratio for the association between genetic variants and medication use in the cases is equivalent to the synergy index on a multiplicative scale for a case–control study.
- The synergy index is the odds ratio for medication use versus the outcome of interest in those with the variant alleles divided by the odds ratio for medication use versus the outcome in those without the variant alleles–see Table 14.3 footnote.

Strengths

- Eliminates the need to identify controls, which is often a major methodological and logistical challenge in case–control studies.
- Can result in greater precision in estimating interactions compared with case–control analyses.
- Possible to use the case-only approach to estimate interactions between genes and medications in large-scale registries of people with diseases or disease outcomes.

Limitations

- Relies on the assumption that the use of the medication is unrelated to the genotype. It is certainly possible that the genotype, by altering response to medications targeted at a specific disease, could affect the medications being prescribed to patients.
- Does not allow assessment of the independent effects of medication use or genotype on outcome.
- Interaction can only be interpreted on a multiplicative scale.

Key points

- Case-only studies can be used to measure the interaction between genetic variants and medications.
- Case-only studies eliminate the difficulty and inefficiency of including a control group.
- Case-only studies rely on the assumption of independence between medication use and genetic variants among those without disease, an assumption that may not be met.
- Case-only studies can be used within the context of a case-control study or using large-scale databases.

Type I error and replication

The chance of type I error (concluding there is an association when one does not exist in fact) increases with the number of statistical tests performed on any one data set (see also Chapter 3). Replication of association studies is required to conclude that a candidate gene is biologically causally plausible and also has a meaningful etiological effect. One of the reasons cited for nonreplication of study findings in molecular pharmacoepidemiology is type I error.

One approach to assessing for possible type I error is the use of "genomic controls." This approach uses the distribution of test statistics obtained for unlinked markers (genotypes at loci that lie in regions other than the location of the gene of interest) to adjust the usual chi square test for the association of interest. For example, if 20 unlinked markers are studied in addition to the candidate gene of interest, none of these 20 should be associated with disease if they are truly random markers with no biological effect. If one or more of these unlinked markers is associated with disease, this implies that the association represents a type I error because associations of these unlinked markers cannot be causally associated with disease, and therefore can only represent false positive associations. Therefore, the observation of associations with the unlinked markers is a measure of the potential for type I error. This approach is also useful for assessing for possible population admixture, as discussed below.

Type II error

Reducing type II error (concluding that there is no association when one does exist in fact) essentially involves a logistical need to ensure adequate sample size (see also Chapter 3). One approach to increasing the sample size of molecular pharmacoepidemiologic studies is to perform large, multicenter collaborative studies. Another is to combine multiple, separately performed cohorts.

Another potential solution to minimizing type II error is through meta-analysis, whereby smaller studies, which are, individually, not powered to detect specific associations (such as interactions) are combined in order to improve the ability to detect such associations (see Chapter 19).

Confounding by population admixture

Although population stratification is unlikely to be a significant source of bias in epidemiologic association studies, this assumes adequate adjustment for race. A number of analytical approaches exist to either circumvent problems imposed by population genetic structure or that use this structure in gene identification. The "structured association" approach identifies a set of individuals who are drawing their alleles from different background populations or ethnicities. This approach uses information about genotypes at loci that lie in regions other than the location of the gene of interest (i.e., "unlinked markers") to infer their ancestry (often referred to as ancestry informative markers) and learn about population structure. It further uses the data derived from these unlinked markers to adjust the association test statistic. By adjusting for these ancestry informative markers, one can adjust for differences in ancestry.

The future

Scientific and clinical developments in biology and molecular biology, particularly in the field of genomics and other biomarkers, have and will continue to affect the field of pharmacoepidemiology in a significant way. Translating biomarkers from the lab and experimental studies to clinical practice has been a difficult path. Often, initial promising findings on drug-gene interactions to predict clinical drug responses could not be replicated in subsequent studies. For sure, the ability of genes and other biomarkers to improve patient care and outcomes will need to be tested in properly controlled studies, including randomized controlled trials in some circumstances. The positive and negative predictive value of carrying a genetic variant will be important determinants of the ability of the variant to improve outcomes. Those genetic variants with good test characteristics may still need to be evaluated in properly controlled trials. Such studies could examine several ways to incorporate genetic testing into clinical practice, including the use of genetic variants in dosing algorithms, in selection of a specific therapeutic class of drug to treat a disease, and in avoidance of using specific medications in those at high risk for adverse drug reactions. These scientific advances are also finding their way into drug discovery and development in order to rationalize drug innovation and to identify good and poor responders, both in terms of efficacy and safety, of drug therapy in an earlier phase. The cost-effectiveness of such approaches is also of great interest because the addition of genetic testing adds cost to clinical care (see also Chapter 17). Research will be needed to determine the cost-effectiveness of new biomarker and genetic tests as they are developed.

What this all means for the future pharmacoepidemiology is a challenging question. Genotype data will increasingly become available and will enrich pharmacoepidemiologic analysis. New methods (e.g., sequencing) will provide new opportunities but also new challenges to analyzing pharmacoepidemiologic data. Further, although it is useful to characterize the three different pathways of how drug-gene interactions may occur as was done in this chapter, this stratification is most likely an oversimplification of the large plethora of possible mechanisms of how drugs, genes, and patient outcomes are interrelated. All these may have consequences for how molecular pharmacoepidemiologic studies are designed, conducted, and analyzed. In addition, the more that genotype testing is applied in clinical practice, the more drug exposure will be influenced by such tests, making genotype and drug exposure non-independent factors.

Finally, just as for all research, the ethical, legal, and social implications of genetic testing must be considered and addressed (see also Chapter 15). Pharmacogenetic testing raises issues of privacy concerns, access to health care services, and informed consent. For example, concern has been raised that the use of genetic testing could lead to targeting of therapies to only specific groups (ethnic or racial) of patients, ignoring others, and to loss of insurance coverage for certain groups of individuals. There also is a concern that medicines will be developed only for the most common, commercially attractive, genotypes, leading to "orphan genotypes."

All of these issues are challenges to overcome as we continue to reap the benefits of the tremendous strides made in determining the molecular basis of disease and drug response.

Key points

- Genes can affect a drug response via: alteration of drug pharmacokinetics, pharmacodynamic effects on drug targets, and gene–drug interactions in the causal pathway of disease.
- Molecular pharmacoepidemiology is the study of the manner in which molecular biomarkers (often, but not exclusively, genes) alter the clinical effects of medications in populations.
- Molecular pharmacoepidemiology answers questions related to: the population prevalence of SNPs and other genetic variants; evaluating how these SNPs alter disease outcomes; assessing the impact of gene–drug and gene–gene interactions on disease risk; and evaluating the usefulness and impact of genetic tests in populations exposed, or to be exposed, to drugs.
- Identifying genes that alter drug response for molecular pharmacoepidemiology studies can use a candidate gene approach or a genome-wide approach; these approaches are really complementary, not mutually exclusive.
- The methodological challenges of molecular pharmacoepidemiology are closely related to issues of statistical interactions, type I and type II errors, and confounding.
- Case-only studies can be used to measure the interaction between genetic variants and medications and eliminate the difficulty and inefficiency of including a control group. However, they rely on the assumption of independence between medication use and genetic variants among those without disease, an assumption that may not be met.
- Given concerns of type I error (along with other methodological concerns such as uncontrolled confounding and linkage disequilibrium), a key issue in molecular epidemiology is the ability to replicate association study findings.
- Because genetic variability leading to phenotypic expression of complex diseases results from the

relatively small effects of many relatively low prevalence genetic variants, the ability to detect a gene–response relationship is likely to require relatively large sample sizes to avoid type II error. Methods to ensure adequate sample sizes include the use of large, multicenter collaborative studies; assembly and genotyping of large, relatively homogenous populations for multiple studies; and meta-analysis.

• Population stratification can distort the gene–medication response association. Although unlikely to be a significant source of bias in well-controlled epidemiological association studies, a number of analytical approaches exist to either circumvent problems imposed by population genetic structure or that use this structure in gene identification.

• The ability of genes and other biomarkers to improve patient care and outcomes needs to be tested in properly controlled studies, including randomized controlled trials in some cases. Similarly, the cost-effectiveness of such approaches must be justifiable given the additional costs of genetic testing in clinical care.

• The ethical, legal, and social implications of genetic testing must be considered and addressed, just as they must be considered for all research.

Further reading

Aithal GP, Day CP, Kesteven PJ, Daly AK (1999) Association of polymorphisms in the cytochrome P450 CYP2C9 with warfarin dose requirement and risk of bleeding complications. *Lancet* **353**: 717–19.

Borges S, Desta Z, Li L, Skaar TC, Ward BA, Nguyen A, *et al.* (2006) Quantitative effect of CYP2D6 genotype and inhibitors on tamoxifen metabolism: implication for optimization of breast cancer treatment. *Clinical Pharmacology & Therapeutics* **80** (1): 61–74.

Botto LD, Khoury MJ (2004) Facing the challenge of complex genotypes and gene–environment interaction: the basic epidemiologic units in case–control and case-only designs. In: Khoury MJ, Little J, Burke W, eds, *Human Genome Epidemiology*. New York: Oxford University Press, pp. 111–26.

Caraco Y, Blotnick S, Muszkat M (2008) CYP2C9 Genotype-guided Warfarin Prescribing Enhances the Efficacy and Safety of Anticoagulation: A Prospective Randomized Controlled Study. *Clin Pharmacol Ther* 2008; **83**: 460–70.

Evans WE, McLeod LJ. Pharmacogenomics–drug disposition, drug targets, and side effects. *N Engl J Med* 2003; **348**: 528–49.

Gage BF, Eby D, Johnson JA, Deych E, Rieder MJ, Ridker PM, *et al.* (2008) Use of pharmacogenetic and clinical factors to predict the therapeutic dose of warfarin. *Clin Pharmacol Ther* **84**: 326–31.

Higashi MK, Veenstra DL, Kondo LM, Wittkowsky AK, Srinouanprachanh SL, Farin FM, *et al.* (2002) Association between CYP2C9 genetic variants and anticoagulation-related outcomes during warfarin therapy. *JAMA* **287**: 1690–8.

Israel E, Drazen JM, Liggett SB, Boushey HA, Cherniack RM, Chinchilli VM, *et al.* (2000) The effect of polymorphisms of the beta(2)-adrenergic receptor on the response to regular use of albuterol in asthma. *Am J Respir Crit Care Med* **162**: 75–80.

Khoury MJ, Flanders WD (1996) Nontraditional epidemiologic approaches in the analysis of gene–environment interaction: case–control studies with no controls! *Am J Epidemiol* **144**: 207–13.

Lohmueller KE, Pearce CL, Pike M, Lander ES, Hirschhorn JN (2003) Meta-analysis of genetic association studies supports a contribution of common variants to susceptibility to common disease. *Nat Genet* **33**: 177–82.

Mallal S, Phillips E, Carosi G, Molina JM, Workman C, Tomazic J, *et al.* (2008) HLA-B*5701 screening for hypersensitivity to abacavir. *NEJM* **358**: 568–79.

Manolio TA, Collins FS, Cox NJ, Goldstein DB, Hindorff LA, Hunter DJ, *et al.* (2009) Finding the missing heritability of complex diseases. *Nature* **461**: 747–53.

Phillips KA, Veenstra DL, Oren E, Lee JK, Sadee W (2001) Potential role of pharmacogenomics in reducing adverse drug reactions: a systematic review. *JAMA* **286**: 2270–9.

Psaty BM, Smith NL, Heckbert SR, Vos HL, Lemaitre RN, Reiner AP, *et al.* (2002) Diuretic therapy, the alpha-adducin gene variant, and the risk of myocardial infarction or stroke in persons with treated hypertension. *JAMA* **287**: 1680–9.

Roses AD (2008) Pharmacogenetics in drug discovery and development: a translational perspective. *Nature Reviews Drug Discovery* **7** (10): 807–17.

Schillevoort I, de Boer A, van der WJ, Steijns LS, Roos RA, Jansen PA, *et al.* (2002) Antipsychotic-induced extrapyramidal syndromes and cytochrome P450 2D6 genotype: a case–control study. *Pharmacogenetics* **12**: 235–40.

Siddiqui A, Kerb R, Weale ME, Brinkmann U, Smith A, Goldstein DBM, *et al.* (2003) Association of multidrug resistance in epilepsy with a polymorphism in the drug-transporter gene ABCB1. *N Engl J Med* **348**: 1442–8.

Veenstra DL (2004) The interface between epidemiology and pharmacogenomics. In: Khoury MJ, Little J, Burke W, eds, *Human Genome Epidemiology*. New York: Oxford University Press, pp. 234–46.

Vesell ES (1979) Pharmacogenetics: multiple interactions between genes and environment as determinants of drug response. *Am J Med* **66**: 183–7.

Wacholder S, Rothman N, Caporaso N (2000) Population stratification in epidemiologic studies of common genetic variants and cancer: quantification of bias. *J Natl Cancer Inst* **92**: 1151–8.

CHAPTER 15

Bioethical Issues in Pharmacoepidemiologic Research

Antoine C. El Khoury

Johnson & Johnson Pharmaceutical, Horsham, PA, USA

Introduction

Research ethics is a discipline that defines the set of norms investigators ought to follow when they conduct research. In the past 50 years as medical research has rapidly evolved, the discipline of research ethics has assumed a largely protectionist posture, principally because of a series of unfortunate scandals and the resulting public outcry. As a result, research ethics has focused primarily on protecting human subjects from the risks of research. The goal has been to minimize risks to subjects, rather than minimizing the risks and maximizing the potential benefits for both subjects and society. Themes that run through many of these scandals are scientists' failure to adequately review and disclose research risks and potential benefits, failure to disclose conflicts of interest, and failure to obtain explicit permission from research subjects. As a result of these events, review of research protocols by an institutional review board (IRB) and strict disclosure of funding sources in addition to informed consent have become the foundations for the protection of human subjects from research risks.

These and other requirements have been remarkably effective in defining the limits of ethical research and have made it much less likely that the most egregious ethical errors of the past will be repeated. Overall, they should be viewed as welcome additions to the practice of clinical research. However, serious scientific and ethical problems may arise when the requirements that were developed to guide clinical research (defined here as research requiring direct patient contact and investigator-initiated interventions) are applied to other kinds of research. In particular, standard protections in clinical research are not easily exported and applied to challenges of epidemiologic research. Therefore, as these rules have been applied to pharmacoepidemiologic research, the result has been the parallel development of modifications to the prevailing ethical guidelines and principles, with concomitant increasing consternation and confusion, about how these modifications should be applied beyond clinical settings.

The central problem has been that, while the ethics of human subjects research has been built upon the protection of human subjects, the human subjects involved in many pharmacoepidemiologic studies are quite different. Indeed, it may be difficult to see how the analysis of an existing data set makes the patients whose information contributes to that data set "human subjects" and why this research requires any review by an ethics review board. The idea that a patient can become a subject without his or her knowledge, and without any direct contact with an investigator, is not intuitively clear. Moreover, the risks to the subjects of observational research are not the usual health risks of research that can be balanced against the potential health benefits of research. Harm is not the issue in most pharmacoepidemiologic research. It is almost

Textbook of Pharmacoepidemiology, Second Edition. Edited by Brian L. Strom, Stephen E. Kimmel, and Sean Hennessy.
© 2013 John Wiley & Sons, Ltd. Published 2013 by John Wiley & Sons, Ltd.

always what in law and philosophy are referred to as "wrongs," that is, a violation of a person's rights, privacy, or dignity. While investigators and ethics review boards may be able to balance medical and research risks against medical benefits, they may find balancing these different currencies to be challenging.

In an effort to deal with these problems, investigators, governments, and professional associations have developed regulations and guidelines to provide and disseminate ethical structure to the growing field of epidemiology. Most of these guidelines apply equally well to pharmacoepidemiologic research, although this field has begun to develop its own principles. Guidelines have addressed four broad categories of ethical issues in epidemiologic research: obligations to society, obligations to funders and employers, obligations to colleagues, and obligations to subjects.

Although these guidelines acknowledge a range of ethical obligations, one of these, the investigators' obligations to subjects, has clearly proven to be the most challenging. This is because the procedures of ethical research, like ethics board review and informed consent, may be overly protectionistic or prohibitively difficult in epidemiologic research. Ethical concerns about pharmacoepidemiologic research, have therefore focused on the kinds of research that require ethics board review and the kinds of research that require the subject's informed consent.

Investigators face a considerable challenge. They must protect patients' privacy and confidentiality in a way that accomplishes research goals accurately and efficiently. This challenge lies at the heart of the ethics of most pharmacoepidemiologic research.

National and international organizations have created principles that provide a backdrop to the research framework, the most well established being those adopted by the Organization for Economic Cooperation and Development (OECD) in 1980 and more recently by the American College of Epidemiology and the International Society for Pharmacoepidemiology. These recommendations suggest that limits to the collection of data should be sought, especially when it relates to data identifiers, that the quality of data is important, that data

use should be specified in advance, and that investigators should adhere to prespecified uses as determined in the protocol. Finally, the OECD suggests a requirement of "openness"–that is, a requirement that goals, uses, and access to data should be a matter of public record, and that individuals should be able to determine whether and how data about them are being used. Despite general agreement about these and other principles, the international community has failed to achieve a consensus about the proper balance of protections and research progress.

A key goal of this chapter is to present the challenges that arise when the principles of research ethics are applied to issues surrounding privacy and confidentiality. This chapter also will focus on observational research, which makes up a large proportion of the research in pharmacoepidemiology.

Clinical problems to be addressed by pharmacoepidemiologic research

Pharmacoepidemiologic research

In its summary statement (the Belmont Report), the US National Commission for the Protection of Human Subjects defined "research" as any activity designed to "develop or contribute to generalizable knowledge."

The major difficulty arises from the definition itself. What is meant by "generalizable knowledge" and how generalizable should the knowledge be before the study or project is considered research? For instance, data may be gathered as part of a health care organization's drug surveillance program, the intent of which is to define the patterns of medication use in a local population. This study may generate results that can be used in the local population and the results may be generalized to the local population. However, these same results may not apply to other populations within the same country. Would this study still be considered research? It is not clear, given the definition based on "generalizable knowledge," whether this project should be construed as research, clinical care, or even as a quality improvement activity. These distinctions are important because once a project is identified as "research," investigators must meet a series of requirements designed to protect the patients, who are now human subjects.

This definition of research is particularly problematic in pharmacoepidemiology, because it is often hard to distinguish the routine practice of pharmacoepidemiology from research. The extremes are evident. The paradigmatic *practice* of epidemiology is public health case finding and surveillance, for adverse drug reactions or drug utilization as examples. This is a social good that we do not, generally, consider being research, although the activities are conducted for the purpose of creating generalizable knowledge upon which to base public health decisions. Analogous would be the quality assurance activities of health plans or hospitals, seeking to improve the use of medications in their settings. These sorts of investigations proceed, and sometimes even produce publishable data, without review by ethics review boards. These activities differ from more "research oriented" pharmacoepidemiologic investigations designed to test hypotheses about drug adverse event associations, drug-drug interactions, drug adherence, or efficacy. These investigations may be identified as research and may be required to undergo review by ethics review boards. However, the difference between these two types of activities can be difficult to demarcate.

Human subjects

Although it is important that any discussion of research and research ethics be clear about the definition of a research subject, this definition is as elusive as the definition of research, on which it depends. A useful definition comes from the United States "Common Rule," the set of Federal regulations first promulgated in 1981 that govern research ethics. The Common Rule defines a "research subject" as "a living individual, about whom an investigator conducting research obtains either: (1) data through intervention or interaction with the individual, or (2) identifiable private information" (US Code of Federal Regulations 46.102f)." For pharmacoepidemiologists, the key

issue here is that the use of information that can be linked to an individual constitutes a contact between an investigator and a human subject. This is true even if the information was gathered in the past and no contact occurs between the investigator and the person. A fundamental issue, then, becomes whether information can be linked to an individual.

Although this may not be a universally accepted definition, the Common Rule applies, at a minimum, to all research carried out by US investigators using Federal funds. In addition, its influence is far greater because the vast majority of institutions that accept these Federal funds have signed an agreement, called a Federal Wide Assurance (FWA), to abide by the Common Rule requirements in all research, regardless of the source of funding. Therefore, the Common Rule serves as *de facto* law governing research at the most productive research institutions in the US and offers a reasonable working definition. Further, even when research is performed outside the United States, if it is done with US Federal support or at an institution with FWA, then it must conform to American regulations governing research ethics.

Privacy and confidentiality

In pharmacoepidemiologic research, the concepts of privacy and confidentiality are of paramount concern. Although they are often discussed together, they are distinct concepts. Privacy is the most basic, and confidentiality is, in a sense, derivative.

Privacy, in the setting of research, refers to security from unwanted intrusion into physical and personal space including personal information and handling of waste materials from a person. In the case of much epidemiologic research, privacy refers to each individual's right to prevent access to his or her medical records. The right to privacy, and others' corresponding obligation to respect privacy, is justified in part by each individual's right to be left alone. Viewed in this light, a right to privacy is a precondition for social interaction and cooperation because it allows and requires a degree of trust.

Confidentiality is a derivative right that is based upon the right to privacy. When individuals choose to allow a health care provider access to personal medical information, they have chosen to waive their right to privacy. Individuals may choose to exercise this right with the expectation, either implicit or explicit, that no one else will have access to that information without the patient's permission. This right to limit the transfer of information, to control the secondary use of information by others, is the right to confidentiality. Like the right to privacy, the right to confidentiality is also based on a basic right to a freedom from interference, in the sense that a right to confidentiality is not possible unless there is an underlying right to privacy. However, the right to confidentiality also engenders a responsibility on the part of the person who has information about another person. The expectation that someone will not disclose the information to a third party creates a fiduciary relationship. This means that confidentiality may be more highly specified by arrangements that may be made at the time that an individual initially grants access to information. For instance, patients may have specific expectations about ways in which the information they divulge may be used. These expectations may include transfer to a third party in either identifiable or unidentifiable form, access to particular kinds of information within a medical record, or limits as to the period of time that information may be available to others.

The fundamental issue is whether information that was gathered in a clinical setting, where rules of confidentiality apply, can be used for reasons, such as research, that were not part of the conditions of that relationship. Both the law and research regulations are ambiguous over what constitutes a substantive violation of confidentiality. Does the use of records without prior authorization constitute a violation of confidentiality? Or does it constitute a risk of a violation that depends on how those records are used, and on what is done with the information?

In general, society has not articulated clear answers to these questions, in large part because the questions engage well-formed but conflicting political and philosophical views about how society should organize the exchange of information. For example, proponents of communitarianism argue that the good of the individual is inextricably tied to the public good. Thus, ethical dichotomies that pit individuals against society (such as the unauthorized use of a person's clinical information for research) must be resolved with attention to both personal and public goods.

However, proponents of liberalism, or a rights-based individualism, disagree. From this perspective, what is right exists prior to what is good. This means that any unauthorized use of a person's information threatens to violate a fundamental right to privacy and the potential good derived from that use is not a proper condition to balance against that violation.

Informed consent

The most disturbing feature of many of the research scandals in recent history has been the total disregard for informed consent. Informed consent is a legally documented procedure that ensures patients are made aware of all the risks that they may incur and the benefits that they may receive when choosing or not choosing a certain therapy or treatment. Every nation which has addressed the subject recognizes that subjects, or for incompetent patients, their surrogates, are to be told about the nature of research and alternatives to participation, and offered the chance to volunteer to participate or not participate. It is not surprising, therefore, that research ethics guidelines, recommendations, and regulations have stressed the procedural requirement of a subject's informed consent. In order for a subject's consent to be informed, he or she must understand the research and must agree to participate voluntarily, without inducement or coercion.

The regulations governing research informed consent in the US, while not universal, are illustrative of these features (CFR 46.116). The US regulations convey the feature of understanding by requiring that the investigator explain the research risks, benefits, and alternatives of research participation; the confidentiality of any information obtained; and the procedures for compensation and for contacting a person responsible for the research. Voluntariness is expressed by the requirement that investigators tell subjects that participation in the research study is voluntary, and that subjects have the right to discontinue participation at any time. In some situations, informed consent may be modified to be verbal instead of written, or even may not need to be obtained at all. Whether informed consent must always be obtained, and in what form consent should be documented, have been the subject of vigorous debate.

The US guidelines offer a helpful perspective on the complexities that this issue raises. The Common Rule requires that written informed consent be obtained in most research situations (CFR 46.116). However, it makes two notable exceptions. First, written documentation of informed consent is not required if the principal risk of the research is a breach of confidentiality and if the written record is the only link between personal data and the subject's identity (CFR 46.117.c). In this case, whether or not a written informed consent document is used depends on each subject's preferences regarding whether he/she wishes to sign a consent document that could be used to link data with identifiable information. Second, informed consent can be entirely waived if the research meets four conditions (CFR 46.116):

1. the research involves no more than minimal risk to the subjects;

2. the waiver or alteration will not adversely affect the rights and welfare of the subjects;

3. the research could not practicably be carried out without the waiver or alteration; and

4. whenever appropriate, the subjects will be provided with additional pertinent information after participation.

These criteria are often applied to pharmacoepidemiologic research. The controversial conditions here are whether the research risks are minimal and whether a waiver of informed consent will adversely affect the subjects' rights and welfare. These are controversial, because in research that involves the use of medical records, the principal risk is the violation of the subjects' confidentiality. A consensus about the proper application of these conditions requires a consensus about whether access to the patient's medical record without the patient's permission is a violation of confidentiality that is greater than minimal risk and violates the subject's rights and welfare.

There are two competing answers to this question. The first relies upon a strict adherence to the principle of respect for autonomy. Accordingly, any unauthorized use of records violates confidentiality, presents more than minimal risk, and adversely affects subjects' rights and welfare. Hence, in all human subjects research, the subject's informed consent could be perceived as an absolute requirement. Although this view follows from strict adherence to some research ethics codes, this is not the view held by most contemporary researchers and ethicists.

Instead, a second interpretation allows for flexibility in the priority of the principle of respect for autonomy. Accordingly, some potential or even actual violations of confidentiality do not adversely affect the subject's rights and welfare or present more than minimal risk. This interpretation requires that we be able to determine to which kinds of information, if any, most people would be willing to grant access. Reasonable people can and do disagree about the magnitude of harm and impact upon rights caused by unauthorized use of information. There are two useful ways to settle this disagreement. The first is to assure that the ethics board review is truly multidisciplinary so that a variety of reasonable views are heard. The second is to require that researchers take steps to minimize the risks and adverse effect upon rights if patient confidentiality is violated. These methods are addressed in the next section.

Minimal risk

Although the general goal of research is to produce knowledge that will benefit society, investigators must also minimize the risks to subjects. It is axiomatic that, as risks to subjects increase, the degree of subject protections, such as ethics review and informed consent, increases as well. The concept of minimal risk attempts to operationalize a risk threshold, above which protections should be stricter. Although the concept of minimal risk is relatively straightforward and would apply to most pharmacoepidemiologic protocols, its definition is problematic.

According to US regulations stated in the Common Rule, research risks are "minimal" if "the probability and magnitude of harm or discomfort are not greater in and of themselves than those ordinarily encountered in daily life or during the performance of routine physical or psychological examinations or tests" (CFR 46.102.i). In most situations, this concept is difficult to operationalize. This is in large part because the definition lacks a clear standard against which to compare the research risks: the daily lives of healthy or "normal" persons, or the daily lives of persons who might be subjects of the research. In pharmacoepidemiologic research where the risk is a potential violation of confidentiality, there is the additional problem of deciding whether any such violation is ordinarily encountered during daily life, such that a violation in the course of research is "minimal risk."

Ethics review boards

In many countries over the past 30 years, ethics review boards have become central to the practice of research. This requirement reflects the consensus that scientists, and science, could benefit from independent review of research protocols. This idea first appeared in the World Medical Association's Declaration of Helsinki in 1964, which requires that an independent committee review all protocols. These recommendations have been taken up rapidly, and review boards have become widespread. Their authority has been clarified as well, and these committees typically have the power to review and reject all research that takes place in their institution or in which their institution's investigators are involved. In addition, there have been several independent institutional review boards established across the US to review protocols for pharmaceutical companies, contract research organizations, and independent researchers.

In the US, while some states have enacted legislation governing human subjects research, the formal system of review has evolved primarily in a manner that links Federal authority and funding. A committee, referred to as an Institutional Review Board (IRB), is required to review all research that is funded by all Federal government branches that have signed on to the "Common Rule." In most other countries, research regulations are not limited by provisions regarding funding but, instead, apply to all research conducted in that country.

The composition of these review boards varies widely across international boundaries. However, a consistent feature is the need for inclusion of expertise from outside the scientific community. For instance, the US regulations mandate the inclusion of at least one member who is not affiliated with the institution, and one member who may be affiliated but who represents law, ethics, or another nonscience discipline (Code of Federal Regulations (CFR) 46.107). Australian regulations mandate a committee's composition by requiring a mix of genders, and by extending the inclusion of nonscience representatives. The purpose of these requirements is to introduce accountability to society and minimize conflicts of interest among scientists who act as research reviewers.

Although review boards have become a commonplace feature on the research landscape, even under US Federal guidelines, not all research requires review. Certain kinds of research can receive expedited review, that is, review by the IRB chair or a designated member of the IRB instead of the full committee, and some may be exempt from IRB review. This is a means to assure that the research risks are truly minor and the research fulfills basic subject protections without using unnecessary IRB resources. Research that does not require IRB review is any project that does not involve human subjects (CFR 46.101). For example, when investigators use data in which nothing would permit the investigator to identify the individual from whom the data came (e.g., medical records without identifiers), ethics board review is not required. In addition, according to the Common Rule, research may be eligible for expedited review if it poses no more than minimal risk and the research involves "existing data," which means a retrospective analysis of records that exist as of the date the research is proposed (CFR 46.110). Most European nations have similar provisions for expediting the review of research that poses no more than minimal risks to subjects.

Methodological problems to be addressed by pharmacoepidemiologic research

There are several procedures available that can protect patient confidentiality. These methods allow patients to control who has access to information.

At the time that clinical data are gathered, such as upon enrollment in a health system, a patient can provide a "universal consent" to determine whether his or her medical record can be used for research. This term should not be interpreted to mean an informed consent to participate in research, because the patient is simply consenting to the generic use of his or her records and not whether to participate in actual protocols. A variation on this method is that patients can shield some aspects of their medical records from use in research. This is possible in some electronic record management systems. For example, patients could place into an electronic "black box" records of certain medications, such as antidepressants. Finally, at the time of the research, patients can be contacted to provide informed consent for the use of their archived records. However, there are two problems in applying these methods to pharmacoepidemiologic research.

First, they may not really protect privacy to the degree that investigators and ethics review boards would hope. For instance, if individuals must be contacted each time their records may be used in a particular study, the individual may consider such contact intrusive. Furthermore, individuals might consider that their confidentiality has been violated if researchers access research information and contact them directly in order to obtain consent for the use of otherwise de-identified records. Individuals may also refuse participation if contacted for a study they consider irrelevant to their health. An individual may also become alarmed if asked to consent for records to be used in such a study of a disease for which she has not been diagnosed (e.g., a control subject in a case–control study of patients with and without breast cancer).

Second, they may erode the validity of the research findings, and therefore utility for the population that stands to benefit from the research. Validity is a necessary precondition for all ethical research, and research should not be done if it cannot answer the hypothesis it claims to test. In pharmacoepidemiologic studies that use archival records, methods that allow patients to control who has access to data can severely limit the validity of the research to be done. For instance, consider the procedure of universal consent, in which each patient is given the opportunity to remove his or her electronic medical records (such as Medicaid data) from use for research. It is certain that at least some patients will opt out. The problem is that willingness to provide consent is generally not random and varies in ways that may bias study results. In addition, when researchers attempt to contact all patients in a database to seek informed consent, some patients may be unavailable to provide consent because they have died, moved, or changed health plans. Those patients also are likely to be distributed in a nonrandom fashion. The potential bias was demonstrated using data from the Mayo Clinic Rochester Epidemiology Project. Data available from all patients over a 50-year period showed a decrease in the population incidence of hip fracture. Data from only those patients known to be alive and able to give consent would produce results showing an increasing risk of hip fracture over time. This consent issue poses particular challenges in studies requiring long periods of exposure or follow-up, studies evaluating events of long latency, and the evaluation of intergenerational effects of medications.

An additional problem is encountered in the conduct of large, multi-institutional case–control studies in which access to a large amount of data must be reviewed in order to identify the cases and controls prior to contacting the appropriate patients for consent. Ethics review boards typically waive the requirement for consent in the initial case-finding review of records, and evaluate the consent used when patients are invited to participate in the study. Applying the current Common Rule framework to these studies requires separate review by ethics review boards from each participating institution of the same protocol. Issues raised by these ethics review boards and encountered in the review process may relate less to true local differences in the research environment than to the administrative differences of each institution's ethics review board process. Absent a more streamlined approach to the current ethics review board process, the time and cost of seeking multiple approvals discourage the conduct of these studies that may have important public health implications.

These issues are even more complex when attempting to conduct studies across multiple countries in which ethics requirements, consent procedures, and data confidentiality regulations may differ substantially. Harmonizing study procedures to accommodate differences in cultural norms, medical care practice patterns, and regulatory oversight while maintaining the integrity of the research design requires significant involvement of individuals at the global, regional and local levels.

Currently available solutions

The challenges discussed above pose considerable obstacles to the conduct of pharmacoepidemiologic research. For records-based studies using data not directly identifying subjects, investigators have relied on the confidentiality policies governing the use of information in the individual institution. For studies using identifiable records, investigators receive guidance and direction, if they receive it at all, through a process of negotiation with local ethics review boards, whose task is to balance the requirements of the research design with the rights and welfare of prospective subjects. Because the tension between ethics requirements and the exigencies of pharmacoepidemiologic research require this balancing process, in a very real sense the ethics of pharmacoepidemiologic research is a negotiated agreement between investigators and one or more review boards. The available solutions to the methodological challenges therefore depend upon two factors. First, they depend upon the steps investigators can take in gathering and handling data. Second, they depend upon the degree to which review boards can and should be involved in research, and on their ability to review research in a manner that is both competent and efficient.

The approach taken both in the US and internationally has tended towards legislative protections for data privacy. These legislative approaches to protect the confidentiality of medical data provide potentially strong protections and safeguards on the creation and reuse of confidential information.

For instance, the European Union (EU) Directive that went into effect October, 1998 covers all information that is either directly identifiable or information from which identity could be inferred. The EU Directive requires consent for all uses of information beyond that for which the information was originally collected. Safeguards on the use and transfer of information are required as well. Each institution must have a data controller/data privacy officer, who is accountable for appropriate procedures and use of data within the institution. In addition, data cannot be transferred from a member state of the EU to another country outside the EU unless that country has safeguards at least as stringent as those of the EU. Notably, however, member states may grant deviations from some provisions of the Directive for activities of substantial public interest. All research would presumably: (i) be conducted with explicit consent, (ii) be conducted only with delinked records, or (iii) be exempted by a specific member state as a type of activity of substantial public interest.

For pharmacoepidemiology, a number of implications of the Directive are of concern. For example, pharmacovigilance activities currently must be conducted using identifiable data. A requirement for patient consent would stifle the collection of a substantial proportion of cases and therefore hinder the ability to identify signals of drug safety problems. Furthermore, analysis of secondary information (from clinical trials or administrative databases) for research questions not anticipated at the time patients signed consent would not be possible without additional consent. Very little research could be conducted using secondary files from which direct patient identifiers have been deleted. This restriction is due to the broad definition in the Directive of identifiable and "indirectly identifiable" data.

In the US, the Health Insurance Portability and Accountability Act (HIPAA) of 1996 called for Congress to pass legislation on medical data privacy, and for the Department of Health and Human Services to promulgate regulations if Congress failed to act. While Congress considered numerous bills that promised stricter scrutiny of research and tighter protections, none was passed. Therefore, the Privacy Rule went into effect in

2003 and offers greater protections of privacy, restrictions on the uses to which existing data can be put, and requirements that individuals must be able to determine who and why others may have access to their personal data in many cases outside of standard medical practice. The rule applies to "covered entities" or organizations that generate and manage personally identifiable health data. While some researchers may not be directly covered by the rule, they generally must obtain access to information from organizations considered covered entities.

Of specific interest for pharmacoepidemiologists are the strategies for protecting confidentiality and enabling researchers to access existing data sets. Under the rule, data sets that are de-identified can be disclosed and used freely. The Privacy Rule defines de-identified data as: (i) a data set from which 18 specified items that could be considered identifiers have been removed, and (ii) a data set which the covered entity knows will not be used alone or with other data for the purpose of subsequently identifying individuals. The covered entity can alternatively use a satisfactory statistical method to de-identify the data set while maintaining some of the 18 elements.

However, investigators would rarely find a data set stripped of these 18 elements appropriate for research because the elements include some items that are essential for research. For example, any specific date field related to an individual would have to be removed. Specific dates are usually required to evaluate sequence and timing of drug exposures and adverse events.

There are several methods researchers can use to gain access to a data set that has not been completely de-identified. First, patient authorization can be obtained. Second, the requirement for patient authorization can be waived by either an IRB or a Privacy Board (which is defined in the rule) if certain conditions are met, such as limits on access to the data, and assurances that the research could not be conducted without the waiver. Third, a "limited data set," that contains some of the 18 elements considered identifiers (e.g., dates and geocodes) can be provided to a researcher if a "data use agreement" has been signed by the researcher

assuring the appropriate use and disclosure of the information for research.

There are two additional features of the Privacy Rule that are important in protecting research. A data set can be considered to be de-identified even though a covered entity maintains a code by which the de-identified database can be relinked to personally identifiable data. The ability to relink a data set to original data in order to supplement a de-identified data set with information on risk factors, outcomes, or extended follow-up time can be critically important in pharmacoepidemiologic studies. In addition, the Privacy Rule has preserved access by researchers to patient information in certain circumstances for activities "preparatory for research." For example, a preliminary review of medical records is often important to identify patients potentially eligible for a study prior to approaching a patient for consent. Researchers may have access under the Privacy Rule only if the identifiable data are necessary for the preparatory work, and the identifiable information may not be removed from the covered entity as it is reviewed.

In 2009, the Institute of Medicine Committee on Health Research and the Privacy of Health Information published a report (Beyond the HIPAA Privacy Rule: Enhancing Privacy, Improving Health Through Research) summarizing major events post-HIPAA and describing how the HIPAA Privacy Rule affected health related research. The Committee concluded that "the HIPAA Privacy Rule does not protect privacy as well as it should, and that, as currently implemented, the HIPAA Privacy Rule impedes important health research." It issued three major recommendations: (1) Congress should allow Health and Human Services and other federal agencies to develop a new approach to protect health related research; (2) revise the current Privacy Rule in order to address the issues related to the Rule; and (3) implement changes at the Health and Human Services and US institutions level to protect the security of health related research data, to provide sound protection against civil suits for Institutional Review Board members and to disseminate more information and educate the public about health related research (see also Case example 15.1).

In addition, the Department of Health and Human Services issued a proposal in 2011 to revisit and update the Common Rule in order to address issues of ambiguity and changes that have occurred since the current regulation governing human subjects research have been developed.

There are also opportunities to improve and maybe standardize the ethics board review process. Ethics review varies widely from country to country, and, depending on each country's culture and needs, there may be differences between countries or even within one country. Certainly, sensitivity to local issues may be a desirable feature for the ethical review of research, particularly if institutions have special populations or circumstances that warrant special scrutiny of protocols. However, this variability may also be the result of variability in the quality of the ethics review board's skills and resources. Standardizing the basic ethics board review processes may be more efficient and effective especially when researchers are involved in multicountry pharmacoepidemiologic studies. In existing guidelines there is general agreement that protocol review by ethics review boards is valuable in principle. However, there is considerably less agreement about what kinds of pharmacoepidemiologic research require this review.

The ability of ethics review boards to review research in a manner that is both competent and efficient addresses issues of the training and certification of membership and resources for handling the volume of new and renewing research protocols. In general, the requirements for the skills and knowledge needed for ethics review board membership are handled by the local ethics review board. No certification exists to assure that ethics review board members possess adequate understanding of research ethics and regulation. Finally, ethics review boards are funded through indirect means, such as the general pool of indirect funds generated from grants. Potential ways to improve the quality and efficiency of ethics board review include training and certification of board members, reduction in the amount of paperwork for

routine monitoring of protocols, and explicit funding that is proportionate to an ethics review board's workload.

Conclusion

The variability and quality of ethics board review pose significant challenges for pharmacoepidemiologic investigators. These should be the focus of future efforts to harmonize research regulations and set minimum standards for ethics review board competency and funding. However, these solutions do not adequately address a larger problem. Although ethics review boards may offer a reasonable procedural solution to ethics review, it is less clear how ethics review boards should balance ethical and methodological requirements. Without a careful consideration of this balancing process, any efforts at regulation, and particularly efforts to standardize ethics board review and boost their resources, will achieve only limited success.

The idea of balancing is not new. Traditional approaches to balancing the ethical and methodological requirements of research typically use the research risks as their guide. The problem, though, is that this relationship is too simple for the situation of pharmacoepidemiologic research. The risks to the subjects of most pharmacoepidemiologic research are not the usual health risks of research that can be balanced against the potential health benefits of research. They are instead largely risks of violation of confidentiality, which is really a civil, rather than a medical, risk.

Investigators and ethics review boards should consider an additional factor in this relationship: the value of the knowledge to be gained. An ethical justification for this position begins, first, with the example of social services research. United States research regulations currently include an exception for studies designed to evaluate social programs (CFR 46.101). The implicit argument for this exception is that these social programs offer clear and evident value. They contribute in an important way to the social good. Studies designed to evaluate them, even if these studies bear all of the markings of "research," are considered to be exempt from the requirements of ethics board review and subject to informed consent that govern the ethical conduct of research. In a sense, the requirements of ethical research are suspended for studies that offer significant and generally agreed upon value.

This is an extreme case of balancing value against research risks. This example is informative not only because it is so extreme, but also because studies of social programs have a great deal in common with pharmacoepidemiologic research. Pharmacoepidemiology's goals of studying medication use and identifying adverse drug reactions are directed as much toward the preservation of the public's health as they are toward the production of generalizable knowledge. The value of pharmacoepidemiologic research is therefore as clear and as readily evident as it is in studies designed to evaluate social programs. On these grounds alone, a compelling argument might be made that some kinds of pharmacoepidemiologic projects, like projects to evaluate important social programs, should be exempt from research review.

Of course, this argument may not be equally cogent and convincing for all pharmacoepidemiologic research because pharmacoepidemiologic research, like any research, spans a continuum. Certainly studies of adverse drug reactions resemble closely the example of social program research. Another example is a study of adverse drug reactions among individuals taking a certain medication. Results of this research would have immediate consequences for the health of the patients, or "subjects," for whom data are gathered. Other studies may be done for private companies or organizations following rigorous methodological standards but where the findings would not be made public or shared with anyone outside the sponsoring organization. It is difficult to know how to balance concerns for privacy against the desire of private entities to obtain pharmacoepidemiologic data. Studies like these should arguably be held to a different ethical standard because they do not hold the immediate possibility of clinically relevant knowledge that could be applicable to the people involved. The problem is that no public and national body exists to decide what kinds of research achieve this level of value.

The central ethical issue in pharmacoepidemiologic research is deciding what kinds of projects will generate generalizable knowledge that is widely available and highly valued, and do this in a manner that protects individuals' right to privacy and confidentiality. The problem is that these two ends differ in kind. The knowledge generated by pharmacoepidemiology is health-related knowledge about such things as the risks and benefits of medicines. In contrast, individuals' right to privacy is a matter of civil law. Although the two are frequently cast as in need of balancing, it may not be possible to weigh a certain amount of knowledge to be gained against a certain amount of confidentiality and privacy to be lost. Instead, perhaps the most productive approach will be to determine what kinds of procedures and practices warrant crossing thresholds of confidentiality and privacy in the pursuit of valuable knowledge.

If the ethical requirement of informed consent is absolute and inviolable, then any balancing would be indefensible. However, this is not a tenable solution, nor is it a solution that would be consistent with the way that society responds to a need for valuable information in other settings. Further public discussion is needed to identify ways in which the policies and procedures for the protection of privacy and the maintenance of confidentiality are fair and consistent with the requirements imposed on other sectors of society.

Acknowledgement

The author would like to thank Kevin Haynes, Jason Karlawish, and Elizabeth Andrews for their contribution to the chapter on bioethical issues in pharmacoepidemiology research that was published in the first edition of the book and that has been adapted in writing the content of this chapter, and Kosuke Kawai for his help with editing the case example.

Key points

• Much like all human subjects research, the risks involved in pharmacoepidemiology studies

---

Case Example 15.1: The HIPAA authorization form and effects on survey response rates, nonresponse bias, and data quality: a randomized community study (Beebe *et al.*, 2007)

Background

- The Health Insurance Portability and Accountability Act (HIPAA) Privacy Rule provides federal protections for personal health information held by health care provider organizations ("covered entities"). The compliance with the Privacy Rule was required as of April 2003. The HIPAA Privacy Rule permits "covered entities" to use and disclose individually identifiable health information for research purposes only with individual authorization. The Privacy Rule does not apply if all 18 HIPAA identifiers (such as zip code or birth dates) are removed from the data sets. Little is known whether the HIPAA authorization has adversely affected clinical research.

Question

- Does including a HIPAA authorization form (HAF) affect response rate, nonresponse bias, and data quality?

Approach

- Investigators conducted a community randomised study among Olmsted County, Minnesota residents. A total of 6939 cases were randomly assigned to receive either a mailed survey packet with the HAF or a mailed survey packet without the HAF.

Results

- Inclusion of the HIPAA authorization form significantly reduced response by 15% (39.8% in the HAF group versus 55.0% in the No HAF group; $p < 0.0001$).

- To examine the presence of nonresponse bias, investigators compared the age, gender, race/ethinicity, and education of respondents to those characteristics in the Olmsted County population. Females, younger, nonwhite, and lower educated residents were under-represented in both the HAF and No HAF groups compared with the population. However, these differences were negligible.

- Reports of general health and the percentage of respondents indicating that they were nonsmokers were both significantly lower in the No HAF group than in the HAF group. The HAF may force the selection of a slightly healthier population into the responding sample.

Strengths

- The investigators used a randomized experimental design to examine the effect of the HIPAA authorization form.

Limitations

- The typical HAF form may be 2 pages or longer. The version of the HAF used in the study was only 1 page long, therefore, their results may be underestimating the potential effect of HAF.

- The Olmsted County population is a unique population and may be more likely to see the value of medical records research. Hence, the generalizability of the findings may be limited.

- The study did not determine why participants refused and did not follow-up on nonresponders to determine why they did not provide authorization.

Key points

- Although the HAF is crucial to protect personal health information; its inclusion in epidemiologic studies may affect response rates and may have implications related to the selection of the study sample.

- Researchers may opt to remove the HIPPA requirement if they do not collect all 18 HIPPA identifiers. However, doing so may affect the number and nature of variables that can be collected in the study.

---

span from risks that require an investigator to obtain subjects' informed consent to risks that are accepted as part of public health surveillance and do not require additional oversight or protection.

- Violation of privacy and confidentiality are the most important risk in most pharmacoepidemiology studies.
- Ethics boards and investigators must gain the knowledge and expertise to review the risks of

pharmacoepidemiology studies in order to develop subject protections that are appropriate to the study's methods.

Further reading

Advisory Committee on Human Radiation Experiments (1995) Final Report, no. 00000848-9, vol. 061. Washington, DC: Government Printing Office.

Andrews E (1999) Data privacy, medical record confidentiality, and research in the interest of the public health. *Pharmacoepidemiol Drug Saf* **8**: 247–60.

Beauchamp TL, Cook RR, Fayerweather WE, Raabe GK, Thar WE, Cowles SR, *et al.* (1991) Ethical guidelines for epidemiologists. *J Clin Epid* **44**: 151S–69S.

Beebe TJ, Talley NJ, Camilleri M, Jenkins SM, Anderson KJ, Locke GR III (2007) The HIPAA authorization form and effects on survey response rates, nonresponse bias, and data quality: a randomized community study. *Medical Care* **45** (10): 959–65.

Beecher HK (1966) Ethics and clinical research. *N Engl J Med* **274**: 1354–60.

Brett A, Grodin M (1991) Ethical aspects of human experimentation in health services research. *JAMA* **265**: 1854–7.

Brody BA (1998) *The Ethics of Biomedical Research: An International Perspective.* New York: Oxford University Press.

Epstein M (2008) Guidelines for good pharmacoepidemiology practices (GPP). *Pharmacoepidemiol Drug Saf* **17**: 200–8.

Grisso T, Appelbaum PS (1998) *Assessing Competence to Consent to Treatment.* New York: Oxford University Press.

Hodge J, Gostin LO (2004) Public Health Practice Vs. Research: A Report for Public Health Practitioners Including Case Studies and Guidance. Available at: http://www.cste.org/pdffiles/newpdffiles/CSTEPHRes-RptHodgeFinal.5.24.04.pdf (accessed on May 10, 2012).

Levine RJ (1986) *Ethics and Regulation of Clinical Research,* 2nd edn. Baltimore, MD: Urban & Schwartzenberg.

McKeown RE, Weed DL, Kahn JP, Stoto MA (2003) American College of Epidemiology ethics guidelines: Foundations and dissemination. *Science and Engineering Ethics* **9**: 207–14.

Nas SJ, Levit LA, Gostin LO (2009) *Beyond the HIPAA Privacy Rule: Enhancing Privacy, Improving Health Through Research.* The National Academies Press, Washington DC.

National Commission for the Protection of Human Subjects of Biomedical and Behavioral Research (1979) The Belmont Report. *Ethical Principles and Guidelines for the Protection of Human Subjects of Research.* Washington, DC: US Government Printing Office.

Nuremberg Code. Reprinted in. Brody H (1998) *The Ethics of Biomedical Research. An International Perspective.* New York: Oxford University Press, p. 213.

Organization for Economic Cooperation and Development (1980) Guidelines on the Protection of Privacy and Transborder Flow of Personal Data. Recommendation of the OECD Council, September 1980.

Warren S, Brandeis L (1890) The right to privacy. *Harv Law Rev* **4**: 193–220.

CHAPTER 16

The Use of Randomized Controlled Trials for Pharmacoepidemiologic Studies

Samuel M. Lesko[1] and Allen A. Mitchell[2]

[1]*Northeast Regional Cancer Institute, and The Commonwealth Medical College, and Pennsylvania State University College of Medicine, Scranton, PA, USA*
[2]*Slone Epidemiology Center at Boston University, Boston, MA, USA*

Introduction

Because they provide unbiased estimates of effect, randomized controlled trials (RCTs) are considered the gold standard for demonstrating the effectiveness of a new medication (see Chapter 2). While RCTs are generally used to evaluate beneficial drug effects, the advantages of this study design also make it ideal for obtaining an unbiased estimate of the risk of adverse outcomes.

During the premarketing phases of drug development, RCTs involve highly selected subjects and in the aggregate include at most a few thousand patients. These studies are designed to be sufficiently large to provide evidence of a beneficial clinical effect and to exclude large increases in risk of common adverse clinical events. However, premarketing trials are rarely large enough to detect relatively small differences in the risk of common adverse events or to estimate reliably the risk of rare events. Identification and quantification of these potentially important risks require large studies, which typically are conducted after a drug has been marketed. Because of design complexity and costs, large controlled trials are not generally conducted in the postmarketing setting. The authors' search for the best method to assess the risk of serious but rare adverse reactions to pediatric ibuprofen and the resulting experience serves as the basis for this chapter (see Case example 16.1) and may prompt others to consider randomized trials for the postmarketing assessment of drug safety.

Clinical problems to be addressed by pharmacoepidemiologic research

Pharmacoepidemiologic methods are used to quantify risks and benefits of medications that could not be adequately evaluated in studies performed during the premarketing phase of drug testing. While this chapter considers only the assessment of the risks of medications, the principles involved also apply to the postmarketing evaluation of the benefits of medications.

As noted in Chapters 1 and 3, premarketing studies are typically too small to detect modest differences in the incidence rates (e.g., relative risks of 2.0 or less) for common adverse events or even large differences in the incidence rates for rare events, such as those that affect 1 per 1000 treated patients. Modest differences in risk of non-life-threatening adverse events can be of substantial public health importance, particularly if the medication is likely to be used by large numbers of

Textbook of Pharmacoepidemiology, Second Edition. Edited by Brian L. Strom, Stephen E. Kimmel, and Sean Hennessy.
© 2013 John Wiley & Sons, Ltd. Published 2013 by John Wiley & Sons, Ltd.

Case Example 16.1

Background

- The use of nonsteroidal anti-inflammatory drugs is associated with an increased risk of GI bleeding and renal failure in adults.
- In 1989, ibuprofen suspension (an NSAID) was approved for use in children by prescription only.
- The risk of rare but serious adverse events among children treated with ibuprofen suspension must be documented before this medication can be considered for a switch from prescription to over-the-counter use in children.
- Confounding by indication is likely in observational studies of prescription ibuprofen use in children.

Question

- Is the use of ibuprofen suspension in children associated with an increased risk of rare but serious adverse events?

Approach

- Conduct a large simple randomized trial of ibuprofen use in children.
- A randomized trial involving nearly 84 000 children 12 years of age and younger with a febrile illness was conducted.

Results

- The risk of rare but serious adverse events (hospitalization for GI bleeding, acute renal failure, anaphylaxis and Reye syndrome) was not significantly greater among children treated with ibuprofen compared to those treated with acetaminophen.

Strengths

- The large sample size allowed evaluation of rare events.
- Randomization effectively controlled for confounding, including confounding by indication.

Limitations

- The use of an active control treatment (acetaminophen) precludes using these data to compare the risk of ibuprofen to that of placebo in febrile children.
- Because medication exposure was limited to the duration of an acute illness, this study cannot be used to assess the risk of long-term ibuprofen use in children.

Key points

- When confounding by indication is likely, a randomized controlled trial may be the only study design that will provide a valid estimate of a medication's effect.
- Large, simple, randomized controlled trials can be successfully conducted to evaluate medication safety.
- By keeping the study simple, it is possible to conduct a large, practice-based study and collect data that reflects current ambulatory medical practice.

---

patients. If there are postlicensing questions about the safety of a drug, large observational studies are typically used to satisfy the sample sizes needed to identify (or rule out) the relevant risks. However, potential confounding is a major concern for virtually every observational study, and uncontrolled or incompletely controlled confounding can easily account for modest associations between a drug and an adverse clinical event (see Chapters 2 and 21).

Weak associations deserve particular attention with respect to uncontrolled confounding. Although there are important exceptions, the general view is that the stronger the association, the more likely the observed relationship is causal. This is not to say that a weak association (e.g., a relative risk ≤ 1.5) can never be causal; rather, it is more difficult to infer causality because such an association, even if statistically significant, can more likely be an artifact of confounding. As an example, consider an analysis where socioeconomic status is a potential confounder and education is used as a surrogate for this factor. Because the relation between years of education completed (the surrogate) and socioeconomic status (the potential confounder) is, at best, imperfect, analyses controlling for years of education can only partially control for confounding. Thus, it is advisable to use extreme caution in making causal inferences from small relative risks derived from observational studies. When there is concern about residual confounding prior to embarking on an observational study, one may wish to consider using a non-observational study design.

Methodological problems to be solved by pharmacoepidemiologic research

Confounding by indication (also referred to as indication bias, channeling, confounding by severity, or contraindication bias) may be a particular problem for postmarketing drug studies. According to Slone *et al.*, confounding by indication exists when "patients who receive different treatments differ in their risk of adverse outcomes, independent of the treatment received." In general, confounding by indication occurs when an observed association between a drug and an outcome is due to the underlying illness (or its severity) and not to any effect of the drug (see also Chapter 21). As with any other form of confounding, one can, in theory, control for its effects if one can reliably measure the severity of the underlying illness. In practice, however, this often is not easily done.

Confounding by indication is a particular concern in a number of settings (see Chapter 21). In general, observational studies are most informative when patients receiving different medications are similar with respect to their risks of adverse events. When there is a single therapy for an illness, and all patients receive that therapy (i.e., are "channeled" to the treatment), it is not possible to control for confounding in an observational study simply because no patients are left untreated to serve as controls. Cohort studies will be compromised if there is no reasonable alternative to the study treatment, including no treatment, to serve as a control. Case–control studies may be infeasible if one cannot identify controls that, aside from any effect of the exposure, are equally at risk of having the outcome diagnosed as the cases.

When there is at least one alternate treatment option and it is possible to control for obvious confounding, observational studies can contribute to our understanding of a medication's risks, particularly where the adjusted relative risk is large. However, as discussed above, a small relative risk (e.g., 1.3) can easily be an artifact of confounding by an unknown factor or by incomplete control of a recognized confounder, as can a large relative risk if the outcome is rare.

When confronted with the task of assessing the safety of a marketed drug product, the pharmacoepidemiologist must evaluate the specific hypothesis to be tested, estimate the magnitude of the hypothesized association, and determine whether confounding by indication is possible. If incomplete control of confounding is likely, it is important to consider performing an RCT. There is nothing inherent in an RCT that precludes a pharmacoepidemiologist from designing and carrying out these studies. To the contrary, the special skills of a pharmacoepidemiologist can be very useful in performing large-scale RCTs after a drug is marketed.

Overview of classic RCTs

As noted above, RCTs are most commonly used during the premarketing phases of drug development to demonstrate a drug's efficacy (and to gather general information concerning safety). By randomization, one hopes to equalize the distributions of confounding factors, whether they are known or unknown. Therefore, the assigned treatment is the most likely explanation for any observed difference between treatment groups in the clinical outcomes (improvement in the illness or the occurrence of adverse clinical events). By definition, participants in observational studies are not assigned treatment at random. In clinical practice, the choice of treatment may be determined by the stage or severity of the illness or by the patient's poor response to or adverse experience with alternative therapies, any of which can introduce bias.

Sample size

In homogeneous populations, balanced treatment groups in RCTs can be achieved with relatively small study sizes. In heterogeneous populations (e.g., children less than 12 years of age), a large sample size may be required to insure the equal distribution of uncommon confounders among study groups (e.g., infants versus toddlers versus school-age children). Study size is determined by the need to assure balance between treatment groups and the magnitude of the effect to be detected (see Chapter 3). Large randomized studies minimize the chance that the treatment groups are different with respect to potential confounders and permit the detection of small differences in common clinical outcomes or large differences in uncommon ones (see Chapter 3).

Blinding

Blinding is used to minimize detection bias and is particularly important where the outcome is subjective. Reporting of subjective symptoms by study participants and the detection of even objectively defined outcome events may be influenced by knowledge of the medications used. For example, if a patient complains of abdominal pain, a physician may be more likely to perform a test for occult blood in the stool if that patient was being treated with an NSAID rather than acetaminophen. Thus, follow-up data collection will only be unbiased if both parties (patient and investigator) are unaware of the treatment assigned. Blinding may be difficult to achieve and maintain, particularly if either the study or control medication produces specific symptoms (i.e., side effects) or easily observable physiologic effects (e.g., nausea or change in pulse rate).

Choice of control treatment

The hypothesis being tested determines the choice of control treatment. Placebo controls are most useful for making comparisons with untreated disease but may not represent standard of care and have been challenged as unethical. Further, it may be difficult to maintain blinding in placebo-controlled studies, as noted above. Studies employing an active control typically utilize usual drug treatments, which frequently represent the standard of care. Although often considered more ethical and easier to keep blinded because the illness and symptoms are not left untreated, these studies do not permit comparison with the natural history of the illness.

Data collection

Data collection in a premarketing clinical trial is generally resource intensive. Detailed descriptive and clinical data are collected at enrollment, and extensive clinical and laboratory data are collected at regular and often frequent intervals during follow-up. In addition to the data needed to test the hypothesis of a clinical benefit, premarketing trials of medications must also assess general safety and therefore must collect extensive data on symptoms, physical signs, and laboratory evaluations.

Data analysis

In observational studies, data analyses may be quite complex because of the need to adjust for potential confounders. In contrast, analysis of the primary hypothesis in many clinical trials is straightforward and involves a comparison of the outcome event in different groups. Analyses involving repeated measures, subgroups of study subjects, or adjustment to control for incomplete or ineffective randomization may be performed, albeit adding complexity.

Generalizability of results

The usual clinical trial conducted during the premarketing evaluation of a drug almost always involves highly selected patients; as a consequence, the results of the trial may not be generalizable to the large numbers of patients who may use the medication after licensing. Observational studies offer an advantage in that they can reflect the real-world experience of medication use and clinical outcomes, and because their modest costs permit studies involving large numbers of patients.

Limitations of RCTs

Methodological strengths notwithstanding, there are several features of the classic RCT that limit its use as a postmarketing study design. First, it may be unethical to conduct a study in which patients are randomly assigned a potentially harmful treatment. For example, an RCT to test the hypothesis that cigarette smoking increases the risk of heart disease would not be acceptable. Second, the complexity and cost of traditional premarket RCTs, with their detailed observations and resource-intensive follow-up, make very large studies of this type generally infeasible. However, if the study can be simplified and use the epidemiologist's tools to track patients and collect follow-up data, it may be possible to both control costs and make a large study feasible.

Currently available solutions

Large simple trials

Large, simple trials (LSTs) may be the best solution when it is not possible to completely control confounding by means other than randomization, and the volume and complexity of data collection can be kept to a minimum. The US Salk vaccine trial of the 1950s is an early example of a very large trial. More recently, large randomized trials have been used to test the efficacy of therapeutic interventions, especially in cardiology, or to evaluate dietary supplements or pharmaceuticals for primary prevention of cardiovascular disease and cancer. This approach has also been used successfully to evaluate the risk of adverse drug effects when the more common observational designs have been judged inadequate. LSTs are just very large randomized trials made simple by reducing data collection to the minimum needed to test only a single hypothesis (or at most a few hypotheses). Randomization of treatment assignment is the key feature of the design, which controls for confounding by both known and unknown factors, and the large study size provides the power needed to evaluate small risks of common events as well as large risks of rare events.

It is useful to note that while LSTs may appear to be similar to pragmatic trials, they can differ in important ways. Both are randomized studies; pragmatic studies are intended to provide widely generalizable results and while they may be large, that is not always the case; by definition, LSTs are large to assess rare events and small relative risks but may not be generalizable. The two designs share similarities when LSTs may have so few exclusion criteria as to make them "pragmatic" (generalizable).

How simple is simple?

Yusuf *et al.* (1984) suggest that very large randomized studies of treatment-related mortality collect only the participants' vital status at the conclusion of the study. Because the question of drug safety frequently concerns outcomes less severe than mortality, these ultra simple trials may not be sufficient. Hasford has suggested an alternative in which "large trials with lean protocols" include only *relevant* baseline, follow-up, and outcome data. Collecting far fewer data than is common in the usual RCT is the key feature of both approaches. With simplified protocols that take advantage of epidemiologic follow-up methods, very large trials can be conducted to test hypotheses of interest to pharmacoepidemiologists.

Power/sample size

Study power is a function of the number of events observed during the course of the study, which in turn is determined by the incidence rate for the event, the sample size, and the duration of observation or follow-up (see Chapter 3). Power requirements can be satisfied by studying a population at high risk, enrolling a large sample size, or conducting follow-up for a prolonged period. The appropriate approach will be determined by the goal of the study and the hypothesis to be tested. Allergic or idiosyncratic events may require a very large study population, and events with long latency periods may be best studied with long duration follow-up. However, power is not the only factor to consider. For example, while an elderly population may be at high risk for gastrointestinal bleeding or cardiovascular events, a study limited to this group may lack generalizability and would not provide information on the risk of these events in younger adults or children.

Data elements

The data collection process can be kept simple by examining primary endpoints that are objective, easily identified, and verifiable. Because confounding is controlled by randomization, data on potential confounders need not be collected. Rather, a few basic demographic variables can be collected at enrollment in order to characterize the population and to confirm that randomization was achieved.

Data collection

The data collection process itself can be simplified; follow-up data can be collected by mail or web-based questionnaires, or telephone interviews conducted with the study participants. Because the study will involve clear and objective outcomes (see below), which can be confirmed by medical record review or other means, self-report by the study participants can be an appropriate source of follow-up data. Other sources of follow-up data could include electronic medical records (e.g., for LSTs conducted among subscribers of a large health insurance plan, see Chapter 9) or vital status records for fatal outcomes (e.g., the US National Death Index).

The primary advantage of simplicity is that it allows very large groups of study participants to be followed at reasonable cost. However, a simple trial cannot answer all possible questions about the safety of a drug but must be limited to testing, at most, a few related hypotheses.

When is a large simple randomized trial appropriate?

LSTs are appropriate when all of the conditions in Table 16.1 apply.

Important research question

Although a simple trial will cost less per subject than a traditional clinical trial, the total cost of a large study (in money and human resources) will still be substantial. The cost will usually be justified only when there is a clear need for a reliable answer to a question concerning the risk of a serious outcome. A minor medication side effect such as headache or nausea may not be trivial for the individual patient but may not warrant the

Table 16.1 Conditions appropriate for the conduct of a large simply randomized trial.

---

(1) The research question is important.
(2) Genuine uncertainty exists about the likely results.
(3) The outcome risk is small.
   (a) The absolute risk is small and confounding by indication is likely, or
   (b) The relative risk is small, regardless of the absolute risk.
(4) Important effect modification (interaction) is unlikely.

---

expense of a large study. On the other hand, if the question involves the risk of premature death, permanent disability, hospitalization, or other serious events, the cost may well be justified.

Uncertainty must exist

An additional condition has been referred to as the "uncertainty principle." Originally described by Gray *et al.* as a simple criterion to assess subject eligibility in LSTs, it states that "both patient and doctor should be *substantially uncertain* about the appropriateness, for this particular patient, of each of the trial treatments. If the patient and doctor are *reasonably certain* that one or other treatment is inappropriate then it would not be ethical for the patient's treatment to be chosen at random" (italic in the original). This principle should be applied to determine the appropriateness of performing all RCTs, including an LST of an adverse clinical event. Very large randomized trials are justified only when there is true uncertainty about the risk of the treatment in the population. Apart from considerations of benefit, it would not be ethical to subject large numbers of patients to a treatment that was reasonably believed to place them at increased risk, however small, of a potentially serious or permanent adverse clinical event. The concept of uncertainty can thus be extended to include a global assessment of the combined risks and benefits of the treatments being compared. One treatment may be known to provide superior therapeutic benefits, but it may be unknown whether the risks of side effects outweigh this advantage. For example, the antiestrogen tamoxifen may improve breast cancer survival, but may do so only at the cost of an increased risk of endometrial cancer. Appropriately, a randomized trial was undertaken to resolve uncertainty in this situation.

Power and confounding

LSTs will only be needed if: (i) the *absolute* risk of the study outcome is small and there are concerns about confounding by indication, *or* (ii) the *relative* risk is small (in which case, there are inherent concerns about residual confounding from any source). By contrast, LSTs would not be necessary if the *absolute* risk were large, because premarket or other conventional RCTs should be adequate, or where uncontrollable confounding is not an issue, because observational studies would suffice; also, if the *relative* risk were large (and confounding by indication and other potential biases inherent in observational studies are not concerns), observational studies would be appropriate.

No interaction between treatment and outcome

An additional requirement for LSTs is that important interactions between the treatment and patient characteristics (effect modification) are unlikely. In other words, the available evidence should suggest that the association will be qualitatively similar in all patient subgroups. Variation in the strength of the association is acceptable among subgroups, but there should be no suggestion that the effect would be completely reversed in any subgroup. Because of the limited data available in a truly simple trial, it may not be possible to test whether an interaction has occurred, and the data collected may not be sufficient to identify relevant subgroups. Because randomization only controls confounding for comparisons made between the groups that were randomized, subsets of these groups may not be strictly comparable with respect to one or more confounding factors. Thus, if clinically important interaction is considered likely, additional steps must be taken to permit the appropriate analyses (e.g., stratified randomization). This added complexity may result in a study that is no longer a truly simple trial.

When is an LST Feasible?

LSTs are feasible when all of the conditions in Table 16.2 are met.

Table 16.2 Conditions which make a large, simple randomized trial feasible.

(1) The study question can be expressed as a simple testable hypothesis.
(2) The treatment to be tested is simple (uncomplicated).
(3) The outcome is objectively defined (e.g., hospitalization, death).
(4) Epidemiologic follow-up methods are appropriate.
(5) A cooperative and motivated population is available for study.

Simple hypothesis

LSTs are best suited to answer focused and relatively uncomplicated questions. For example, an LST can be designed to test the hypothesis that the risk of hospitalization for any reason, or for acute gastrointestinal bleeding, is increased in children treated with ibuprofen. However, it may not be possible for a single LST to answer the much more general question, "Is ibuprofen safe with respect to all possible outcomes in children?"

Simple treatments

Simple therapies (e.g., a single drug at a fixed dose for a short duration) are most amenable to study with LSTs. They are likely to be commonly used, so that it will be feasible to enroll large numbers of patients, and the results will be applicable to a sizeable segment of the population. Complex therapeutic protocols are difficult to manage, can reduce patient adherence, and by their very nature may not be compatible with the simple trial design.

Objective and easily measured outcomes

The outcomes to be studied should be objective and easy to define ("simple"), identify, and recall. An example might include hospitalization for acute gastrointestinal bleeding. Study participants may not correctly recall the details of a hospital admission, or even the specific reason for admission, but they likely will recall the fact that they were admitted, the name of the hospital, and at least the approximate date of admission. Medical records can be obtained to document the details of the clinical events that occurred. Events of this type can be reliably recorded using epidemiologic follow-up methods (e.g., questionnaires, telephone interviews, or linkage with public vital status records). On the other hand, clinical outcomes that can be reliably detected only by detailed in-person interviews, physical examinations, or extensive physiologic testing may not be amenable for study in simple trials.

Cooperative population

A cooperative and motivated study population will greatly increase the probability of success. Striking examples are the large populations in the

Physicians' and Women's Health Studies; the success of these studies is at least partly due to the willingness of large numbers of knowledgeable health professionals to participate. Because of the participants' knowledge of medical conditions and symptoms and participation in the US health care system, relatively sophisticated information was obtained using mailed questionnaires, and even biologic samples were collected.

Logistics of conducting an LST

An LST may be appropriate and feasible, but it will only succeed if all logistical aspects of the study are kept simple as well. In general, LSTs are "multicenter" studies involving a group of primary investigators who are responsible for the scientific conduct of the study, a central data coordinating facility, and a network of enrollment sites (possibly the offices of collaborating physicians or other health care providers). Health care professionals (e.g., physicians, nurse practitioners, and pharmacists) can participate by identifying eligible patients and by facilitating contact between patients and the investigators. Registration of study subjects can also be accomplished online using a secure Internet connection to the coordinating center, which allows for immediate confirmation of eligibility and randomization. Because success depends on the cooperation of multiple health care providers and a large number of patients, it is best to limit the demands placed on each practitioner (or his/her clinical practice).

To facilitate patient recruitment and to maximize generalizability of the results, minimal restrictions should be placed on patient eligibility. Patients with a medical contraindication or known sensitivity to either the study or control drug should not, of course, be enrolled, but other restrictions should be kept to a minimum and should ideally reflect only restrictions that would apply in a typical clinical setting.

Substantial bias can be introduced if either physician or patient can choose not to participate after learning (or guessing) which treatment the patient has been assigned. Therefore, patients should be randomized only after eligibility has been confirmed and the enrollment process completed.

Importance of complete follow-up

Because dropouts and losses to follow-up may not be random but may be related to adverse treatment effects, it is important to make every effort to obtain follow-up data on all subjects. A study with follow-up data on even tens of thousands of patients may not be able to provide a valid answer to the primary study question if this number represents only a modest proportion of those randomized. The duration of the follow-up period can affect the completeness of follow-up data collection. If it is too short, important outcomes may be missed (i.e., some conditions may not be diagnosed until after the end of the follow-up period). On the other hand, as the length of the follow-up period increases, the number lost to follow-up or exposed to the alternate treatment (contaminated exposure) increases. In the extreme, a randomized trial becomes an observational cohort study because of selective dropouts in either or both of the treatment arms. Beyond choosing a motivated and interested study population, the investigators can minimize losses to follow-up by maintaining contact with all study participants. Regular mailings of supplies of medication, a study newsletter, or email reminders can be helpful, and memory aids such as medication calendar packs or other devices may help maintain adherence with chronic treatment schedules.

Follow-up data collection

Follow-up data collection is the responsibility of the central study staff. Busy health care providers cannot be expected to commit the time required to obtain systematically even minimal follow-up data from large numbers of subjects. However, the clinician who originally enrolled the subject may be able to provide limited follow-up data (e.g., vital status) or a current address or telephone number for the occasional patient who would otherwise be lost to follow-up. A questionnaire delivered by mail, supplemented by telephone interviews when needed, is effective. The response rate will likely be greatest if the questions are both simple and direct and minimal time is required to complete the questionnaire. Medical records can be reviewed to verify important outcomes, such as rare adverse events, and the work needed to obtain and abstract the relevant records should be manageable. If there is a need to confirm a diagnosis or evaluate symptoms, a limited number of participants can be referred to their enrolling health care provider for examination or to have blood or other studies performed, although as previously noted this can make the trial far more complex. In addition, a search of public records (e.g., the National Death Index in the US) can identify study subjects who have died during follow-up.

Analysis

Primary analysis

Analyses of the primary outcomes are usually straightforward and involve a simple comparison of incidence rates between the treatment and control groups. Under the assumption that confounding has been controlled by the randomization procedure, complex multivariate analyses are not necessary (and may not be possible because only limited data on potential confounders are available). Descriptive data collected at enrollment should be analyzed by treatment group to test the randomization procedure; any material differences between treatment groups suggest an imbalance despite randomization. As noted above, it is assumed that there is no material interaction between patient characteristics and medication effects, thus eliminating the need for complex statistical analyses to test for effect modification.

Subgroup analyses

It is important to remember that confounding factors will be distributed evenly only among groups that were randomized; subgroups which are not random samples of the original randomization groups may not have similar distributions of confounding factors. For example, participants who have remained in the study (i.e., have not dropped out or been lost to follow-up) may not be fully representative of the original randomization groups and may not be comparable with respect to confounders among the different groups. Despite all efforts, complete follow-up is rarely achieved, and because only the original randomization groups

can be assumed to be free of confounding, at least one analysis involving all enrolled study subjects (i.e., an intention-to-treat analysis) should be performed. Also, unless a stratified randomization scheme was used, one cannot be certain that unmeasured confounding variables will be evenly distributed in subgroups of participants, and the smaller the subgroup, the greater the potential for imbalance. Therefore, subgroup analyses will be subject to the same limitations as observational studies (i.e., the potential for uncontrolled confounding).

Data monitoring/interim analyses

Because of the substantial commitment of resources and large number of patients potentially at risk for adverse outcomes, it is appropriate to monitor the accumulating data during the study. A study may be ended prematurely if participants experience unacceptable risks, if the hypothesis can be satisfactorily tested earlier than anticipated, or if it becomes clear that a statistically significant result cannot be achieved, even if the study were to be completed as planned. A data monitoring committee, independent of the study investigators, should conduct periodic reviews of the data using an appropriate analysis procedure.

The future

With accelerated approval of new medications and rapid increases in their use, we may see a greater need for large, randomized postmarketing studies to assess small differences in risk. This is particularly the case for medications considered for over-the-counter switch, because the risks of rare and unknown events that would be acceptable under prescription status might be unacceptable when the drug is self-administered by much larger and more diverse populations. In the absence of techniques that reliably control for confounding by indication in observational studies, there will be a growing need for LSTs to evaluate larger relative risks. Because of few restrictions on participant eligibility, LSTs are more likely than classical randomized clinical trials to reflect the true benefits and risks of medications when used in actual clinical practice. The generalizability of the results of LSTs and other pragmatic clinical trials makes these studies particularly attractive to regulators and policy-makers and may lead to increased use of these studies.

One possible approach that may improve efficiency in large studies would be to conduct trials involving patients who receive care from very large health delivery systems with automated medical records (see Chapters 8 and 9). If reliable data concerning relevant outcomes (e.g., hospitalization for gastrointestinal bleeding) were available in automated medical records for all study participants, it would be theoretically possible to eliminate the need to contact patients to collect follow-up data. It would still be necessary to identify eligible subjects, obtain consent, and randomize treatment. In addition, assurance would have to be provided that events were not missed by patients presenting to out-of-plan providers. In settings where there is no appropriate control treatment and it is not ethical to randomize between active drug and placebo, an alternative to an LST might be to enroll and follow a single cohort of perhaps the first 10 000 users of a new medication. However, the absence of a comparison group would make it impossible to determine whether the observed risks were due to the drug, the disease, or other factors, although it would at least be possible to accurately estimate the absolute risk of important events among exposed subjects. Where feasible, patients could be randomized to receive different doses, and a dose–response relationship could be sought.

It is clear that very large simple controlled trials of drug safety can be successfully carried out. It is less clear, however, how frequently the factors that indicate the need for a very large trial (Table 16.1) will converge with those that permit such a trial to be carried out (Table 16.2). As a discipline, pharmacoepidemiology is well suited to conduct LSTs and to develop more efficient methods of subject recruitment and follow-up data collection that can make these studies a more common option for the evaluation of small but important risks of medication use.

Key points

• Randomization usually controls for confounding, including confounding by indication.
• A large study allows assessment of small to modest associations of common events and large associations with rare events and assures that randomization produces balanced treatment groups.
• Large randomized controlled trials are feasible if data collection is kept simple and outcome events are objective and verifiable.

Further reading

Brass EP. The gap between clinical trials and clinical practice: the use of pragmatic clinical trials to inform regulatory decision making. *Clin Pharm Ther* **87**: 351–5.

Connolly SJ, Ezekowitz MD, Yusuf S, Eikelboom J, Oldgren J, Parekh A, *et al.* (2009) Dabigatran versus warfarin in patients with atrial fibrillation. *N Engl J Med* **361** (12): 1139–51.

DeMets DL (1998) Data and safety monitoring boards. In: Armitage P, Colton T, eds *Encyclopedia of Biostatistics*. Chichester: John Wiley & Sons, Ltd, pp. 1067–71.

Fisher B, Costantion JP, Wickerham DL, Redmond CK, Kavannah M, Cronin W.M. *et al.* (1998) Tamoxifen for prevention of breast cancer: report of the National Surgical Adjuvant Breast and Bowel Project P-1 Study. *J Natl Cancer Inst* **90**: 1371–88.

Francis T Jr, Korns R, Voight R, Boisen M, Hemphill F, Napier J. *et al.* (1955) An evaluation of the 1954 poliomyelitis vaccine trials: summary report. *Am J Public Health* **45** (suppl): 1–50.

Gray R, Clarke M, Collins R, Peto R (1995) Making randomized trials larger: a simple solution? *Eur J Surg Oncol* **2**: 137–9.

Hasford J, Bussmann W-D, Delius W, Koepcke W, Lehmann K, Weber E (1991) First dose hypotension with enalapril and prazosin in congestive heart failure. *Int J Cardiol* **31**: 287–94.

Hasford J (1994) Drug risk assessment: a case for large trials with lean protocols. *Pharmacoepidemiol Drug Saf* **3**: 321–7.

Hennekens CH, Buring JE (1989) Methodologic considerations in the design and conduct of randomized trials: the U.S. Physicians' Health Study. *Control Clin Trials* **10**: 142S–50S.

Hennekens CH, Buring JE, Manson JE, Stampfer M, Rosner B, Cook N.R. *et al.* (1996) Lack of effect of long-term supplementation with beta carotene on the incidence of malignant neoplasms and cardiovascular disease. *N Engl J Med* **334**: 1145–9.

Lee IM, Cook NR, Manson JE, Buring JE, Hennekens CH (1999) Beta-carotene supplementation and incidence of cancer and cardiovascular disease: the Women's Health Study. *J Natl Cancer Inst* **91** (24): 2102–6.

Lesko SM, Mitchell AA (1995) An assessment of the safety of pediatric ibuprofen: a practitioner-based randomized clinical trial. *JAMA* **273**: 929–33.

Mitchell AA, Lesko SM (1995) When a randomized controlled trial is needed to assess drug safety: the case of pediatric ibuprofen. *Drug Saf* **13**: 15–24.

O'Brien PC (1998) Data and safety monitoring. In: Armitage P, Colton T, eds *Encyclopedia of Biostatistics*. Chichester: John Wiley & Sons, Ltd, pp. 1058–66.

ONTARGET Investigators, Yusuf S, Teo KK, Pogue J, Dyal L, Copland I, Schumacher H, *et al.* (2008) Telmisartan, ramipril, or both in patients at high risk for vascular events. *N Engl J Med* **358** (15): 1547–59.

Rothman KJ, Michels KB (1994) The continuing unethical use of placebo controls. *N Engl J Med* **331**: 394–8.

Santoro E, Nicolis E, Grazia Franzosi M (1999) Telecommunications technology for the management of large scale clinical trials: the GISSI experience. *Comput Methods Programs Biomed* **60**: 215–23.

Slone D, Shapiro S, Miettinen OS, Finkle WD, Stolley PD (1979) Drug evaluation after marketing. A policy perspective. *Ann Intern Med* **90**: 257–61.

Yusuf S (1993) Reduced mortality and morbidity with the use of angiotensin-converting enzyme inhibitors in patients with left ventricular dysfunction and congestive heart failure. *Herz* **18** (suppl): 444–8.

Yusuf S, Collins R, Peto R (1984) Why do we need some large, simple randomized trials? *Stat Med* **3**: 409–20.

CHAPTER 17

Pharmacoeconomics: Economic Evaluation of Pharmaceuticals

Kevin A. Schulman[1], Henry A. Glick[2], Daniel Polsky[2], and Shelby D. Reed[3]

[1]*Duke University, Durham, NC, USA*
[2]*Perelman School of Medicine at the University of Pennsylvania, Philadelphia, PA, USA*
[3]*Duke University School of Medicine, Durham, NC, USA*

Conventional evaluation of new medical technologies includes consideration of efficacy, effectiveness, and safety. Health care researchers from a variety of disciplines have developed techniques for the evaluation of the economic effects of clinical care and new technologies. In this chapter, we briefly review the methods of pharmacoeconomics and discuss some methodological issues that have confronted researchers investigating the economics of pharmaceuticals.

Clinical problems to be addressed by pharmacoeconomic research

The cost of drugs is not limited to their purchase price. The accompanying costs of preparation, administration, monitoring for and treating side effects, and the economic consequences of successful disease treatment are all influenced by the clinical and pharmacologic characteristics of pharmaceuticals. Thus, in addition to differences in efficacy and safety, differences in efficiency (or the effectiveness of the agent in actual clinical practice compared to its cost) distinguish drugs from one another.

A large number of national governments now require the presentation of pharmacoeconomic data at the time of product registration for pharmaceuticals to qualify for reimbursement through the national health insurance systems. Clinical economics research is being used increasingly by managed care organizations and value-based insurance plans in the United States to inform funding decisions for new therapies. Decision makers increasingly are interested in guidance regarding the cost-effectiveness of new medical technologies such as pharmaceuticals. This guidance can be provided by clinical economic analyses.

Trends in pharmacoeconomic research

The biotechnology revolution in medical research has added another challenge to pharmacoeconomic research. Pharmacoeconomics is increasingly being used to help determine the effect on patients of new classes of therapies before they are brought to the marketplace and to help determine appropriate clinical and economic outcomes for the clinical development program. The challenge is twofold: (1) understanding the potential effect of a therapy, and (2) understanding the transition from efficacy to efficiency in clinical practice. These challenges span the clinical development spectrum. As we learn more about the potential effect and use of a new product, these issues can be re-addressed in an iterative process. Finally, more firms are beginning to use economic models to help guide the business planning process and the new product development process to address the economic issues

Textbook of Pharmacoepidemiology, Second Edition. Edited by Brian L. Strom, Stephen E. Kimmel, and Sean Hennessy.
© 2013 John Wiley & Sons, Ltd. Published 2013 by John Wiley & Sons, Ltd.

surrounding new therapies at the beginning of the product development cycle.

Pharmacoeconomic studies are designed to meet the different information needs of health care purchasers and regulatory authorities. Economic data from Phase III studies are used to support initial pricing of new therapies and are used in professional educational activities by pharmaceutical firms. Postmarketing economic studies are used to compare new therapies with existing therapies and increasingly to confirm the initial Phase III economic assessments of the product.

Economic evaluation and the drug development process

The development of economic data as part of a clinical trial requires integrating pharmacoeconomics into the clinical development process. Economic analysis requires the establishment of a set of economic endpoints for study, review of the clinical protocol to ensure that there are no economic biases in the design of the clinical trial–such as requirements for differential resource use between the treatment arms of the study—and the development of the economic protocol. Ideally, the economic study will be integrated into the clinical protocol and the economic data will be collected as part of a unified case report form. Two examples of cost analyses within clinical trials are provided in Case Examples 17.1 and 17.2.

Methodological problems to be addressed by pharmacoeconomic research

In considering economic analysis of medical care, there are three dimensions of such analysis with which readers should become familiar—type of analysis, perspective of the analysis, and types of costs. (Figure 17.1).

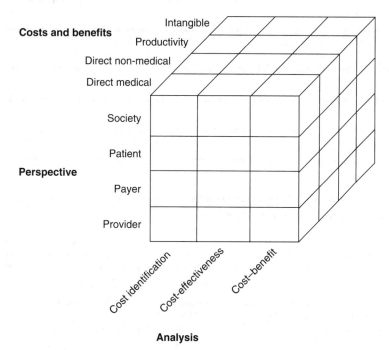

Figure 17.1 The three dimensions of economic evaluation of clinical care. Reproduced from Bombardier and Eisenberg (1985) with permission from *The Journal of Rheumatology*.

Case Example 17.1: Economic evaluation of high-dose chemotherapy plus autologous stem cell transplantation for metastatic breast cancer

Background

- A clinical trial of high-dose chemotherapy plus autologous hematopoietic stem cell transplantation versus conventional-dose chemotherapy in women with metastatic breast cancer found no significant differences in survival between the two treatment groups. Thus, the economic evaluation would provide decision makers with important additional information about the two therapies.

Question

- What were the differences between the two treatment groups with regard to course of treatment and resources consumed?

Approach

- The researchers abstracted the clinical trial records and oncology department flow sheets retrospectively to document resource use.
- Each patient's course of treatment and resource use was analyzed in four phases. Based on these clinical phases, patients were grouped into one of three clinical "trajectories."
- Costs were estimated using the Medicare Fee Schedule for inpatient costs and average wholesale prices for medications.
- Sensitivity analyses examined changes in the discount rate, hospital costs, and the number of cycles of the chemotherapeutic drugs paclitaxel and docetaxel.

Results

- Patients undergoing transplantation used more resources, mostly due to inpatient care.
- The investigators also found differences by clinical trajectory, and these differences were not consistent between treatment groups.
- High-dose chemotherapy plus stem-cell transplantation was associated with greater morbidity and economic costs with no improvement in survival.
- Results of the sensitivity analyses suggested that the findings were robust even when important cost assumptions varied.

Strengths

- By studying resource use and estimating costs, the authors were able to quantify the economic burden associated with the two treatments.
- The study allowed the investigators to provide novel information about the "clinical trajectories" of patients with metastatic breast cancer.
- The economic evaluation did not place any additional data collection burden on investigators, but yielded important secondary findings.
- Economic evaluation allowed the researchers to quantify the economic burden associated with interventions.

Limitations

- Collection of resource use data from the clinical trial records may have resulted in underestimation of treatment costs.
- Resource costs were estimated rather than directly observed.

Key points

- By studying resource use and estimating costs, the authors were able to quantify the economic burden associated with the two treatments and to provide information about the "clinical trajectories" of patients with metastatic breast cancer.
- Sensitivity analyses are crucial in studies that rely on numerous estimates and assumptions.
- Economic analysis can provide important additional information to decision makers in cases where no differences were observed between treatment groups on the primary clinical endpoint.

Case Example 17.2: Multinational economic evaluation of valsartan in patients with chronic heart failure

Background

- Clinical investigators found no differences in mortality in a clinical trial of ACE inhibitor with the addition of either valsartan or placebo for patients with heart failure.

Question and issue

- Economic data were collected prospectively as part of the multinational clinical trial.
- What challenges are presented in a multinational economic evaluation?

Approach

- Resource use data were collected at regular intervals in the case report form.
- Hospital and outpatient cost estimates were based on Medicare reimbursement rates for US patients and on the estimates of local health economists for patients outside the US (based on national fee schedules or hospital accounting systems).
- Cost estimates were converted to 1999 US dollars using purchasing power parties from the Organization for Economic Cooperation and Development.

Results

- Mean cost of a hospitalization for heart failure was $423 less for patients in the valsartan group, compared to patients in the placebo group.
- Much of the savings was offset by higher costs for non-heart-failure hospitalizations among patients in the valsartan group, yielding a nonsignificant decrease in inpatient costs of $193 for patients in the valsartan group.
- Overall within-trial costs, including outpatient costs and the cost of valsartan, were $545 higher for patients in the valsartan group. Thus, there was no finding of dominance.
- However, the subgroup of patients who received valsartan and were not taking an ACE inhibitor at baselines had $929 lower costs compared to their counterparts receiving placebo, even after including the cost of valsartan. Thus, in this subgroup, valsartan was the dominant strategy.

Strengths

- Data were collected prospectively.
- The study capitalized on the randomized design of the clinical trial to detect unbiased treatment effects.
- The study demonstrated the relative shift in costs incurred caused by the treatment effect of valsartan.

Limitations

- Practice patterns, resource use, and costs can vary significantly between countries, affecting the generalizability of the findings.

Key points

- In multinational economic evaluations, methods of cost-estimation are available that maintain the relation between relative costs and resource use within countries.
- Additional evaluations may be necessary to account for country-specific practice patterns, cost differences, and sociopolitical context.
- Treatment strategies can still be considered dominant even if they increase overall costs.

Types of analysis

There are three general types of economic analysis of medical care–cost–benefit, cost-effectiveness, and cost identification. In this chapter, we focus on the most common type, cost-effectiveness analysis.

Cost-effectiveness analysis

In cost-effectiveness analysis, cost generally is calculated in terms of dollars spent, and effectiveness is determined independently and may be measured only in clinical terms, such as number of lives saved, complications prevented, or diseases cured. Health outcomes can also be reported in terms of a change in an intermediate clinical outcome, such as cost per percent change in blood cholesterol level. These results generally are reported as a ratio of costs to clinical benefits, with costs measured in monetary terms but with benefits measured in the units of the relevant outcome measure (for example, dollars per year of life saved). When several outcomes result from a medical intervention, cost-effectiveness analysis may consider these outcomes together only if a common measure of outcome can be developed.

Cost-effectiveness analysis compares a treatment's incremental costs and incremental effectiveness, resulting in an estimate of the additional effect per additional treatment dollar spent. Programs that cost less and demonstrate improved or equivalent treatment outcomes are said to be dominant and should be adopted. Programs that cost more and are more effective should be adopted if their incremental cost-effectiveness ratios fall below an acceptable threshold. If there is a budgetary constraint, this must also be factored into the adoption decision. Programs that cost less and have reduced clinical outcomes may be adopted depending upon the magnitude of the changes in cost and outcome. Programs that cost more and have worse clinical outcomes are said to be dominated and should not be adopted.

Sensitivity analysis

Most cost-effectiveness studies require large amounts of data that may vary in reliability and validity, and could affect the overall results of the study. Sensitivity analysis is a set of procedures in which the results of a study are recalculated using alternate values for some variables to test the sensitivity of the conclusions to these altered specifications. In general, sensitivity analyses are performed on variables that have a significant effect on the study's conclusions but for which values are uncertain.

Types of costs

Economists consider three types of costs: direct, productivity, and intangible. Direct medical costs usually are associated with monetary transactions

and are incurred during the provision of care, such as payments for purchasing a pharmaceutical product, payments for physicians' fees, or purchases of diagnostic tests. Because charges may not accurately reflect the resources consumed, accounting or statistical techniques may be needed to determine direct costs.

Direct nonmedical costs are incurred because of illness or the need to seek medical care. They include, for example, the cost of transportation to the hospital or physician's office, the cost of hotel stays for receiving medical treatment at a distant medical facility, and the cost of special housing. Direct nonmedical costs, which are generally paid out of pocket by patients and their families, are just as much direct costs as are expenses that are typically covered by third-party insurance plans.

In contrast to direct costs, productivity costs do not stem from transactions for goods or services. Instead, they represent the cost of morbidity (e.g., time lost from work) or mortality (e.g., premature death leading to removal from the work force). They are costs because they represent the loss of opportunities to use a valuable resource, a life, in alternative ways.

Intangible costs are those of pain, suffering, and grief. These costs result from medical illness itself and from the services used to treat the illness. They are difficult to measure as part of a pharmacoeconomic study and are often omitted in clinical economics research.

Perspective of analysis

The third dimension of economic analysis is the perspective of the analysis. Costs and benefits can be calculated with respect to society's, the patient's, the payer's, and the provider's points of view. The perspective determines which costs and benefits are included. Because costs will differ depending on the perspective, the economic impact of an intervention will vary across different perspectives. It has been recommended that, as a base case, all analyses adopt a societal perspective. If an intervention is not good value for money from the societal perspective, it would not be a worthwhile intervention for society, even if the intervention may have economic advantages for other stakeholders.

Methodological issues in the pharmacoeconomic assessment of therapies

The basic approach for performing economic assessments of pharmaceuticals has been adapted from the general methodology for cost-effectiveness analysis. This section reviews some of the issues commonly confronted in the design, analysis, and interpretation of pharmacoeconomic evaluations.

Clinical trials versus common practice

Clinical trials are useful for determining the efficacy of therapeutic agents. However, their focus on efficacy rather than effectiveness and their use of protocols for testing and treating patients pose problems for cost-effectiveness analysis. One difficulty in assessing the economic impact of a drug as an endpoint in a clinical trial is the performance of routine testing to determine the presence or absence of a study outcome.

First, the protocol may induce the detection of extra cases–cases that would have gone undetected if no protocol were used in the usual care of patients. These cases may be detected earlier than they would have been in usual care. This extra or early detection may also reduce the average costs for each case detected, because subclinical cases or those detected early may be less costly to treat than clinically detected cases.

Second, protocol-induced testing may lead to the detection of adverse drug effects that would otherwise have gone undetected. The average costs of each may be less because the adverse effects would be milder. However, their frequency would be higher than severe adverse effects, and they could result in additional testing and treatment.

Third, protocol-induced testing may lead to the occurrence of fewer adverse events from the pharmaceutical product than would occur in usual care. The extra tests done in compliance with the protocol may provide information that otherwise would not have been available to clinicians, allowing them to take steps to prevent adverse events and their resulting costs. This potential bias would tend to lower the overall costs of care observed in the trial compared to usual care.

Fourth, outcomes detected in trials may be treated more aggressively than they would be in usual care. In trials, it is likely that physicians will treat all detected treatable clinical outcomes. In usual care, physicians may treat only those outcomes that in their judgment are clinically relevant. This potential bias would tend to increase the costs of care observed in the trial compared to usual care.

Fifth, protocol-induced testing to determine the efficacy of a product or to monitor the occurrence of all side effects generally will increase the costs of diagnostic testing in the trial. Alternatively, the protocol may reduce these costs in environments where there is overuse of testing. In teaching settings, for example, some residents may normally order more tests than are needed, and this excess testing may be limited by the protocol's testing prescriptions.

Sixth, clinical protocols may offer patients additional resources that are not routinely available in clinical practice. These additional resources may provide health benefits to patients. This could result in a bias in the study design if there are differences in the amount of services provided to patients in the treatment and control arms of a trial.

Seventh, patients in trials often are carefully selected and the result of the trial may not be readily generalizable to substantially older or younger populations (see Chapter 16). Similarly, exclusion criteria in clinical protocols may rule out many kinds of patients with specific clinical syndromes. These exclusions further limit the generalizability of the findings.

Routinely appending economic evaluations to clinical trials will likely yield "cost-efficacy" analyses, the results of which may be substantially different from the results of cost-effectiveness analyses conducted in the usual care setting. Clinical economics must explicitly recognize the complexity of having different resource-induced costs and benefits derived from clinical protocols and from observing patients in different health care systems in multicenter clinical trials.

Possible solutions

One possible solution to this problem is the inclusion of a "usual care" arm of the clinical trial. In such a study, patients randomized to the usual care arm of the study would be treated as they would be outside of the trial, rather than as mandated by the study protocol, and economic and outcomes data from usual care could thus be collected. These data would make it possible to quantify the number of outcomes that likely would be detected in usual care and the costs of these outcomes.

A second method that has been used to overcome these problems is to collect data from patients who are not in the trial but who would have met its entry criteria, using these data to estimate the likely costs and outcomes in usual care. These patients could have received their care prior to the trial (historical comparison group) or concurrent with it (concurrent comparison group). In either case, some of the data available in the trial may not be available for patients in the comparison groups. Thus, investigators must insure comparability between the data for usual care patients and trial patients.

However, two problems arise when using a concurrent comparison group to project the results of a trial to usual care. First, as with the randomization scheme above, the use of a protocol in the trial may affect the care delivered to patients who are not in the trial. If so, usual care patients may not receive the same care they would have received if the trial had not been performed. Thus, the results of the trial may lose generalizability to other settings. Second, the trial may enroll a particular type of patient (e.g., investigators may "cream-skim" by enrolling the healthiest patients), possibly leaving a biased sample for inclusion in the concurrent comparison group. This potential bias would tend to affect the estimate of the treatment costs that would be experienced in usual care.

Adoption of a historical comparison group would offset the issue of contamination. Because the trial was not ongoing when these patients received their care, it could not affect how they were treated. A historical comparison group would also tend to offset the selection bias: the subset of patients who would have been included in the trial if it had been carried out in the historic period will be candidates for the comparison group. However, use of a historical comparison group is unlikely to offset this bias entirely. Because this group is identified retrospectively, its attributes likely will reflect those of the average patients eligible for the trial, rather than those of the subset of patients that would have been enrolled in the trial. In addition, temporal trends in the rates of disease outcomes and therapeutic strategies can make historical controls problematic.

Issues in the design of prospective pharmacoeconomic studies

Despite their difficulty, prospective pharmacoeconomic studies are often the only opportunity to collect and analyze information on new therapies before decisions are made concerning insurance reimbursement and formulary inclusion for these agents. Table 17.1 outlines the steps required for developing an economic analysis plan.

Sample size

The sample required to address the economic questions posed in a trial may differ from that needed for the primary clinical question. In some cases, the sample size required for the economic analysis is smaller than that required to address the clinical question. More often, however, the opposite is

Table 17.1 Steps in an economic analysis plan.

1. Study design/summary
2. Study hypothesis/objectives
3. Definition of endpoints
4. Covariates
5. Prespecification of time periods of interest
6. Statistical methods
7. Types of analyses
8. Hypothesis tests
9. Interim analyses
10. Multiple testing issues
11. Subgroup analyses
12. Power/sample size calculations

true, in that the variances in cost and patient preference data are larger than those for clinical data. Then one needs to confront the question of whether it is either ethical or practical to prolong the study for longer than need be to establish the drug's clinical effects. Power calculations can be performed, however, to determine the detectable differences between the arms of the study given a fixed patient population and various standard deviations around cost and patient preference data.

Participation of patients

Protocols should allow prospective collection of resource consumption and patient preference data, while sometimes incorporating a second consent to allow access to patients' financial information. This second consent would be important if the primary concern was the possibility of patient selection bias in the analysis of clinical endpoints. However, given the low rates of refusal to the release of financial information, a single consent form should be preferred for all trial data. The single consent avoids the possibility of selection bias in the economic endpoints relative to the clinical endpoints.

Data collection

While some prospective data collection is required for almost all pharmacoeconomic studies, the amount of data to be collected for the pharmacoeconomic evaluation is the subject of much debate. There is no definitive means of addressing this issue. Phase II studies can be used to develop data that will help determine which resource consumption items are essential for the economic evaluation. Without this opportunity for prior data collection, however, we have to rely upon expert opinion to suggest major resource consumption items that should be monitored within the study. Duplicate data collection strategies (prospective evaluation of resource consumption within the study's case report form with retrospective assessment of resource consumption from hospital bills) can be used to ensure that data collection strategies do not miss critical data elements. However, one should develop a plan *a priori* to address any potential inconsistencies between information coming from different sources.

Multicenter evaluations

The primary result of economic evaluations usually is a comparison of average, or pooled, differences in costs and differences in effects among patients who received the therapies under study. It is an open question, however, whether pooled results are representative of the results that would be observed in the individual centers or countries that participated in the study. There is a growing literature that addresses the transferability of a study's pooled results to subgroups.

Economic data

Analysts generally have access to resource utilization data such as length of stay, monitoring tests performed, and pharmaceutical agents received. When evaluating a therapy from a perspective that requires cost data rather than charge data, however, it may be difficult to translate these resources into costs. For example, does a technology that frees up nursing time reduce costs, or are nursing costs fixed in the sense that the technology is likely to have little or no effect on the hospital payroll? Economists taking the societal perspective would argue that real resource consumption has decreased and thus nursing is a variable cost. Accountants or others taking the hospital perspective might argue that, unless the change affects overall staffing or the need for overtime, it is not a saving. This issue depends in part on the temporal perspective taken by the analyst. In the short term, it is unlikely that nursing savings are recouped; in the long term, however, there probably will be a redirection of services. This analysis may also be confounded by the potential increase in the quality of care that nurses with more time may be able to provide to their patients.

Measurement and modeling in clinical trials

The types of data available at the end of the trial will depend upon the trial's sample size, duration, and clinical endpoint. There are two categories of clinical endpoints considered in pharmacoeconomic analysis: intermediate endpoints and final endpoints. An intermediate endpoint is a clinical parameter, such as systolic blood pressure, which varies as a result of therapy. A final endpoint is an outcome variable, such as change in survival or quality-adjusted survival. Such final endpoint variables are often common in clinical trials, and thus allow for comparisons of economic data across clinical studies.

The use of intermediate endpoints to demonstrate clinical efficacy is common in clinical trials, because it reduces both the cost of the clinical development process and the time needed to demonstrate the efficacy of the therapy. Intermediate endpoints are most appropriate in clinical research if they have been shown to be related to the clinical outcome of interest, as in the Framingham Heart Study, which used changes in blood cholesterol levels to demonstrate the efficacy of new lipid lowering agents.

Ideally, a clinical trial would be designed to follow patients throughout their lives, assessing both clinical and economic variables, to allow an incremental assessment of the full impact of the therapy on patients over their lifetimes. Of course, this type of study is almost never performed. Instead, most clinical trials assess patients over a relatively short period of time. Thus, most pharmacoeconomic assessments must utilize data collected from within the clinical trial in combination with an epidemiologic model to project the clinical and economic trial results over an appropriate period of a patient's lifetime.

In projecting results of short-term trials over patients' lifetimes, it is typical to present at least two of the many potential projections of lifetime treatment benefit. A one-time effect model assumes that the clinical benefit observed in the trial is the only clinical benefit received by patients. Given that it is unlikely that a therapy will lose all benefits as soon as one stops measuring them, this projection method generally is pessimistic compared to the actual outcome. A continuous-benefit effect model assumes that the clinical benefit observed in the trial is continued throughout the patients' lifetimes. Under this model, the conditional probability of disease progression for treatment and control patients continues at the same rate as that measured in the clinical trial. In contrast to the one-time model, this projection of treatment benefit most likely is optimistic compared to the treatment outcome.

Analysis plan for cost data

Analysis of cost data shares many features with analysis of clinical data. One of the most important is the need to develop an analysis plan before performing the analysis. The analysis plan should describe the study design and any implications the design has for the analysis of costs (e.g., how one will account for recruiting strategies such as rolling admission and a fixed stopping date). The analysis plan should also specify the hypothesis and objectives of the study, define the primary and secondary endpoints, and describe how the endpoints will be constructed (e.g., multiplying resource counts measured in the trial times a set of unit costs measured outside the trial). In addition, the analysis plan should identify the potential co-variables that will be used in the analysis and specify the time periods of interest. Also, the analysis plan should identify the statistical methods that will be used and how hypotheses will be tested. Further, the plan should prespecify whether interim analyses are planned, indicate how issues of multiple testing will be addressed, and predefine any subgroup analyses that will be conducted. Finally, the analysis plan should include the results of power and sample size calculations.

If there are separate analysis plans for the clinical and economic evaluations, efforts should be made to make them as consistent as possible (e.g., shared use of an intention-to-treat analysis, shared use of statistical tests for variables used commonly by both analyses, etc.). At the same time, the outcomes of the clinical and economic studies can differ (e.g., the primary outcome of the clinical evaluation might focus on event-free survival while the primary outcome of the economic evaluation might focus on quality-adjusted survival). Thus, the two plans need not be identical.

The analysis plan should also indicate the level of blinding that will be imposed on the analyst. Most, if not all, analytic decisions should be made while the analyst is blinded to the treatment groups. Blinding is particularly important when investigators have not precisely specified the models that will be estimated, but instead rely on the structure of the data to help make decisions about these issues.

Methods for analysis of costs

When one analyzes cost data derived from randomized trials, one should report means of costs for the groups under study as well as the difference in the means, measures of variability and precision such as the standard deviation and quantiles of costs (particularly if the data are skewed), and an indication of whether or not the costs are likely to be meaningfully different from each other in economic terms.

Traditionally, the determination of a difference in costs between the groups has been made using Student's t-tests or analysis of variance (ANOVA) (univariate analysis) and ordinary least squares regression (multivariable analysis). More recently, analysts have moved toward the use of generalized linear models to improve the predictive power of multivariable analyses.

Uncertainty in economic assessment

There are a number of sources of uncertainty surrounding the results of economic assessments. One source relates to sampling error (stochastic uncertainty). The point estimates are the result of a single sample from a population. If we ran the experiment many times, we would expect the point estimates to vary. One approach to addressing this uncertainty is to construct confidence intervals both for the separate estimates of costs and effects as well as for the resulting cost-effectiveness ratio.

A common method for deriving 95% confidence intervals for cost-effectiveness ratios is the non-parametric bootstrap method. In this method, one re-samples from the study sample and computes cost-effectiveness ratios in each of the multiple samples. To do so, the analyst (1) draws a sample of size n with replacement from the empiric distribution and uses it to compute a cost-effectiveness ratio; (2) repeats this sampling and calculation of the ratio (by convention, at least 1000 times for confidence intervals); (3) orders the repeated estimates of the ratio from "lowest" to "highest"; and (4) identifies a 95% confidence interval from this rank-ordered distribution. The percentile method is one of the simplest means of identifying a confidence interval, but it may not be as accurate as other methods. When using 1000 repeated estimates, the percentile method uses the 26th and 975th ranked cost-effectiveness ratios to define the confidence interval.

In addition to addressing stochastic uncertainty, one may want to address uncertainty related to parameters measured without variation (e.g., unit cost estimates, discount rates, etc.), whether or not the results are generalizable to settings other than those studied in the trial, and, for chronic therapies, whether the cost-effectiveness ratio observed within the trial is likely to be representative of the ratio that would have been observed if the trial had been conducted for a longer period. These sources of uncertainty are often addressed using sensitivity analysis.

The future

This is a challenging period for the field of clinical economics. Many of the earlier methodological challenges of the field have been addressed, and researchers have gained experience in implementing economic evaluations in a multitude of settings. This experience has raised new questions for those interested in the development of new clinical therapies and in the application of economic data to the decision-making process.

With the increasing importance of multinational clinical trials in the clinical development process, many of the problems facing researchers today involve the conduct of economic evaluations in multinational settings. Foremost among these is the problem of generalizability. There is little consensus among experts as to whether the findings of multinational clinical trials are more generalizable than findings from trials conducted in single countries. This question is even more problematic for multinational economic evaluations, because the findings of economic evaluations reflect complex interactions between biology, epidemiology, practice patterns, and costs that differ from country to country.

As physicians are asked simultaneously to represent their patients' interests while being asked to deliver clinical services with parsimony, and as reimbursement for medical services becomes more centralized in the United States and other countries, decision makers must turn for assistance to collaborative efforts of epidemiologists and economists in the assessment of new therapeutic agents. Through a merger of epidemiology and economics, better information can be provided to the greatest number of decision makers, and limited resources can be used most effectively for the health of the public.

Key points

- Ideally, in economic evaluations of clinical trials, the economic study is integrated into the clinical protocol and the economic data are collected as part of a unified case report form for both clinical and economic variables.
- In general, programs that cost more and are more effective (and perhaps even some programs that cost less and have reduced clinical outcomes) should be adopted if both their cost-effectiveness and incremental cost-effectiveness ratios fall within an acceptable range.
- To address concerns about their reliability and validity, all economic evaluations should include sensitivity analyses of variables that have a significant effect on the study's conclusions but for which values are uncertain.
- Results of an economic analysis are just one component of the decision-making process regarding the adoption of an intervention; social, legal, political, and ethical issues, among others, are also important.

Further Reading

Bombardier C, Eisenberg J (1985) Looking into the crystal ball: can we estimate the lifetime cost of rheumatoid arthritis? *J Rheumatol* **12**: 201–4.

Brown M, Glick HA, Harrell F, Herndon J, McCabe M, Moinpour C, et al. (1998) Integrating economic analysis into cancer clinical trials: the National Cancer Institute—American Society of Clinical Oncology Economics workbook. *J Natl Cancer Inst Monogr* **24**: 1–28.

Cook JR, Drummond M, Glick H, Heyse JF (2003) Assessing the appropriateness of combining economic data from multinational clinical trials. *Stat Med* **22**: 1955–76.

Detsky AS, Naglie IG (1990) A clinician's guide to cost effectiveness analysis. *Ann Intern Med* **113**: 147–54.

Drummond MF, Stoddart GL, Torrance GW (1987) *Methods for the Evaluation of Health Care Programs*. New York: Oxford Medical Publications.

Eddy DM (1992) Cost-effectiveness analysis: is it up to the task? *JAMA* **267**: 3342–8.

Efron B, Tibshirani RJ (1993) *An Introduction to the Bootstrap*. New York: Chapman & Hall.

Eisenberg JM (1989) Clinical economics: a guide to the economic analysis of clinical practices. *JAMA* **262**: 2879–86.

Finkler SA (1982) The distinction between cost and charges. *Ann Intern Med* **96**: 102–9.

Glick HA (2011) Sample size and power for cost-effectiveness analysis (part 1). *Pharmacoeconomics* **29**: 189–98.

Gold MR, Siegel JE, Russell LB, Weinstein MC, eds. (1996) *Cost-Effectiveness in Health and Medicine*. New York: Oxford University Press.

Granneman TW, Brown RS, Pauly MV (1999) Estimating hospital costs. *J Health Econ* **5**: 107–27.

Laska EM, Meisner M, Seigel C (1999) Power and sample size in cost-effectiveness analysis. *Med Decis Making* **19**: 339–43.

Polsky DP, Glick HA, Willke R, Schulman K (1997) Confidence intervals for cost-effectiveness ratios: a comparison of four methods. *Health Econ* **6**: 243–52.

Reed SD, Anstrom KJ, Bakhai A, Briggs AH, Califf RM, Cohen DJ, et al. (2005) Conducting economic evaluations alongside multinational clinical trials: toward a research consensus. *Am Heart J* **149**: 434–43.

Reed SD, Friedman JY, Gnanasakthy A, Schulman KA (2003) Comparison of hospital costing methods in an economic evaluation of a multinational clinical trial. *Int J Technol Assess Health Care* **19**: 396–406.

Schulman KA, Lynn LA, Glick HA, Eisenberg JM (1991) Cost effectiveness of low-dose zidovudine therapy for asymptomatic patients with human immunodeficiency virus (HIV) infection. *Ann Intern Med* **114**: 798–802.

Willan AR (2001) Analysis, sample size, and power for estimating incremental net health benefit from clinical trial data. *Control Clin Trials* **22**: 228–37.

Willke RJ, Glick HA, Polsky D, Schulman K (1998) Estimating country-specific cost-effectiveness from multinational clinical trials. *Health Econ* **7**: 481–93.

CHAPTER 18

Using Quality-of-Life Measurements in Pharmacoepidemiologic Research

Holger J. Schünemann[1], Bradley C. Johnston[1,2,3], Roman Jaeschke[1,4], and Gordon H. Guyatt[1,4]

[1]*McMaster University, Hamilton, Ontario, Canada*
[2]*University of Toronto, Toronto, Ontario, Canada*
[3]*The Hospital for Sick Children Research Institute, Toronto, Ontario, Canada*
[4]*St. Joseph's Hospital, Hamilton, Ontario, Canada*

Introduction

One may judge the impact of drug interventions by examining a variety of outcomes. In some situations, the most compelling evidence of drug efficacy may be found as a reduction in mortality (β-blockers after myocardial infarction), rate of hospitalization (neuroleptic agents for schizophrenia), rate of disease occurrence (antihypertensives for strokes), or rate of disease recurrence (chemotherapy after surgical cancer treatment). Alternatively, clinicians frequently rely on direct physiological or biochemical measures of the severity of a disease process and the way drugs influence these measures—for example, left ventricular ejection fraction in congestive heart failure, spirometry in chronic airflow limitation, or glycosylated hemoglobin level in diabetes mellitus.

However, clinical investigators have recognized that there are other important aspects of the usefulness of the interventions which these epidemiologic, physiologic, or biochemical outcomes do not address. These are typically patient-reported outcomes. These areas encompass the ability to: function normally; be free of pain and physical, psychological, and social limitations or dysfunction; and be free from iatrogenic problems associated with treatment. On occasion, the conclusions reached when evaluating different outcomes may

differ: physiologic measurements may change without people feeling better, a drug may ameliorate symptoms without a measurable change in physiologic function, or life prolongation may be achieved at the expense of unacceptable pain and suffering. The recognition of these patient-important (versus disease-oriented) and patient-reported areas of well-being led to the introduction of a technical term: Health-Related Quality-of-Life (HRQL).

HRQL is a multifactorial concept that, from the patient's perspective, represents the final common pathway of all the physiological, psychological, and social influences of the therapeutic process. It follows that, when assessing the impact of a drug on a patient's HRQL, one may be interested in describing the patient's status (or changes in the patient status) on a whole variety of domains, and that different strategies and instruments are required to explore separate domains.

Clinical problems to be addressed by pharmacoepidemiologic research

HRQL effects may be pertinent in investigating and documenting both beneficial as well as harmful aspects of drug action. The knowledge of these

Textbook of Pharmacoepidemiology, Second Edition. Edited by Brian L. Strom, Stephen E. Kimmel, and Sean Hennessy.
© 2013 John Wiley & Sons, Ltd. Published 2013 by John Wiley & Sons, Ltd.

drug effects may be important, not only to the regulatory agencies and physicians prescribing the drugs, but to the people who agree to take the medication and live with both its beneficial actions and detrimental side effects. Investigators must, therefore, recognize the clinical situations where a drug may have an important effect on HRQL. This requires careful examination of data available from earlier phases of drug testing and, until now, has usually been performed in the latter stages of Phase III testing. For example, Croog and colleagues studied the effect of three established antihypertensive drugs—captopril, methyldopa, and propranolol—on quality-of-life, long after their introduction into clinical practice. Their report, which showed an advantage of captopril in several HRQL domains, had a major impact on drug prescription patterns at the time of its publication. The earlier in the process of drug development potential effects on quality-of-life are recognized, the sooner appropriate data might be collected and analyzed.

Methodological problems to be addressed by pharmacoepidemiologic research

Researchers willing to accept the notion of the importance of measuring HRQL in pharmacoepidemiologic research and ready to use HRQL instruments in postmarketing (or, in some cases, premarketing) trials, face a considerable number of challenges. Investigators must define as precisely as possible the aspects of HRQL in which they are interested (e.g., a specific domain or general HRQL).

Having identified the purpose for which an investigator wishes to use an HRQL instrument, one must be aware of the measurement properties required for it to fulfill its purpose. An additional problem occurs if researchers developed the original instrument in a different language, because one cannot assume the adequate performance of an instrument after its translation. When one has dealt satisfactorily with these problems, the investigator has to ensure—as in any measurement—the rigorous fashion (standardized, reproducible, unbiased) with which to obtain the measurements

(interviews or self- or computer-administered questionnaires). Finally, one is left with the chore of interpreting the data and translating the results into clinically meaningful terms.

Currently available solutions

Quality-of-life measurement instruments in investigating new drugs: potential use and necessary attributes

In theory, any HRQL instrument could be used either to discriminate among patients (either according to current function or according to future prognosis), or to evaluate changes occurring in the health status (including HRQL) over time. In most clinical trials, the primary objective of quality-of-life instruments is the evaluation of the effects of therapy, expressing treatment effects as a change in the score of the instrument over time. Occasionally, the intended use of instruments is to discriminate among patients. An example would be a study evaluating the effect of drug treatment on functional status in patients after myocardial infarction, where the investigators may wish to divide potential patients into those with moderate versus poor function (with a view toward intervening in the latter group).

The purpose for which investigators use an instrument dictates, to some degree, its necessary attributes. Each HRQL measurement instrument, regardless of its particular use, should be valid. The *validity* of an instrument refers to its ability to measure what it is intended to measure. This attribute of a measurement instrument is difficult to establish when there is no gold standard, as is the case with the evaluation of HRQL. In such situations, where so-called *criterion validity* cannot be established, the validity of an instrument is frequently established in a step-wise process including examination of *face validity* (or sensibility) and *construct validity*.

Face validity (sensibility) relies on an intuitive assessment of the extent to which an instrument meets a number of criteria, including applicability, clarity and simplicity, likelihood of bias, comprehensiveness, and whether redundant items have been included. *Construct validity* refers to the extent to which results from a given instrument relate to other measures in a manner consistent with theoretical hypotheses. It is useful to distinguish between *cross-sectional construct validity* and *longitudinal construct validity*. To explain the former, one could hypothesize that scores on one HRQL instrument should correlate with scores on another HRQL instrument or a physiological measure when measured at one point in time. For example, for identification of patients with chronic airflow limitation who have moderate to severe functional status impairment, an instrument measuring patient-reported dyspnea should show correlation with spirometry. In contrast, one would anticipate that spirometry would discriminate less well between those with worse and better emotional function than it does between those with worse and better physical function. To exemplify longitudinal construct validity, one could hypothesize that *changes* in spirometry related to the use of a new drug in patients with chronic airflow limitation should bear a close correlation with *changes* in functional status of the patient and a weaker correlation with *changes* in their emotional status.

The second attribute of an HRQL instrument is its ability to detect the "signal," over and above the "noise" which is introduced in the measurement process. For *discriminative instruments*, which measure differences among people at a single point in time, this "signal" comes from differences among patients in HRQL. In this context, the way of quantifying the signal-to-noise ratio is called *reliability*. If the variability in scores among subjects (the signal) is much greater than the variability within stable subjects (the noise), an instrument will be deemed reliable. Reliable instruments will generally demonstrate that stable subjects show more or less the same results on repeated administration. The reliability coefficient (in general, most appropriately an intraclass correlation coefficient), which measures the ratio of between-subject variance to total variance (which includes both between- and within-subject variance), is the statistic most frequently used to measure signal-to-noise ratio for discriminative instruments.

Classical reliability focuses on each observation or test score with a single true score, which belongs to one family of parallel observations, and yields a single reliability coefficient. Cronbach and colleagues introduced generalizability theory (G theory) as a framework for conceptualizing, investigating, and designing reliable observations in response to limitations of the true-score-model of classical reliability theory. G theory acknowledges that in any measurement situation, there are multiple, perhaps infinite, sources of error variance. It involves the same assumptions as classical test theory, but is simply an extension that allows for a linear model including multiple sources of error. Application of G theory focuses on identifying and measuring these error variances.

For *evaluative instruments*, those designed to measure changes within individuals over time, the "signal" comes from the differences in HRQL within patients associated with the intervention. The way of determining the signal-to-noise ratio is called *responsiveness* and refers to an instrument's ability to detect change. If a treatment results in an important difference in HRQL, investigators wish to be confident they will detect that difference, even if it is small. The responsiveness of an instrument is directly related to: (i) the magnitude of the difference in score in patients who have improved or deteriorated (the capacity to measure this signal can be called *changeability*), and (ii) the extent to which patients who have not changed obtain more or less the same scores (the capacity to minimize this noise can be called *reproducibility*). It follows that, to be of use, the ability of an instrument to show change when such change occurs has to be combined with its stability under unchanged conditions.

Another essential measurement property of an instrument is the extent to which one can understand the magnitude of any differences between treatments that a study demonstrates—the instrument's *interpretability*. If a treatment improves HRQL score by 3 points relative to control, what are we to conclude? Is the treatment effect very large, warranting widespread dissemination in clinical practice, or is it trivial, suggesting the new treatment should be abandoned? This question highlights the importance of being able to interpret the results of our HRQL questionnaire scores.

Researchers have developed a number of strategies to interpret HRQL scores, referred to as anchored-based methods. Successful strategies have three common attributes. First, they require an independent standard of comparison. Second, this independent standard must itself be interpretable. Third, there must be at least a moderate relationship between changes in questionnaire score and changes in the independent standard. The authors of this chapter have found that a correlation of 0.5 approximates the boundary between an acceptable and unacceptable relationship for establishing interpretability.

We have often used global ratings of change (patients classifying themselves as unchanged, or experiencing small, medium, and large improvements or deteriorations) as the independent standard. We construct our disease-specific instruments using 7-point scales with an associated verbal descriptor for each level on the scale. For each questionnaire domain, we divide the total score by the number of items so that domain scores can range from 1 to 7. Using this approach to framing response options, we have found that the smallest difference that patients consider important is often approximately 0.5 per question. A moderate difference corresponds to a change of approximately 1.0

per question, and changes of greater than 1.5 can be considered large. So, for example, in a domain with four items, patients will consider a one-point change in two or more items as important. This finding seems to apply across different areas of function, including dyspnea, fatigue, and emotional function in patients with chronic airflow limitation; symptoms, emotional function, and activity limitations in both adult and child asthma patients, and parents of child asthma patients; and symptoms, emotional function, and activity limitations in adults with rhinoconjunctivitis.

Another anchor-based approach uses HRQL instruments for which investigators have established the minimal important difference (MID, see Case Example 18.1). Investigators can apply regression or other statistical methods to compute the changes on a new instrument that correspond to those of the instrument with the established MID. For example, using the established MID of the CRQ, we computed the MID for two other instruments that measure HRQL in patients with chronic airflow limitation, the feeling thermometer and the St George's Respiratory Questionnaire. Similar to the anchor-based approach using transition ratings, investigators should ensure that the strength of the correlation between the change scores of these instruments exceeds a minimum (for example, a correlation coefficient of 0.5).

Case Example 18.1: Interpreting results of clinical trials focusing on HRQL outcomes

Background

- Clinical studies in patients with chronic obstructive pulmonary disease (COPD) rely on measuring health-related quality-of-life because physiological measures do not correlate highly with how patients feel. Investigators used a health-related quality-of-life instrument to measure whether patients with COPD had improved dyspnea after a drug intervention. They measured a mean change of 0.8 on the 7 point scale of the chronic respiratory questionnaire (CRQ) dyspnea domain in the intervention group and no change in the control group.

Question

- What have researchers done to help readers and clinicians answer the question "What does a change of 0.8 on the 7 point scale of the CRQ mean"?

Approach

- Investigators have used several techniques to investigate the interpretability of the CRQ and other health-related quality-of-life instruments. They have determined what constitutes the minimal important difference (MID) using comparisons with global ratings of change, with other instrument for which interpretability is known, and distribution-based statistical methods.

Results

- A change of 0.5 or more on the CRQ dyspnea domain indicates that patients, on average, have experienced an important change. The majority of patients in this study who received the intervention experienced an important improvement.

Strengths

- Multiple methods have shown a similar magnitude for the MID on the CRQ.
- Clinicians can interpret changes on health-related quality-of-life instruments if they know what constitutes an important change.

Limitations

- There is no gold standard for measuring health-related quality-of-life and to measuring interpretability.

Key points

- Health-related quality-of-life is a key outcome in chronic disease, such as COPD.
- Clinicians need to be able to interpret results of health-related quality-of-life outcomes.
- Several techniques exist that facilitate interpretation of health-related quality-of-life changes, including methods that have extended the interpretation of quality-of-life data based on risk difference and MID units in the context of meta-analysis.

Investigators have proposed distribution-based methods to determine the interpretability of HRQL instruments. Distribution-based methods differ from anchor-based methods in that they interpret results in terms of the relation between the magnitude of effect and some measure or measures of variability in results. The magnitude of effect can be the difference in an individual patient's score before and after treatment, a single group's score before and after treatment, or the difference in score between treatment and control groups. If an investigator used the distribution-based approach, the clinician would see a treatment effect reported as, for instance, 0.3 standard deviation units. The great advantage of distribution-based methods is that the values are easy to generate for almost any HRQL instrument because there will always be one or more measures of variability available. The problem with this methodology is that the units do not have intuitive meaning to clinicians.

Cohen addressed this problem in a seminal work by suggesting that changes in the range of 0.2 standard deviation units represent small changes, those in the range of 0.5 standard deviation units represent moderate changes, and those in the range of 0.8 standard deviation units represent large changes. Thus, one would tell a clinician that if trial results show a 0.3 standard deviation difference between treatment and control, then the patient can anticipate a small improvement in HRQL with treatment. However, this approach has statistical limitations (the same effect will appear different if population heterogeneity differs). Thus 0.2, 0.5, and 0.8 standard deviation units do not consistently represent small, medium, and large effects.

The standard error of measurement (SEM) presents another distribution-based method. It is defined as the variability between an individual's observed score and the true score, and is computed as the baseline standard deviation multiplied by the square root of 1 minus the reliability of the QOL measure.

Clinicians and investigators tend to assume that if the mean difference between a treatment and a control is appreciably less than the smallest change that is important, then the treatment has a trivial effect. This may not be so. Let us assume that a randomized clinical trial (RCT) shows a mean difference of 0.25 in a questionnaire with an MID of 0.5. One may conclude that the difference is unimportant, and the result does not support administration of the treatment. This interpretation assumes that every patient given treatment scored 0.25 better than they would have, had they received the control. However, it ignores possible heterogeneity of the treatment effect. Depending on the true distribution of results, the appropriate interpretation may be different.

Consider a situation where 25% of the treated patients improved by a magnitude of 1.0, while the other 75% of the treated patients did not improve at all. Summary measures would yield a mean change of 0.25 in the treated patients, and median change of 0 in this group, suggesting minimal effect. Yet, 25% of treated patients obtained moderate benefit from the intervention. Using the number needed to treat (NNT), a methodology developed for interpreting the magnitude of treatment effects, investigators have found that clinicians commonly treat 25–50 patients, and often as many as 100, to prevent a single adverse event. Thus, the hypothetical treatment with a mean difference of 0.25 and an NNT of 4 proves to have a powerful effect.

We have shown that this issue is much more than hypothetical. In a crossover randomized trial in asthmatic patients comparing the short-acting inhaled β-agonist salbutamol to the long-acting inhaled β-agonist salmeterol, we found a mean difference of 0.3 between groups in the activity dimension of the Asthma Quality-of-Life Questionnaire (AQLQ). This mean difference represents slightly more than half the minimal important difference in an individual patient. Knowing that the minimal important difference is 0.5 allows us to calculate the proportion of patients who achieved benefit from salmeterol—that is, the proportion who had an important improvement (greater than 0.5 in one of the HRQL domains) while receiving salmeterol relative to salbutamol. For the activity domain of the AQLQ, this proportion proved to be 0.22 (22%). The NNT is simply the inverse of the proportion who benefit, in this case 4.5. Thus, clinicians need to treat fewer than five patients with salmeterol to ensure that one patient obtains an important improvement in their ability to undertake activities of daily living.

Quality-of-life measurement instruments: taxonomy and potential use

We have also suggested a taxonomy based on the domains of HRQL which an instrument attempts to cover. According to this taxonomy, a HRQL instrument may be categorized as generic or specific. *Generic instruments* cover the complete spectrum of function, disability, and distress of the patient, and are applicable to a variety of populations and conditions. Within the framework of generic instruments, health profiles and utility measures provide two distinct approaches to measurement of global quality-of-life. In contrast, *specific instruments* are focused on disease or treatment issues particularly relevant to the disease or condition of interest.

Generic instruments

Health profiles

Health profiles are single instruments that measure different aspects of quality-of-life. They usually provide a scoring system that allows aggregation of the results into a small number of scores and sometimes into a single score (in which case, it may be referred to as an index). As generic measures, they are designed for use in a wide variety of conditions. For example, one health profile, the Sickness Impact Profile (SIP), contains twelve "categories" which can be aggregated into two dimensions and five independent categories, and also into a single overall score. Increasingly, a collection of related instruments from the Medical Outcomes Study have become the most popular and widely used generic instruments. Particularly popular is one version that includes 36 items, the SF-36. The SF-36 is available in over 40 languages, and normal values for the general population in many countries are available.

Because health profiles are designed for a wide variety of conditions, one can potentially compare the effects on HRQL of different interventions in different diseases. The main limitation of health profiles is that they may not focus adequately on the aspects of quality-of-life specifically influenced by a particular intervention or particular disease. This may result in an inability of the instrument to detect a real effect in the area of importance (i.e., lack of responsiveness). In fact, disease-specific instruments offer greater responsiveness compared with generic instruments.

Utility measurement

Economic and decision theory provides the underlying basis for *utility measures*. The key elements of a utility instrument are, first, that it is preference-based, and second, that scores are tied to death as an outcome. Typically, HRQL can be measured as a utility measure using a single number along a continuum from dead (0.0) to full health (1.0). The use of utility measures in clinical studies requires serial measurement of the utility of the patient's quality-of-life throughout the study.

There are two fundamental approaches to utility measurement in clinical studies. One is to ask patients a number of questions about their function and well-being. Based on their responses, patients are classified into one of a number of categories. Each category has a utility value associated with it, the utility having been established in previous ratings by another group (ideally a random sample of the general population). This approach is typified by three widely used instruments: the Quality of Well-Being Scale, the Health Utilities Index, and the Euroqol (EQ5).

The second approach is to ask patients to make a single rating that takes into account all aspects of their quality-of-life. This rating can be made in many ways. The "standard gamble" asks patients to choose between their own health state and a gamble in which they may die immediately or achieve full health for the remainder of their lives. Using the standard gamble, patients' utility or HRQL is determined by the choices they make, as the probabilities of immediate death or full health are varied. Another technique is the "time trade-off," in which subjects are asked about the number of years in their present health state they would be willing to trade-off for a shorter life span in full health. A third technique is the use of a simple visual analogue scale presented as a thermometer, the "feeling thermometer." When completing the feeling thermometer, patients choose the score on the thermometer that represents the value they place on their health state. The best state is full health (equal to a score of 100) and the worst state is dead (a score of 0).

A major advantage of utility measurement is its amenability to cost–utility analysis. In cost–utility analysis, the cost of an intervention is related to the number of quality-adjusted life-years (QALYs) gained through application of the intervention. Cost per QALY may be compared and provides a basis for allocation of scarce resources among different health care programs.

However, utility measurement also has limitations. Utilities can vary depending on how they are obtained, raising questions on the validity of any single measurement. Utility measurement does not allow the investigator to determine which aspects of HRQL are responsible for changes in utility and they may not be responsive to small but still clinically important changes.

Specific instruments

An alternative approach to HRQL measurement is to focus on aspects of health status that are specific to the area of primary interest. The rationale for this approach lies in the increased responsiveness that may result from including only those aspects of HRQL that are relevant and important in a particular disease (e.g., for chronic lung disease, for rheumatoid arthritis, for cardiovascular diseases, for endocrine problems), a population of patients (e.g., the frail elderly, who are afflicted with a wide variety of different diseases), a certain function (e.g., emotional or sexual function), or to a given condition or problem (e.g., pain) which can be caused by a variety of underlying pathologies.

Like generic instruments, disease-specific instruments may be used for discriminative purposes. They may aid, for example, in evaluating the extent to which a primary symptom (for example, dyspnea) is related to the magnitude of physiological abnormality (for example, exercise capacity). Whatever approaches one takes to the construction of disease-specific measures, a number of head-to-head comparisons between generic and specific instruments suggest that the latter approach will fulfill its promise of enhancing responsiveness.

In addition to the improved responsiveness, specific measures have the advantage of relating closely to areas routinely explored by the physician. For example, a disease-specific measure of quality-of-life in chronic lung disease focuses on dyspnea during day-to-day activities, fatigue, and areas of emotional dysfunction, including frustration and impatience. Specific measures may, therefore, appear clinically sensible to the clinician.

The disadvantages of specific measures are that they are (deliberately) not comprehensive, and cannot be used to compare across conditions or, at times, even across programs. This suggests that there is no one group of instruments that will achieve all the potential goals of HRQL measurement. Thus, investigators may choose to use multiple instruments. However, use of multiple instruments requires caution on how to interpret results if they differ between instruments and because of multiple testing of statistical hypotheses.

The future

The considerations we have raised suggest a step-by-step approach to addressing issues of HRQL in pharmacoepidemiology studies. Clinicians must begin by asking themselves if investigators have addressed all the important effects of treatment on patients' quantity and quality-of-life. If they have not, clinicians may have more difficulty applying the results to their patients.

If the study has addressed HRQL issues, have investigators chosen the appropriate instruments? In particular, does evidence suggest the measures used are valid measures of HRQL? If so, and the study failed to demonstrate differences between groups, is there good reason to believe the instrument is responsive in this context? If not, the results may be a false negative, failing to show the true underlying difference in HRQL.

Whatever the differences between groups, the clinician must be able to interpret their magnitude. Knowledge of the difference in score that represents small, medium, and large differences in HRQL will be very helpful in making this interpretation. Clinicians must still look beyond mean differences between groups, and consider the distribution of differences. The NNT for a single patient to achieve an important benefit in HRQL offers one way of expressing results that clinicians are likely to find meaningful. More recently,

methods including risk difference and MID have been published for improving the interpretation of quality-of-life data at the systematic review level.

Key points

- Health-related quality-of-life has become an established outcome measure in clinical research.
- The *validity* of an instrument refers to its ability to measure what it is intended to measure, while *responsiveness* determines the signal-to-noise ratio and refers to an instrument's ability to detect change.
- *Discriminative instruments* aim to measure differences among patients at one point in time, while *evaluative instruments* aim to measure changes over time.
- *Interpretability* is a key measurement property of an instrument and relates to the extent to which one can understand the magnitude of any differences between treatments that a study demonstrates.

Further reading

Bennett K (1996) Measuring health state preferences and utilities: rating scale, time trade-off, and standard gamble techniques. In: Spilker B (ed.), *Quality-of-life and Pharmacoeconomics in Clinical Trials*. Philadelphia, PA: Lippincott-Raven, p. 259.

Cohen J (1988) *Statistical Power Analysis for the Behavioral Sciences*, 2nd edn. Hillsdale, NJ: Lawrence Erlbaum Associates.

Croog S, Levine S, Testa M (1986) The effects of antihypertensive therapy on the quality-of-life. *N Engl J Med* **314**: 1657–64.

Guyatt GH, Berman LB, Townsend M, Pugsley SO, Chambers LW (1987) A measure of quality-of-life for clinical trials in chronic lung disease. *Thorax* **42** (10): 773–8.

Guyatt GH, Feeny D, Patrick D (1993) Measuring health-related quality-of-life: basic sciences review. *Ann Intern Med* **70**: 225–30.

Guyatt GH, Juniper E, Walter S, Griffith L, Goldstein R (1998) Interpreting treatment effects in randomized trials. *BMJ* **316**: 690–3.

Guyatt GH, Thorlund K, Oxman AD, Walter SD, Patrick D, Furukawa TA, Johnston BC, Karanikolas P, Vist G,

Kunz R, Brozek J, Meerpohl J, Akl EA, Christensen R, Schünemann HJ (2012) Preparing summary of findings tables: continuous outcomes. *J Clin Epidemiol* (in press).

Guyatt GH, Zanten SVV, Feeny D, Patrick D (1989) Measuring quality-of-life in clinical trials: a taxonomy and review. *Can Med Assoc J* **140**: 1441–7.

Jaeschke R, Guyatt G, Keller J, Singer J (1989) Measurement of health status: ascertaining the meaning of a change in quality-oflife questionnaire score. *Control Clin Trials* **10**: 407–15.

Jaeschke R, Singer J, Guyatt G (1991) Using quality-of-life measures to elucidate mechanism of action. *Can Med Assoc J* **144**: 35–39.

Johnston BC, Thorlund K, Schünemann HJ, Xie F, Murad HM, Montori VM, Guyatt GH (2010) Improving the interpretation of health-related quality of life evidence in meta-analyses: The application of minimal important difference units. *BMC Health Qual Life Outcomes* **11** (8): 116.

Schünemann HJ, Guyatt GH (2005) Commentary—goodbye M(C)ID! Hello MID, where do you come from? *Health Serv Res* **40** (2): 593–7.

Wiebe S, Guyatt G, Weaver B, Matijevic S, Sidwell C (2003) Comparative responsiveness of generic and specific quality-of-life instruments. *J Clin Epidemiol* **56**: 52–60.

CHAPTER 19

The Use of Meta-analysis in Pharmacoepidemiology

Jesse A. Berlin and M. Soledad Cepeda
Janssen Research & Development, LLC, Johnson & Johnson, Titusville, NJ, USA

Introduction

Definitions

Meta-analysis has been defined as "the statistical analysis of a collection of analytic results for the purpose of integrating the findings." Meta-analysis is used to identify sources of variation among study findings and, when appropriate, to provide an overall measure of effect as a summary of those findings. While epidemiologists have been cautious about adopting meta-analysis because of the inherent biases in the component studies and the great diversity in study designs and populations, the need to make the most efficient and intelligent use of existing data prior to (or instead of) embarking on a large, primary data collection effort has dictated a progressively more accepting approach.

The distinguishing feature of meta-analysis, as opposed to the usual qualitative literature review, is its systematic and structured presentation and analysis of available data. The traditional review has been increasingly recognized as being subjective, whereas meta-analysis can be approached as a more rigorous scientific endeavor with the same requirements for planning, prespecification of definitions, use of eligibility criteria, etc., as any other research. In recent years, the terms "research synthesis" and "systematic review" have been used to describe the structured review process in general, while "meta-analysis" has been reserved for the quantitative aspects of the process. For the purposes of this chapter, we shall use "meta-analysis" in the more general sense.

This chapter summarizes many of the major conceptual and methodological issues surrounding meta-analysis and offers the views of the authors about possible avenues for future research in this field.

Clinical problems to be addressed by pharmacoepidemiologic research

There are a number of reasons why a pharmacoepidemiologist might be interested in conducting a meta-analysis. These include the study of uncommon adverse outcomes of therapies, the exploration of reasons for inconsistencies of results across previous studies, and the exploration of subgroups of patients in whom therapy may be more or less effective.

Meta-analysis, by combining results from multiple *randomized* studies, can potentially address the problem of rare events and rectify the associated lack of adequate statistical power in a setting free of the confounding and bias of nonexperimental studies. When reports of several investigations of a specific suspected adverse drug reaction disagree, whether randomized or nonexperimental in design, meta-analysis can also be used to help resolve these disagreements. These disagreements among studies

Textbook of Pharmacoepidemiology, Second Edition. Edited by Brian L. Strom, Stephen E. Kimmel, and Sean Hennessy.
© 2013 John Wiley & Sons, Ltd. Published 2013 by John Wiley & Sons, Ltd.

may arise from differences in the choice of endpoints, the exact definition of exposure, the eligibility criteria for study subjects, the methods of obtaining information, other differences in protocols, or a host of other reasons possibly related to the susceptibility of the studies to bias. The exploration of the reasons for heterogeneity among study results may at least provide valuable guidance concerning the design of future studies.

Among the key recommendations from the Safety Planning, Evaluation, and Reporting Team (SPERT, formed by the Pharmaceutical Research and Manufacturers of America) was that sponsors plan a series of repeated meta-analyses of the safety data obtained from the studies conducted within a drug development program. Leading up to these meta-analyses, sponsors need to develop clear definitions of adverse events of special interest and to standardize various aspects of data collection and study design in order to facilitate combining studies and the interpretation of the combined analyses. By following a proactive approach during development, including periodic updating of cumulative meta-analyses, potential harms may be identified earlier in the development process.

Evidence-based medicine requires the use of the best evidence available in making decisions about the care of patients. Traditional meta-analyses, which have been one of the cornerstones of evidence-based medicine, often focus on placebo controlled trials because head-to-head comparisons of medications are generally unavailable. But what health care providers, patients, and policy-makers need to make better informed decisions is an analysis that provides a comprehensive look at all available evidence—how a specific pharmacological treatment compares with other available treatments in terms of safety and efficacy for the specific condition. Extended meta-analytic techniques such as indirect comparisons and multiple treatment meta-analyses can combine all available evidence in a single analysis. These techniques provide estimates of the effect of each intervention relative to every other, whether or not they have been directly compared in trials, allowing ranking of treatments in terms of efficacy and safety. The main drawback of these analyses is that the validity

of the findings depends on whether homogeneity and consistency assumptions, which we describe below, are met.

Methodological problems to be addressed by pharmacoepidemiologic research

Susceptibility of the original studies to bias

Early work in meta-analysis used the term "study quality." More recent efforts have adopted language that refers to susceptibility to bias or likelihood of bias. We adopt that new terminology in the remainder of this chapter. Many articles on "how to do a meta-analysis" and the PRISMA (Preferred Reporting Items for Systematic reviews and Meta-Analyses) guidelines, recommend that the meta-analyst assess the susceptibility to bias of the studies being considered in a meta-analysis.

Combinability of studies

Clearly, no one would suggest combining studies that are so diverse that a summary would be nonsensical. Should studies with different patient populations be combined? How different can those populations be before it becomes unacceptable to combine the studies? Should nonrandomized studies be combined with randomized studies? Should nonrandomized studies ever be used in a meta-analysis? Should studies with active drugs as comparators be combined with studies with placebos as comparators? These are questions that cannot be answered without generating some controversy.

Publication bias

Unpublished material cannot be retrieved by literature searches and is likely to be difficult to find referenced in published articles. *Publication bias* occurs when study results are not published, or their publication is delayed, because of the results. The usual pattern is that statistically significant results are more likely to be published than nonsignificant results. While one could simply decide not to include unpublished studies in a meta-analysis since those data have often not been peer-reviewed, unpublished data can represent a large proportion of all available data. If the results of unpublished studies are systematically different from those of published studies, particularly with respect to the magnitude and/or direction of the findings, their omission from a meta-analysis would yield a biased summary estimate.

Other forms of bias, related to publication bias, have also been identified. These include reference bias, i.e., preferential citation of significant findings; language bias, i.e., exclusion of studies in languages other than English; and bias related to source of funding. The selective reporting of some outcomes within a study, but not others, because of the direction of the results has also been identified as a major problem. Considerable efforts to reduce publication bias have been made. For example, to be considered for publication, many journals require that clinical trials were publicly registered prior to participant enrolment. In addition, the FDA Amendments Act of 2007 requires that protocols for all clinical trials involving FDA-regulated drugs and biologics be registered in a publicly accessible registry. This law also requires the registration of trial results within 1 year of trial completion.

Bias in the abstraction of data
Meta-analysis, by virtue of being conducted after the data are available, is a form of retrospective research and is thus subject to the potential biases inherent in such research.

In a number of instances, more than one meta-analysis has been performed in the same general area of disease and treatment. A review of 20 of these instances showed that, for almost all disease/ treatment areas, there were differences between two meta-analyses of the same topic in the acceptance and rejection of papers to be included. The acceptance or rejection of different sets of studies can drastically change conclusions. Despite efforts to make meta-analysis an objective, reproducible activity, there is evidently some judgment involved. In a meta-analysis of gastrointestinal side effects of NSAIDs, Chalmers and colleagues examined over 500 randomized studies. They measured the agreement of different reviewers and found disagreements on 10–20% of the items evaluated.

Currently available solutions

This section will first present the general principles of meta-analysis and a general framework for the methods typically employed in a meta-analysis. In the second part of this section, specific solutions to the methodological issues raised in the previous section are presented. Finally, case studies of applications that should be of interest to pharmacoepidemiologists will be presented, illustrating approaches to some of the clinical and methodological problems raised earlier.

Steps involved in performing a meta-analysis (Table 19.1)

Define the purpose
While this is an obvious component of any research, it is particularly important to define precisely the primary and secondary objectives of a meta-analysis. A well-formulated question should have a clearly defined patient population, intervention, comparator, and outcome of interest. This framework is called PICO and stands for *p*atient, *i*ntervention, *c*omparison, and *o*utcome. The important primary question might be "Are NSAIDs used for the treatment of pain associated with an increased risk of gastrointestinal side effects, compared with placebo?" It is important to consider that questions defined too broadly could lead to the criticism of "mixing apples and oranges" and that questions focused too narrowly could lead to finding no, or limited data, or the inability to generalize the study results.

Perform the literature search
Several studies have examined problems with the use of electronic searches. Use of search terms that are too nonspecific can result in large numbers of

Table 19.1 General steps involved in conducting a meta-analysis.

---

1. Define purpose
2. Perform literature search
3. Establish inclusion/exclusion criteria
4. Collect the data
5. Perform statistical analysis
6. Formulate conclusions and recommendations

---

mostly irrelevant citations that need to be reviewed to determine relevance. Use of too many restrictions can result in missing a substantial number of relevant publications. Search strategies to identify specifically reports of all definite or possible randomized or quasi-randomized trials have been developed.

Other methods of searching, such as review of the reference sections of retrieved publications found to be relevant, and manual searches of relevant journals, are also recommended.

Establish inclusion/exclusion criteria

A set of rules for including and excluding studies from the meta-analysis should be defined during the planning stage of the meta-analysis and should be based on the specific hypotheses being tested in the analysis. If broad inclusion criteria are established, then a broad, and perhaps more generalizable, hypothesis may be tested. The use of broad entry criteria also permits the examination of the association between research design and outcome (e.g., do randomized and nonrandomized studies tend to show different effects of therapy?) or the exploration of subgroup effects.

A key point is that exclusion criteria should be based on *a priori* considerations of design of the original studies and completeness of the reports and, specifically, should *not* be based on the results of the studies. To exclude studies solely on the basis of results that contradict the majority of the other studies will clearly introduce bias into the process. Such exclusions made after having seen the data, and the effect of individual studies on the pooled result, may form the basis for legitimate sensitivity analyses, but should not be viewed as primary exclusion criteria.

Collect the data

When the relevant studies have been identified and retrieved, the important information regarding study design and outcome needs to be extracted. The data collection should include an assessment of the likelihood of bias. The argument has been made, however, that general quality scoring systems are arbitrary in their assignment of weights to particular aspects of study design, and that such systems risk losing information, and can even be misleading. Jüni and colleagues, for example,

examined studies comparing low molecular weight heparin with standard heparin with respect to prevention of postoperative thrombosis. They used 25 different quality assessment scales to identify high quality trials. For six scales, the studies identified as being of "high quality" showed little to no benefit of low molecular weight heparin, while for seven scales, the "high quality" studies showed a significant advantage of low molecular weight heparin. This apparent contradiction raised questions about the validity of such scales as methods for stratifying studies. These data suggest that the use of summary quality scores to identify trials of high quality should be avoided and that relevant methodological aspects of study design should be assessed individually, and their influence on effect size explored, e.g., whether or not the assessment of outcome is blinded to treatment status and whether the presence or absence of such blinding is related to the magnitude of the treatment effect.

Thus, in a given meta-analysis, one might wish to examine *specific* aspects of study design that are unique to that clinical or statistical situation. For example, Schulz and colleagues found that trials in which the concealment of randomized allocation was inadequate, on average, produced larger estimates of treatment effects, compared with trials in which allocation was adequately concealed.

The Cochrane Collaboration recommends six domains to determine the quality of each one of the studies included in the analysis. These domains are: the method used to generate the allocation sequence; whether allocation concealment was implemented; whether blinded assessment of outcomes was performed; the degree of completeness of outcome data; whether selective outcome reporting is likely; and "other" dimensions when researchers identify problems that could put the study at a high risk of bias and are not part of the above framework.

Two procedural recommendations have been made regarding the actual techniques for data extraction. One is that studies should be read independently by two readers. The justification for this comes from meta-analyses in which modest but important inter-reader variability has been demonstrated. A second recommendation is that readers be masked to certain information in studies, such as the identity of the authors and the institutions at which a study was conducted, and masked to the specific treatment assignments. While masking has a high degree of intuitive appeal, the effectiveness of masking in avoiding bias has not been demonstrated. Only one randomized trial examined the issue of the effect of masking on the results of meta-analyses. The masked and unmasked teams produced nearly identical results on a series of five meta-analyses, lending little support to the need for masking.

Perform statistical analyses

Choice of Effect Measurement

There are three summary measures of effect size that can be used in meta-analysis when the outcome of interest is binary (e.g., proportion of subjects with pain relief): relative risk (RR), odds ratio (OR), or risk difference (RD). Although, the summary measure used does not typically affect the statistical significance of the results, the choice of effect measure could affect the transferability of results of the meta-analysis into clinical practice. Which summary measure to select depends on the ease of interpretation, the mathematical properties, and the consistency of the results when the particular effect measure is used. We focus here on the aspects that are specifically relevant to meta-analysis.

When the baseline (untreated) risk is constant across studies, or is assumed to be constant, the RD also allows calculation of relevant public health measures (e.g., number of events prevented or caused by a given treatment). A disadvantage of using RDs in meta-analysis is that, in an empirical study of a large number of meta-analyses, RDs displayed more heterogeneity than ORs, i.e., the results from study to study appeared more inconsistent with RDs. RR and OR are more consistent than RD and therefore are preferred from this perspective.

Choice of Statistical Method

In most situations, the statistical methods for the actual combination of results across studies are fairly straightforward, although a great deal of literature in recent years has focused on the use of increasingly sophisticated methods. If one is interested in combining odds ratios or other estimates of relative risk across studies, for example, some form of weighted average of within-study results is appropriate, and several of these exist. A popular example of this is the Mantel–Haenszel procedure, in which odds ratios are combined across studies with weights proportional to the inverse of the variance of the within-study odds ratio. Other approaches include inverse-variance weighted averages of study-specific estimates of multivariate-adjusted relative risks and exact stratified odds ratios.

One basic principle in many analytic approaches is that the comparisons between treated (exposed) and untreated (unexposed) patients are typically made within a study prior to combination across studies. In the combination of randomized trial results, this amounts to preserving the randomization within each study prior to combination. In all of the procedures developed for stratified data, "study" plays the role of the stratifying variable. In general, more weight is assigned to large studies than to small studies because of the increased precision of larger studies.

A second basic principle to note is that some of these methods assume that the studies are all estimating a single, common effect, e.g., a common odds ratio. In other words, the underlying treatment effect (whether beneficial or harmful) that all studies are estimating is assumed to be the same for all studies. Any variability among study results is assumed to be random and is ignored in producing a summary estimate of the effect. One may wish to use methods for combining studies that do not make the assumption of a common treatment effect across all studies. These are the so-called "random-effects" models, which allow for the possibility that the underlying true treatment effect, which each study is estimating, may not be the same for all studies, even when examining studies with similar designs, protocols, and patient populations. Hidden or unmeasured sources of among-study variability of results are taken into account by these random-effects models through the incorporation of such variability into the weighting scheme when computing a weighted average summary estimate.

One usual practical consequence of the random-effects models is to produce wider confidence intervals than would otherwise be produced by the traditional methods. This approach is considered particularly useful when there is heterogeneity among study results, and exploratory analyses have failed to uncover any known sources of observed heterogeneity. However, random-effects models should not be viewed as a panacea for unexplained heterogeneity. One danger is that a summary measure of heterogeneous studies may not really apply to any particular study population or study design; i.e., they lose information by averaging over potentially important study and population characteristics.

Assess and analyze variability among study results: heterogeneity is your friend

The underlying question in any meta-analysis is whether it is clinically and statistically reasonable to estimate an average effect of therapy, either positive or negative. If one errs on the side of being too inclusive, and the studies differ too greatly, there is the possibility that the average effect may not apply to any particular subgroup of patients. Conversely, diversity of designs and results may provide an opportunity to understand the factors that modify the effectiveness (or toxicity) of a drug.

The assessment of the degree of variation can involve statistical tests. An important word of caution is that statistical tests of heterogeneity suffer from a notorious lack of statistical power. Thus, a finding of significant heterogeneity may safely be interpreted as meaning the studies are not all estimating the same parameter. A lack of statistical significance, however, may not mean that heterogeneity is not important in a data set or that sources of variability should not be explored.

The I^2 statistic has become a widely adopted approach to statistical quantification of the among-study variability. It estimates the proportion of variability in point estimates due to heterogeneity rather than sampling error.

With respect to how one should approach the search for sources of heterogeneity, a number of options are available. One might stratify the studies according to patient characteristics or study design

features and investigate heterogeneity within and across strata. To the extent that the stratification explains the heterogeneity, the combined results would differ between strata and the heterogeneity within the strata would be reduced compared to the overall result. In addition to stratification, regression methods such as weighted least squares linear regression (termed "meta-regression") could be used to explore sources of heterogeneity.

Analysis of Rare Events

We have mentioned that, by combining results of many trials, meta-analysis can address the problems of rare events. However, the analysis of rare events in meta-analysis is still challenging. Many of the methods to combine data in meta-analysis are based on large sample approximations and therefore may be unsuitable when events are uncommon. In addition, the results could vary substantially depending on the method used to combine the data. Recommendations as to what method to use under which circumstances are based on studies that have used simulations in which the "truth" is generated by the investigators. The results of these studies show that fixed effect models should be used over random effect methods and that the inverse-variance-average should be avoided.

When dealing with rare events, many studies may have no events in any of the treatment arms, and relative measures such as relative risk or odds ratios cannot be calculated. If relative measures are used, studies with no events in either treatment arm will be excluded by virtue of the mathematics, not because the meta-analyst chooses to exclude them. However, in these circumstances, risk differences can be estimated. The problem is that risk differences models in the presence of rare events produce biased results and have very limited power.

Relative measures in cases when there are no events in *one* arm can be calculated. Many of the methods require "continuity corrections," i.e., adding a small value to all cells in a two-by-two table. The Mantel-Haenszel method often uses this approach. Traditionally, 0.5 is added to each of the cells and some statistical packages do this automatically. However, such continuity correction leads to bias in the presence of rare events, and is not necessary, even for the Mantel-Haenszel method. Smaller continuity corrections such as the reciprocal of the sample size of the opposite treatment arm, in contrast with the traditional continuity correction, produce unbiased results.

There are methods that do not require using any continuity correction, such as the Peto method and Bayesian methods. The Peto method, also known as the "one-step" model, is a fixed effect model that focuses on the observed number of events in the experimental intervention and compares it with the expected number of events. Since it uses the expected number of events, it can deal with individual groups in individual trials with no observed events, as long as there is at least one event in at least one of the arms in the trial. The Peto method produces unbiased results provided there is no substantial imbalance between treatment and control group sizes within trials, and provided the treatment effects are not exceptionally large (less than an OR of 5). The Bayesian methods often use prior distributions that are noninformative, so as not to impose an assumption about the anticipated effect, and use Markov chain Monte Carlo techniques that are capable of including trials that have no events in one of the arms. The Bayesian fixed effect models produce unbiased results independently of the imbalance in the allocation of treatment groups and therefore are recommended when dealing with rare events.

When a meta-analysis of rare events is contemplated, a thorough sensitivity analysis using different methods to combine studies is recommended and the results of such analyses should be reported so that the readers can assess the robustness of the results.

Other Considerations

Formulate Conclusions and Recommendations
As with all research, the conclusions of a meta-analysis should be clearly summarized, with appropriate interpretation of the strengths and weaknesses of the meta-analysis. Authors should clearly state how generalizable the results are and how definitive they are and should outline the areas that need future research. Any hypotheses generated by the meta-analysis should be stated as such, and not as conclusions.

Publication Bias
As discussed above, when the primary source of data for a meta-analysis is published data, the possibility needs to be considered that the published studies represent a biased subset of all the studies that have been done. In general, empirical studies have found that it is more likely that studies with statistically significant findings will be published than studies with nonsignificant findings. A practical technique for determining the potential for publication bias is the "funnel plot," first proposed by Light and Pillemer. This method involves plotting the effect size (e.g., the risk difference) against a measure of study size, such as the sample size or the inverse of the variance of the individual effect sizes. If there is no publication bias, the points should produce a kind of funnel shape, with a scatter of points centered around the true value of the effect size, and with the degree of scatter narrowing as the variances decrease. If publication bias is a problem, the funnel would look as though a bite had been taken out, with very few (if any) points around the point indicating no effect (e.g., odds ratio of 1.0) for studies with large variances. This method requires a sufficient number of studies to permit the visualization of a funnel shape to the data. It is important to note that publication bias is only one possible explanation for funnel plot asymmetry, so that the funnel plot should be seen as estimating "small study effects," rather than necessarily publication bias.

An additional methodological caution generated by publication bias relates to the use of random-effects models for combining results. When the results of the studies being analyzed are heterogeneous and a random-effects model is being used to combine those results, one of the properties of the model, described above, is to assign relatively higher weights to small studies than would otherwise be assigned by more traditional methods of combining data. If publication bias is a problem in a particular data set, one consequence implied by the funnel plot is that small studies would tend to show larger effects than large studies. Thus, if publication bias is present, one of the reasons for heterogeneity of study results is that the small studies show systematically larger effects than the large studies. The assignment of higher relative weights to the small studies could, when publication bias is present, lead to a biased summary result.

Indirect comparison and simultaneous comparison of treatments available for specific conditions

What health care providers, patients, policy-makers, and payers often need in order to make informed decisions is to understand how pharmacologic treatments compare to other pharmacologic treatments, even in the absence of direct evidence (head-to-head comparisons). When the treatments of interest have been compared to a common comparator, for example placebo, it is possible to get comparative information via indirect evidence.

Indirect evidence involves using data from trials that have compared medication "A" vs medication "B," and from trials that have compared medication "A" vs medication "C," to draw conclusions about the effect of medication "B" relative to medication "C" (Figure 19.1). It is crucial that when an indirect comparison is estimated, the analysis respect the randomization. This means that the analysis must be based on treatment differences within each trial. Pooling the results from the various treatment arms of the clinical trials, by simply collapsing results for that treatment arm across studies, ignores the randomization and produces biased and overly precise estimates. To correctly assess how medication B compares with medication C, one needs to analyze all the trials that have compared medication A with medication B and calculate (in the case of dichotomous outcome) the appropriate meta-analytic OR and do the same for the trials that have compared medication A with medication C, and then divide

these two ORs, i.e., OR (B vs. C) = OR (A vs. B) / OR (A vs. C).

There is, however, a cost in terms of precision. Specifically, indirect evidence estimates are less precise than direct estimates because the variance of the indirect comparison of B vs. C is the sum of the variances of the two comparisons estimated above (A vs. B and A vs. C).

When what is needed is a comparison of all available treatments for a specific condition, more flexible analyses are appropriate. An extended meta-analytic method, such as a mixed treatment comparison, a network meta-analysis, or a multiple treatment meta-analysis permit the pharmacoepidemiologist to perform simultaneous comparisons of all treatments. These techniques also permit the assessment of inconsistency, i.e., the disagreement between direct and indirect evidence. These methods can also provide a probabilistic ranking of treatments.

Assumptions

The validity of the indirect comparisons and the extended methodologies we just described depend on meeting assumptions, which are similar to the assumptions of the traditional meta-analysis.

The first assumption is homogeneity. For example if treatment A in our example is placebo, the results of the placebo-controlled trials that evaluated treatment B should be homogeneous enough to be combined, and the results of the placebo-controlled trials that evaluated treatment C should be homogeneous enough to be combined as well.

The second assumption is similarity. All factors that affect the response to a treatment, effect modifiers, must be similarly distributed across the entire set of trials. This requires that the trials in the network are clinically similar with respect to patient

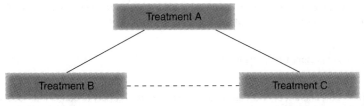

Figure 19.1 Indirect evidence involves using data from trials that have compared medication "A" vs medication "B", and from trials that have compared medication "A" vs medication "C," to draw conclusions about the effect of medication "B" relative to medication "C" (dotted line).

characteristics, settings, follow up, and outcomes evaluated, and that the trials are methodologically similar, as well.

The last assumption to assure validity of the results is consistency, i.e., agreement between direct (head-to-head) and indirect evidence. It requires that before combining direct and indirect estimates, the consistency of these estimates needs to be checked.

Currently available solutions

Investigation of adverse effects

As mentioned earlier, the investigation of adverse or unwanted effects of existing therapies is an important application of meta-analysis. Adverse events associated with pharmaceutical products are often so uncommon as to be difficult to study. In particular, the usual premarketing randomized studies frequently have too few patients to provide any useful information on the incidence of uncommon adverse events (see Chapter 3). By the same token, individual studies may have low statistical power to address particular questions. Meta-analysis provides the benefit of increased statistical power to investigate adverse events.

Differential effects among subgroups of patients (see Case Example 19.1)

Antidepressant labels warn about an increased risk of suicidality in children and adolescents during treatment. To assess this risk in adults, the FDA

Case Example 19.1: Risk of suicidality in clinical trials of antidepressants in adults: analysis of proprietary data submitted to US Food and Drug Administration (Stone *et al.*, 2009)

Background

• Antidepressants labels warn about an increased risk of suicidality in children and adolescents during treatment.

• Risk in adults was unknown.

Question

• What is the risk of suicidality in adults exposed to antidepressants?

Approach

• Individual patient data meta-analysis

• Industry sponsors of antidepressant products were asked by the FDA to provide individual data from all completed double blind RCTs of their products.

Results

• For subjects with nonpsychiatric indications, suicidal behavior and ideation were extremely rare.

• For those with psychiatric indications, the relative risk of suicidality, associated with treatment, was different for different age groups; risk was elevated in young adults and was decreased in the oldest age group.

Strengths

• This meta-analysis shows the power of individual data meta-analysis to identify subgroups of patients at higher risk of developing adverse events, and the process of adjudicating adverse events that need to be followed when the outcome of interest has not been prespecified or has not been reported in publications.

Limitations

• Risk of suicidality was not prespecified in the trials.

Key points

• The example illustrates the amount of effort and regulatory authority necessary to gather individual data from a great number of RCTs and multiple industry sponsors to assess whether a drug class increases the risk of a rare but serious outcome.

performed an individual patient data meta-analysis. Eight industry sponsors of 12 antidepressant products were asked to provide individual data from all completed double blind randomized controlled trials (RCTs) of their products, for any indication in adults, with at least 20 participants per arm. Trials limited to known drug responders, such as those using randomized withdrawal designs, were excluded.

Industry sponsors were asked to search their electronic databases for adverse events reported during the double blind phase of treatment, using text strings. All events identified by this search were considered possibly related to suicidality, unless they were identified as false positive. The sponsors adjudicated the events.

Events were classified into seven mutually exclusive categories: 1. completed suicide, 2. suicide attempt, 3. preparatory acts towards imminent suicidal behavior, 4. suicidal ideation, 5. self injurious behavior, intent unknown, 6. not enough information (fatal), and 7. not enough information (nonfatal). The primary outcome was suicidal ideation or worse (categories 1, 2, 3, or 4). The secondary outcome was suicidal behavior (categories 1, 2, or 3).

All the analyses were conditioned on (i.e., stratified by) study. The authors calculated ORs and RDs using conditional logistic regression and other methods, such as exact stratified methods, Mantel-Haenszel, Bayesian, and unconditional and random effects logistic regression. These multiple methods were used to test the robustness of the findings to the choice of statistical approach. To assess the effect of age on the risk of suicidality, the investigators included age and the interaction of treatment with age as both categorical and continuous variables (in separate models).

The analysis included a total of 99 231 participants in 372 trials. It is worth noting that most of the studies included were unpublished and, for those that were published, the authors found that they seldom contained information concerning suicidality in the publication.

All the methods to combine the data provided similar results. For participants with non-psychiatric indications, suicidal behavior and ideation were extremely rare. For those with psychiatric indications, the relative risk of suicidality, associated with treatment, was different for different age groups. The relative risk was higher in participants under 25, neither elevated nor reduced in those aged 25 to 64, and reduced in those aged 65 and older.

This meta-analysis nicely illustrates the amount of effort and regulatory authority necessary to coordinate and gather individual data from a great number of RCTs, involving many drugs and multiple industry sponsors, to assess whether or not a drug class increases the risk of a rare but serious outcome and whether or not the increase in risk varies with the characteristic of the subjects exposed. This meta-analysis shows the power of individual data meta-analysis to identify subgroups of patients at higher risk of developing adverse events, and the process of adjudicating adverse events that need to be followed when the outcome of interest has not been prespecified in the trials or has not been reported in publications.

Cumulative meta-analysis as a tool to detect harm signals earlier (see Case Example 19.2)

One prominent group has advocated the routine use of what they have termed "cumulative meta-analysis," i.e., performing a new meta-analysis each time the results of a new clinical trial are published. Cumulative meta-analysis could be used as a tool to detect safety signals earlier. Rofecoxib, a cyclo-oxygenase-2 inhibitor, was withdrawn from the market in September 2004 because of cardiovascular adverse effects. A cumulative meta-analysis of RCTs was performed to establish whether robust evidence on the adverse effects of rofecoxib was available before its removal. The authors searched bibliographic databases and relevant files of the FDA and included all RCTs in patients with chronic musculoskeletal disorders that compared rofecoxib with other NSAIDs or placebo. Myocardial infarction was the primary outcome.

The authors identified 18 randomized controlled trials and found that by the end of 2000 (four years before the withdrawal), the relative risk was 2.30 (95% CI 1.22–4.33), and one year later it was 2.24 (1.24–4.02). The authors found no evidence that

---

Case Example 19.2: Risk of cardiovascular events and rofecoxib: cumulative meta-analysis (Juni *et al.*, 2004)

Background

- Rofecoxib, a cyclo-oxygenase-2 inhibitor, was withdrawn from the market because of cardiovascular adverse effects.

Question

- Can cumulative meta-analysis of RCTs establish whether evidence on the adverse effects of rofecoxib was available before its removal?

Approach

- The authors searched bibliographic databases and FDA files and included all RCTs in patients with chronic musculoskeletal disorders that compared rofecoxib with other NSAIDs or placebo. Myocardial infarction was the outcome assessed.

Results

- The adverse cardiovascular effects of rofecoxib could have been identified several years earlier.

Strengths

- Cumulative meta-analysis potentially can detect harm earlier than traditional meta-analysis.

Limitations

- The validity of pooling of trials that were not clinically homogeneous. The authors combined the results of trials with dissimilar control arms (placebo, naproxen and non-naproxen NSAIDs).
- The authors excluded trials that evaluated Alzheimer's disease. In this case, the inclusion of such a trial would have made the early signal disappear.

Key points

- Cumulative meta-analysis is a tool to evaluate the safety of health interventions.

---

the relative risk differed depending on the type of control group (placebo, non-naproxen NSAID, or naproxen) or trial duration. They concluded that the adverse cardiovascular effects of rofecoxib could have been identified several years earlier, and appropriate action taken.

Cumulative meta-analysis for the evaluation of safety signals brings to light potential methodological problems that are also shared by traditional meta-analysis. First, one might question the validity of pooling of trials that are not clinically homogeneous. For example, the authors combined the results of trials with dissimilar control arms (placebo, naproxen, and non-naproxen NSAIDs).

Second, the validity of excluding trials that assessed the intervention of interest, but for other indications, can also be questioned. For example, the authors concentrated on trials that evaluated

chronic musculoskeletal pain and excluded trials that evaluated Alzheimer's disease. In this case, the inclusion of such a trial would have made the early signal disappear.

Third, one can ask whether efficacy and safety should be evaluated with the same methodological standards. For efficacy, there are concerns that multiple looks at the data will lead to false positive results and that p-values should be adjusted accordingly. When evaluating safety, it could be argued that adjustments to p-values should not be as large as they are for efficacy analyses.

Fourth, it is uncertain whether cumulative meta-analysis can systematically detect harm earlier. Rare adverse events, or the adverse events that occur late after exposure, will likely be absent in RCTs performed during drug development, and therefore cumulative meta-analysis would not always be expected to detect harms earlier.

Indirect comparisons and simultaneous evaluation of treatment therapies for the same indication

The efficacy and acceptability of new generation antidepressants for the treatment of major depression were assessed using multiple treatment meta-analyses. Authors of this meta-analysis included randomized controlled trials that compared 12 new antidepressants. Overall, there was consistency between direct and indirect evidence. The authors concluded that not all the antidepressants were equally efficacious or equally well tolerated; they provided a matrix that simultaneously compared the twelve antidepressants for efficacy and acceptability and reported the ranking of antidepressants for efficacy or acceptability.

It is not surprising that studies of this nature generate a lot of attention. One of the main criticisms was that excluding placebo-controlled data and including only one dose group when multiple doses were evaluated would lead to selection bias that could affect the rank-order of antidepressants. In fact, the ranks were different from those calculated in other studies.

FDA's regulatory role

In recent years, the FDA has used meta-analysis to investigate adverse events associated with the use of certain drugs. The findings from those meta-analyses were used to support a regulatory decision to mandate a labelling change.

As an example similar to the antidepressant and suicidality analysis described above, to review the possible association of suicidality events with antiepileptic drugs, the FDA contacted all sponsors of antiepileptic drugs and requested that they submit placebo-controlled trial data from all of their studies. The FDA statistical review of 199 placebo-controlled trials from 11 antiepileptic drugs found that there were 1.9 per 1000 (95% CI: 0.6, 3.9) more antiepileptic drug patients than placebo patients who experienced suicidal behavior or ideation compared to the placebo patients. Based on the findings, the FDA requested the sponsors of antiepileptic drugs, except for those indicated for short-term use, to include new information in the product labelling about an increased risk of suicidal thoughts or actions and to develop a Medication Guide to help patients understand this risk. The rarity of the outcome made it essential to combine data across multiple compounds and indications.

Not only does meta-analysis sometimes support the decision to change or update the current labelling of approved drugs, it can also provide evidence as to whether or not to keep a drug on the market for continued use in patients.

The future

Meta-analysis plays an increasingly important role in the formulation of treatment and policy recommendations. But, there are areas in meta-analysis that need further research.

One relates to the appropriate approach to evaluating safety during drug development. In particular, how the issue of multiplicity should be addressed is not resolved. During drug development, multiplicity arises in one sense because there are an enormous number of adverse events that are routinely collected. If cumulative meta-analyses are updated each time a trial is completed during development, the repeated testing (even of events prespecified for formal testing) generates the possibility of generating an excessive number of false positive signals. Although "compromise" corrections have been proposed, these tend to focus mostly on p-values, ignoring direct consideration of the magnitude of effects and the clinical importance of the events in question.

The question of how to respond, from a sponsor or regulatory perspective, in the presence of heterogeneous results, is also an open one. When there is little or no heterogeneity of results among trials, one might be willing to accept meta-analytic evidence. It is less obvious what to do with the results of a meta-analysis when there is substantial unexplained heterogeneity. How should results be interpreted when some trials show harm and others show no effect of drug. Is this an indication that treatment is harmful in some, but not all, situations? Does such a situation simply reflect random variability? The threshold for action in the face of heterogeneity of findings may well be different for safety endpoints than for efficacy endpoints, but work is needed to establish transparent criteria by which to evaluate such situations.

As the focus of policy and clinical decisions moves in the direction of comparative effectiveness, there are serious questions about how to define research agendas. In principle, one might wish to make direct comparisons across all drugs (or therapies) for a given indication. The principles defining validity of indirect comparisons have been described. Work is needed, however, to explore in practice, the conditions under which indirect comparisons, or mixed treatment comparisons, may be both valid and useful. Indirect comparisons often, but not always, agree with direct comparisons and how and when to incorporate studies that are not head-to-head comparisons needs further empirical study.

The inclusion of non-experimental observational studies in meta-analyses, particularly of serious but uncommon adverse events, will almost certainly be a necessity. To the extent that clinical trials performed in support of new drug approvals tend to include populations that are different from the population in which the drug will be used after approval, safety assessments done during development will need to be supplemented with studies done in actual clinical practice. Sample sizes during development also tend to be limited, making it necessary to study large populations to evaluate risks of uncommon but serious adverse events.

Key points

• Meta-analysis, if carefully done, is a powerful method that can be used to identify sources of variation among studies and provide an overall measure of effect.
• Combining evidence across diverse study designs and study populations may lead to generalizable results.
• Publication bias, and flaws in the design of component studies, should lead to careful interpretation of meta-analyses.
• Extended meta-analytic techniques such as indirect comparisons and multiple treatment meta-analyses can potentially strengthen the inference

regarding a treatment because the results are based on more data.
• Meta-analysis plays an increasingly important role in safety assessment.

Further reading

Bradburn MJ, Deeks JJ, Berlin JA, Russell LA (2007) Much ado about nothing: a comparison of the performance of meta-analytical methods with rare events. *Stat Med* **26**: 53–77.

Bucher HC, Guyatt GH, Griffith LE, Walter SD (1997) The results of direct and indirect treatment comparisons in meta-analysis of randomized controlled trials. *J Clin Epidemiol* **50**: 683–91.

Cochrane Collaboration (2010) The Cochrane Collaboration's tool for assessing risk of bias. Available from: URL: http://www.ohg.cochrane.org/forms/Risk%20of %20bias%20assessment%20tool.pdf

Colditz GA, Burdick E, Mosteller F (1995) Heterogeneity in meta-analysis of data from epidemiologic studies: a commentary. *Am J Epidemiol* **142**: 371–82.

DerSimonian R, Laird N (1986) Meta-analysis in clinical trials. *Controlled Clin Trials* **7**: 177–88.

Dias S, Welton NJ, Caldwell DM, Ades AE (2010) Checking consistency in mixed treatment comparison meta-analysis. *Stat Med* **29**: 932–44.

Greenland S (1994) Quality scores are useless and potentially misleading. *Am J Epidemiol* **140**: 300–1.

Higgins J, Green S.Cochrane (2009) *Handbook for Systematic Reviews of Interventions Version 5.0.2.* Available from: URL: www.cochrane-handbook.org.

Juni P, Nartey L, Reichenbach S, Sterchi R, Dieppe PA, Egger M (2004) Risk of cardiovascular events and rofecoxib: cumulative meta-analysis. *Lancet* **364**: 2021–9.

Juni P, Witschi A, Block R, Egger M (1999) The hazards of scoring the quality of clinical trials: lessons for meta-analysis. *JAMA* **282**: 1054–60.

Liberati A, Altman DG, Tetzlaff J, Mulrow C, Gotzsche PC, Ioannidis JP, et al. (2009) The PRISMA statement for reporting systematic reviews and meta-analyses of studies that evaluate health care interventions: explanation and elaboration. *Ann Intern Med* **151**: W65–W94.

Light RJ, Pillemer DB (1984) *Summing Up: The Science of Reviewing Research.* Cambridge, MA: Harvard University Press.

Song F, Loke YK, Walsh T, Glenny AM, Eastwood AJ, Altman DG (2009) Methodological problems in the use of indirect comparisons for evaluating healthcare interventions: survey of published systematic reviews. *BMJ* **338**: b1147.

Stone M, Laughren T, Jones ML, Levenson M, Holland PC, Hughes A, et al. (2009) Risk of suicidality in clinical trials of antidepressants in adults: analysis of proprietary data submitted to US Food and Drug Administration. *BMJ* **339**:b2880. doi: 10.1136/bmj.b2880.:b2880.

Sterne JAC, Egger M, Smith GD (2001) Investigating and dealing with publication and other biases in meta-analysis. *BMJ* **323**: 101–5.

Sweeting MJ, Sutton AJ, Lambert PC (2004) What to add to nothing? Use and avoidance of continuity corrections in meta-analysis of sparse data. *Stat Med* **23**: 1351–75.

CHAPTER 20

Studies of Medication Adherence

Trisha Acri[1] and Robert Gross[2]

[1]*Temple University School of Medicine, Philadelphia, PA, USA*
[2]*Perelman School of Medicine at the University of Pennsylvania, Philadelphia, PA, USA*

Introduction

In this chapter, we describe the importance of adherence measurement in pharmacoepidemiologic research, the methods by which medication adherence can be measured, methodologic issues that arise once adherence has been measured, and future directions for the field. We use many drug–disease examples in this chapter but focus on examples from antiretroviral therapy for HIV disease because it has been at the forefront of recent adherence research.

As many as half of all patients do not take all of their medication as prescribed, resulting in an estimate of more than $100 billion of avoidable hospitalizations. However, the problem will remain underappreciated and poorly addressed unless accurate adherence measurement is incorporated into research and clinical practice.

The definitions used to describe the behavior of interest can be confusing. *Compliance* has been defined as "the extent to which the patient's dosing history conforms to the prescribed regimen." The idea of a patient passively "conforming" may impose a judgmental framework on the problem; therefore, the term *adherence* has supplanted the term compliance. *Adherence* conveys the idea of a treatment alliance where the patient implements the provider's recommendations.

Adherence encompasses several steps that result in the patient actually consuming the medication. *Acceptance* denotes initial engagement with the prescribed medication. *Persistence* refers to how long the patient continues to follow the regimen.

Execution represents how well the patient follows the prescribed regimen during treatment engagement. Failure to perform any of these steps results in nonadherence. These terminologies highlight the fact that the patient who never fills a prescription, perhaps because of medication cost, differs from the patient who forgets to take an occasional dose, and differs from the patient who begins the therapy and initially executes it well but discontinues it over time. Defining these three patients as nonadherent based on the average percentage of medication consumed over a certain time period ignores the likelihood that each might have different treatment outcomes and would require different interventions to improve upon adherence.

The actual behaviors involved in taking a prescribed medication as directed become much more complicated when each step of the process is considered. This is just one of many limitations encountered in the study of adherence and why measuring adherence and attempts to enhance adherence are so difficult. Regardless, practical approaches to measuring and analyzing adherence have been developed. We discuss the utility of various approaches and the remaining challenges.

Clinical problems to be addressed by pharmacoepidemiologic research

Adherence measurement is essential to address several issues in the interpretation of studies of beneficial and adverse effects of medications. In

Textbook of Pharmacoepidemiology, Second Edition. Edited by Brian L. Strom, Stephen E. Kimmel, and Sean Hennessy.
© 2013 John Wiley & Sons, Ltd. Published 2013 by John Wiley & Sons, Ltd.

randomized controlled trials, adherence can be an important factor affecting the outcome of the trial and estimates of medication efficacy and safety. Poor adherence to the drug can lead to underestimates of the efficacy of the drug being tested. Further, adherence information allows for a more accurate assessment of the incidence of toxicity because toxicity cannot occur if the drug was not taken. Since perfect adherence cannot be expected all the time, even in clinical trial participants, adherence measurement can inform whether a drug is not effective because it did not work or because it was not taken.

Clinical trial volunteers are probably more motivated to take medication than those treated in clinical practice. Therefore, measuring adherence in observational studies of drug effectiveness and toxicity may be even more important than in clinical trials. Furthermore, assessing adherence in observational studies provides a more realistic estimate of adherence in clinical populations than in the artificial clinical trial setting. Moreover, since it is a major determinant of treatment outcome for chronic diseases managed with efficacious medications, adherence itself can be the focus of pharmacoepidemiologic research.

Nonadherence can be volitional or unintentional. Observational studies over the past several decades have identified many potential barriers to adherence. These can be categorized as patient-level factors, system-level factors, and medication-specific factors. Common patient barriers are forgetting to take the medication, missing doses to avoid side effects, and psychosocial factors such as depression and lack of social support. Common system barriers include logistical difficulty in obtaining the medication from the dispenser and sporadic drug unavailability ("stock outs"). Common medication-specific barriers are dosing frequency and adverse effects. Patients in observational settings miss doses for the same reasons as participants in clinical trials, but may also be affected more by lack of trust or lack of motivation because they differ from clinical trials volunteers. Further, patients may decide on a dose-by-dose basis whether to take medicine as prescribed for a variety of reasons. For example, patients may take doses intermittently to avoid side effects at particular times (e.g., avoidance of diarrhea when needing to take public transportation). In addition, adherence may wane over time and post-marketing observational studies may demonstrate pill fatigue when patients are followed for longer periods of time than is typical for clinical trials. Thus, adherence studies in observational settings can provide unique data not available from trials.

While missing doses is the more common adherence problem, taking extra doses can also be an issue in some settings. An example is warfarin for anticoagulation. Of course, patients may take extra doses of narcotics prescribed for the treatment of pain because of inadequate pain relief or for recreational purposes.

Adherence is important not only for the patient's clinical outcome, but can also impact public health, particularly regarding infectious diseases. In tuberculosis and HIV, nonadherence modifies the disease itself by selecting for organisms resistant to the treatment. Since these diseases are transmissible, and transmitted resistance has been confirmed, the measurement of nonadherence and interventions to improve it for the individual take on greater public health importance.

Adherence measurement can also be useful for determining the threshold of how much medication must be taken to obtain the desired clinical outcome. In hypertension, for example, taking 80% of prescribed medication is an acceptable standard. Yet in HIV, this standard is often insufficient for treatment success. Unfortunately, such detailed information is not available for most drugs and diseases. Therefore, the default goal should be to encourage the patient to take as many of the prescribed doses as possible.

Methodologic problems to be solved by pharmacoepidemiologic research

Challenges in adherence measurement

The gold standard for measuring adherence to pharmacotherapy is directly observed therapy. However, this approach is only practical in limited settings, such as the administration of a novel agent in a controlled environment. Provider predictions of adherence are usually no better than chance and should not be used. Knowledge that one's adherence is being monitored, unless done unobtrusively, risks influencing the behavior it is meant to measure (i.e., a Hawthorne effect). In addition, tracking of a daily activity can be burdensome whether or not individuals are aware of their own nonadherence. Therefore, adherence measurement requires creative approaches to assess a daily activity performed at different times per day for different individuals.

Challenges in the analysis of adherence data

Once adherence is measured, the best approach to data analysis becomes central. In clinical trials, adjusting results for adherence is complicated by the fact that adherence itself is related to better health outcomes, irrespective of receiving active drug or placebo. For example, in the Beta-Blocker Heart Attack Trial (BHAT), a randomized double-blind placebo-controlled trial of propranolol after myocardial infarction, the odds ratio of mortality in poor adherers compared with good adherers was the same within the active arm and the placebo arm. Presumably, adherence to the medication, whether propranolol or placebo, was strongly associated with other factors (e.g., lifestyle) related to mortality. This is particularly relevant in the setting where other uncontrolled factors, like diet and exercise, play a role in determining outcome.

Other analytic challenges include the duration and timing of adherence measurement. Adherence behavior varies over time. Therefore, for chronic treatments, an individual may be adherent for part of the observation period and nonadherent for another. For example, individuals on HIV therapy are prescribed lifelong regimens. In any one year, initial adherence may differ from adherence over the final 12 weeks. Simply summing adherence over the entire interval provides an average amount of adherence for the treatment course. Yet, short periods of nonadherence can have a major impact on outcome. Further, whatever the interval chosen, the summation of the adherence data during that interval can be accomplished in many different ways. The simplest, percent of doses taken, may not be the most clinically relevant metric. Depending on the pharmacokinetics and pharmacodynamics, duration of gaps and variability in adherence over time may be more important. Defining the duration of the adherence interval, determining which intervals are likely to be related to the treatment outcome, and defining the metrics of interest are key issues in the analysis of this phenomenon.

Additionally, many diseases, like hypertension and tuberculosis, are treated with combination therapy. While the effects of these drugs are often studied in combination, weighting differential adherence among the drugs is challenging.

Currently available solutions

Specific techniques for measuring adherence

Self-reports

Self-reports of medication adherence are simple, relatively inexpensive, feasible, and commonly used in clinical practice (see Case example 20.1). They can be obtained over the telephone, in person, or with paper or electronic surveys. Several methods have been validated for measuring self-reported adherence. The Adult AIDS Clinical Trials Group instrument queries subjects about missed doses of each medication for the last four days, missed doses on weekends, the last missed dose, and adherence to dietary instructions. A simpler but still comprehensive measure validated in a large cohort of patients with HIV that is used for other medications is the Simplified Medication Adherence Questionnaire. It contains specific questions about forgetfulness or carelessness about taking medications and missed doses over the previous 24 hours, the past week, the last weekend, and the last three months. Other studies have used a single measure such as a visual analog scale, asking participants to mark a point on a line from 0% to 100% to indicate the amount of medication taken over a specified recent time period. Still others ask participants to estimate numerically how much medication they have taken. These methods, which can be self-administered in high-literacy patients or can be conducted by an interviewer, are all limited by a patient's ability to recall missed doses and biased by social desirability (reporting conformity with physician instructions to avoid embarrassment). Social desirability can be mitigated by using permissive statements like, "We know that it is sometimes difficult to take all your medications on time as directed."

Simple interview techniques are potentially limited by multiple factors including language barriers, literacy, provider time, social desirability, and difficulty with communication of complicated regimens and medication names. Use of audio computer-assisted self-administered interview (ACASI) can reduce these barriers. ACASI utilizes an audio track to read instructions and questions and can include high-resolution medication photographs to assist participants with lower literacy. Empirical data suggest that computer-aided self-reports are less likely to overestimate adherence but do not eliminate the issue of faulty recall.

Refill data

Pharmacy refill data has been widely used to measure adherence in various chronic diseases. The high quality of pharmacy refill data is predicated on a pair of positive and negative incentives for its accuracy. If refills are dispensed, but not recorded, the dispenser does not get reimbursed for the medication. If refills are recorded, but not dispensed, the dispenser is guilty of fraud. In contrast to self-reports, the pharmacy refill measure is less susceptible to deception, not biased by poor recall, can be obtained from computerized records, and can be assessed retrospectively.

The pharmacy refill measure of adherence estimates the amount of medication an individual has in possession during a given time period without assessing actual pill-taking behavior, either on average or day-to-day. As such, it cannot be used when the timing of missed doses during the interval is pivotal. However, the technique is a valid measure of adherence for chronic medications where measuring exposure between refills is clinically relevant. For example, a time-to-refill measure of adherence has

been associated with changes in HIV viral load and changes in hypertensive blood pressure. Furthermore, the measure provides additional information to self-reported adherence data. In a study of antiretroviral therapy, individuals self-reporting 100% adherence varied in their treatment response dependent upon their refill adherence. As expected, those with higher adherence on the refill measure had higher rates of treatment response, despite self-reports of perfect adherence in both groups.

This adherence measure only yields estimates of a person's maximum possible adherence since it is based on the amount of medication in their possession. The measure is most feasible when prescription refills are obtained from a single pharmacy or the information is obtained centrally in a data repository such as may be used with managed care insurance. The accuracy of pharmacy refill data for measuring adherence can also be limited by the possibility that patients obtain medication from other sources like friends or family, or during hospitalization. Prescribed dosages also may change during the time of monitoring. Notably, it is not useful when refills are automatically mailed to patients without request to the dispenser.

The pharmacy refill measure of adherence has been described and used with several different definitions. The approaches each assume that all doses from the prior bottle have been consumed before a new refill is obtained. Further, it requires that the medication be prescribed for chronic use with refills of the initial prescription. In the most commonly applied approach, the proportion of doses taken over the interval is calculated using the following formula: days' supply/(last day of refill minus first day of refill). Other approaches include calculating the number of refills obtained divided by the number of refills expected over the time frame, or calculating the excess amount of time between refills as a gap in adherence. Although easier to calculate, the simpler measures have more limited utility. For example, the number of 1-month refills divided by the number of months of follow-up over time is difficult to use over a shorter time period. More specifically, three 30-day refills are expected when assessing a 3-month refill interval. In this situation, adherence can only be categorized as 100% (3/3), 66% (2/3),

33% (1/3) or 0% (0/3). The patient who returns for the last refill one day late would be assigned 66% adherence. The time-to-refill approach addresses this issue. Over a three-month time period during which 3 refills of 30 days' supply each would be expected, the patient's adherence would be 90/91 or 99%, a much better reflection of actual medication consumption than 66%. This measure gives greater precision, and can be particularly useful when adherence between 66% and 100% is crucial, as in HIV disease outcomes. This problem becomes less important when longer intervals are assessed.

Refill-based measures must always address the issue of non-refill. This measurement technique requires that the days' supply be determined and then divided by the time period of interest. However, if the patient stops taking the medication, the recorded stop date is either inaccurate or unavailable. In this scenario, it is necessary to artificially assign a refill date for the last refill to close the time interval. Potential approaches include setting it at the end of follow-up or at a fixed point after the last refill (e.g., 2 months late for a 1-month supply). Whichever method is chosen, sensitivity analyses in which this artificial stop date is assigned different times are important to assess the robustness of the results.

Pill counts

Adherence can also be measured by pill counts. Pill counts are similar to pharmacy refill data in that percent adherence is calculated by dividing the days supply consumed by the number of days observed. Like refill data, pill counts cannot determine if the medication was actually taken or the pattern of medication taking. However, they do provide direct evidence that the medication was not taken when pills are left over. Pill counts are more susceptible to patient deception since "dumping" pills on the way to the pill count visit is simple and can be done impulsively before a visit. Unannounced pill counts, in person or by telephone, are alternatives to mitigate this type of misclassification.

The potential disadvantages of the method are the time and annoyance for both the staff who do the counting and the participants who bring their pill bottles, adding an additional source of error.

Reinforcing the importance of accuracy with the staff is vital for this measure to be valid.

Medication diaries

Although the measures described above yield a global amount of drug taken over a specified time period, they give no detail on the timing of missed doses and medication-taking. Based on the pharmacokinetics and pharmacodynamics, missing doses several days during a month may have different consequences depending on whether consecutive doses were missed or if doses were sporadically missed throughout the month. This specificity may be vital to the adherence classification. Medication diaries are a technique where participants keep a record of the date and time of each medication dose and whether it was taken with or without food. They can provide this critical information to interpret results of studies of drugs such as insulin that are difficult to track using other measures.

Medication diaries are susceptible to both overreporting and underreporting of adherence. Social desirability can lead patients to report doses that were not taken. This potential for deception is lessened somewhat by the burden of creating a detailed falsified record. In fact, the burden of tracking each dose actually increases the risk of underreporting since medications may be taken without recording in the diary.

Electronic drug monitors

Electronic drug monitors (EDMs) feature the same advantages as the medication diaries, without susceptibility to deception, forgetting, or avoiding recording the dose data. Multiple hardware options are available, but all electronic drug monitors employ electronic date/time stamp technology that is triggered by opening the container or puncturing a blister pack to obtain the dose. The data are downloaded to a computer for analysis. It is thought to be the rare subject who will game the system by opening and closing the monitor to record medication-taking events over long periods of time without actually taking the medication. EDMs are also less susceptible to underreporting than medication diaries because they often do not require the subject to do anything other than take the prescribed medication. Additionally, they can be used as medication diaries even when the medication is not kept in the container.

The packaging of EDMs can be burdensome. They often preclude the use of pill boxes and require that the medication remain in the package until taken. Therefore, they are susceptible to underestimating adherence (e.g., a one-week supply of doses taken from the container at one time will appear as one dose taken). Another limitation of this approach is the cost of purchasing the monitors and the hardware and software to analyze the data, and this limits their use in clinical practice.

Drug concentrations

Identification of a drug in plasma or other tissues provides evidence of drug ingestion. However, the use of drug concentrations to measure adherence is limited by variability between patients in drug processing (i.e., absorption, distribution, metabolism, and clearance–see Chapters 4 and 14). The more variable those steps are between patients, the weaker the relation between drug concentration and adherence. Further, if the drug has a short half-life in the compartment (e.g., plasma), then the measurement only captures short-term use. Thus, this approach is limited by the issue of interval censoring between measurements.

Measurement of drug concentrations in hair assessed by liquid chromatography and confirmed by tandem mass spectrometry can be a useful indicator of long-term exposure to medication. For example, antiretroviral drug levels in hair give an average of the exposure to drug over the past weeks to months and operate better than serum drug levels to predict HIV viral response. The duration of exposure to drug measured by hair drug concentrations and serum drug levels is analogous to the relationship between hemoglobin A1C and a single serum glucose measurement. Hair concentrations have also been used to determine exposure to nonprescription drugs of abuse.

Unfortunately, many of these assays are unavailable commercially. Furthermore, for other drugs, the serum drug level is not the relevant measure because the site of action is elsewhere. Additionally, unless these assays are done with short turnaround time, they are not useful clinically. Assessment of combination regimens is difficult because assays for each drug may not be available, and adherence classification is difficult if the drug concentrations are differential.

Another approach to assessing drug concentrations is to use a marker drug that is easily added to a formulation and can be measured more easily than the actual drug of interest. The primary example here is the incorporation of riboflavin into active drugs as a urine metabolite drug marker to assess adherence to medication in clinical trials. Fluorescence spectrophotometry is used to assess the concentration. Of course, this strategy is only relevant in settings where control over the formulation is in the hands of the researchers (e.g., clinical trials).

Adherence to non-pill formulations

Medication diaries and self-reports can be used to monitor adherence to non-pill formulations of medication therapy with the same considerations described above. Particular circumstances raise several unique challenges to measuring non-pill formulation adherence. For example, measuring adherence to injectable pegylated interferon for the treatment of hepatitis C is feasible using pharmacy refill dates and the number of interferon syringes dispensed with each refill, because the days supply is fixed and/or syringes are pre-filled. However, when an injectable medication like insulin is administered based on a sliding scale, with doses adjusted as needed, measuring adherence using refill data may be invalid.

Topical treatments pose a particular challenge. For transdermal formulations in patches (e.g., nicotine, testosterone), because the supply is typically fixed, refill adherence is a viable option. However, for creams and ointments, because the amount used at each application varies by the size of the lesion being treated or the size of the individual or other characteristics, self-reports and medication diaries may be the only viable options at present.

Electronic Drug Monitors (EDMs) have been used for metered dose inhalers and ophthalmologic solutions. The monitors do increase the bulk of the packaging. However, unlike pills, these formulations cannot be taken out of the package. Thus, the patient burden of needing to keep pill formulations in the monitored package is not relevant for these formulations.

Analysis issues

Use of adherence data in the interpretation of clinical trials

In clinical trials, missed doses typically make the active drug less effective and diminish the observed difference in comparison to placebo. To compensate for this effect, trials may inflate sample sizes to account for variability in drug exposure. Clinical trials may also incorporate run-in periods to minimize poor adherence (see Chapter 16).

In analyzing trials when nonadherence occurs, the standard approach remains intention-to-treat. This approach limits the introduction of bias and makes the results more generalizable to clinical practice (see Chapter 16). Secondary analyses can be done, limiting inclusion exclusively to the adherent subset. Unfortunately, in the setting in which lifestyle changes serve as co-interventions with medication (e.g., studies of treatment of congestive heart failure), such secondary analyses only tease out the effect of the drug over and above lifestyle change and are not true measures of drug efficacy. Most importantly, the benefits of randomization are negated and results can be difficult to interpret.

Inclusion of adherence data in analyses of trials is particularly important when a treatment fails. Reasons for failure might include lack of biological effect or lack of adherence. Unless adherence is measured and identified as the cause of failure, the results of the trial will be only partly useful. While regulators will only approve a drug for the studied indication if it is shown to result in improved outcomes, it is important for the drug developer to know if the compound retains any potential for further use. For example, in the Lipid Research Clinics Coronary Primary Prevention Trial, rates of coronary heart disease events were compared in participants with hypercholesterolemia who were randomized to receive either cholestyramine to decrease lipid levels or a placebo. Adherence in the treatment group was lower than in the placebo group due to side effects in the treatment arm. Low adherence attenuated the lipid-lowering response and the decrease in cardiac events in the treatment group, and the difference in event rates in a comparison between the two groups was less than it could have been with higher adherence. Because adherence was measured, it was possible to determine that the high rate of intolerable side effects resulted in lower adherence and, perhaps, lower treatment effectiveness.

Time-varying nature of adherence and duration of adherence intervals

Adherence is a dynamic phenomenon. Therefore, categorizing an individual as adherent or not requires that the time interval of interest be specified. As previously discussed, using a single adherence metric to categorize adherence to chronic medications over long time periods may not be relevant. For example, an individual on antiretroviral therapy who interrupts treatment for as little as 2 weeks is likely to experience virologic failure. However, adherence metrics summarized over a year would yield very small deviations from perfect adherence (50 weeks adherent/52 weeks of observation=96%). In contrast, if one-month intervals were chosen, the individual would have 11 months of perfect adherence and one month of 50% adherence. This low adherence month would explain the treatment failure more clearly than does 96% adherence.

The selection of the duration of an adherence interval depends on two important factors: the pharmacokinetics/pharmacodynamics and the granularity of the adherence measurement. For drugs with short half-lives and short off-set of action, short intervals are likely to be more clinically relevant than when the drugs have long half-lives and longer off-sets of action. For adherence measures that can accurately assess adherence over short periods of time such as electronic drug monitors, shorter intervals can be calculated. In contrast, when pharmacy refill measures are used, intervals can only be as short as the expected time between fills (e.g., 30 days).

The relation between adherence and outcome has been well described in antiretroviral therapy and oral contraceptives. Using refill data, intervals of adherence as long as 1 year and as short as 30 days have been associated with viral load outcomes with antiretroviral therapy. In a direct comparison, a 90-day measure was found to be more strongly associated with viral load than a 30-day measure. For oral contraceptives, two consecutive days of nonadherence resulted in an unacceptably high rate of treatment failure.

Unfortunately, for the vast majority of medications, the duration of a relevant adherence interval is unknown. Much research is needed to optimize the assessment of adherence in chronic diseases such as diabetes, hypertension, and hypercholesterolemia. While the choice of interval length depends on the goals of the research, in general, monitoring adherence over shorter intervals is desirable. The shorter the adherence interval monitored the more readily barriers to adherence can be assessed and the more rapidly interventions can be implemented. But, this advantage comes at the expense of decreased accuracy regarding true adherence behavior. By way of illustration, in the extreme case, the time interval could be 1 day in which one missed dose would categorize an individual as nonadherent. Clearly, such a short interval is prone to misclassification of biologically relevant adherence status. But without information on the relation between adherence to the medication of interest and treatment outcome, investigators must choose without direct guidance. In these cases, choices for an adherence interval should be made based on pharmacokinetics and pharmacodynamics data (see Chapter 4).

Adherence metrics

The simplest approach to summarizing adherence is the percent of doses taken. However, this metric does not capture potentially relevant patterns of adherence. Other approaches are possible, particularly for electronic monitors and refill data. For electronic monitors, because the timing of each dose is available, percent of doses taken "on time," standard deviation of time between doses, duration of maximum time gap between doses, and many other metrics can be calculated. For refill data, metrics focus on either the percentage of available medication or the duration of gaps between refills. Self-reports focus on the proportion of doses the patients have taken or the time since the last dose was missed.

Whichever metric is used, adherence can be a continuous or dichotomous variable; the choice depends on the question. Threshold levels must take into account both the likelihood and the clinical consequences of treatment failure. Few thresholds have been evidence-based. Rather, 80% of doses taken is frequently quoted to categorize good vs. poor adherence based upon expert opinion. In other settings, higher magnitudes of adherence have been more closely associated with treatment success or failure. Combination therapy potentially complicates this issue significantly. Since nonadherence can differ between drugs in the regimen, the categorization of an individual's adherence can be essentially infinite. Fortunately, evidence suggests that for medications taken simultaneously, adherence to one is highly collinear with adherence to the other. Yet, differential nonadherence has been documented.

Determining whether an individual is nonadherent or that the medication was discontinued by the physician can be difficult for all measurement methods. A record of the physician recommendation to discontinue the medication is needed to determine if such an individual is nonadherent. Further, even when records are available and the recommendation is documented, the exact date can be difficult to determine.

Future directions

Once-daily therapies have not solved the problem of nonadherence, simple interventions have not worked, and no accurate and reproducible predictive model for nonadherence exists. Therefore, better methods for detecting nonadherence and better methods for addressing it will be welcome developments.

Regarding adherence measurement, novel strategies use microelectronic technology, often linked with communication systems that both identify and report nonadherence. Mobile telephone technology has resulted in numerous developments for tracking adherence and intervening, including short message system (SMS or "text messaging") and interactive voice messaging. Refinements to currently available electronic monitors will likely include more convenient packaging that can both enhance adherence (e.g., a reminder or organizer system) and electronically track adherence. In addition, these systems have the potential to include two-way communication to both gather data and provide automated customized feedback.

Completely novel approaches are likely to emerge as well. Researchers have designed an ingestible sensor which coats the medication and is activated by stomach fluids. It sends a signal to a device worn by the patient which records the event. Another novel approach is the use of a marker in the pill coating that can be detected on the breath by sensor.

Many challenges remain. Objective measurement of adherence to non-pill formulations is difficult, especially for liquids and topical treatments. Regarding analyses, the optimal adherence metric for virtually every drug–disease dyad remains unknown. This is further complicated by the enormous number of possible combinations of partial adherence to drugs in combination regimens. Hopefully, greater recognition of the importance of nonadherence will lead to more research over the next several decades to solve some of these problems and to develop better approaches to improving adherence so that efficacious medications can ultimately be maximally effective.

Key points

• Nonadherence occurs in as many as half of patients, resulting in an estimate of over $100 billion of avoidable hospitalizations. Accurate adherence measurement must be incorporated into research and clinical practice or the problem will remain underappreciated and poorly addressed.
• Potential barriers to adherence can be categorized as patient-level factors, system-level factors, and medication-specific factors.

• While missing doses is the more common adherence problem, taking extra doses can also be an issue in some settings, including anticoagulation and pain medication.
• Adherence is important not only for the patient's clinical outcome, but can also impact public health, particularly regarding the transmission of resistance to infectious diseases like tuberculosis and HIV.
• Measurement of adherence can be used to determine the threshold of how much medication must be taken to obtain the desired clinical outcome.
• Measuring adherence unobtrusively is a challenge requiring creative approaches to assess a daily behavior performed at different times per day for different individuals.
• Currently available techniques for measuring adherence include self-reports, pharmacy refill measures, pill counts, medication diaries, electronic drug monitors, and drug concentrations. Measuring adherence to non-pill formulations has special challenges.
• Because adherence behavior varies over time, analysis of data requires consideration of the appropriate duration, time period, and metrics for adherence.
• The use of adherence data in planning for clinical trials and analysis of trial results has special challenges including controlling for co-factors related to adherence and the potential for introduction of bias and limitation of generalizability. Inclusion of adherence data in analyses of clinical trials is particularly important when a treatment fails.
• Once-daily therapies have not solved the problem of nonadherence, simple interventions have not worked, and no accurate and reproducible predictive model for nonadherence exists. Therefore, better methods for detecting nonadherence and better methods for addressing it will be welcome developments.

Further Reading

Acri T, Grossberg R, Gross R (2010) How long is the right interval for assessing antiretroviral pharmacy refill adherence? *JAIDS* **54** (5): e16–e18.

Amico KR, Fisher WA, Cornman DH, Shuper PA, Redding CG, Konkle-Parker DJ, et al. (2006) Visual analog scale of ART adherence: association with 3-Day self-report and adherence barriers. *Journal of Acquired Immune Deficiency Syndromes* **42**: 455–9.

Chesney MA, Ickovics JR, Chambers DB, Gifford AL, Neidig J, Zwickl B, et al. (2000) Self-reported adherence to antiretroviral medications among participants in HIV clinical trials: the AACTG adherence instruments. *AIDS Care* **12**: 255–6.

Coronary Drug Research Group (1980) Influence of adherence to treatment and response of cholesterol on mortality on the coronary drug project. *New Engl J Med* **302**: 1038–41.

Cutler DM, Everett W (2010) Thinking outside the pillbox–medication adherence as a priority for health care reform. *New Engl J Med* **362**: 1553–5.

Feldman HI, Hackett M, Bilker W, Strom BL (1999) Potential utility of electronic drug compliance monitoring in measures of adverse outcomes associated with immunosuppressive agents. *Pharmacoepidemology and Drug Safety* **8**: 1–14.

Gross R, Bilker WB, Friedman HM, Strom BL (2001) *Effect of adherence to newly initiated antiretroviral therapy on plasma viral load. AIDS* **15**: 2109–17.

Grossberg R, Zhang Y, Gross R (2004) A time-to-prescription-refill measure of antiretroviral adherence predicted changes in viral load in HIV. *Journal of Clinical Epidemiology* **57**: 1107–10.

Haynes RB, Taylor DW, Sackett DL (eds) (1979) *Compliance in Health Care*. Baltimore: Johns Hopkins University Press.

Horwitz RI, Horwitz SM (1993) Adherence to treatment and health outcomes. *Arch Intern Med* **153**: 1863–8.

Ickovics JR, Meisler AW (1997) Adherence in AIDS clinical trials: a framework for clinical research and clinical care. *J Clin Epidemiol* **50**: 385–91.

Lipid Research Clinics Program (1984) The lipid research clinics coronary primary prevention trial results: Reduction in incidence of coronary heart disease *J Am Med Assoc* **251**: 351–64.

Low-Beer S, Yip B, O'Shaughnessy MV, Hogg RS, Montaner JS (2000) Adherence to triple therapy and viral load response. *Journal of Acquired Immune Deficiency Syndromes* **23**: 360–1.

Lu M, Safren SA, Skolnik PR, Rogers WH, Coady W, Hardy H, et al. (2008) Optimal recall period and response task for self-reported HIV medication adherence. *AIDS Behav* **12**: 86–94.

Osterberg L, Blaschke T (2005) Adherence to medication. *New Engl J Med* **353**: 487–97.

Simoni JM, Kurth AE, Pearson CR, Pantalone DW, Merrill JO, Frick PA (2006) Self-report measures of antiretroviral therapy adherence: a review with recommendations for HIV research and clinical management. *AIDS Behav* **10**: 227–45.

Steiner JF, Earnest MA (2000) The language of medication-taking. *Ann Intern Med* **132**: 926–30.

Steiner JF, Koepsell TD, Fihn SD, Inui TS (1988) A general method of compliance assessment using centralized pharmacy records: description and validation. *Medical Care* **8**: 814–23.

Thompson MA, Mugavero MJ, Amico KR, Cargill VA, Chang LW, Gross R, et al. (2012) Guidelines for improving entry into and retention in care and antiretroviral adherence for persons with HIV: evidence-based recommendations from an International Association of Physicians in AIDS Care Panel. *Ann Intern Med*. Mar 5. (Epub ahead of print.).

Urquhart J (2000) Defining the margins for errors in patient compliance. *Pharmacoepidemiology and Drug Safety* **9**: 565–8.

CHAPTER 21

Advanced Approaches to Controlling Confounding in Pharmacoepidemiologic Studies

Sebastian Schneeweiss[1] and Samy Suissa[2]

[1]*Harvard Medical School and Brigham & Women's Hospital, Boston, MA, USA*
[2]*McGill University and Lady Davis Research Institute, Jewish General Hospital, Montreal, Quebec, Canada*

The past two decades have witnessed advances in the design and analysis of epidemiologic studies. In this chapter, we introduce some of these approaches with a focus on confounding control, one of the major methodological challenges in pharmacoepidemiology.

Clinical problems to be addressed by pharmacoepidemiologic research

Pharmacoepidemiologic analyses are in principle not different from analyses in other subject areas within epidemiology. They are concerned with valid estimation of the causal effects. Some issues specific to pharmacoepidemiology stem from the constraints of secondary data sources, in particular large electronic longitudinal healthcare databases (see Chapter 9). Another difference is the close interdependency of treatment choice with health status, severity of disease, and prognosis. Pharmacoepidemiologists try to reduce bias by appropriate choices of study design and analytic strategies. This chapter provides an overview of selected options that fit typical pharmacoepidemiologic data sources and study questions.

Methodological problems to be addressed by pharmacoepidemiologic research

The availability of large longitudinal patient-level healthcare databases make the new-user cohort design a natural design choice as a starting point that mimics the classical parallel group controlled trial, except of course for the randomized treatment assignment (Figure 21.1). Efficient sampling within such cohorts, including case-control, case-cohort, and 2-stage sampling designs are important extensions.

Bias can be reduced by appropriate design choices. Considerations about the sources for exposure variation will lead to decisions on the appropriate study design. In a hypothetical causal experiment, one would expose a patient to an agent and observe the outcome, then rewind time, leave the patient unexposed, and keep all other factors constant to establish a counterfactual experience. Since this experiment is impossible, the next logical expansion is to randomly introduce or observe exposure variation within the same patient but over time (Figure 21.2). If we observe sporadic drug use resulting in fluctuations of exposure status within a patient over time, if that drug has a short washout period, and if the adverse event of interest has a rapid onset,

Textbook of Pharmacoepidemiology, Second Edition. Edited by Brian L. Strom, Stephen E. Kimmel, and Sean Hennessy.
© 2013 John Wiley & Sons, Ltd. Published 2013 by John Wiley & Sons, Ltd.

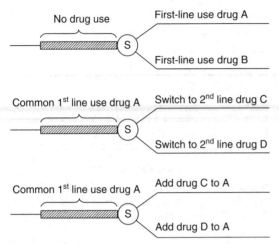

Figure 21.1 Principle of the new user design and its variations when studying second line therapies. Reproduced from Schneeweiss (2010) with permission from John Wiley & Sons Ltd.

then we may consider a case-crossover design or related approach (see below). Another option is random allocation of treatments between different patients. For most pharmacoepidemiologic studies, we utilize variation in exposure among individual patients, and we will therefore use a cohort study design. Exposure variation among higher-level entities (provider, region, etc.) can be exploited using instrumental variable analyses (described below).

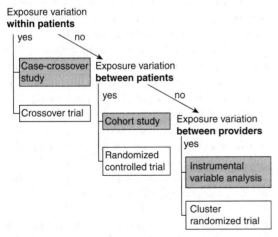

Figure 21.2 Study design choice by source of exposure variation. Reproduced from Schneeweiss (2010) with permission from John Wiley & Sons Ltd.

In a cohort design, there are several advantages to identifying patients who start a new drug. As patients in both the study group and the comparison group have been newly started on medications, they have been evaluated by physicians who concluded that these patients might benefit from the newly prescribed drug. This makes treatment groups more similar in characteristics. The clear temporal sequence of confounder ascertainment before treatment initiation in an incident user design also avoids mistakenly adjusting for consequences of treatment. Studying new users is also useful when studying comparing newly marketed to existing medications, which is prone to bias because patients who stay on treatment for a longer time may be less susceptible to the study outcome.

A common criticism of the incident user design is that excluding prevalent users reduces study size. While true, researchers should be aware that by including prevalent users they might gain precision at the cost of validity. Identifying incident users in secondary databases is not costly. In some situations, particularly studies of second-line treatments in chronic conditions, we can only study patients who switch from one drug to another, as very few patients will be treatment naive. Such switching is often not random. A fairer treatment comparison may be achieved by comparing new switchers to the study drug with new switchers to a comparison drug (Figure 21.1).

Even with appropriate designs, however, all observational pharmacoepidemiologic studies still must consider carefully how to approach potential confounding.

Currently available solutions

The solutions available to minimize confounding in pharmacoepidemiologic database studies can be broadly categorized into: (1) approaches that collect more information on potential confounders and apply efficient sampling designs to reduce the time and resources it takes to complete the study, and (2) analytic approaches that try to make better use of the existing data with the goal of improved control of confounding.

Efficient sampling designs within a cohort study

In any cohort study, the resources needed to collect data on all cohort members can be prohibitive. Even with cohorts formed from computerized databases, there may be a need to supplement and validate data with information from hospital records and other sources. When the cohort size is large, such additional data gathering can become a formidable task. Moreover, even if no additional data are needed, the data analysis of a cohort with multiple and time-dependent drug exposures can be technically infeasible, particularly if the cohort size and number of outcome events are large.

To counter these constraints, designs based on sampling subjects within a cohort exist. These designs are based on the selection of all cases with the outcome event from the cohort, but differ in the selection of a small subset of "noncases." Generally, they permit the precise estimation of relative risk measures with negligible losses in precision. Below, we discuss structural aspects of cohorts and present three sampling designs within a cohort: nested case–control, multi-time case-control, and case–cohort.

Structures of cohorts

Figure 21.3 illustrates a hypothetical cohort of 21 newly diagnosed diabetics over the period 1995 to 2010. This cohort is plotted in terms of *calendar time*, with subjects ranked according to their date of entry, which can correspond to the date of diagnosis or treatment initiation. An alternative depiction of

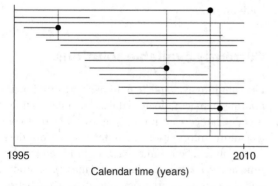

1995   2010
Calendar time (years)

Figure 21.3 Illustration of a *calendar-time* cohort of 21 subjects followed from 1978 to 1990 with 4 cases (•) occurring and related risk-sets (—).

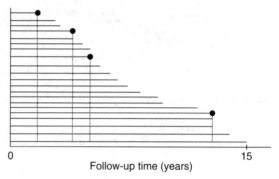

0   15
Follow-up time (years)

Figure 21.4 Illustration of *follow-up-time* cohort representation after rearranging the cohort in Figure 21.1, with the new risk-sets (—) for the 4 cases.

this same cohort could be based on disease onset. In this instance, the illustration given in Figure 21.4 for the same cohort, using follow-up time as the new time axis, is significantly different from the previous one. In these *follow-up-time* cohorts, the same subjects are ranked according to the length of follow-up time in the study with zero-time being the time of diagnosis or treatment start.

The question of which of the two forms one should use rests on one's judgment of the more relevant of the two time axes. This decision is important, since it affects the demarcation of "risk-sets," which are fundamental to the analysis of data from cohorts and consequently the sampling designs within cohorts. A risk-set is formed by the members of the cohort who are at-risk of the outcome event at a given point in time, namely they are free of the outcome and members of the cohort at that point in time called the index date. Drug exposure measures are then anchored at this index date. It is clear that Figures 21.3 and 21.4 produce distinct risk-sets for the same cases in the same cohort, as illustrated by the different sets of subjects crossed by the vertical broken line for the same case under the two forms of the cohort. In Figure 21.3, for example, the first chronological case to occur has in its risk-set only the first 6 subjects to enter the cohort, while in Figure 21.4, all 21 cohort members belong to its risk-set at the time that the first case arises. While the second form based on disease duration is often used, because drug exposure can vary substantially over calendar time, the first form may be as relevant for the formation of risk-sets and data analysis as the second form. Regardless, an advantage of having data on the entire cohort is that the primary time axis can be changed according to the study question, using calendar time for one analysis, duration of disease or drug exposure for another, with respective adjustment in the analysis for the effect of the other time axis.

The nested case–control design

The modern nested case-control design involves four steps:
1. defining the cohort time axis, as above;
2. selecting all cases in the cohort, i.e., all subjects with an outcome event of interest;
3. forming a risk-set for each case; and
4. *randomly* selecting one or more controls from each risk-set.

Figure 21.5 illustrates the selection of a nested case–control sample from a cohort, with one control per case (1:1 matching). It is clear from the definition of risk-sets that a future case is eligible to be a control for a prior case, as illustrated in the figure for the fourth case (the circle occurring last in time), and that a subject may be selected as a control more than once. Bias is introduced if controls are forced to be selected only from the noncases and subjects are not permitted to be used more than once.

This property leading to subjects possibly being selected more than once in the sample may be challenging when the exposure and covariate factors are time-dependent, particularly when the data are obtained by questionnaire where the respondent would have to answer questions regarding multiple time points in their history. (See also Chapter 12.)

The nested case–control design is used primarily to compare exposures to different drugs. At times, however, it is of interest to contrast exposure to drugs versus no exposure, so external comparisons are performed, comparing the rate of outcome in the cohort to that of an external population. The resulting measure is usually called the standardized mortality ratio (SMR) or the standardized incidence ratio (SIR). Calculating such measures directly from a nested case–control design is not appropriate, because subjects are sampled with regard to outcome. Indeed, it is evident from Figure 21.3 that cohort members with the longest follow-up have a greater chance of being selected in the nested case–control sample, since they belong to all the risk-sets. The appropriate method to perform external comparisons using data from a nested case–control design has been developed and uses knowledge about the sampling structure to yield an unbiased estimate of the standardized rate.

The case–cohort design

The case–cohort design involves two steps:
1. selecting all cases in the cohort, i.e., all subjects with an adverse event; and
2. randomly selecting a sample of predetermined size of subjects from the cohort, irrespective of case or control status.

Figure 21.6 depicts the selection of a case–cohort sample of six subjects from the illustrative cohort. Note that it is possible that some cases selected in

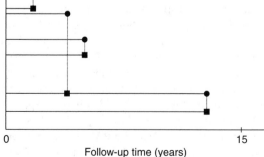

Figure 21.5 Nested case-control sample of one control (■) per case (●) from cohort in Figure 21.4.

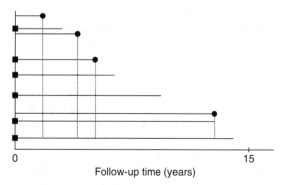

Figure 21.6 Case-cohort sample with six controls (■) from cohort in Figure 21.4.

step 1 are also selected in the step 2 sample, as illustrated in the figure for the third case.

The case–cohort design resembles a reduced version of the cohort, with all cases from the full cohort included. The method of analysis for a case–cohort sample takes into account the overlap of cohort members between successive risk-sets induced by this sampling strategy.

The first advantage of the case–cohort design is its capacity to use the same sample to study multiple types of events. In contrast, the nested case–control design requires different control groups for each type. For example, a nested case-control study of the risks of β-agonists had two distinct control groups, one of size 233 for the 44 asthma deaths, the other of size 422 for the 85 asthma near-deaths. Another useful advantage is that the case–cohort design permits one to change the primary time axis of analysis from calendar to disease time and vice versa, depending on either the assumed model or the targeted outcome. This is not possible with the nested case–control study, where the primary time axis must be set *a priori* to permit the risk-set construction. Yet another advantage is its simplicity in sampling, which has benefits in both comprehensibility and computer programming.

The nested case–control design does have some advantages over the case-cohort design. The first is the simplicity of statistical power calculation. The nested case–control design is independent of the size of the cohort, while for the case–cohort design knowledge about overlap in risk-sets is essential, thus greatly complicating these calculations. Second, data on time-dependent exposure and covariates need only be collected up to the time of the risk-set for the nested case–control study, while the collection must be exhaustive for the case–cohort.

Within-subject designs

When dealing with the study of transient effects on the risk of acute adverse events, Maclure asserts that the best representatives of the source population that produced the cases would be the case subjects themselves: this is the premise of the case-crossover design. This is a design where comparisons between exposures are made within subjects, thus removing confounding by factors that remain

constant within subject. An extension to the case–crossover design, the case–time–control design is also presented here.

The case-crossover design

The case-crossover study is simply an observational crossover study *in the cases only*. The subjects alternate at varying frequencies between exposure and non-exposure to the drug of interest, until the adverse event occurs, which happens for all subjects in the study sample, since all are cases by definition. With respect to the timing of the adverse event, each case is investigated to determine whether exposure was present within the presumed effect period. This occurrence is then classified as having arisen either under drug exposure or non-exposure on the basis of the presumed effect period. Thus, for each case, we have either an exposed or unexposed status, which represents for data analysis the first column of a 2×2 table, one for each case. Since each case will be matched to itself for comparison, the analysis is matched and thus we must create separate 2×2 tables for each case.

With respect to control information, the data on the average drug use pattern are necessary to determine the typical probability of exposure during the time window of effect. This is done by obtaining data for a sufficiently stable period of time. For example, we may wish to study the risk of ventricular tachycardia in association with the use of inhaled beta-agonists in asthma, where prolonged Q-T intervals were observed in patients in the 4-hour period following drug absorption. Table 21.1 diplays data for 10 cases of ventricular tachycardia, including the average number of times a day each case has been using β-agonists in the past year. Note that there are six 4-hour periods (the duration of the effect period) per day. Such data determines the proportion of time that each asthmatic is usually spending in the effect period and thus potentially "at risk" of ventricular tachycardia. This proportion is then used to obtain the expected exposure on the basis of time spent in these "at risk" periods, for comparison with the actual exposure in the cases observed during the last 4-hour period. This is done by forming a 2×2 table for each case, with the corresponding control data as

Table 21.1 Hypothetical data for 10 subjects with ventricular tachycardia included in a case-crossover study of the risk of ventricular tachycardia in asthma associated with the four-hour period after β-agonist exposure.

Case #	β-agonist use in last 4 hours[*] (E_i)	Usual β-agonist use in last year	Periods of exposure (N_{1i})	Periods of no exposure (N_{0i})
1	0	1/day	365	1825
2	1	6/year	6	2184
3	0	2/day	730	1460
4	1	1/month	12	2178
5	0	4/week	208	1982
6	0	1/week	52	2138
7	0	1/month	12	2178
8	1	2/month	24	2166
9	0	2/day	730	1460
10	0	2/week	104	2086

[*]Inhalations of 200 mcg: 1 = yes, 0 = no.
Note: Rate ratio estimator is $(\sum E_i N_{0i})/(\sum (1 - E_i)N_{1i})$.

defined above, and combining the tables using the Mantel–Haenszel technique.

To carry out a case-crossover study, three critical points must be considered. First, the study outcome must be an acute event that is hypothesized to be the result of a transient drug effect. Thus, drugs with chronic or regular patterns of use which vary only minimally between and within individuals are not amenable to this design. Nor are latent adverse events. Second, since a transient effect is under study, the presumed effect period must be precisely stated. For example, in a study of the possible acute cardiotoxicity of inhaled β-agonists in asthmatics, this effect period can be hypothesized to be 4 hours after having taken the usual dose. An incorrect specification of this time window can have important repercussions on the relative risk estimate. Third, one must be able to obtain reliable data on the usual pattern of drug exposure for each case, over a sufficiently long period of time.

The case–time–control design

One of the limitations of the case-crossover design is the assumption of the absence of a time trend in the exposure prevalence. An approach that adjusts for such time trends is the case–time–control design, an extension of the case-crossover analysis that uses, in addition to the case series, a series of control subjects to adjust for exposure time trends. By using cases and controls of a conventional case–control study as their own referents, the *case–time–control design* addresses the time trend assumption.

The approach is illustrated with data from the Saskatchewan Asthma Epidemiologic Project, conducted to investigate the risks associated with the use of inhaled β-agonists. Using a cohort of 12,301 asthmatics followed during 1980–87, 129 cases of fatal or near-fatal asthma and 655 controls were identified. The amount of β-agonist used in the year prior to the index date was used for exposure. Table 21.2 displays

Table 21.2 Illustration of a case-time-control analysis of data from a case-control study of 129 cases of fatal or near-fatal asthma and 655 matched controls, and current beta-agonist use.

	Cases		Controls		OR	95% CI
	high	low	high	low		
Current beta-agonist use (case-control)	93	36	241	414	3.1[*]	1.8–5.4
Discordant[a] use (case-crossover)	29	9			3.2	1.5–6.8
Discordant[a] use (control-crossover)			65	25	2.6	1.6–4.1
Case-time-control	29	9	65	25	1.2	0.5–3.0

[*]Adjusted estimate from case-control analysis
[a]Discordant from exposure level during reference time period.

the data comparing low ($\leq$12 canisters per year) with high (>12) use of β-agonists. The crude odds ratio for high β-agonist use was 4.4 (95% CI: 2.9–6.7). Adjustment for all available markers of severity lowered the odds ratio to 3.1 (95% CI: 1.8–5.4).

To apply the case–time–control design, exposure to β-agonists was obtained for the one-year current period and the one-year reference period prior to the current period. First, a case-crossover analysis was performed using the discordant subjects among the 129 cases, namely the 29 who were current high users of β-agonists and low users in the reference period, and the 9 cases who were current low users of β-agonist and high users previously. This analysis is repeated for the 655 controls, of whom there were 90 discordant in exposure; that is, 65 were current high users of β-agonists and low users in the reference period, and 25 were current low users of β-agonists and high users previously. The case–time–control odds ratio, using these discordant pairs frequencies for a paired-matched analysis, is given by (29/9)/(65/25) = 1.2 (95% CI: 0.5–3.0). This estimate, which does not account for potential confounding by asthma severity that varies over time, indicates a minimal risk for these drugs.

The case–time–control approach can provide an unbiased estimate of the odds ratio in the presence of confounding by time-invariant factors, including indication, despite the fact that the indication for drug use (in our example, intrinsic disease severity) is not measured, because of the within-subject analysis. It also controls for time trends in drug use. Nevertheless, its validity is subject to several assumptions, including the absence of time-varying confounders, such as increasing asthma severity over time (an important problem, since new drugs may be more likely to be implemented when disease is most severe), so that caution is recommended in its use.

Analytic approaches for improved confounding control

Balancing patient characteristics
Confounding caused by imbalance of patient risk factors between treatment groups is a known threat to validity in nonrandomized studies. Many options for reducing confounding are available. Several

approaches fit key characteristics of longitudinal healthcare databases well and address important concerns in pharmacoepidemiologic analyses.

Propensity score analyses
Propensity score analysis has emerged as a convenient and effective tool for adjusting large numbers of confounders. In an incident user cohort design, a propensity score (PS) is the estimated probability of starting medication A versus starting medication B, conditional on all observed pretreatment patient characteristics. Propensity scores are a multivariate balancing tool that balance large numbers of covariates in an efficient way even if the study outcome is rare, which is frequent in pharmacoepidemiology. Estimating the propensity score using logistic regression is uncomplicated, and strategies for variable selection are well described. Variables that are only predictors of treatment choice but are not independent predictors of outcome will lead to less precise estimates and in some extreme situations to bias. Selecting variables based on p-values is not helpful as this strategy depends on study size. Once a propensity score is estimated based on observed covariates there are several options to utilize it in a second step to reduce confounding. Typical strategies include adjustment from quantiles of the score with or without trimming, regression modeling of the PS, or matching on propensity scores. Matching illustrates the working of propensity scores well.

Fixed ratio matching on propensity scores like 1:1 or 1:4 matching has several advantages that may outweigh its drawback of not utilizing the full dataset in situations where not all eligible patients match. Such matching will exclude patients in the extreme PS ranges where there is little clinical ambivalence in treatment choice (Figure 21.7). These tails of the PS distribution often harbor extreme patient scenarios that are not representative for the majority in clinical practice and may be due to residual confounding. Trimming these extreme PS values will generally reduce residual confounding. Another advantage is that the multivariate balance of potential confounders can be demonstrated by cross-tabulating observed patient characteristics by actual exposure status after fixed ratio matching. Matching with a fixed ratio in

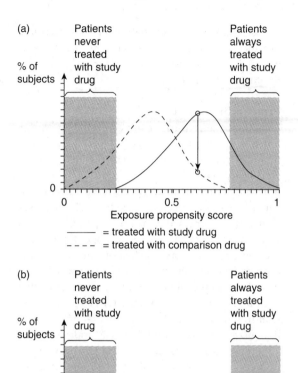

Figure 21.7 Two hypothetical propensity score distributions before and after matching. A: Before matching: two propensity score distributions partially overlap indicating some similarities between the comparison groups in a multivariate parameter space. B: After 1:1 matching on propensity score: Not all patients found matches that were similar enough in their multivariable characteristics. Areas of non-overlap between PS distributions drop out entirely. Reproduced from Schneeweiss (2010) with permission from John Wiley & Sons Ltd.

cohort studies does not require matched analyses, but variable ratio matching does. Analytic techniques that condition on the matching sets and may be used in this setting include conditional logistic regression or stratified Cox regression, depending on the data model.

In summary, propensity score analyses are convenient tools to adjust for many covariates when study outcomes are rare. Extensive confounding adjustment is central in most pharmacoepidemiologic applications, and in secondary healthcare databases we can often define many covariates. In contrast to traditional outcome models, PS matching allows the investigator to achieve covariate balance achieved in the final study sample. PS estimation is well developed for comparing two agents using logistic regression to predict treatment choice. When more than two agents or several dose categories are compared, multinomial regression models are used to estimate the propensity score and either pragmatic pairwise matching to a common reference group or multidimensional matching is applied. Of importance, PS anlyses still can only adjust for measured variables, although they can be used to adjust for many at the same time. Further, one loses the ability to see the effects of adjusting for one variable at a time.

In situations where exposure is rare, disease risk scores, an alternative to propensity score analysis, might be more suitable. They estimate the association between patient factors and the study outcome in an unexposed population using multivariate regression and summarize the relationship in each patient's estimated probability of the outcome independent of exposure.

Focusing on the analysis of comparable patients

Restriction is a common and effective analytic tool to make drug user groups more comparable by making populations more homogeneous, which leads to less residual confounding. Some restrictions are quite obvious since they are made by explicit criteria, for example, limiting the study population to elderly patients with dementia to study the safety of antipsychotic medications used to control behavioral disturbances in this population. Other restrictions are more implicit and blur the line between design and analytic strategies.

Choice of comparator group: picking a comparator group is arguably the most fundamental choice in a pharmacoepidemiologic study design and may influence results dramatically. Ideally, we want to restrict the comparison population to patients who have the identical indication as the users of the study agent. Rosiglitazone and pioglitazone are such a medication pair. They were marketed around the same time, were both indicated for second line treatment of diabetes, come from the same class of compound, and in the early marketing phase were thought to have a similar effectiveness and safety profiles. This should make treatment choice largely random with regard to patient characteristics and treatment groups comparable by design, resulting in almost overlapping propensity score distributions and little confounding.

Limiting to incident users: By restricting the study population to new users of the study agent or a comparator agent we implicitly require that both groups have been recently evaluated by a physician. Based on this evaluation the physician has decided that the indicating condition has reached a state where a pharmacologic treatment should be initiated. Therefore, such patients are likely to be more similar in observable and unobservable characteristics than comparing incident users versus non-users or versus ongoing users of another drug.

Matching on patient characteristics: Multivariate propensity scores demonstrate areas of non-overlap where no referent patients with comparable baseline characteristics can be identified. It is recommended to remove those patients from the analysis as they do not contribute to the estimation and may introduce bias. Such a restriction can be achieved by trimming these patients from the study population (see Figure 21.7b) or by matching patients on the propensity score or on specific key patient characteristics of importance.

While restriction is an important tool to improve internal validity it will reduce generalizability of findings. However, in pharmacoepidemiology we usually place higher value on internal validity even if that comes at the price of reduced external validity. Investigators need to be aware of this tradeoff and make choices accordingly.

Unobserved patient characteristics and residual confounding

Once a study is implemented, strategies to reduce confounding further are limited to observable disease risk factors. Secondary data, like electronic healthcare databases often lack critical details on health state and risk factors, which can lead to residual confounding.

Proxy adjustment

Longitudinal electronic health care databases are as much a description of medical sociology under financial constraints as they are records of delivered health care and can be analyzed as a set of proxies that indirectly describe the health status of patients. This status is presented through the lenses of health care providers recording their findings and interventions via coders and operating under the constraints of a specific health care system. For example, old age serves as a proxy for many factors including comorbidity, frailty, and cognitive decline; use of an oxygen canister is a sign of frail health; having regular annual check-ups is indicative of a health-seeking lifestyle and increased adherence. Adjusting for a perfect surrogate of an unmeasured factor is equivalent to adjusting for the factor itself. Frequently used proxies in pharmacoepidemiologic analyses are the number of prescription drugs dispensed, the number of physician visits, and hospitalizations before the index drug exposure. Such measures of healthcare intensity are useful proxies for general health and access to care and have been shown to meaningfully help adjust for confounding.

Proxy adjustment can be exploited by algorithms that systematically search through recorded codes for diagnoses, procedures, equipment purchases, and prescription drug dispensings before the initiation of study drug use to identify potential confounders or proxies thereof. The hundreds of proxies that will be identified can then be adjusted for in a large propensity score model. Collinearity may likely occur but is irrelevant, as the individual parameters estimated in the large propensity score regression will not be interpreted but only used for predicting treatment. Such a high-dimensional propensity score approach has been shown empirically to improve confounding adjustment in many settings, although it is not yet fully evaluated. Although adjusting for variables that are only related to the exposure and not to the outcome (an instrumental variable) could theoretically introduce bias, in practical scenarios the advantage of adjusting for potential confounders outweighs the risk of adjusting for the rare instrument.

Exploiting random aspects in treatment choice via instrumental variable analysis

As explained above, we are interested in identifying residual random exposure variation after adjusting for observable confounders to more completely account for confounding. However, in secondary data, not all clinically relevant risk factors of the outcome may be recorded. To attempt to address this limitation, we can try to identify naturally occurring quasi-random treatment choices in routine care. Factors that determine such quasi-random treatment choices are called instrumental variables (IVs), and IV analyses can result in unbiased effect estimates even without observing all confounders if several assumptions are fulfilled (discussed further below).

An instructive example of an instrument is a hospital drug formulary. Some hospitals list only drug A for a given indication and other hospitals list only drug B. It is a reasonable assumption that patients do not choose their preferred hospital based on its formulary but rather based on location and recommendation. Therefore, the choice of drug A versus drug B should be independent of patient characteristics in the hospitals with these restricted formularies. Thus, comparing patient outcomes from drug A hospitals with patient outcomes from drug B hospitals should result in unbiased effects of drug A versus drug B, using the appropriate analytic tools. An example of such a study is a study on the risk of death from aprotinin, an antifibrinolytic agent given to reduce bleeding during cardiac surgery. The study identified surgeons who always used aprotinin and compared their outcomes to surgeons who always used aminocaproic acid, an alternative drug. If physician skill level and performance are on average equal between institutions, independent of drug use, this will result in valid findings. On the other hand, of course, such an assumption may not be valid, e. g., if academic hospitals allow less restrictive formularies, are more likely to see sicker patients, and have skilled physicians, all of which may be true.

Instrumental variable analyses rely on the identification of a valid instrument, a factor that is assumed to be related to treatment, but neither directly nor indirectly related to the study outcome. As such, an IV is an observed variable that causes (or is a marker of) variation in the exposure similar to random treatment choice. Typically the following three assumptions need to be fulfilled for valid IV estimation: (1) an IV should affect treatment or be associated with treatment choice by sharing a common cause. The strength of this association is also referred to as the instrument strength; (2) an IV should be a factor that is as good as randomly assigned, so that it is unrelated to patient characteristics; and (3) an IV should not be related to the outcome other than through its association with treatment. As such, an IV analysis sounds very much like a randomized trial with noncompliance. The flip of a coin determines the instrument status (treat with A vs. treat with B) and the amount of random noncompliance determines the strength of the instrument. In nonrandomized research, however, identifying valid instruments is difficult and successful IV analyses are infrequent. In principle, treatment preference can be influenced by time if treatment guidelines change rapidly and substantially. A comparison of patient outcome before versus after a sudden change in treatment patterns may then be a reasonable instrument.

Sensitivity analyses

A series of sensitivity analyses can help investigators to better understand how robust a study's findings are to a set of structural assumptions. Some of the sensitivity analyses suggested below are generic and others are specific to database analyses.

An important but underutilized diagnostic tool for the impact of unobserved confounders on the validity of findings in nonrandomized studies is quantitative sensitivity analyses. Basic sensitivity analyses of residual confounding try to determine how strong and how imbalanced a confounder would have to be among drug categories to explain the observed effect. Such an "externally" adjusted relative risk (RR_{adj}) can be expressed as a function of the unadjusted relative risk (RR_{unadj}), the independent RR of the unmeasured confounder on the disease outcome (RR_{CD}), and the prevalence of the confounder in both drug exposure categories ($P_{C|E}$):

$$RR_{adj.} = \frac{RR_{unadj}}{\left[\frac{P_{C|E=1}(RR_{CD} - 1) + 1}{P_{C|E=0}(RR_{CD} - 1) + 1}\right]}$$

A recent cohort study could not find the expected association between use of TNF alpha inhibitors, an immunomodulating agent, in treating rheumatoid arthritis, and the incidence of serious bacterial infections. There was a concern that physicians may have prescribed the agent selectively in patients with more progressive disease. A sensitivity analysis demonstrated the direction and strength of any such bias and concluded that it would be unlikely to change the clinical implications of the study. This type of sensitivity analysis is particularly helpful in database studies, but is underutilized. Spreadsheet software is available for easy implementation of such sensitivity analyses (drugepi.org). Lash and Fink proposed an approach that considers several systematic errors simultaneously, allowing sensitivity analyses for confounding, misclassification, and selection bias in one process.

When using retrospective databases, it is usually cumbersome or impossible to contact patients and ask when they began using a drug for the first time in order to implement an incident user cohort design. Therefore, incident users are identified empirically by a drug dispensing that was not preceded by a dispensing of the same drug for a defined time period. This washout period is identical for all patients. A typical length is 6 months. In sensitivity analyses, this interval could be extended to 9 and 12 months. In a study on the comparative safety of antidepressant agents in children in British Columbia this interval was extended from 1 year to 3 years to ensure that the children in the study were treatment-naïve before their first use, which helped balance comparison groups and reduce confounding. Although increasing the length of the washout increases the likelihood that patients are truly incident users, it also reduces the number of patients eligible for the study. This tradeoff is particularly worth noting in health plans with high enrollee turnover.

There is often uncertainty about the correct definition of the exposure risk window based on the clinical pharmacology of the study agent. This is further complicated in healthcare databases, since the discontinuation date is imputed through the days' supply of the last dispensing/prescription. Varying the exposure risk window is therefore insightful and easy to accomplish in cohort studies.

Conclusion

Minimizing confounding in pharmacoepidemiologic research is an ongoing development. While great progress has been made in analyzing longitudinal healthcare databases, much remains to be improved to reliably achieve unbiased estimates that will carry the weight of medical decision making. Several developments are promising. One is the use of instrumental variable analyses utilizing the multilevel structure of healthcare systems. Another is the expanded use of propensity score methods including its combination with data mining activities for high-dimensional proxy adjustment. A development that is gaining importance is the enrichment of existing data environments with supplemental clinical data linked from electronic medical records, from disease registries, from patient surveys, and/or from laboratory test result repositories. While this information will provide an opportunity for improved confounding adjustment, it comes with equally large methodological challenges, as information is collected in routine care and may have been requested/recorded selectively in patients who were thought to benefit most. Clearly there is still plenty of work to be done to find satisfactory solutions for the control of confounding.

Key points

- Pharmacoepidemiologic studies must be efficient by offering rapid information of the utmost validity.
- Computerised databases provide valuable data sources for pharmacoepidemiologic studies with unique methodological challenges.

- Epidemiologic designs such as nested case-control and case-crossover are efficient approaches to assess the risks and benefits of drugs if additional data is collected.
- Confounding bias can be assessed efficiently using subsets of the data.

Case Example 21.1

Background

- The occurrence of relapses in multiple sclerosis is highly variable and unpredictable. Vaccines, particularly for hepatitis B, have been suspected to induce relapses in multiple sclerosis.

Question

- Does vaccination increase in the rate of relapse in multiple sclerosis?

Approach

- A case-crossover study within the European Database for Multiple Sclerosis network. Cases with a relapse after a 12-month relapse-free period were questioned on vaccinations. Exposure to vaccination in the two-month risk-period immediately preceding the relapse was compared with that of the four previous two-month control periods to estimate the relative risk.

Results

- The prevalence of exposure during the two-month risk period was similar to that of the four control periods.
- The relative risk of relapse associated with exposure to any vaccination was thus unity.

Strengths

- Large clinical population with extensive computerized information.
- Efficient study design using only cases for this acute event and transient drug exposure.
- Confounding factors that do not change over time are inherently controlled for by the within-subject matched analysis.

Limitations

- Low vaccination prevalence in this clinical population does not permit assessment of the risk for shorter effect periods, such as a week.
- Confounding by factors that change over time, such as infections, could not be controlled for.

Key points

- Multiple sclerosis is highly variable over time and thus not easily amenable to cohort or case-control study designs.
- The case-crossover design is an efficient approach to study vaccine safety.

Case Example 21.2

Background

- A meta-analysis of randomized placebo-controlled trials has shown an increased risk of suicides among children initiating antidepressants (AD), however, the study could not elucidate the comparative safety, i.e. whether this risk varies meaningfully between antidepressant agents.

Question

- Do tricyclic antidepressants have similar risk of suicidal actions including completed suicide compared with selective serotonin reuptake inhibitors (SSRIs).

Approach

- A propensity score-matched new user cohort study of children and young adults (10–18 years of age) using health care utilization databases from the province of British Columbia linked with vital statistics information. Suicidal actions were defined as emergency hospitalizations for intentional self harm and completed suicides. First exposure to a tricyclic AD with no AD exposure in previous 3 years was compared to new use of fluoxetine. Follow-up started the day after the first AD dispensing and ended 14 days after their last exposure to the cohort-qualifying drug exposure.

Results

- Unadjusted and insufficiently adjusted analyses showed a spurious up to 50% relative risk decrease for tricyclic ADs compared with SSRIs, suggesting that tricyclic agents are avoided in patients with suicidal thoughts as they are known to be poisonous in high doses.
- There was no difference in the risk for suicidal actions between tricyclic ADs and fluoxetine after nonparsimonious high-dimensional propensity scores matching.

Strengths

- Large stable population of children and young adults with information on all health service encounters and vital statistics.
- The new users design ensures that all patient characteristics are assessed before exposure starts and that suicidal actions shortly after initiation will be accounted for and the duration of use-dependent risk function can be plotted and illustrate the depletion of the most susceptible patients.
- Confounding factors may bias results due to strong channeling of sicker patients to the safer SSRIs but nonparsimonious adjustment with high-dimensional propensity scores can remedy the issue in this example.

Limitations

- Despite the large population size the number of outcomes remains limited leading to less precise estimates and making adjustment for many potential confounders in outcome regression models perilous.

- Confounding by outcome risk factors that channel patients into the treatment groups can be strong and hard to control.

Key points

- Two major antidepressant classes have similar risks of suicidal actions in newly treated children and young adults.

- The new user cohort design is a flexible and robust approach for studies that rely entirely on secondary healthcare databases when combined with nonparsimonious propensity score adjustment.

Further reading

Blais L, Ernst P, Suissa S (1996) Confounding by indication and channelling over time: the risks of beta-agonists. *Am J Epidemiol* **144**: 1161–9.

Brookhart MA, Rassen JA, Schneeweiss S (2010) Instrumental variable methods in comparative safety and effectiveness research. *Pharmacoepidemiol Drug Saf* **19**: 537–54.

Brookhart MA, Schneeweiss S, Rothman KJ, Glynn RJ, Avorn J, Sturmer T (2006) Variable selection for propensity score models. *Am J Epidemiol* **163**: 1149–56.

Collet JP, Schaubel D, Hanley J, Sharpe C, Boivin JF (1998) Controlling confounding when studying large pharmacoepidemiologic databases: a case study of the two-stage sampling design. *Epidemiology* **9**: 309–15.

Confavreux C, Suissa S, Saddier P, Bourdès V, Vukusic S for the Vaccines in Multiple Sclerosis Study Group (2001) Vaccinations and the risk of relapse in multiple sclerosis. *New Engl J Med* **344**(5): 319–26.

Farrington CP, Nash J, Miller E (1996) Case series analysis of adverse reactions to vaccines: a comparative evaluation. *Am J Epidemiol* **143**: 1165–73.

Hallas J (1996) Evidence of depression provoked by cardiovascular medication: a prescription sequence symmetry analysis. *Epidemiol* **7**: 478–84.

Maclure M (1991) The case-crossover design: a method for studying transient effects on the risk of acute events. *Am J Epidemiol* **133**: 144–53.

Ray WA (2003) Evaluating medication effects outside of clinical trials: new-user designs. *Am J Epidemiol* **158**: 915–20.

Rothman KJ, Greenland S, Lash TL (eds) (2008) *Modern Epidemiology*. 3rd edn. Philadelphia, PA: Lippincott Williams & Wilkins.

Schneeweiss S (2010) A basic study design for expedited safety signal evaluation based on electronic healthcare data. *Pharmacoepidemiol Drug Saf* **19**: 858–68.

Schneeweiss S, Avorn J (2005) A review of uses of health care utilization databases for epidemiologic research on therapeutics. *J Clin Epidemiol* **58**: 323–37.

Schneeweiss S, Patrick AR, Sturmer T, Brookhart MA, Avorn J, Maclure M, *et al.* (2007) Increasing levels of restriction in pharmacoepidemiologic database studies of elderly and comparison with randomized trial results. *Med Care* **45** (10 Suppl 2): S131–42.

Schneeweiss S, Rassen JA, Glyn RJ, Avorn J, Mogun H, Brookhart MA (2009) High-dimensional propensity score adjustment in studies of treatment effects using health care claims data. *Epidemiology* **20**: 512–22.

Schneeweiss S, Seeger JD, Maclure M, Wang PS, Avorn J, Glynn RJ (2001) Performance of comorbidity scores to control for confounding in epidemiologic studies using claims data. *Am J Epidemiol* **154**: 854–64.

Spitzer WO, Suissa S, Ernst P, Horwitz RI, Habbick B, Cockcroft D, *et al.* (1992) The use of beta-agonists and the risk of death and near death from asthma. *N Engl J Med* **326**: 501–6.

Sturmer T, Rothman KJ, Avorn J, Glynn RJ (2010) Treatment effects in the presence of unmeasured confounding: dealing with observations in the tails of the propensity score distribution–a simulation study. *Am J Epidemiol* **172**: 843–54.

Suissa S (1995) The case–time–control design. *Epidemiology* **6**: 248–53.

Suissa S, Edwardes MD, Boivin JF (1998) External comparisons from nested case–control designs. *Epidemiology* **9**: 72–8.

Wacholder S (1991) Practical considerations in choosing between the case–cohort and nested case–control designs. *Epidemiology* **2**: 155–8.

Walker AM (1996) Confounding by indication. *Epidemiology* **7**: 335–6.

PART IV
Special Applications

CHAPTER 22

Special Applications of Pharmacoepidemiology

The following individuals contributed to writing sections of this chapter:

David Lee[1], Sumit R. Majumdar[2], Helene L. Lipton[3], Stephen B. Soumerai[4], Claudia Vellozzi[5], Robert T. Chen[5], Jason Glanz[6], Danica Marinac-Dabic[7], Sharon-Lise T. Normand[8], Art Sedrakyan[9], Allen A. Mitchell[10], Gerald J. Dal Pan[7], Stella Blackburn[11], Claudia Manzo[7], Hanna M. Seidling[12], David W. Bates[13], Melissa A. Robb[7], Rachel E. Sherman[7*], Brian L. Strom[14], Rita Schinnar[14], and Sean Hennessy[14]*

[1] Center for Pharmaceutical Management, Management Sciences for Health, Arlington, VA, USA
[2] Faculty of Medicine and Dentistry, University of Alberta, Edmonton, Alberta, Canada
[3] Schools of Medicine and Pharmacy, University of California at San Francisco, San Francisco, CA, USA
[4] Harvard Medical School and Harvard Pilgrim Health Care Institute, Boston, MA, USA
[5] Centers for Disease Control and Prevention, Atlanta, GA, USA
[6] School of Public Health, Denver, CO, USA
[7] US Food and Drug Administration, Silver Spring, MD, USA
[8] Harvard Medical School and Harvard School of Public Health, Boston, MA, USA
[9] New York Presbyterian Hospital and Weill Cornell Medical College, New York, NY, USA
[10] Boston University Schools of Public Health and Medicine, Boston, MA, USA
[11] European Medicines Agency, London, UK
[12] Cooperation Unit Clinical Pharmacy, University of Heidelberg, Heidelberg, Germany
[13] Brigham and Women's Hospital and Harvard Medical School, Boston, MA, USA
[14] Perelman School of Medicine at the University of Pennsylvania, Philadelphia, PA, USA

In this chapter, we will present selected special applications of pharmacoepidemiology, which include studies of drug utilization; evaluating and improving physician prescribing; special methodological issues in pharmacoepidemiology of vaccine safety; pharmacoepidemiologic studies of devices; studies of drug-induced birth defects; pharmacoepidemiology and risk management; the use of pharmacoepidemiology to study medication errors; FDA's Sentinel Initiative; and comparative effectiveness research. Again, we present this information using a standard format, focusing on clinical and methodological problems, examples of solutions, and perspectives on the future. Each application section then ends with a case example and key points.

Studies of drug utilization

Introduction

Drug utilization was defined by the World Health Organization (WHO) as the "marketing, distribution, prescription and use of drugs in a society, with special emphasis on the resulting medical, social, and economic consequences." Studies of drug utilization address not only the medical and nonmedical aspects influencing prescribing, dispensing, administration, and taking of medication, but also the effects of drug utilization at all levels of the health care system.

Drug utilization studies may be *quantitative* or *qualitative* (Table 22.1). In the former, the objective

*The views expressed are those of the authors and do not necessarily represent those of the US Food and Drug Administration.

Table 22.1 Drug utilization studies in perspective: operational concepts.

	Drug statistics	Drug utilization study	Drug utilization review program
Synonyms (therapeutic)	Drug utilization data	Drug utilization review or drug utilization review study	Drug audit
Quantitative approach	Yes	Usually	Usually
Qualitative approach	No	Maybe	Yes
Continuous (ongoing)	Usually	No	Yes

is to quantify the present state, developmental trends, and time course of drug usage at various levels of the health care system, whether national, regional, local, or institutional. Routinely compiled *drug statistics* or drug utilization data that result from such studies can be used to estimate drug utilization in populations by age, sex, social class, morbidity, and other characteristics, and to identify areas of possible over- or underutilization. They also can be used as denominator data for calculating rates of reported adverse drug reactions (see Chapter 7); to monitor the utilization of specific therapeutic categories where particular problems can be anticipated (e.g., narcotic analgesics, hypnotics and sedatives, and other psychotropic drugs); to monitor the effects of informational and regulatory activities (e.g., adverse events alerts, delisting of drugs from therapeutic formularies); as markers for very crude estimates of disease prevalence (e.g., antiparkinsonian drugs for Parkinson's disease); to plan for drug importation, production, and distribution; and to estimate drug expenditures.

Qualitative studies assess the appropriateness of drug utilization, usually by linking prescription data to the reasons for drug prescribing. Explicit predetermined criteria are created against which aspects of the quality, medical necessity, and appropriateness of drug prescribing may be compared. Drug use criteria may be based upon such parameters as indications for use, daily dose, and length of therapy, or others such as: failure to select a more effective or less hazardous drug if available, use of a fixed combination drug when only one of its

components is justified, or use of a costly drug when a less costly equivalent drug is available. In North America, these studies are known as *drug utilization review* (DUR) or *drug use evaluation (DUE) studies*. For example, a large number of studies have documented the extent of inappropriate prescribing of drugs, particularly antibiotics, and the associated adverse clinical, ecological, and economic consequences.

DUR and DUE *studies*, aimed at problem detection and quantification, are usually one-time projects, not routinely conducted, provide for only minimal feedback to the involved prescribers and, most importantly, do not include any follow-up measures to ascertain whether any changes in drug therapy have occurred (Table 22.1). A DUR or DUE *program*, on the other hand, is an intervention in the form of an authorized, structured, and ongoing system for improving the quality of drug use within a given health care institution (Table 22.1).

Clinical problems to be addressed by pharmacoepidemiologic research

For a drug to be marketed, it must be shown that it can effectively modify the natural course of disease or alleviate symptoms when used appropriately– that is, for the right patient, with the right disease, in the proper dosage and intervals, and for the appropriate length of time. Used inappropriately, drugs fail to live up to their potential, with the potential for consequent morbidity and mortality. Even when used appropriately, drugs have the potential to cause harm. However, many of their adverse effects are predictable and preventable.

Adverse drug reactions (particularly Type A reactions) and nonadherence to therapy are important causes of preventable adult and pediatric hospital admissions. The situations that may lead to preventable adverse drug reactions and drug-induced illness include the use of a drug for the wrong indication; the use of a potentially toxic drug when one with less toxicity risk would be as effective; the concurrent administration of an excessive number of drugs, thereby increasing the possibility of adverse drug interactions; the use of excessive doses, especially for pediatric or geriatric patients; and continued use of a drug after evidence becomes available concerning important toxic effects. Many contributory causes have been proposed: excessive prescribing by the physician, failure to define therapeutic endpoints for drug use, the increased availability of potent prescription and nonprescription drugs, increased public exposure to information about drugs, the availability of illicit preparations, and prescribers' lack of knowledge of the pharmacology and pharmacokinetics of the prescribed drugs. Medication error (discussed in the "Medication Errors" section of this chapter), poor patient adherence (Chapter 20), discontinuation of therapy, and problems in communication resulting from modern day fragmentation of patient care also may contribute to increased morbidity and mortality.

Therapeutic practice, as recommended by relevant professional bodies, academic researchers, and opinion leaders is initially based on data from premarketing clinical trials. Complementary data from clinical experience and studies in the postmarketing period may result in changes in indication (e.g., an antibiotic no longer a choice due to antimicrobial resistance), treatment duration (e.g., short-course antibiotic treatment of community-acquired pneumonia in children under 5 years old), regimen (e.g., changes due to tolerance to oral hypoglycemic agents), and precautions and contraindications (e.g., gastrointestinal bleeding with nonsteroidal anti-inflammatory agents) among others. As therapy recommendations are updated through guidelines and other approaches, drug utilization studies must address the relationship between therapeutic practice as recommended and actual clinical practice.

Methodological problems to be addressed by pharmacoepidemiologic research

Drug use data may be obtained from several sources, and their usefulness depends on the purpose of the study at hand. All have certain limitations in their direct clinical relevance. For quantitative studies, the ideal is a count of the number of patients in a defined population who ingest a drug of interest during a particular time frame. The data available are only approximations of this, and raise many questions about their presentation and interpretation. For qualitative studies, the ideal is a count of the number of patients in a defined population who use a drug inappropriately during a particular time frame among all those who received the drug in that population during that time frame. Available drug exposure and diagnosis data are suboptimal. Also, the criteria to be used to define "appropriate" are arbitrary.

Since most drug consumption statistics were compiled for administrative or commercial reasons, the data are usually expressed in terms of cost or volume. Data on drug utilization can be available in several different quantities: One is *total costs or unit cost*, such as cost per package, tablet, dose, or treatment course. Although such data may be useful for measuring and comparing the economic impact of drug use, these units do not provide information on the amount of drug exposure in the population. Moreover, cost data are influenced by price fluctuations over time, distribution channels, inflation, exchange rate fluctuations, price control measures, etc.

Another quantity, *volume data*, are available from manufacturers, importers, or distributors, as the overall weight of the drug sold or the unit volume sold (e.g., the number of tablets, capsules, or doses sold). This is closer to the number of patients exposed. However, tablet sizes vary, making it difficult to translate weight into the number of tablets. Prescription sizes also vary, so it is difficult to translate number of tablets into the number of exposed patients.

The *number of prescriptions* is the measure most frequently used in drug utilization studies. However, different patients receive a different number of prescriptions in any given time interval.

To translate the number of prescriptions into the number of patients, one must divide by the average number of prescriptions per patient, or else distinctions must be made between first prescriptions and refill prescriptions. The latter is, of course, better for studies of new drug therapy, but will omit individuals who are receiving chronic drug therapy. Additional problems may be posed by differences in the number of drugs in each prescription. Finally, it should be noted that all these units represent approximate estimates of true consumption. The latter is ultimately modified by the patients' actual drug intake (i.e., degree of adherence, Chapter 20).

From a quality of care perspective, to interpret drug utilization data appropriately, it is necessary to relate the data to the reasons for the drug usage. Data on morbidity and mortality may be obtained from national registries (general or specialized); national samples where medical service reimbursement schemes operate; ad hoc surveys and special studies; hospital records, physician records; and patient or household surveys. "Appropriateness" of use must be assessed relative to indication for treatment, patient characteristics (age-related physiological status, sex, habits), drug dosage (over- or under-dosage), concomitant diseases (that might contraindicate or interfere with chosen therapy), and the use of other drugs (interactions). However, no single source is generally available for obtaining all this information. Moreover, because of incompleteness, the medical record may not be a very useful source of drug use data.

Examples of currently available solutions

Current data sources

Because of the importance of studying drug utilization, many computer databases have been used for DUR studies in Europe and North America (Table 22.2). Many of these data sources lack information on morbidity and are mostly used for generating drug statistics and descriptive studies of drug consumption patterns. Some collect data in the form of drug sales, drug movement at various levels of the drug distribution channel,

pharmaceutical or medical billing data, or all prescriptions dispensed.

Although the use of health insurance databases has also been reported in countries outside North America and Europe, medical and pharmaceutical databases are generally not available in most developing countries. The International Network for Rational Use of Drugs (INRUD) and WHO have developed an approach that uses standardized criteria/indicators to measure changes in medicines prescribing, dispensing, and patient care, which has facilitated the study of drug utilization in developing countries. It includes recommendations on core and complementary indicators, minimum sample sizes, sampling methods, and data collection techniques, depending on study objectives.

Units of measurement

The defined daily dose (DDD) methodology was developed in response to the need to convert and standardize readily available volume data from sales statistics or pharmacy inventory data to medically meaningful units and to make crude estimates of the number of persons exposed to a particular medicine or class of medicines. The DDD is the assumed average daily maintenance dose for a drug for its main indication in adults. Expressed as DDDs per 1000 inhabitants per day, for chronically used drugs, it can be interpreted as the proportion of the population that may receive treatment with a particular medicine on any given day. For use in hospital settings, the unit is expressed as DDDs per 100 bed-days (adjusted for occupancy rate); it suggests the proportion of inpatients that may receive a DDD. For medicines that are used for short-term periods, such as antimicrobials, the unit is expressed as DDDs per inhabitant per year; this provides an estimate of the number of days for which each person is treated with a particular medication in a year.

The DDD methodology is useful for working with readily available gross drug statistics and is relatively easy and inexpensive to use. However, the DDD methodology should be used and interpreted with caution. The DDD is not a recommended or a prescribed dose, but a technical unit of comparison;

Table 22.2 Some computer databases for drug utilization studies.

Not diagnosis-linked	Diagnosis-linked
North America	
National Prescription Audit[a]	National Disease and Therapeutic Index[a]
US Pharmaceutical Market—Drugstores[a]	Kaiser Permanente Medical Plan[a]
US Pharmaceutical Market—Hospitals[a]	Group Health Cooperative[b]
Medicaid Management Information Systems	The Slone Survey[c]
Saskatchewan Health Plan[b]	
Europe	
Swedish National Corporation of Pharmacies	Sweden's Community of Tierp Project
Sweden's County of Jämtland Project	United Kingdom's General Practice Research Database
Norwegian Institute of Public Health	The Netherlands' Integrated Primary Care Information Database
	PHARMO Record Linkage System
United Kingdom's Prescription Pricing Authority	
Spain's Drug Data Bank (National Institute of Health)	
Denmark's Odense	
Pharmacoepidemiologic Database	
Denmark's County of North Jutland	
Pharmacoepidemiologic Prescription Database	
Danish Registry of Medicinal Product Statistics	
Finnish Prescription registry	
Norwegian Prescription database	
Swedish Prescribed Drug Register	
Icelandic Pharmaceutical Database	

[a]IMS America, Ltd.
[b]Patient-specific data available for longitudinal studies.
[c]Reason for use.

it is usually the result of literature review and available information on use in various countries. Thus, DDDs may be high or low relative to actual prescribed doses. Since children's doses are substantially lower than the established DDDs, if unadjusted, this situation will lead to an underestimation of population exposures, which may be significant in countries with a large pediatric population. Pediatric DDDs have also been proposed, but the concept and its applicability have not been incorporated into the WHO methodology. Finally, DDDs do not take into account variations in adherence.

The prescribed daily dose (PDD) is another unit, developed as a means to validate the DDDs. The PDD is the average daily dose prescribed, as obtained from a representative sample of prescriptions. Problems may arise in calculating the PDD due to a lack of clear and exact dosage indication in the prescription and dosage alteration via verbal instructions between prescribing events. For certain groups of drugs, such as the oral antidiabetics, the mean PDD may be lower than the corresponding DDDs. Up to twofold variations in the mean PDD have been documented in international comparisons. Although the DDD and the PDD may be used to estimate population drug exposure "therapeutic intensity," the methodology is not useful to estimate incidence and prevalence of drug use or to quantify or identify patients who receive doses lower or higher than those considered effective and safe.

Classification systems

Classification systems are used to categorize drugs into standardized groups. For example, the Anatomic Therapeutic Chemical (ATC) classification system is generally used in conjunction with the DDD methodology. The ATC system consists of five hierarchical levels: a main anatomical group, two therapeutic subgroups, a chemical–therapeutic subgroup, and a chemical substance subgroup. Medicinal products are classified according to the main therapeutic indication for the principal active ingredient. Use of the ATC classification system is recommended for reporting drug consumption statistics and conducting comparative drug utilization research. The WHO International Drug Monitoring Program uses the system for drug coding in adverse drug reaction monitoring, and some developing countries have begun to use the ATC system to classify their essential drugs, which may eventually lead to preparation of drug utilization statistics.

The US uses the Iowa Drug Information System (IDIS), which is a hierarchical drug coding system based on the three therapeutic categories of the American Hospital Formulary Society (AHFS), to which a fourth level was added to code individual drug ingredients. Other coding systems, such as the National Drug Code and the Veterans' Administration Classification, do not provide unique codes for drug ingredients.

The future

From a public health perspective, the observed differences in national and international patterns of drug utilization require much further study. The medical consequences and the explanations for such differences are still not well documented. Analysis of medicine use by gender and age group may suggest important associations. The increasing availability of population-based data resources will facilitate studies of incidence and prevalence of medicine use by age and gender.

Numerous studies have addressed factors influencing drug prescribing. However, the relative importance of the many determinants of appropriate prescribing still remains to be adequately elucidated. Many strategies aimed at modifying prescribing behavior have been proposed and adopted. Current evidence indicates that mailed educational materials alone are not sufficient to modify prescribing behavior. For interventions shown to be effective in improving drug prescribing, there is a need to further define their relative efficacy and proper role in a comprehensive strategy for optimizing drug utilization. Questions yet to be addressed through proper methodology deal with the role of printed drug information such as drug bulletins; the duration of effect of educational interventions such as group discussions, lectures, and seminars, each in the outpatient and inpatient settings; and the generalizability of face-to-face methods.

More clinically applicable approaches to drug utilization review programs, such as the computerized screening of patient-specific drug histories in outpatient care to prevent drug-induced hospitalizations, still require further development and assessment. Patient outcome measures and process measures of quality of drug utilization have to be included in such studies.

The availability of large computerized databases that allow the linkage of drug utilization data to diagnoses is contributing to expand this field of study. The WHO/INRUD indicator-based approach to drug utilization studies facilitates the conduct of drug utilization research in developing and transitional countries. Drug utilization review programs, particularly approaches that take into primary consideration patient outcome measures, merit further rigorous study and improvement. Opportunities for the study of drug utilization are still underexplored, but the political issue regarding the

---

Case Example 22.1: For prevalence of potentially suboptimal medication use in older men and association with adverse outcomes

Background

Medication-related symptoms often underlie presentations to primary care services and emergency departments and are a common cause of hospital admission, morbidity and mortality. Among frail older people, falls and confusion (geriatric syndromes) and hip fractures may be medicine-use related. Adverse drug reactions and polypharmacy are also common in the elderly.

Question

• How prevalent is suboptimal use of medicines in men over 65 years old and is this associated with adverse outcomes?

Approach

• Prospective cohort study of community-dwelling older men.

• Use of a comprehensive population-based data linkage system, combined with self-reported retrospective data from a health-in-men survey that included biochemical and hormone analysis of blood samples.

• Adverse outcomes included self-reported or documented history of falls and database-recorded hospital admissions due to geriatric syndromes, cardiovascular events, and death.

• Markers of suboptimal medication use were defined for potential over-utilization, potential under-utilization, and potentially inappropriate medicines use.

Results

• Use of potentially inappropriate medicines (48.7%), polypharmacy ($\geq$5 medications, 35.8%), and potential under-utilization (56.7%) were highly prevalent, and overall 8.3% of participants reported some form of potentially suboptimal medication use.

• Polypharmacy was associated with all cause admission to hospital, cardiovascular events, and all cause mortality over 4.5 years of follow-up.

• Potential medication under-utilization was associated with subsequent cardiovascular events.

• Reported use of one or more potentially inappropriate medicines was associated with greater hazard of admission to hospital.

• Hospital admissions for falls were not associated with any of the markers of suboptimal prescribing.

Strengths

• Community-based sampling of study population.

• Large sample size.

• Reliable data on selected morbidity and mortality endpoints captured through comprehensive data linkage system.

Limitations

• Study was based on volunteers, recruited from randomly selected subjects of a previous population-based study.

• Potential underestimation of adverse events; e.g., falls that do not result in hospitalization were not captured in the comprehensive database, and may not be recalled in self-reports.

• Accuracy of self-reported medication histories was not validated.

• Unavailability of medication dosage data limits determining inappropriateness due to excessive dosing.

• Potential underutilization focused only on certain cardiovascular conditions and treatments.

• Medication use variables did not account for all valid medication indications/contraindications.

Key points

• Additional data collection approaches may be combined with use of comprehensive data linkage systems.

• Study results suggest that both medication overuse and underuse occur frequently in older men and may be associated with significant adverse clinical outcomes.

• Reducing under-utilization is just as important as reducing over-utilization and inappropriate medication use.

confidentiality of medical records and limitations in funds and manpower will determine the pace of growth of drug utilization research.

Key points for studies of drug utilization

• Drug utilization studies can be performed to quantify and identify problems in drug utilization, monitor changes in utilization patterns, or evaluate the impact of interventions.

• Drug utilization studies may be conducted on an on-going basis in programs for improving the quality of drug use.

• Assessing appropriateness of drug utilization requires data on indication for treatment, patient characteristics, drug regimen, concomitant diseases, and concurrent use of other medications. Even then, the criteria to be used to define "appropriate" are arbitrary.

• When assessing quality of care, drug utilization studies must often rely on multiple sources of data.

Evaluating and improving physician prescribing

One of the most important, but perhaps underappreciated, goals of pharmacoepidemiology is to foster ways to improve evidence-based prescribing. It is clear, however, that there is a significant disconnect between the available evidence for treatment ("what we know") and everyday clinical practice ("what we do"). This so called *care-gap* in prescribing needs to be urgently addressed. If physicians and other health practitioners fail to update their knowledge and practice in response to new evidence about the outcomes of specific prescribing patterns, then pharmacoepidemiologic research may have little impact on clinical practice. Thus, the science of assessing and improving prescribing has grown rapidly; much of the growth is based on the recognition that passive knowledge dissemination (e.g., publishing articles, distributing practice guidelines, traditional continuing medical education) is generally insufficient to improve clinical practices without supplemental behavioral change interventions based on relevant theories of

diffusion of innovations, persuasive communications, adult learning theory, and knowledge translation.

Clinical problems to be addressed by pharmacoepidemiologic research

Issues related to underuse, overuse, and misuse of medications all belong in the domain of prescribing "errors." Factors responsible for suboptimal prescribing include failure of clinicians to keep abreast of new evidence; excessive promotion by the pharmaceutical industry; errors of omission; patient demands; and clinical inertia. Such diverse influences suggest the need for tailoring intervention strategies to the key factors affecting any given behavior based on models of knowledge translation. Poor adherence to medications is another important factor contributing to the care-gap (discussed in Chapter 20).

Methodological problems to be addressed by pharmacoepidemiologic research

Internal validity

Uncontrolled studies of medication prescribing interventions (e.g., one-group post-only or pre–post designs without a control group) can produce misleading (and usually exaggerated) estimates of effect. Many nonintervention factors can affect medication use over time. Indeed, the "success" of many uncontrolled studies is often due preexisting secular or temporal trends in practice rather than to the intervention under study. This tends to occur because quality of prescribing does tend to improve over time—it just does so too slowly or too haphazardly. Because randomized controlled trials (RCTs) are sometimes not feasible (e.g., contamination of controls within a single institution) or ethical (e.g., withholding quality assurance programs from controls), other quasi-experimental designs (e.g., interrupted time-series with or without comparison series, pre–post with concurrent comparison group studies) should be used instead of relying on weak one-group post-only or pre–post designs that do not generally permit causal inferences.

Regression toward the mean

The tendency for observations on populations selected on the basis of exceeding a predetermined threshold level to approach the mean on subsequent observations is a common and insidious problem. This argues once again for the need to conduct RCTs and well-controlled quasi-experiments to establish the effectiveness of interventions before they become a routine part of quality improvement programs.

Unit of analysis

A common methodological problem in studies of physician behavior is the incorrect use of the patient as the unit of analysis. This violates basic statistical assumptions of independence because prescribing behaviors for individual patients are likely to be correlated within an individual physician's practice. Such hierarchical "nesting" or statistical "clustering" often leads to accurate point estimates of effect but exaggerated significance levels and inappropriately narrow confidence intervals compared with the correct unit of analysis, such as the physician or practice or facility. Consequently, interventions may appear to lead to "statistically significant" improvements in prescribing when no such claim is warranted. Fortunately, methods for analyzing clustered data are available that can simultaneously control for clustering of observations at the patient, physician, and facility levels.

Ethical and medico-legal problems hindering the implementation of randomized clinical trials

It has been argued that there are ethical and medico-legal problems related to "withholding" interventions designed to improve prescribing. This explicitly assumes that the proposed interventions will be beneficial. In fact, the effectiveness of many interventions is the very question that should be under investigation. Some have argued that mandating interventions without adequate proof of benefit is unethical. What is important is to demonstrate that such interventions are safe, efficacious, and cost-effective *before* widespread adoption.

Detecting effects on patient outcomes

Few large well-controlled studies have linked changes in prescribing to improved patient outcomes, e.g., a link between improvements in process and patient outcomes such as mortality. Sample sizes may need to be enormous to detect even modest changes in patient outcomes. However, process outcomes (e.g., use of recommended medications for acute myocardial infarction from evidence-based practice guidelines) are often sensitive, clinically reasonable, and appropriate measures of the quality of care and there have been several recent empiric demonstrations that improvements in processes of care are directly associated with better clinical outcomes.

Examples of currently available solutions

Conceptual framework

A useful starting point for designing an intervention to improve prescribing is to develop a framework for organizing the clinical and non-clinical factors that could help or impede desired changes in clinical behaviors. There are many such extant frameworks, such as the "Theory of Planned Behavior" or "PRECEDE" (Predisposing, Reinforcing, and Enabling Constructs in Educational Diagnosis and Evaluation). This latter model—PRECEDE—was developed for adult health education programs, and proposes factors influencing three sequential stages of behavior change: predisposing, enabling, and reinforcing factors. *Predisposing* variables include such factors as awareness of a guideline, knowledge of the underlying evidence, or beliefs in the efficacy of treatment. However, while a mailed drug bulletin may predispose some physicians, behavior change may be impossible without new *enabling* skills (e.g., skills in administering a new therapy or overcoming patient or family demand for unsubstantiated treatments). Once a new pattern of behavior is tried, multiple and positive *reinforcements* (e.g., through point-of-care reminders or audit and feedback) may be necessary to establish fully the new behavior. Such a framework explains a common observation:

namely, that multifaceted interventions that encompass all stages of behavior change are more likely to improve physician prescribing than are uni-dimensional interventions that only predispose, enable, or reinforce.

Empirical evidence on the effectiveness of interventions to improve prescribing

There are numerous research syntheses that have evaluated the effectiveness of the most commonly studied interventions, including: dissemination of educational materials and guidelines; group education; profiling, audit, and feedback; reminders and computerized decision support systems; opinion leaders or educationally influential physicians; face-to-face educational outreach; financial incentives and penalties; and so on.

Distributing printed educational materials aimed at improving prescribing practice remains the most ubiquitous form of prescribing education. Unfortunately, use of disseminated educational materials alone may affect some predisposing variables (e.g., knowledge or attitudes), but have little or no effect on actual prescribing practice. Group education methods traditionally involve large-group didactic continuing medical education, but they are less effective than small group discussions conducted by clinical leaders.

Another popular approach to improving physician performance is providing physicians with clinical feedback regarding their prescribing practices, either in the form of comparative practice patterns with peers or predetermined standards such as practice guidelines, or in the form of patient-level medication profiles intended to highlight excessive, duplicative, or interacting medication use. Most types of feedback have a minimal effect on prescribing and medication profiles are generally ineffective. On the other hand, computerized reminders enable physicians to reduce errors of omission by issuing alerts to perform specific actions in response to patient-level information such as laboratory findings or diagnoses. However, excessive reminders may create "reminder-fatigue." In addition, while studies of reminders have generally been positive, this does not extend to rigorously examined computerized decision support systems that attempt to move beyond the "secretarial" function of reminders. (See Case example 22.2.)

Identifying local opinion leaders is another approach to help in the adoption of new pharmacological agents. In addition to opinion-leader involvement, this approach includes brief orientation to research findings, printed educational materials, and encouragement to implement guidelines during informal "teachable moments" that occur naturally in their ongoing collegial associations.

Academic detailing programs combine professionally illustrated materials with brief face-to-face visits by university-based pharmacists or peers, and have been consistently successful in reducing prescribing of contraindicated or marginally effective therapy. What sets academic detailing apart from industry detailing is that the messengers and the messages of the former are independent and based on the totality of the available evidence.

Finally, using financial incentives has been shown by numerous observational studies to affect the way that physicians practice medicine, and to be more powerful than using penalties—unfortunately, there have been no adequately controlled randomized trials showing that such methods are effective or even safe and without unintended consequences.

The future

In general, it is clear that long-term changes in practice depend on inclusion of multiple strategies that predispose, enable, and reinforce desired behaviors. The following characteristics recur in successful interventions:

• use of theoretical or conceptual frameworks to help identify key factors that influence prescribing decisions, informed by surveys or focus groups;
• targeting physicians in need of education (e.g., review of prescribing data);
• recruitment and participation of local opinion leaders;
• use of credible and objective messengers and materials;
• face-to-face interaction, especially in primary care settings;

Case Example 22.2: For evaluating and improving physician prescribing

Background

- Because many experts assume that computerized decision support will be the magic bullet that improves physician prescribing, vast resources are being committed to widespread implementation before rigorous evaluation.

Question

- Can computerized decision support improve quality of ambulatory care for chronic conditions such as ischemic heart disease or asthma?

Approach

- Cluster randomized controlled trial of 60 primary care practices in the United Kingdom; 30 practices randomized to heart disease and 30 to asthma, with each practice acting as a control for the non-assigned condition. Practices already had computerized health records and many had electronic prescribing.

- Compared about 40 measures of guideline adherence (prescribing, testing, patient reported outcomes) between intervention and control practices one year after implementation of decision support.

Results

- No effect of computerized decision support on any measure of guideline adherence for either heart disease or asthma.

- Hypothesized reason for lack of effect was extremely low levels of use of, and dissatisfaction with, the decision support tools by physicians.

Strengths

- Cluster randomized trial design eliminated selection and volunteer bias, while controlling for any secular improvements in quality of care.

- Overcomes almost all of the flaws in design and analysis of previous studies of computerized decision support.

- Conducted in a "real world" setting rather than with housestaff or within academic practices or in the hospital setting.

Limitations

- Newer technologies or better delivery systems may be more acceptable to primary care physicians.

- Inadequate attention may have been paid to the nontechnological factors that influence the acceptability and use of an intervention (e.g., lack of up-front buy in from end-users, lack of incentives for using the system, lack of participation in the actual guideline development process).

Key points

- Just as with any drug or device, interventions to improve prescribing should be tested in controlled studies before widespread adoption.

- Results of interventions (including decision support) conducted at specialized academic centers or in the hospital setting may not necessarily be applicable to the "real world" of busy primary care practice.

- audit and feedback (*if it is used at all*) that incorporates achievable benchmarks, comparisons with peers, and patient-specific data;
- repetition and reinforcement of a limited number of messages at one time;
- brief educational materials to predispose and reinforce messages;
- use of multiple strategies to address multiple barriers to best practice;
- an emphasis on the goal of improvement in the quality of prescribing and patient safety, not just cost minimization in the guise of quality improvement.

Currently, we know that prescribing problems exist, but we know little about their prevalence or determinants. This paucity of data is all the more remarkable considering three-quarters of all physician visits end in the prescription of a drug. Future research efforts need to describe in greater detail the nature, prevalence, rate of prescribing, and severity of prescribing problems associated with the overuse, misuse, and underuse of medications (as discussed in the previous section on "Drug utilization" in this chapter). Finally, studies examining the relationship between interventions and clinical outcomes would advance the field.

There is also a tremendous need for carefully controlled research of some existing and new methods for improving prescribing, and how best to combine various evidence-based strategies to allow for rapid local implementation of prescribing guidelines. New models are needed to predict the most effective types of intervention for specific problem types and various broader questions still need to be answered, including issues related to opportunity costs and cost-effectiveness.

Important effects of medications on many health outcomes have been demonstrated in clinical trials; therefore, it is reasonable to hypothesize that more appropriate use of some medications could reduce morbidity and mortality, increase patient functioning, and improve quality-of-life. Whether improved prescribing is a surrogate measure, or an outcome in its own right, it remains a critically important but relatively neglected area for rigorous study and investigation.

Key points for evaluating and improving physician prescribing

• Quality problems in prescribing exist at the level of medication overuse (e.g., antibiotics for viral respiratory tract infections), misuse (e.g., NSAIDs without gastric protection for patients at very high risk of upper gastrointestinal bleeding), and underuse (e.g., bisphosphonates in the secondary prevention of osteoporosis-related fractures or inhaled corticosteroids for reactive airways disease).

• The vast majority of prescribing problems are related to underuse of proven effective treatments.

• Passive interventions, such as dissemination of printed or emailed guidelines, drug utilization reviews and medication profiles, or traditional continuing medical education lectures, are unlikely to improve practice.

• More active intervention strategies (e.g., point-of-care reminders, educational outreach, achievable benchmarks with audit and feedback), especially when combined together to overcome barriers at the level of the system, the physician, and the patient, are able to modestly improve the quality of prescribing.

• Just as with the adoption of drugs and devices, interventions to improve physician prescribing need to be tested in rigorous controlled trials before widespread and expensive implementation. In particular, investigators should consider "mixed-method" evaluations (i.e., quantitative data, prescriber surveys, qualitative inquiry about barriers and facilitators to adoption) of their interventions to better understand what works or does not work - and why.

Special methodological issues in pharmacoepidemiologic studies of vaccine safety

Vaccines are among the most cost-effective public health interventions available, however no vaccine is perfectly safe or effective. Concerns over adverse events following immunizations (AEFIs) have often threatened the stability of immunization programs. As such programs "mature" and there is high vaccine coverage, with near elimination of target vaccine-preventable diseases, there may be increased prominence of vaccine-induced and vaccine-coincidental AEFI's, particularly in the modern media.

Clinical problems to be addressed by pharmacoepidemiologic research

The tolerance for AEFI's to vaccines given to healthy persons—especially healthy babies—is lower than for medical products administered to persons due to ill health. A higher standard of safety is required for vaccines because of the large number of persons who are exposed, some of whom are compelled to do so by law or regulation for public health reasons. These issues are the basis for strict regulatory control and other oversight of vaccines by the Food and Drug Administration

(FDA) and the World Health Organization (WHO). These concerns also often lead to investigation of much rarer adverse events following vaccinations than for pharmaceuticals. However, the cost and difficulty of studying AEFI's increase with their rarity, and it is difficult to provide definitive conclusions from epidemiologic studies of such rare events. Furthermore, high standards of accuracy and timeliness are needed because vaccine safety studies may have important impact on vaccination policies.

Unlike many classes of drugs for which other effective therapy may be substituted, vaccines generally have few alternative choices, and the decision to withdraw a vaccine from the market may have wide ramifications. Establishing associations of adverse events with vaccines and prompt definition of the attributable risk are critical in placing AEFI's in the proper risk/benefit perspective. Vaccines are relatively universal exposures, therefore, despite the relative rarity of serious true vaccine reactions, the number of total reports of AEFI's received annually in the US now averages ~27 000 (~8% are serious), although few reports can be causally linked to vaccination. Vaccine safety monitoring is a dynamic balancing of risks and benefits. As vaccine preventable diseases approach eradication, information on complications due to vaccination relative to that of the disease (that the vaccine prevents) may lead to a perception that the vaccine complications outweigh the benefits and therefore to a discontinuation or decreased use of the vaccine.

Research in vaccine safety can help to distinguish true vaccine reactions from coincidental events, estimate an attributable risk, identify risk factors that can inform the development of valid precautions and contraindications, and if the pathophysiologic mechanism becomes known, develop safer vaccines.

Methodological problems to be addressed by pharmacoepidemiologic research

An Institute of Medicine (IOM) review of vaccine safety in 1991 found that the US knowledge and research capacity has been limited by: (i) inadequate understanding of biologic mechanisms underlying adverse events; (ii) insufficient or inconsistent information from case reports and case series; (iii) inadequate size or length of follow-up of many population-based epidemiologic studies; and (iv) limitations of existing surveillance systems to provide persuasive evidence of causation. These limitations were cited again in a more recent IOM review (2011), *Adverse Events of Vaccines: Evidence and Causality*. This report noted that even very large epidemiologic studies may not detect or rule out rare events, and using case reports was complicated by the wide variation of available information often insufficient to rule out other potential causes of the adverse event. To overcome these limitations, epidemiology and creative methodology have been vital in providing a rigorous scientific approach for assessing the safety of vaccines.

Signal detection

High profile vaccine adverse events, such as intussusception following rotavirus vaccination (see Case example 22.3), demonstrate the need for surveillance systems able to detect potential aberrations in a timely manner. However, some factors make identification of true signals difficult; for example, many vaccines are administered early in life, at a time when the baseline risk for many adverse health outcomes is constantly evolving. Until the recent advent of systematic analyses of automated data including data mining of spontaneous reports, identification of a vaccine safety signal occurred as much due to a persistent patient as from data analysis.

Assessment of causality

Assessing whether any adverse event was actually caused by vaccine is generally not possible unless a vaccine-specific clinical syndrome (e.g., myopericarditis in healthy young adult recipients of smallpox vaccine), recurrence upon rechallenge (e.g., alopecia and hepatitis B vaccination), or a vaccine-specific laboratory finding (e.g., Urabe mumps vaccine virus isolation) can be identified. When the adverse event also occurs in the absence of vaccination (e.g., seizure), epidemiologic studies are necessary to assess whether vaccinated persons are at higher risk than unvaccinated persons. The latter is

Case Example 22.3: For special methodological issues in pharmacoepidemiologic studies of vaccine study

Background

- Intussusception was reported among recipients of a rhesus-human rotavirus reassortant-tetravalent vaccine (RRV-TV), RotaShield® (Wyeth Laboratories, Inc).

Question

- Is a vaccine containing 4 live viruses, a rhesus rotavirus (serotype 3) and three rhesus-human reassortant viruses (serotypes 1, 2, and 4), associated with intussusception in RRV-TV vaccine recipients?

Approach

- Analyze Vaccine Adverse Event Reporting System (VAERS) spontaneous reporting surveillance for reports of intussusception.
- Conduct a case-control and cohort study on RRV-TV recipients.
- Conduct postmarketing vaccine surveillance.
- Quantify risk associated with RRV-TV receipt and intussusception.

Results

- 15 initial VAERS reports (total of 112 VAERS intussusception reports from licensure on August 31, 1998 to December 31, 1999) with 95 confirmed intussusception cases following RRV-TV (confirmed by medical record review).
- Case-control study found infants receiving RRV-TV were 37 times more likely to have intussusception 3–7 days after the first dose than infants who did not receive RRV-TV (95% confidence interval (CI) = 12.6–110.1).
- Retrospective cohort study among 463 277 children in managed care organizations demonstrated that those receiving the vaccine, 56 253 infants, were 30 times more likely to have intussusception 3–7 days after the first dose than infants who did not receive the vaccine (95% CI = 8.8–104.9).
- Causal link between RRV-TV receipt and intussusception established in postmarketing period at a frequency detectable by current surveillance tools (approximately 1/5000–1/10 000 vaccinees).

Strengths

- Multiple studies confirmed association between RRV-TV and intussusception.
- Two different study designs found similar results and validated the signal in the spontaneous reporting system.
- Despite the limitations of passive surveillance, VAERS successfully provided a vaccine adverse event alert.

Limitations

- Passive surveillance systems such as VAERS are subject to multiple limitations, including underreporting and biased reporting, reporting of temporal associations or unconfirmed diagnoses, lack of denominator data, and unbiased comparison groups; VAERS cannot usually assess causality.

Key points

- CDC recommended temporarily suspending use of RRV-TV following initial 15 VAERS reports.
- No case of RRV-TV-associated intussusception occurred among infants vaccinated after the recommendation was issued on July 16, 1999.
- When the VAERS findings were substantiated by preliminary findings of the more definitive studies, the manufacturer voluntarily recalled the vaccine.
- The US Advisory Committee on Immunization Practices recommendations for RRV-TV vaccination were withdrawn in October 1999.
- A new "rapid cycle" initiative for more timely detection of vaccine safety signals has been formed by the CDC Vaccine Safety Datalink (VSD) project; this project successfully simulated and retrospectively "detected" the RRV-TV intussusception signal within the VSD by mid-May 1999.
- Subsequent clinical trials and post-marketing studies of next generation rotavirus vaccine used standardized Brighton Collaboration case definition for intussusception to show these new vaccines are safer than RotaShield[1]

complicated by limited unvaccinated populations (particularly among children), potential confounding due to differences between those vaccinated and not vaccinated, and determining whether events are attributable to particular vaccines since frequently combination vaccines or more than one vaccine are administered together.

Measurement accuracy

Misclassification of exposure status (vaccination) may occur if there is poor documentation of vaccinations. Documentation of exposure status has been fairly good through school age, but difficulty has been encountered in ascertaining vaccination status in older persons. Misclassification of outcomes can also occur in observational studies that rely on ICD-9 codes from computerized databases. Such diagnosis codes are often validated with a manual medical records review.

Sample size

Because concerning adverse health events (e.g., encephalopathy) are often extremely rare, it may be a challenge to identify enough cases for a meaningful study. The difficulty with adequate study power is further compounded in assessing rare events in populations less frequently exposed (e.g., subpopulations with special indications). For studies of rare outcomes, case-control and self-control designs are the most efficient. Case-control designs typically sample the source population of cases, identify an appropriate control group, and assess the exposure status of both groups to estimate the risk associated with exposure (see Chapter 2). The self-control design usually finds vaccinated cases in the source population and compares incidence rates of postvaccination adverse events during defined periods following vaccination (also known as the risk interval) with the rates of the adverse event in the same person during varying control periods (either pre- or postvaccination) which do not occur in close relationship to the time of vaccination.

Confounding and bias

Because childhood vaccines are generally administered on schedule and children may have developmental dispositions to particular events, age may confound exposure-outcome relations, e.g., MMR vaccine and febrile seizures or pneumococcal vaccine and sudden infant death syndrome (SIDS). Consequently, such factors must be controlled in the study design and analysis, often done by matching.

More difficult to control are factors leading to delayed vaccination or nonvaccination. Such factors (e.g., low socioeconomic status) may confound studies of AEFIs and lead to underestimates of the true relative risks. Those who have not been vaccinated may differ substantially from the vaccinated population in risks of AEs and thus be unsuitable as a reference group in epidemiologic studies. The unvaccinated may be persons for whom vaccination is medically contraindicated, or they may have other risks for the outcome being studied (e.g., they may be members of low socioeconomic groups). Similarly, vaccinated persons may be preferentially targeted for vaccination because of their underlying medical condition, potentially over-estimating the true relative risk. In addition, some children may be unvaccinated due to parental choice. These children may have different health care utilization patterns than fully vaccinated children, which in turn could bias study results.

Examples of currently available solutions

Signal detection

Identifying a potential new vaccine safety problem ("signal") requires a mix of clinical and epidemiologic expertise. Data mining is often used to assess disproportional reporting in spontaneous reporting systems. One disproportionality assessment tool for comparing safety profiles of vaccines involves comparing the proportions of particular symptoms out of the total number of symptoms reported for a given vaccine to that observed among reports for another vaccine or group of vaccines. Due to the ease of implementation and interpretation, this proportional reporting rate ratio (PRR) has been widely used for vaccine safety signal detection in spontaneous reporting systems such as the US Vaccine Adverse Event Reporting System (VAERS, see Chapter 7). However, there are several methods of statistical data mining or disproportionate reporting analysis commonly used. Of course, any signals need to be confirmed in formal epidemiologic studies.

Epidemiologic studies

Historically, ad hoc epidemiologic studies have been employed to assess potential AEFI's. However, automated, large-linked databases provide a more flexible framework for hypothesis testing than ad hoc epidemiologic studies. More recently new methodology has evolved allowing the use of large-linked databases for vaccine safety surveillance as well as hypothesis testing. The Centers for Disease Control and Prevention (CDC) initiated the Vaccine Safety Datalink (VSD) project in 1990 and this has become the standard for vaccine safety surveillance and research. The VSD project prospectively collects vaccination, medical outcome (e.g., hospital discharge, outpatient visits, emergency room visits, and deaths), and covariate data (e.g., birth certificates, census) under joint protocol at multiple medical care organizations (MCOs) (see "Health maintenance organizations / health plans" in Chapter 9). The VSD project provides near-real time surveillance using data sets that are updated weekly or monthly. This surveillance is usually employed to monitor newly licensed vaccines and existing vaccines that may have new recommendations. Prespecified events of interest (usually chosen based on prelicensure clinical trials, signals from other sources, or historical concerns, such as Guillain-Barre Syndrome) are tested at regular intervals (weekly or monthly) for increased risk of an event following the vaccine under surveillance using an appropriate comparison group, either historical data or a concurrent cohort. The VSD can also validate surveillance findings and test new ad hoc vaccine safety hypotheses using traditional epidemiologic methods and recently more frequent use of self-control designs that can avoid potential confounding from person-level factors and comorbidities (assuming they do not change over time). Due to the high coverage attained in the MCOs for most vaccines, few nonvaccinated controls are available, and thus the VSD is limited in its capacity to assess associations between vaccination and adverse events with delayed or insidious onset (e.g., neurodevelopmental or behavioral outcomes).

The VSD provides an essential, powerful, and relatively cost-effective complement to ongoing evaluations of vaccine safety in the US. Similar systems have since been developed in countries such as Denmark, the UK, and Taiwan.

The future

Although considerable progress has been achieved in vaccine safety monitoring and research there are still several challenges, both scientific and non-scientific. One analytic challenge is identifying optimal risk windows following vaccination which requires understanding the biologic mechanisms of the AEFI but can be somewhat arbitrary; data-driven approaches to defining risk intervals are underway. Detecting lifetime dose responses to multiple exposures of the same vaccine or vaccine components, determining the feasibility of studying vaccine safety of combined and simultaneous vaccinations, and data-mining for unknown AEFI using electronic medical records are all challenging areas in vaccine safety research. Vaccine safety science also faces the challenge of credibility; as vaccine preventable diseases continue to decline, many are skeptical about the need for vaccination and are suspicious of the motives of both governments (since many vaccines are mandated) and manufacturers. Faulty research may arise from those seeking to prove the motives for vaccination are questionable. Furthermore, proving that an AEFI may be coincidental can be difficult, particularly when the event is rare. Vaccine safety surveillance and research requires persistence in providing rigorous science, educating the public, and providing reassurance that robust vaccine safety systems are in place.

Key points for special methodological issues in pharmacoepidemiologic studies of vaccine study

- There are still substantial gaps and limitations to our knowledge of many vaccine safety issues.

• A high standard of safety is required for vaccines due to the large number of persons who are exposed, some of whom are compelled to do so by law or public health regulations.

• New research capacity, such as the Vaccine Safety Datalink, provides powerful tools to address many safety concerns.

Epidemiologic studies of implantable medical devices

Recent decades have witnessed a dramatic growth in medical device technology—the US medical device market exceeded $100 billion in 2008, representing roughly 42% of the worldwide market. In addition to new generations of conventional devices, groundbreaking innovations in nanotechnology, telemedicine, minimally invasive/non-invasive procedures, and sophisticated health information technology continue to offer new diagnostic and therapeutic options to patients and clinicians.

The expansion of such a diverse technology has created unprecedented demands for valid approaches to study the benefits and risks of devices. Medical device epidemiology is well suited to study the utilization of medical devices as well as the incidence of certain outcomes. Methodology to integrate information from a growing body of heterogeneous data is needed.

What is a medical device and how is it different from a drug?
The US government defines a medical device as

> an instrument, apparatus, implement, machine, contrivance, implant, in vitro reagent or other similar or related article, including any component part or accessory which is: (1) recognized in the official National Formulary or United States Pharmacopeia or any supplement of them; (2) intended for use in the diagnosis of disease or other conditions or in the cure, mitigation, treatment or prevention of disease in men or other animals; or (3) intended to affect the structure or any function of the body of man or other animals, and which does not achieve its primary

intended purposes through chemical action within or on the body of man or other animals and which is not dependent upon being metabolized for the achievement of any of its principal intended purposes.

While there are similarities among countries regarding medical device definitions and classifications, differences exist in requirements for approval. For example, before a medical device is allowed to enter the US market, a reasonable assurance of its safety and effectiveness must be established. Based on the level of benefit/risk, devices are classified into three regulatory classes. Class I devices present minimal potential for harm to the patient and require neither clinical testing nor special controls (e.g., elastic bandages, gloves, manual surgical instruments). Class II devices are higher-risk and are subject to additional regulatory control including special controls and clinical testing (e.g., infusion pumps, diagnostic ultrasound machines). Medical devices with the highest level of risk are categorized as class III. The effectiveness and safety of these devices have to be determined based on valid scientific evidence (e.g., implantable deep brain stimulators, coronary stents, and hip resurfacing systems). We concentrate on implantable devices class II and class III because of their significant public health impact, high risk for adverse events, and uncertainties surrounding the long-term exposure.

Implantable devices often have a long (years or even decades) product life cycles (from design to device removal) although incremental changes occur over time. Implantable devices may consist of multiple components (such as a total hip implant) or a single component (such as a pacemaker lead). Exposure to such devices is typically chronic, with the onset of exposure clearly defined at time of implantation. Exposure ends at the time of device removal, but may not be discrete if part of the device remains in the human body (e.g., silicone leakage from ruptured breast implants).

Outcomes associated with implantable devices are affected not only by underlying patient factors and device factors (such as biomaterials), but also by user interface (e.g., operator technique, operator experience). Adverse effects of implantable devices are typically localized but may sometimes be systemic (e.g., secondary to toxic, allergic, auto-immune effects). Additional hazards may be related to human factors (e.g., improper programming of pacemakers) and interference (e.g., magnetic reso-nance imaging interaction with deep brain stimula-tor leads). Lastly, malfunctions may derive from several sources, including manufacturing prob-lems, design-induced errors, and anatomic or engi-neering effects.

Clinical problems to be addressed by medical device epidemiologic research

Diffusion of medical device technology is influ-enced by many factors including device complexity, relative advantage compared to existing treat-ments, positions of opinion-leading organizations, health care reimbursement decisions, commercial competition, and practice guidelines. Accordingly, adoption of new devices often follows different and sometimes unpredictable patterns. These patterns may contribute to variations in patient outcomes and the frequency of adverse events. Epidemiologic assessment of factors that influence the adoption can inform regulatory science. Additionally, two important issues should be considered to inform regulatory science:

1. assessment of benefits and harms in real world settings, and
2. assessment of long-term outcomes

Benefits and harms profile in a real word setting

The national interest in comparative effectiveness research (CER) facilitated by the 2009 American Recovery and Reinvestment Act (see "Comparative effectiveness research" section in this chapter) and subsequent health care reform legislation have focused national attention on building methods and infrastructure for real world evaluative research. The real world implantable device evalu-ation will predominantly rely on observational research methods. One of the main reasons for such focus is related to limitations of RCTs. In the RCTs of surgical devices, the participating operators are typically early adopters, highly skilled, and

quick learners, which affects the "learning curve." Traditionally, the learning curve is studied using observational studies of the volume-outcome rela-tionship. In the past, some volume-outcome stud-ies have demonstrated that increased surgical volume has an inverse linear relationship with the incidence of adverse outcomes; while others have identified a volume threshold for procedures above which increasing volume is no longer associated with improved outcomes. There are three distinct components of the volume-outcome relationship that can be studied: (1) lifetime experience (oper-ator's volume), (2) operator's volume per unit of time (e.g., year), and (3) hospital volume where operators practice. Other factors related to learning curve might include type of procedure and practice setting (e.g., academic hospital). Adequate study of learning curves can establish thresholds for profi-ciency based on background expertise related to physicians' specialties. For example, thresholds for stenting of carotid artery vary by operator across specialties (e.g., radiologists, cardiologists, and neurosurgeons).

In addition to highly-selected clinicians, RCTs often involve homogeneous nonrepresentative patient populations (see Chapters 2 and 16). Pre-marketing device trials often lack sufficient repre-sentation of important patient populations (women, children, elderly, racial and ethnic minor-ities, etc.), which diminishes the generalizability of results. Well-designed observational studies can provide more information on device performance in the sub-populations of interest in routine care. The utility of observational studies has been increasing with advances in medical device data capture in medical records, electronic databases, and prospective registries, and with the develop-ment of and dissemination of analytical tools.

Long-term safety and effectiveness

Device premarketing clinical trials are typically of short duration, and generate limited information on long-term safety and effectiveness. Because of the inherent complexity of implantable devices, it is often difficult to predict device long-term safety and effectiveness based solely on the preclinical testing and premarketing clinical trials. In the US,

FDA's postmarketing attention is increasingly directed towards ensuring that studies of sufficient size and follow-up duration are conducted in the postmarketing setting to better predict and understand problems occurring long-term. Several other countries have established national registries of procedures involving implanted medical devices that collect long-term patient outcomes and device performance (e.g., Sweden, United Kingdom, Australia, and Canada).

Methodological problems solved by medical device epidemiologic research

As noted before, evidence generation for implantable medical devices requires accounting for issues that do not arise when examining drugs. Such issues include the interaction of device, operator, and the interventional area in which the device is being used. The device design, its complexity, and its specific mechanical characteristics can be as important as the clinical details such as type of the lesion being treated, severity of the disease, and concomitant therapy provided. In the commonly used research databases these details are often only partially observed or missing.

Challenges in individual patient exposure assessment

There are two major obstacles to ascertaining individual exposure to a medical device. First, unlike pharmaceuticals where the National Drug Code (NDC) Directory was established, there is no common medical device nomenclature utilized by all stakeholders. The routine capture of device information, such as manufacturer name, brand, or model, linked to device group terms, would allow proper identification and easier data management. Second, devices are frequently approved or used as systems involving several components; device components are often used in combination with components of the same or different brand. Capturing complete device exposure information is thus far more complex for devices than for drugs. Once adopted, a robust, widely incorporated medical device nomenclature will advance safety and effectiveness surveillance of medical devices.

Challenges in national population exposure assessment

The challenges include incorporation of unique device identifiers (UDIs) into data systems, including electronic health records, and routine documentation of device use and patient problems associated with that use. In the US surveillance environment, population medical device exposure data must be derived from a variety of sources including administrative claims data, registries, national surveys, nationally representative samples of health providers, and marketing data. These data sources differ in their level of device specific granularity, design (retrospective versus prospective), and data collection (patient reports, sales, etc.). While these sources differ in the level of completeness and reliability, they may complement each other.

Challenges in comparative studies

Epidemiologic research relies on non-experimental data to develop evidence about safety and effectiveness of medical products. While limitations of non-randomized (vs randomized) studies are well-known, two facts must be recognized. First, of the methodological approaches that are recognized as key components of high internal validity in pharmaceutical studies (e.g., randomization, allocation concealment, masking/blinding, withdrawal/follow-up, and intention-to-treat analyses), only some can be applied to evidence development for medical devices. Aside from recognized limitations of clinical trials (e.g., select study subjects, small sample sizes, short duration), the need for data observed in routine care arises because of learning curve issues, product modifications, and risks of unexpected adverse events related to mechanical failure of the products.

Addressing sample size and real world performance issues

Premarketing clinical trials are designed to have sufficient statistical power for effectiveness outcomes. Powering the RCTs for less common or rare but serious side effects is not feasible in most instances (see Chapter 3). RCTs of devices, because of small sample size and participant selection, often lack *generalizability (or external validity)*, which is defined as the extension of research findings and conclusions from a study conducted on a sample population to the population at large.

Systematic reviews with meta-analyses (see Chapter 19) attempt to capitalize on the detailed data collection within each study. Systematic reviews are one mechanism to address the small study problems of the RCTs. Systematic reviews with meta-analysis assume that most of the individual RCTs of devices and surgery carefully record relevant clinical outcomes and offer a good opportunity to conduct evidence appraisal and synthesis when a reasonable number of studies are available.

Well-designed observational studies are often large and involve consecutive patient enrollment and comprehensive data collection. They are the best suited tools to evaluate the safety and effectiveness of devices in routine care. With large observational studies, one can evaluate relevant subgroup effects as well as rare safety and effectiveness endpoints that cannot usually be captured by RCTs.

Ensuring comparability of study groups

Cohort designs offer the opportunity to create groups of patients exposed to different devices of interest. Optimally, these designs are based on prospective and consecutive patient enrollment, prospective data collection, and a study that is hypothesis driven. Such observational studies should use statistical approaches to adjust for measured confounders and methods that help characterize the impact of unmeasured confounding on results (see Chapter 21).

We have good tools to address unequal distribution in observed patient characteristics (predictors). Most of the adjustment techniques deal with imbalances in baseline factors among study groups. Several analytical methods are available to handle selection factors and confounding. These methods involve stratification, regression models, or a combination of the two using propensity scores. Each approach relies on a set of statistical assumptions which may or may not be appropriate in the particular setting. When it is felt that there is unmeasured confounding present beyond that

accounted for in the collected information, another potential approach is that of *instrumental variable-based methods* (see Chapter 21) which have assumptions and limitations of their own.

Examples of currently available solutions

Passive surveillance

Once approved, manufacturers must monitor the safety of their products, including forwarding reports of adverse events to regulatory authorities. In the US, manufacturers are required to submit reports of device-related deaths, serious injuries, and malfunctions to the FDA. Healthcare providers and consumers submit reports voluntarily. These reports, obtained through passive surveillance (see Chapter 7) are housed in the Manufacturer and User Facility Device Experience (MAUDE) database, established in 1996. The vast majority of reports in MAUDE (about 200 000 individual per annum) are from manufacturers, with a small percentage from user facilities, voluntary sources, and importers.

Passive reporting systems have notable weaknesses including: (a) data may be incomplete or inaccurate and are typically not independently verified; (b) data may reflect reporting biases driven by event severity or uniqueness or by publicity and litigation; (c) causality generally cannot be reliably inferred from any individual report; and (d) events are generally underreported and this, in combination with lack of denominator (exposure) data, precludes determination of event incidence or prevalence. The latter point is particularly important for implantable devices, because reports may capture device-associated events (such as thrombosis, infection, stroke, revision or replacement) for which estimation of incidence is of paramount importance (see also Chapter 7).

To enhance the usefulness of reported data, statistical tools are used to assist in detecting safety signals. Bayesian and other data mining methods are employed to estimate the relative frequency of specific adverse event–device combinations as compared to the frequency of the event with all other devices in the same group.

Enhanced surveillance

Medical Product Safety Network (MedSun) was established to provide national medical device surveillance based on a representative subset of 350 user facilities in the US In addition, specialty networks such as electrophysiology devices (HeartNet) and pediatric ICU devices (KidNet) have emerged within MedSun to focus on device-specific issues within the relevant clinical specialty. This *enhanced surveillance* network helps amplify potential safety signals in real time through targeted surveys, problem solving, and posting of reports.

Active surveillance

FDA uses *active surveillance* to monitor high risk devices, such as in a national registry of implanted ventricular-assist devices or in *de novo* studies fulfilling post-approval study requirements.

Another evolving active surveillance effort utilizes Data Extraction and Longitudinal Time Analysis (DELTA) surveillance system to monitor outcomes data registry in interventional cardiology. Through collaboration with academia, FDA has applied DELTA to the surveillance of hemostasis devices and coronary stents in the state of Massachusetts and continues to promote utilization of DELTA in the existing national cardiovascular and orthopedic registries.

In addition, FDA effectively utilizes the Consumer Product Safety Commission (CPSC)'s National Electronic Injury Surveillance System (NEISS), a sentinel system designed to capture information on consumer-product and other product-related injuries that are seen in hospital emergency departments (EDs). FDA collaborated with CPSC to use NEISS to establish the first national estimates of device-related adverse events resulting in ED. More recent efforts focused on examining reasons for device-related visits to ED involving pediatric populations.

To provide more robust national medical product surveillance, the FDA launched the Sentinel Initiative in 2008 (see "FDA's Sentinel Initiative" section in this chapter). The principal aim of the Sentinel Initiative is to advance surveillance capabilities with a national integrated electronic healthcare infrastructure for medical product active surveillance.

The surveillance utilizes national distributed data sources (with populations totaling over 130 million), transformed to a common data model, against which FDA queries can be run. In other countries, national registries of procedures involving implanted medical devices have significantly augmented their national surveillance efforts.

Mandated postmarketing studies

FDA has a unique statutory authority to mandate postmarketing studies either as a condition of approval or "for cause" later in the postmarketing period. A major regulatory/public health challenge FDA is facing is to find appropriate balance for obtaining clinical data premarketing to prevent delays in device approval and ensure that only safe and effective devices enter the marketplace. The appropriate postmarketing questions answerable in a mandated post-approval study include long-term safety and effectiveness, a real-world experience of the device as it enters broader user populations (clinicians and patients), effectiveness of training programs and learning curve effects, and the device performance in certain subgroups of patients not well studied in the premarketing clinical trials. Designing scientifically sound but practical studies, and achieving adequate patient and physician recruitment rates though can be challenging for implantable device studies.

In 2005, FDA Center for Devices and Radiological Health (CDRH) established the Medical Device Post-Approval Studies (PAS) Program to consolidate the review, tracking, and oversight functions for all medical device post-approval studies imposed by the PMA order. Since then, the CDRH has significantly raised expectations for the quality of new PAS, established a PAS electronic tracking system and a publicly available website posting the study status, began inspection of selected studies, and instituted routine updates to the Advisory Panels. In parallel, CDRH epidemiologists launched significant efforts to build a robust infrastructure and new innovative epidemiologic methods suitable for PAS.

Statutory and regulatory authority also permit FDA to require postmarketing surveillance study for Class II and Class III devices that are:

(1) intended to be implanted in human body for longer than a year; (2) is life sustaining or life supporting (and used outside of the user facility); (3) failure would reasonably be likely to have serious health consequences; or (4) anticipated to have significant use in pediatric population. Possible study designs vary from detailed review of complaint history and the literature, nonclinical testing, use of registries, observational study designs, and randomized clinical trials.

Registries

Recognition that RCTs cannot fill all the gaps in clinical evidence for implantable devices is not new but has garnered renewed interest as registries have emerged as powerful resources to harness a full potential of observational studies.

The Agency for Healthcare Research and Quality defines a patient registry for evaluating outcomes as "an organized system that uses observational study methods to collect uniform data (clinical and other) to evaluate specified outcomes for a population defined by a particular disease, condition, or exposure, and that serves a predetermined scientific, clinical, or policy purpose(s)."

Patient registries provide important infrastructure for conducting large-scale medical device studies. In the absence of a unique device identification code, the added value of registries for medical devices surveillance include capturing brand/model specific information crucial for signal identification and comparative effectiveness/safety studies. The complexity and scientific rigor of a registry can vary from those designed to evaluate quality of health care delivered, those specifically established to study sustained effectiveness and safety of a specific procedure, and those designed to systematically collect long-term data on many different types of treatment including risk factors, clinical events, and outcomes in a defined population. Once the framework of a registry is in place, studies with various designs can be performed using the registry data (e.g., cohort, case-control, cross sectional, quasi-experimental).

Major limitations of the registries include their often voluntary nature and short duration of follow-up of patients. For implantable medical devices in particular, the modes of follow-up are critical. These registries can be linked to other databases including administrative billing data. The linkage of clinically rich procedural and intra-hospital data captured by the registry to the follow-up data from administrative databases (such as Medicare and Medicaid databases (see Chapter 9)) can substantially augment the value of registries.

Administrative claims data

The use of administrative databases for epidemiologic research has the strengths of studying large numbers of patients with diverse characteristics and wide varieties of clinical settings, as well as inclusion of longitudinal data from the real world clinical care, and good representation of vulnerable populations, leading to increased external validity (generalizability) (see Part II). The large number of diverse patients present opportunities to study device effect heterogeneity and to advance methods such as high-dimensionality propensity scores and instrumental variables. Current limitations of administrative databases include the lack of unique device identifiers, potential inaccuracy of coding of diagnosis, difficulty separating comorbidity from complications, and type of revision procedure performed. The lack of clinical information in the administrative billing data can be supplemented by linking the billing data to data from registries or other clinically rich data from other data sources.

Methodological framework for implantable device outcome evaluation

A methodological framework for implantable device epidemiology and surveillance involves understanding factors impacting the decision to implant the device, identifying the comparison group(s), and estimating the safety and effectiveness of the device compared to the alternative strategies. In the context of multiple clinical issues and methodological challenges noted previously, a critical issue in addressing these goals relates to the multiple sources of variability that exist with implantable devices. These sources relate to systematic and random variations due to the patient, to the surgeon or operator, to the healthcare center, and to the device itself.

Measurable patient characteristics may predict what type of device is implanted as well as clinical and device outcomes (*patient variation*). For instance, in the case of total hip replacements, advanced age, comorbidities such as heart failure and diabetes, and non-elective admissions are associated with inferior patient outcomes. However, advanced age is also associated with increased use of metal-on-polyethylene hip systems compared to hip systems constructed from other bearing surfaces.

Surgeon and surgical center skills (*provider variation*) may have a large impact on the type of implantable device is used, such as type of hip replacement surgery and clinical outcomes. Several features of the surgical procedure in which the device is implanted vary. For example, some orthopedic surgeons may use less invasive approaches/access when implanting a total hip replacement system than other surgeons. Complications and device failures can increase if the surgeon is early in his/her learning curve and annual surgical volumes of the surgeon and of the center may be associated with procedural success.

Several measurable characteristics of devices have been shown to be predictive of device use and outcome (*device variation*). Using the same example of hip replacement systems, the type of bearing surface is related to revision rates. In particular, hard on hard bearing surfaces, such as metal-on-metal or ceramic-on-ceramic, result in higher revision rates (see Case example 22.4). Additionally, large diameter femoral head size may result in lower dislocation rates. The process of implantation fixation to the bone also results in variations in clinical outcomes. Hip systems can be implanted with bone cement that helps position the implant within the bone or the systems may have a porous surface that permits bone to grow into its surface.

The future

Epidemiology and evidence-informed practice and policy

Epidemiology is becoming that essential link between an exploding demand for the knowledge derived from diverse evidence and the decisions made in health care policy and practice settings. In the larger public health context, the imminent future of device epidemiology will be to integrate and infer from massive amounts of heterogeneous and multidimensional data available from disparate data sources. In doing so, medical device epidemiology will continue to draw from advances in electronic health records, electronic data capture, standard taxonomy, unique device identifiers, global patient identifiers, integrated security, and privacy services. Contemporary device epidemiology will be able to mobilize the advances of translational health research sciences through new methods that combine basic science and clinical data, leading to the choice of best available treatment targeted for specific groups of patients.

Epidemiology and regulatory science

In 2010 the FDA launched the Medical Devices Epidemiology Network (MDEpiNet) Initiative, to identify evidence gaps and questions, datasets, and approaches for conducting robust analytic studies to improve understanding of clinical outcomes and performance of medical devices through strategic consortium with academic centers and other stakeholders. This effort is uniquely focused on medical devices and it comes at a particularly opportune time when many recent developments, ranging from establishment of UDI system to creation and expansion of device-based registries to significant strides toward the universal adoption of electronic health records, provide new and promising opportunities for the epidemiologic study of medical devices. The MDEpiNet structure emphasizes the intersection between meeting regulatory responsibilities and addressing the public health needs surrounding medical devices. An important task for the MDEpiNet involves the development and testing of novel methods for the systematic evaluation of all available evidence relevant to a device's risk-benefit profile, including premarketing bench, animal and clinical studies; postmarketing surveillance studies; and adverse event reports. The intent is to have a comprehensive, up-to-date risk-benefit profile of specific medical devices at any point in its life cycle so that we can make optimally informed decisions and provide more useful information to practitioners, patients, and industry.

Case Example 22.4: For pharmacoepidemiologic studies of devices

Background

- Metal-on-metal hip implants were available in the US prior to 1976, but they were rarely used until recently.

- In 2003, ceramic-on-ceramic hips were approved for use in the US.

- In 2010, the British Orthopaedic Association and UK regulatory authority became concerned about adverse reactions to the wear particles in metal-on-metal hips requiring revision hip surgery.

- The FDA initiated a comprehensive review of evidence related to various bearing surfaces.

Issues

- Measure the risk of hip revision surgery for US patients implanted with total artificial hips with various bearing surfaces.

- Determine if revision rates differ by bearing surface type.

- No national registry available in US but a few national registries available outside the US.

- Hospital claims data code for bearing surface was introduced in 2005.

Approach

- Hip implants are expensive and implanted within a hospitalization. The exposure information appears in US hospital claims data. Revision hip surgery also requires hospitalization and is expensive—outcome information appears in US hospital claims data.

- Individuals were required to have continuous insurance coverage or linkable with information on completeness of follow-up.

- Investigated data sources inside and outside the US that could be used to identify strata defined by patient and bearing surface type in which hip revision rates are assumed exchangeable, clinically coherent, and large enough to prevent identification of any individual.

- Distributed specifications to data owners and requested strata-specific summaries.

Results

- Two-year hip revision surgery rates were obtained for 510,944 discharges implanted with hips between 2001 and 2009 for osteoarthritis, using national Medicare billing data and two prospective registries (within the US and Australia).

- Adjusted revision rates varied from 1.72% (95% Posterior Interval: 1.12, 2.43) for males greater than 65 years of age implanted with ceramic-on-polyethylene hips to a high of 2.53% (1.45, 3.62) for females less than 65 years of age implanted with metal-on-metal hips.

- Metal-on-metal, metal-on-polyethylene, and ceramic-on-ceramic hip replacements were each associated with higher 2-year revision surgery risks compared to ceramic-on-polyethylene.

Strengths

- Large and diverse patient population.

- Ability to specify patient and hip subgroups.

- Bearing surface information in billing codes facilitated classification of patients despite some limitations.

Limitations

- Reliability and completeness of bearing surface codes unknown.

- Mixing of designs—billing data information is retrospectively collected whereas the registries used prospective data collection.

- The US data largely influenced by the Medicare population, with information on bearing surface effects for those under 65 years coming mostly from Australia.

Key points

- Even when individual level data are not available and the outcome of interest is rare, medical device studies are possible.

- Globalization of medical devices permits borrowing information from different countries, to better learn about adverse events in any one country.

Epidemiology and international infrastructure

The accelerating pace of emerging medical technologies will continue, and the advances in information science applications will further shape the information technology-based health care worldwide. The future impact of epidemiology on our understanding of implantable devices will depend on technological and policy solutions for international collaboration to achieve consistency between global data sources, regulations, and methodological approaches for medical device implant applications.

Collaborative research efforts can particularly help to fill a major gap in the clinical areas where individual countries are limited in developing a research infrastructure. One example effort is FDA-initiated International Consortium of Orthopedic Registries (ICOR), led by Cornell University. Development of international infrastructure creates opportunities for novel methods developments for epidemiologic studies. The methods for harmonization, sharing, and combining data are not well developed and require innovative approaches. Furthermore, making conclusions and recommendations when device performance varies from country to country is a unique challenge often beyond statistics or current paradigms in epidemiology.

Key points for pharmacoepidemiologic studies of devices

- Medical devices are of great public health importance.
- Medical devices and their users have diverse and unique characteristics, creating different challenges compared with studying pharmaceuticals.
- Existing data sources have limited utility for medical device epidemiology because complete documentation of device use is not routine.
- The lack of a detailed identification system (analogous to the National Drug Code) for medical devices presents a barrier to understanding device performance.
- Due to increasing availability of electronic data sources, methodology for extracting and assessing the information from diverse data sources will be required.

Studies of drug-induced birth defects

Major birth defects, typically defined as those that are life threatening, require major surgery, or present a significant disability, affect approximately 2–4% of liveborn infants. Minor malformations are of lesser clinical importance, and vary considerably in their definition, detection, and prevalence.

Teratogenesis is a unique adverse drug effect, affecting an organism (the fetus) other than the one for whom the drug was intended (the mother). Whatever benefit/risk accrues to the mother, only the fetus is at risk for birth defects.

We are usually completely unaware of a drug's teratogenic potential when it is first marketed. Ignorance about embryologic mechanisms constrain development of predictive *in vitro* tests, and testing in animals is only rarely predictive. Premarketing clinical studies do not provide this information either. Traditionally, women of childbearing age were excluded from clinical studies, specifically because of concerns about potential teratogenicity; newer guidelines encourage their enrolment, but most studies assure that they are at minimal risk of becoming pregnant.

Clinical problems to be addressed by pharmacoepidemiologic research

As noted, the fetus is the "innocent bystander" with respect to its mother's therapy. Further, since roughly half of pregnancies (at least in the US) are unplanned, teratogenic concerns extend to women who might become pregnant while taking a medication. Finally, unlike other adverse outcomes, teratogenic effects can be prevented by avoidance of pregnancy, and the birth of a malformed infant can be avoided by termination of pregnancy. Our understanding of a drug's teratogenic risk, therefore, has important consequences for how a given drug is used clinically.

Drugs known to be teratogenic

Human teratogens tend to fall into two broad categories. Drugs that produce major defects in a high proportion (roughly, 25%) of exposed pregnancies can be considered "high risk" teratogens (e.g., thalidomide and isotretinoin). More common are "moderate risk" teratogens, which increase the rate of specific birth defects by perhaps 5–20-fold (e.g., carbamazepine and neural tube defects). The differences between high-risk and moderate-risk teratogens are relevant to how these drugs are considered in the clinical setting.

Various approaches may be applied to the few drugs known to be human teratogens. Such drugs may be prohibited or removed from the general market, as was the case for thalidomide in the 1960s, given its high teratogenic risk without offsetting therapeutic benefits.

Most known teratogens, such as carbamazepine and valproic acid, pose moderate risks balanced by clinical benefits. Physicians are expected to discuss the benefits and risks with their patients. Sometimes, a drug may be restricted to prescription by selected physicians.

The third, more recent, approach utilizes a formal risk management program (see also the "Pharmacoepidemiology and risk management" section in this chapter) involving education of physicians and patients, and combined, in some cases, with restricted access to the drug (e.g., isotretinoin).

Drugs for which teratogenic risk is unknown

Most prescription and nonprescription drugs fall into a much larger category of drugs with unknown teratogenic risk. Labels may offer a general warning against use in pregnancy, but these hardly contribute to rational drug therapy: Where the true teratogenic risk is nil, these warnings deny potentially useful therapy; where the true risk is elevated, the nonspecific warnings offer little practical discouragement to use in pregnancy.

Drugs for which teratogenesis is alleged, and clinical consequences

At one time or another, many drugs have been alleged to be teratogenic, with profound clinical consequences. For example, about 30 years ago, the widely used antinausea drug Bendectin® (Debendox®, Lenotan®) was alleged to cause various birth defects. Despite the lack of support for these allegations, legal concerns led the

manufacturer to withdraw the drug from the market. Ironically, the aggregate data for Bendectin have provided the strongest evidence of safety for any medication used in pregnancy (see Case example 22.5). Other effects of unproven allegations include overwhelming guilt among women who give birth to a malformed child and anxiety among currently-pregnant women; consequences of the latter can range from consultations with physicians, to diagnostic procedures (e.g., amniocentesis), to elective termination of the pregnancy.

The fallacy of "class action" teratogenesis

While structure/activity relationships shared by members of a given drug class can help predict a given class member's efficacy and adversity in the general population, this cannot be assumed for teratogenesis, because we cannot know whether the responsible component is the "class" or that part of a drug's structure that differentiates one class member from another. Thus, we cannot project the teratogenicity (or safety) of one class member onto others.

Methodological problems to be addressed by pharmacoepidemiologic research

Sample size considerations

"Birth defects" is not a single, homogeneous outcome, and teratogens do not uniformly increase the rates of all birth defects, but rather increase rates of selected defects. Defects vary widely in terms of gestational timing, embryologic tissue of origin, and mechanism of development. Thus, one would predict that malformations produced by a drug would vary according to the timing of exposure, the sensitivity of the end organ (i.e., embryologic tissue), and the teratogenic mechanism.

The need to focus on *specific* birth defects dramatically affects sample size requirements. For example, a cohort study of a few hundred exposed pregnancies might be sufficient to identify a doubling of the overall rate of "birth defects;" ruling out a doubling of the overall rate would require larger numbers, but still within the same order of magnitude. However, any specific defect is rare,

---

Case Example 22.5: For studies of drug-induced birth defects

Background

- In the late 1970s, the antinausea drug Bendectin (Debendox; Lenotan: doxylamine, dicyclomine, and pyridoxine) was widely used to treat nausea and vomiting of pregnancy.
- Legal claims based on allegations of the drug's teratogenicity ultimately resulted in the manufacturer removing it from the market.

Issue

- Concern about the possible teratogenic effects of the drug were raised by studies that suggested increased risks of selected cardiac defects and oral clefts among the babies of mothers who had taken the drug in the first trimester.
- In both studies, exposure among mothers of cases was compared to exposure among mothers of normal infants, and there were questions about the rigor and symmetry regarding collection of exposure information.

Approach

- Utilizing data from an ongoing case-control surveillance program of specific birth defects in relation to medication use in pregnancy, researchers identified cases with selected cardiac defects and cases with two kinds of oral clefts and compared maternal Bendectin exposure among cases to that among mothers of controls with various malformations other than those in the cases.

Results

- Among the 970 malformed controls, the prevalence of first trimester exposure was 21%.
- Case groups ranged in size from 98 to 221 infants.
- Risk estimates ranged from 0.6 to 1.0.
- All upper 95% confidence bounds were 1.6 or less.

Strengths

- The existence of the case-control surveillance database provided sufficient power (for this common exposure) to test the hypotheses without the need for further data collection.
- Sample sizes were large enough to provide tight confidence bounds.
- Direct interviews with mothers of study subjects provided information on important potential confounding variables.
- Use of malformed subjects as controls minimized the risk of biased recall.
- Prevalence of exposure among controls was similar to that identified by sales data.

Limitations

- Malformed controls could include defects caused by the drug of interest.
- The possibility of very small risks could not be excluded.
- The possibility of residual confounding remains.

Key points

- Recall bias can affect findings of case-control studies, particularly in comparisons between malformed and normal infants when exposure information is not rigorously and symmetrically collected.
- Ongoing case-control surveillance approaches, by accruing large numbers of subjects with specific malformations with detailed exposure and covariate data, can efficiently test hypotheses without the need to mount new studies that would take years to complete.
- The impact of false-positive teratogenic studies can be considerable.

---

occurring in 1 per 1000 live births (e.g., oral clefts) to 1 per 10 000 or fewer (e.g., biliary atresia). For a cohort study to *detect* a doubling of risk for a relatively common specific birth defect (e.g., 1/1000) requires over 20 000 exposed pregnancies. To *rule out* a doubling of risk for the same defect, one would need a far larger sample size of exposed pregnancies.

Exposure

Prescribed Drugs

Most pharmacoepidemiologic studies have focused on drugs prescribed immediately before or during pregnancy. While this is indeed an area in need of major research attention, it is often assumed that drugs prescribed or prescriptions filled represent exposure, yet we know from increasingly detailed studies of medication adherence that such is not routinely the case (see Chapter 20). Adherence varies according to many factors, including the condition and drug involved, but whatever the cause, nonadherence creates problems with exposure misclassification. Relatedly, as influenza vaccines have come to be recommended for use in pregnant women, the source of such exposures has expanded from the woman's health care provider to include nontraditional settings such as pharmacies, supermarkets, and occupational health clinics. Without such exposures being recorded in the patient's medical record, medical-record based research will classify many exposed women as unexposed.

While medication adherence has long been recognized as a problem by clinicians and researchers, borrowed prescription medications has only more recently been identified as being surprisingly common, and such exposures are unlikely to be reported to health care providers and thus are unlikely to be recorded in medical records.

Nonprescribed Drugs

Over-the-counter (OTC) drugs present a unique situation. By definition, use of OTC drugs does not require physician involvement. Like other consumers, women of childbearing age view OTC drugs as safer than prescription products, and they may assume the same is true for use of these drugs in pregnancy. Though prescription drugs generally become OTC based on a history of wide use and safety, this history rarely includes systematic information on potential human teratogenicity. This is particularly true for drugs that became available OTC decades ago.

Although the teratogenic effects of OTC drugs have, until recently, been largely unstudied, these agents have been used widely in pregnancy for decades, and the more recent increase in herbal product use among pregnant women has raised additional concerns. These exposures should be a focus of pharmacoepidemiologic research.

Recall Bias

Issues of sample size favor case–control approaches for studying specific birth defects. Deriving exposure information from maternal interviews raises concern about recall accuracy and potential bias (see Chapter 12). Because of feelings of guilt, the mother of a malformed infant may be more likely than the mother of a healthy infant to accurately recall her pregnancy exposures, and the difference in recall accuracy could lead to false positive associations. However, the simple possibility of recall bias does not invalidate interview-based studies, and there are various approaches to minimizing this problem.

Restricting analysis to mothers of malformed infants (whether they are cases or controls) limits the likelihood of false positive results due to biased recall among mothers of malformed infants. The likelihood of a false positive can be further minimized by including a wide range of malformations among controls, since it is unlikely that a drug increases the risk of most specific defects (see Case example 22.5).

Open-ended questions invite differential recall between mothers of malformed and normal infants, whereas focused questions are more likely to yield complete information. Recall is also substantially improved when women are asked about use according to various indications and when drugs are asked by specific names. Post-hoc, if one is studying a medication in relation to a number of birth defects, an observation of appreciable variations in effect estimates (some including the null, others not) would argue against the presence of recall bias, since such bias would likely manifest in consistently increased risks (or possibly decreased risks) for all defects. Still, the *possibility* of recall bias cannot be eliminated completely, either by the use of a malformed control group or by asking specific questions about drug use.

Outcome

Though birth defects are often classified by organ system (e.g., "musculoskeletal"), whenever possible they should be classified on the basis of the embryologic origin for a given defect. For example, neural crest cells form various structures of the face/ears, heart, and neural tube, and it is of note that the retinoid isotretinoin, which interferes with neural crest cell migration/development, produces malformations of the ear, heart, and neural tube.

Confounding

Potential confounders that are routinely considered in teratologic studies include maternal age, race, geography, and socioeconomic status. However, additional potential confounders must be identified based on understanding the epidemiology of specific defects. Prominent among these is exposure to periconceptional folic acid, which is known to reduce the risk of a number of defects (such exposure, typically in the form of multivitamins, should not be confused with exposure to prescribed "prenatal" folate-containing multivitamins, which are typically taken after the critical period for the development of a number of folate-preventable defects). Also, since medication use may be associated with various health behaviors (e.g., vitamin use is more common among nonsmokers), one may need to consider various health behaviors, including smoking, alcohol, and nutrition, in studies of certain exposures and outcomes. Further, it is critically important to separate risks due to the drug from risks associated with the condition for which the drug is taken, known as "confounding by indication."

Finally, there is the important possibility of pregnancy termination. As malformations become detectable at earlier stages of pregnancy (and as more such pregnancies are terminated), studies of liveborn and stillborn infants will increasingly underestimate the prevalence of such defects, and the likelihood of termination may be related both to the outcome under study and the use of a given drug.

Biologic plausibility

How does one evaluate the importance of biologic plausibility for newly observed associations? Unlike other areas of drug safety research, little is known about the mechanisms that lead to birth defects, and it is commonly the case that findings of increased risk following a given exposure cannot be linked to a known biologically plausible mechanism. Indeed, many would argue that such findings, if consistently observed, should prompt studies in other areas (e.g., laboratory experiments) to identify the biologic mechanisms. While a requirement that every observed risk increase have an identifiable biologic mechanism would have led to dismissal of most accepted human teratogens, some aspects of biologic plausibility must be met. For example, it is implausible that a defect could be caused by an exposure that first occurs after the gestational development of the defect. It is also unlikely that an exposure would produce defects that span gestational timing from preconception to late pregnancy and do not share embryologic tissue of origin. Thus, though we cannot dismiss hypotheses simply because they lack a biologically plausible explanation, observations of increased risks in a given study should be considered speculative at best unless they meet certain aspects of biologic plausibility.

Examples of currently available solutions

Cohort and case–control designs are the favored approaches used to generate and test hypotheses regarding drugs and birth defects.

Cohorts

Three types of cohorts relevant to the pharmacoepidemiologic study of birth defects include studies designed to follow large populations exposed to various agents, use of data sets created for other purposes, and follow-up studies of selected exposures. Though many cohorts are sufficiently large to assess risks of birth defects overall, few cohorts have sufficient numbers of exposed subjects with specific defects, most of which have background rates ranging from 1 per 1000 to 1 per 10 000.

Studies Designed to Follow Large Populations Exposed to Various Agents

This approach involves following a population of pregnant women with collection of data on exposures, outcomes, and covariates. An example is the US Collaborative Perinatal Project (CPP), which enrolled over 58 000 women between 1959 and 1965, obtained detailed information on their pregnancies, and followed the children until age 7. The strength of this approach is the prospective, systematic, and repeated collection of information that includes exposure to a wide variety of medications taken by a diverse population, many potential confounding variables, and good outcome information. However, a major weakness of even a cohort this large is the relatively few infants with *specific* malformations. For example, while there were approximately 2200 infants with "major malformations" there were only 31 with cleft palate (CP) and 11 with tracheoesophageal fistula (TEF). This weakness is compounded by limited numbers of women exposed to most drugs. For a drug taken by as many as 10% of the women, the expected number of exposed infants with CP and TEF would be 3 and 1, respectively; if a drug were used by 3%, the expected intercepts would be 1 and 0.3. Such a cohort may be large enough to identify some high-risk teratogens, but power is usually inadequate to identify moderate-risk teratogens among commonly used drugs, and power is routinely inadequate to identify such teratogens among the vast majority of other drugs.

Further, the inordinate costs of such intensive efforts typically limit enrolment and data collection to a few years. Because of changing patterns of drug use over time, the clinical relevance of the available data diminishes.

Use of data sets created for other purposes

Increasing attention has focused on cohorts identified from administrative databases produced for purposes other than epidemiologic research by organizations or governments involved in medical care (see Chapters 8 and 9). The strengths and weaknesses vary with the nature of the specific data set (see Chapters 8 and 9). All have the advantage of identifying exposures independent of knowledge of the outcome, and national, linked, claims-based, and other datasets may include large populations. While some may have good reporting of malformations, in others the quality of diagnosis data is quite limited. Despite their overall size, these databases may contain few subjects with specific malformations who were exposed to a particular drug in utero, and there may be difficulties identifying the onset of pregnancy with sufficient precision to establish meaningful exposure windows during the gestational period. The validity of exposure information may be limited by problems of misclassification, whether due to nonadherence or nonrecorded exposures (e.g., influenza vaccines or medication borrowing). Further, information is almost universally absent on important confounding variables (e.g., periconceptional exposure to folate, smoking, alcohol, diet, OTC drugs). While administrative datasets may have value in identifying high-risk teratogens, their value in identifying the more common moderate-risk teratogens remains to be demonstrated.

Follow-up of selected exposures

Cohorts of women exposed to specific drugs can be developed by enrolling pregnant women in pregnancy registries, either by physicians or by the women themselves. Registries, whether operated by a manufacturer or a teratogen information service, can identify women exposed to a drug of interest early in pregnancy and, most importantly, identify and enroll the women before the pregnancy outcome is known. Registries that are in direct contact with pregnant women can also prospectively collect other information, such as data relating to other exposures and potential confounding variables.

Cohorts of a few dozen to a few hundred exposed pregnancies are highly efficient and effective for identifying–and ruling out–high-risk teratogens. On the other hand, such cohorts are quite limited in their ability to identify a drug as a moderate-risk teratogen or to rule out such an effect.

Registries may be limited by problems of self-referral bias and losses to follow-up. In addition, comparators may be absent or inappropriate, and the registry data may not allow exploration of confounding by indication.

Case–control studies

The rarity of birth defects overall, and particularly specific defects, argues for the use of the case–control design when exposure prevalence is sufficiently high (see Chapter 2). Such studies may be conducted on an ad hoc basis or within the context of case–control surveillance. Examples of the latter include the longstanding Slone Epidemiology Center "Birth Defects Study" and the more recently established National Birth Defects Prevention Study, the latter involving several state birth defects surveillance programs and coordinated by the Centers for Disease Control and Prevention (CDC). From the perspective of specific birth defects, case–control studies can have the statistical power required for the assessment of both risk and safety. By obtaining information directly from the mother, such studies can identify actual exposures (rather than prescriptions issued or filled), and they can similarly identify exposures to borrowed medications, whatever the source. The "direct-to-consumer" approach used in these studies can also capture information on critical covariates that would not be obtained from other sources, such as periconceptional folate exposure, smoking, alcohol, diet, and use of nonprescription drugs.

Statistical power is a major strength of the case–control approach, but power does not assure validity. As noted, a concern with this approach is recall bias; however, the simple *possibility* of such bias does not invalidate a case–control study; rather, its potential requires careful efforts to consider and minimize such bias in the study population.

The future

Integration of epidemiology and biology

Advances in molecular biology and genetics will markedly enhance our ability to classify defects in biologically meaningful categories and facilitate development of biologically plausible hypotheses. Even the most notorious human teratogens do not produce malformations in all (or most) exposed fetuses, and this "incomplete penetrance" is likely due to differences in host susceptibilities, such as the host's handling of drugs. Although we have yet to identify a single gene whose regulation of drug

metabolism accounts for the increased risks of a specific defect following antenatal exposure to a particular drug, we can be optimistic that the rapid advances in genetic research, coupled with the dramatic cost-efficiencies that accompany such advances, will allow identification both of population subsets at increased risk for certain birth defects and of drugs that pose particular risk in subjects with genetic factors that predispose to gene-environment interactions. With this knowledge, it may become possible, in advance of pregnancy, to evaluate the genomes of women to determine if, given exposure to a particular drug, they are genetically at increased risk for their fetus being affected with a specific birth defect. Information of this kind has obvious usefulness in selecting (and avoiding) specific drugs for the treatment of women who are pregnant or at risk for becoming pregnant.

The legal and regulatory climate

Pharmacoepidemiologic studies of teratogenesis require access to information that identifies women who have become pregnant, their medication exposures, and details of the pregnancy outcomes of those pregnancies. Disclosure of such information to researchers has become highly contentious in many countries. For case–control studies in particular, the enrollment of malformed and/or normal subjects requires that identifying information be made available to researchers, who then contact eligible subjects to invite them to participate in an interview.

Though there is little evidence that medical researchers in this area have compromised confidentiality, epidemiologic studies may be compromised or eliminated by privacy/confidentiality regulations (see Chapter 15). It is critical that researchers engage their communities about the public health value of epidemiologic research and the need for balancing privacy concerns with the need to provide critical information on the risks and safety of medications taken in pregnancy.

Hope for an integrated approach

Future studies of birth defects should consider secular changes in use not only related to prescription drugs (including vaccines), but also to OTC and herbal products, and they will undoubtedly focus increased attention on issues of validity and statistical power. Although the thalidomide debacle did much to stimulate research and regulatory attention on the adverse effects of medications, it is ironic that in the 50 years since that teratogenic disaster, drugs have yet to come under systematic study for their potential teratogenic risks. Consequently, information available to pregnant women and their health care providers about the safety of drugs in pregnancy is woefully inadequate. This situation need not persist—systematic approaches to pharmacoepidemiologic research in this important area can be established both by exploring novel uses of data not designed for epidemiologic research and, more simply, by coordinating proven methodologies. In the US, for example, our knowledge of each drug's risk and safety to the fetus can be dramatically improved in a highly cost-efficient manner by taking advantage of existing comprehensive surveillance that combines the complementary strengths of already established cohort and case–control surveillance infrastructures, as has been accomplished for the study of influenza vaccine safety in pregnancy.

Key points for studies of drug-induced birth defects

• Because teratogenesis involves maternal exposures that adversely affect another organism's development, it creates unique issues for pharmacoepidemiologic research.

• Known teratogens do not increase risks of all birth defects, but rather one or several specific defects; with baseline birth prevalence of about 1 per 1000 to 1 per 10 000, specific defects are rare outcomes.

• Pregnancy registries (small cohorts) are useful to identify high risk teratogens (e.g., isotretinoin) but are underpowered to identify lesser risks.

• Large databases (large cohorts) can sometimes provide adequate power but are usually constrained by serious limitations in information available on exposures, outcomes, and covariates.

• Case-control studies and particularly case-control surveillance are well suited to assess risks of birth defects in relation to various antenatal exposures.

• In the absence of knowledge regarding biologic mechanisms for the development of birth defects, a presumably valid and consistently-observed association between an exposure and particular birth defect should not be dismissed because biologic plausibility cannot be demonstrated.

Risk management

Note: The views expressed in this section are those of the authors, and not necessarily those of the US Food and Drug Administration or the European Medicines Agency.

In medicine, risk management is used to ensure that the potential benefits of a medicine exceed its potential risks, and to minimize those risks. Risk management of medicines is not new, though it has received increased attention in the past two decades. Current understanding of the risks of medicines is based on the premise that the risk of a medicine derives not only from the inherent properties of the medicine, but also from the harm that can result from inappropriate use of a medicine in a complex medical care system.

In the context of human medicines in the United States, the Food and Drug Administration (FDA) has defined risk management as

> an iterative process of (1) assessing a product's benefit-risk balance, (2) developing and implementing tools to minimize its risks while preserving its benefits, (3) evaluating tool effectiveness and reassessing the benefit-risk balance, and (4) making adjustments, as appropriate, to the risk minimization tools to further improve the benefit-risk balance. This four-part process should be continuous throughout a product's lifecycle, with the results of risk assessment informing the sponsor's decisions regarding risk minimization.

In Europe, the concept of risk management is established in legislation. Article 1 (28b) of Directive 2001/83 EC as amended, defines a risk management system as: "a set of pharmacovigilance activities and interventions designed to identify, characterize, prevent or minimize risks relating to a medicinal product including the assessment of the effectiveness of those interventions." Thus, in Europe, risk management incorporates (1) an overview of what is known, and not known about the risks of the drug, (2) the planning of pharmacovigilance activities to identify additional risks and also characterize the risks—i.e., seriousness, frequency, risk factors, and public health impact, (3) measures to minimize the risks including the measurement of the effectiveness, and (4) a feedback process so that new information about the risks or risk minimization is incorporated into the overview and pharmacovigilance and risk minimization activities adjusted accordingly.

Clinical problems to be addressed by pharmacoepidemiologic research

All medicines have risks. The traditional tools used to manage the risks of prescription medicines have been the prescription status itself (i.e., whether the drug was approved for prescription only use or whether it could be obtained without a prescription), labeling for healthcare professionals, and the requirement that manufacturers monitor and report to regulatory authorities adverse events that occur with use of the medicine once it is marketed. Additional steps taken over the past twenty years to manage more actively the risks of certain medications have included increased communication to patients as well as to healthcare professionals, and measures to restrict, in various ways, the usage of certain medicines.

The complexities of the medication use system

The medication use system is a complex network of stakeholders, including patients, their families, physicians, nurses, pharmacists, other health professionals, health care organizations and facilities (e.g., hospitals, clinics), payors, manufacturers, and regulatory agencies. Not only does each have a role in ensuring the safe use of a medicine, the interactions among them do as well.

Because not all the risks of a medicine are known at the time the product is approved, risk management efforts must continue throughout the lifecycle of a medicine.

The sources of risk from medical products

There are several sources of risks from medical products. The known risks of a product are based on prior experience or, in some cases, on the pharmacologic or other properties of the medicine. In some cases these risks are preventable, while in others they are not. Preventable risks can occur when a product is administered under a condition of use that imparts a risk that would not be present under a different condition of use. For example, if drug A, when used in combination with drug B, results in an unacceptable risk that is not present when either drug is used alone, this unacceptable risk is preventable by ensuring that drug A and drug B are never coadministered. Contraindicating concomitant use is a regulatory step that can be used to warn against concomitant use; actual avoidance of concomitant prescribing can only be achieved by health professionals' adherence to this recommendation. Risk management efforts can be used to ensure that preventable adverse events are minimized.

Unpreventable risks are those that occur when all the known necessary conditions for safe use of a product are followed. An unpreventable risk may become a preventable risk once risk factors are identified. There will always be some risks, which although known cannot be prevented. In these circumstances, risk minimization activities might be directed towards identifying the adverse consequences as early as possible with the aim of preventing more serious harm. For example, a drug may be known to cause hepatic damage but its occurrence in a specific patient may not be predictable or preventable. Risk minimization activities might be directed towards regular monitoring of hepatic enzyme levels to identify any hepatic damage as early as possible and so prevent serious hepatitis or hepatic failure.

In addition, risk management efforts can be used to ensure that medications are not administered to patients at higher risk for a serious adverse event, or administered only to patients for whom the benefits outweigh the risks, including the unpreventable risks. Removing all risks from the use of all medicines is not the overall goal of managing the risks of medicines, nor is it achievable. Rather, careful consideration of risk-benefit balance both for the individual patient and for the target population is an important consideration of risk management.

Risk management strives to be scientifically driven

The scientific approach to risk management requires integrating data from various studies and disciplines that, when taken together, can promote the safe and effective use of a medicine. The scientific approach also compels manufacturers and regulators to examine, throughout the lifecycle of the medicine, the critical gaps in knowledge that exist. Such gaps may concern the pharmacologic properties of the medicine, clinical outcomes related to its use, including that in higher risk populations, or the way the medicine is used in actual practice. Any of these areas could lead to further post-approval studies, the results of which would lead to changes in labeling or other changes that could enhance the safe and effective use of the medicine. However, changes in labeling do not always result in changes in prescribing practices.

Risk management is a proactive process

Risk management must be proactive to be optimally effective. The ability to identify risks in the pre-approval period allows manufacturers to work with regulators on risk management planning during the drug development phase. A proactive approach in the post-approval phase demands that manufacturers, regulators, and practitioners have in place systems to identify new risks, manage known risks, assess the effectiveness of the risk management efforts, and modify them as needed. A carefully designed risk management plan can identify risks, manage risks, and assess the effectiveness of these efforts in a proactive way.

Risk management is an iterative process involving multiple related activities

Managing the risks of medicines is not a single activity or the province of a single profession or stakeholder group. Rather, it is an iterative process that involves a set of interrelated activities. In broad categories, these activities include risk assessment, risk mitigation, and evaluation of risk mitigation measures. These activities occur throughout the product's lifecycle, and are adjusted and refined as new risk assessments provide new information and as evaluations of risk mitigation activities provide data upon which risk mitigation activities can be improved or modified.

Risk Assessment

Risk assessment consists of identifying, characterizing, and quantifying the risks associated with the use of a medicine. The nature, frequency and severity of the risks are assessed. In addition, if possible, the conditions under which the risk is more likely to occur are identified.

Risk assessment occurs throughout the premarketing and postmarketing phases of a product's life. Premarket, or preapproval, risk assessment, is generally a very extensive process that involves preclinical safety assessments (e.g., animal toxicology testing), clinical pharmacology assessments, and clinical trials.

Because even large clinical development programs cannot identify all risks associated with a product (see Chapters 3 and 16), risk assessment must continue in the post-approval period, when large numbers of persons will be exposed to the medicine, including many with comorbid conditions or on concomitant medications not present in clinical trials. Post-approval risk assessment can be based on either non-experimental data or on clinical trial data. Non-experimental data include individual case reports of suspected adverse drug reactions (spontaneous reports), case series of such reports, databases of spontaneous reports, disease-based registries, drug-based registries, electronic medical records systems, administrative claims databases, drug utilization databases, poison control center databases, and other public health databases that track medication usage.

It is also important for risk assessments to identify medication errors (see also "Medication errors" section in this chapter), and the potential for medication errors, throughout the product's lifecycle.

Risk mitigation

Risk mitigation refers to a set of activities designed to minimize the risks of a medicine while preserving its benefits. The range of risk mitigation activities varies from one country or region to the next, but certain common themes emerge.

For most prescription medicines, the prescription status, professional label, and information directed to patients are sufficient risk mitigation measures to ensure that the benefits of a medicine outweigh its risks. In some cases, additional measures are needed to address one, or at most a few, specific serious risks. These measures generally fall into one of three categories: (1) focused information for patients; (2) additional, focused information for practitioners; and (3) measures that restrict, in some way, the use of the medicine. A risk mitigation strategy may use one or more of these measures.

Because additional risk mitigation measures are focused on only one or a few serious risks, the communications focused both toward healthcare professionals and patients must address these risks in detail, while at the same time putting these specific serious risks in the context of the overall risk-and-benefit profile of the medicine. In some cases, the communication is focused principally on the nature of a serious risk, so that patients and prescribers can make an informed decision if the potential benefits outweigh the potential risks in their individual situation. In other cases, the communication also focuses on specific steps that can be taken to mitigate the risk or to recognize it early.

The measures to restrict the way a medicine is prescribed, dispensed, or used is complex and, more than other risk mitigation efforts, requires complex interactions with the medication distribution and use system.

Because these additional risk mitigation measures are highly focused, it is critical that they have clearly specified and well thought out goals. In the absence of clear goals, proper interventions cannot be designed, and the impact of these interventions cannot be measured.

Evaluation of risk mitigation measures

Evaluation of risk mitigation activities is a critical component of risk management. The evaluation of a risk mitigation activity is closely related to the risk assessment activities, but it also differs in some ways. While traditional risk assessments are designed to identify, characterize, and quantify previously unknown risks, evaluations of risk mitigation activities are designed to examine the impact of these risk mitigation activities. It is thus important that the measures used to evaluate a risk mitigation activity focus on the goals of the risk mitigation plan.

Evaluation of risk mitigation measures can occur at several levels. First, evaluation of risk mitigation activities can assess if certain processes specified by the risk mitigation strategy are being followed. For example, if the risk mitigation strategy consists of providing patients with specific information about measures that can be taken to minimize a particular risk, the assessment could consist of determining the proportion of patients who receive the information. Second, the evaluation can determine if certain behaviors are being followed. In the above example, measurements of behavior could assess if patients read the information they are given, if they understand the information, and if they do the specific things the information recommends. Third, the evaluation can measure the frequency of the health outcome that the risk mitigation strategy is designed to minimize. These three types of evaluation are each quite different from each other, in terms of both the data needed to conduct the evaluations as well as the methods to analyze the data. In some cases, evaluations of adherence to specific processes may be easier to conduct than other types of evaluations. However, it is important that the final health outcome of interest be evaluated, since adherence to process may not guarantee attainment of the health outcome of interest.

Pharmaceutical manufacturers are held responsible for the safety of their products, so it is usually they who conduct or fund risk assessments, put into place risk mitigation strategies, and evaluate the effectiveness of those strategies. Regulators review the results of manufacturers' testing, proposed risk mitigation strategies, and the evaluations of the risk mitigation strategies. Regulators may also conduct independent assessments of drug safety. As the academic field of pharmacoepidemiology has grown, university-based researchers also conduct drug safety research, either independent of manufacturers and regulators or in collaboration with them.

Defining and setting the goals of a risk mitigation strategy presents several challenges, especially because it is critical to define the overall success or failure or a risk mitigation strategy in terms of the actual health outcomes of interest. First, data on the actual frequency of the health outcome of interest may not be readily available or may not be reliable or representative of the entire population taking the medicine. Second, without prior experience with similar risk mitigation strategies, it is difficult to set a quantitative goal for the risk mitigation strategy. The aspirational goal for mitigation of certain avoidable risk is zero, but the complexities of the medication use system, and the reliance on the behavior of so many individuals, make such a goal impractical.

Risk management plans need to be assessed, but current methods of assessing the impact of specific risk mitigation measures and their component parts on processes, behaviors, and most importantly health outcomes need to be developed, so that effective measures can be continued and ineffective ones can be removed.

Some aspects of the risk mitigation measures, especially those that impose restrictions on the use of a medicine, may be burdensome on the healthcare system and may have unintended consequences. One potential unintended consequence is that the burdens imposed by the system will deter practitioners from prescribing a medicine to patients for whom that medicine would be the optimal treatment choice. There are few data at this time to determine the impact of this potential unintended consequence.

Risk communication

Communicating information about the benefits and risk of medicines is central to risk management of medicines. Risk communication is a broad field, and a full discussion is beyond the scope of this chapter. Risk communication has traditionally been directed towards healthcare professionals, but in recent years increasing attention has been paid to communications directed towards patients and consumers.

The principal form of communication to healthcare professionals is the product's approved professional labeling, which is designed to present to the healthcare professional information needed to prescribe the product. In Europe, this professional information is known as the Summary of Product Characteristics (SmPC). To help minimize risks, the professional label contains information on those clinical situations in which the drug should not be used, or should be used only with extreme caution; about the known risks of the medicine; and about the conditions of safe use of the medication, such as the proper dosing (including, when applicable, the dose adjustments needed for renal and hepatic impairment or those based on age), drug–drug interactions, drug–disease interactions, use in pregnant or lactating women, and use in other specific clinical situations. However, changes in labeling do not always result in changes in prescribing practices.

Additional communications to healthcare professionals come in the form of so-called "Dear Healthcare Professional Letters" or "Dear Doctor Letters." These letters are typically issued by a medicine's manufacturer and generally focus on specific, newly-identified safety information. The nature of the risk is explained, and a summary of the changes to the product label is often included. The letter can also highlight actions that the healthcare professional can take in prescribing and dispensing the product, as well as other measures that can help assure the product's safe and appropriate use. Frequently, in Europe, the text of these letters is agreed upon together with the appropriate regulatory authority and, in some cases, its provision to healthcare professionals made a condition of the marketing authorization.

Information to patients can come in a variety of forms. One common form is product-specific information directed towards patients. This can take the form of approved patient labeling, which is developed by the manufacturer and reviewed and approved by FDA. Examples of approved patient labeling include the Medication Guide or a Patient

Package Insert. Labeling directed to patients and consumers highlights basic information necessary for the safe use of the product, and often provides instructions for actions to take when certain symptoms are present.

In Europe, all medicines are required to have a package leaflet (sometimes also referred to as a patient information leaflet) which must be provided to the patient. This leaflet is based upon the information provided to the physician (the Summary of Product Characteristics—SmPC) but written in patient-friendly language. There is a requirement to test the readability of the package leaflet with an appropriate target group of patients/consumers and provide the results to the competent authorities prior to authorization.

Methodological problems to be addressed by pharmacoepidemiologic research

The roles of pharmacoepidemiology in risk management

Pharmacoepidemiology can play several roles in risk management. The most fundamental role is to identify and quantify the risks of a medicine. Identification and quantification of risks can occur using a variety of pharmacoepidemiologic techniques, including clinical trials, spontaneous reports, case series, and observational pharmacoepidemiologic studies. Use of these techniques for risk assessment is described elsewhere in this book.

An important use of pharmacoepidemiology in the development of risk mitigation strategies is to measure how medications are used in practice, especially if they are used under conditions that can lead to adverse outcomes. Examples of pharmacoepidemiologic findings that could signal that a product is not being used appropriately include a finding that a medication is being prescribed concomitantly with a contraindicated medication, a finding that a drug is being used in a population of patients for whom the potential benefits do not outweigh the potential risks, and a finding that a medication is frequently prescribed for a duration of treatment that is associated with an increased risk of serious adverse events.

Another application of pharmacoepidemiology is to provide population-based assessments of the causes and contexts in which known harm from medications can occur. For these analyses, one or more public health databases may be especially helpful to estimate the burden of a given drug-related toxicity in the population. Generally, these databases are more useful for characterizing and quantifying known drug risk, rather than identifying new risks.

Pharmacoepidemiology can play an important role in the assessment of risk mitigation efforts. Of all the ways in which pharmacoepidemiology can be used in risk management, understanding the best ways to assess risk mitigation efforts is the least developed. There are many challenges. First, for an effective evaluation, the risk mitigation activity must have a clearly defined goal that is relevant and measurable, even if prespecified criteria for success or failure are not established. Goals based on vague or imprecise metrics generally cannot be measured, and even if they are measurable, interpretations of the findings would be difficult. Second, as noted above, assessing the effectiveness of a risk mitigation strategy can be conducted at several levels, including processes, behaviors, and health outcomes. While the traditional methods of pharmacoepidemiology may be used to assess the third level (health outcomes), it is quite likely that additional methods, such as those used in social sciences and health policy and management fields, may be needed for the first two levels (process and behavior). Third, it is important to understand the relationship between each component of the risk mitigation strategy and the desired health outcomes. It is possible that practitioners and patients adhere to the processes and exhibit the behaviors desired by the risk mitigation strategy, but that the health outcome of interest is not improved (i.e., the specific risk is not mitigated). Alternatively, it is possible that practitioners and patients do not adhere to the processes or exhibit the desired behaviors, but the desired health outcome (e.g., a reduction in the specific risk) is achieved, perhaps because of other interventions or factors that were not part of the risk mitigation strategy. In either case, a critical examination of the risk mitigation strategy would be necessary. In the final analysis, a risk mitigation strategy is successful only if there is mitigation of the specific risks that are the focus of the strategy.

The assessment of risk communications is a broad endeavor, and can involve many disciplines and approaches. Approaches may include a survey of patients' and healthcare providers' understanding of the risks and safe use of a medicine. Other approaches may include focus groups, questionnaires, interviews, and other methods used to assess readability and/or understanding, though little evidence exists linking risk communication activities to measureable health outcomes.

Examples of currently available solutions

In both the United States and in the European Union, specific legislation has been enacted to formalize managing the risks of medicines. The legal and regulatory frameworks in each of these jurisdictions are beyond the scope of this chapter. In the US, the legislation specifies that FDA can require a risk evaluation and mitigation strategies (REMS) when certain criteria are met. In the European Union, a Risk Management Plan (RMP) is required for drug products. Despite their differences, REMS and RMPs share the common features of being able to use, as appropriate and allowed by law or regulation, communication to patients, communication to healthcare professionals, and certain restrictions to manage the risks of medicines. In the US, it is required that REMS be assessed to ensure that they are meeting their goals. In the EU, measuring the effectiveness of risk minimization activities and interventions is included in the definition of a risk management system.

The future

Managing the risk of medicines is an evolving area involving multiple stakeholders in the complex medication use system and many opportunities for refinements of the current systems that are in place.

One critical area for future development is to measure the impact of risk mitigation strategies.

Measurement of this impact is important, because it allows policy-makers and other stakeholders to determine if the goals of the risk mitigation strategy are being met. The optimal way to measure the impact of risk mitigation strategies is not well developed, and is an area in which pharmacoepidemiology, along with other disciplines, will play an important role. The challenges for this field include developing models to relate risk mitigation strategies to health outcomes, as well as ways to identify the contribution of individual components of the strategy to the overall outcome. A further challenge is to assess if there are negative consequences of risk mitigation strategies.

Risk management plans are often implemented within a complex medication use system. A current challenge for risk management plans is that they be developed in ways that can integrate with minimal difficulty into the current medication use systems. Some aspects of risk management, such as providing information to patients, are already incorporated, at least to some degree, in many medication use systems. Other aspects, of risk mitigation measures, especially those that impose restrictions on the use of a medicine, are not easily incorporated into current medication use systems. If these risk mitigation strategies are to be used more widely than they are today, or if they are to be used for medicines that are widely used, it will be imperative that systems be developed that integrate into the medication use system.

As risk management planning evolves in multiple countries and regions, there is considerable interest in international harmonization of these efforts. At this time, there are many challenges that prevent harmonization from becoming a reality. The diversity of healthcare systems and medication use systems from one country to the next limits the degree to which identical, or even similar, individual risk mitigation strategies can be put into place across several countries. The differences in risk management activities across countries and regions, however, create a natural opportunity for stakeholders to determine the relative impact of different approaches to risk management.

Case Example 22.6: For pharmacoepidemiology and risk management

Background

- Vigabatrin is an anti-epileptic medication that can cause bilateral peripheral visual field constriction in a high percentage of patients. It is indicated as monotherapy for pediatric patients with infantile spasms for whom the potential benefits outweigh the potential risk of visual loss, and as adjunctive therapy for adult patients with refractory complex partial seizures who have responded inadequately responses to several alternative treatments.

Question

- How to manage the risk of potential for visual loss in the US

Approach

- Because of the potential for visual loss, vigabatrin was approved in the US with a a risk evaluation and mitigation strategy (REMS). The goals of the REMS, which are directed at managing the risks of visual loss, are:
  1. to reduce the risk of a vigabatrin-induced vision loss while delivering benefit to the appropriate patient populations;
  2. to ensure that all patients receive a baseline ophthalmologic evaluation; 50% of patients will receive this within 2 weeks of starting vigabatrin and 100% within 4 weeks;
  3. to discontinue vigabatrin therapy in patients who experience an inadequate clinical response;
  4. to detect vigabatrin-induced vision loss as early as possible;
  5. to ensure regular vision monitoring to facilitate ongoing benefit-risk assessments; and
  6. to inform patients/parents or legal guardians of the serious risks associated with vigabatrin, including vision loss.
- The approved REMS consists of the following components:
  1. Communication to patients through a Medication Guide that focuses on the potential for visual loss, including some of the symptoms and instructions to seek medical attention should these symptoms arise.
  2. A communication plan including a Dear Healthcare Professional Letter, directed at ophthalmologists. The letter describes the patterns of visual loss with vigabatrin, the required mandatory vision monitoring for adults and infants treated with vigabatrin, and the challenges of assessing visual field defects in infants.
  3. "Elements to assure safe use," which function as a type of restricted distribution system. The particular elements in this case include the following:
     - certification of healthcare providers who prescribe vigabatrin;
     - certification of pharmacies that dispense vigabatrin;
     - a requirement that vigabatrin be dispensed to patients with evidence or other documentation of safe-use conditions including periodic vision assessments;
     - and enrollment of each patient using vigabatrin in a registry.
  4. An implementation system which describes how operational elements and responsibilities specified in the REMS will be implemented by the drug company.
  5. A timetable for assessments of the effectiveness of the REMS.

Results

- Vigabatrin was approved with the REMS described above, which is now in place. The success of the plan is pending assessments.

Strengths

- Risk management efforts can focus on mitigating specific risks.

Limitations

- The risk management plan can monitor patients for visual loss, but it can not completely prevent it.

Key points

- No risk mitigation strategy can completely eliminate all serious adverse events.
- When the risk of a medication is very serious, but the benefits still outweigh those risks, it is important for health care providers to understand well the nature of the risk and to ensure that the proper pre- and posttreatment monitoring is done.
- The target of communicating the risks of a medication is not only those physicians who will prescribe the medication, but also those who may see the complications of treatment.
- A robust plan must be put into place at the time the risk mitigation strategy is implemented, to determine whether the strategy is effective in mitigating the risk.

Key points for risk management

- The risks of a medicine derive both from its inherent pharmacological properties as well as from the way the medicine is used.
- Because the risks of medicines can occur at any point in the complex medication use system, managing the risks of medicines requires that the entire drug use system be involved.
- Risk management is an iterative process involving multiple, related activities that proceed throughout the product's lifecycle.
- Risk mitigation refers to a set of activities designed to minimize the risks of a medicine while preserving its benefits.
- Risk communication is an important component of risk management.
- It is critical that risk management activities be evaluated.

The use of pharmacoepidemiology to study medication errors

Medications are the most commonly used form of medical therapy today. For adults, about 75% of office visits to general practitioners and internists are associated with the continuation or initiation of a drug, while in the hospital multiple medication orders tend to be written for each patient daily. edication errors have been defined as "any error in the process of ordering, dispensing, or administering a drug" regardless of whether an injury occurred or the potential for injury was present. Mechanistically, medication errors may result from errors in planning actions (i.e., knowledge-based mistakes or rule-based mistakes) or errors in executing correctly planned actions (i.e., action-based slips or memory-based lapses). In clinical practice, a medication error may occur at any stage of drug therapy, including drug prescribing, transcribing, manufacturing, dispensing, administering, and monitoring. Medication errors with potential for harm are called near-misses or potential ADE, and these errors may be intercepted before they reach the patient, or reach the patient without consequence. However, generally about one in ten medication errors results in patient harm. An ADE would be considered preventable if a medication error is associated with the ADE.

Medication errors are frequent, but fortunately only a small proportion result in harm. However, given the prevalence of prescription medication use, it is not surprising that preventable adverse drug events (ADE) are one of the most frequent types of preventable iatrogenic injuries. The IOM report, *To Err Is Human* suggested at least 44 000–98 000 deaths nationally from iatrogenic injury. If accurate, this would mean that there are about 8000 deaths yearly from ADE and 1 million injuries from drug use.

Safety theory

One theory, borrowed from psychology and human engineering, focuses on the man–machine interface, where providers must make decisions using data from multiple monitoring systems while under stress and bombarded by interruptions.

Industrial quality theory suggests that most accidents occur because of problems with the production process itself, not the individuals operating it. This theory suggests that blame for problems can be misplaced, and that although "human errors" occur commonly, the true cause of accidents is often the underlying systems that allow an operator error to result in an accident. *Root cause* analysis can be used to define the cause of the defect. Only relatively infrequently are individuals responsible for clusters of errors, and, most often, errors resulting in harm are made by workers whose overall work is good. To make the hospital a safer place, a key initial step is to eliminate the culture of blame, and build a culture of safety. Errors and adverse outcomes should be treated as opportunities for improving the process of care through system changes, rather than a signal to begin disciplinary proceedings.

Indeed, systems changes for reducing errors can greatly reduce the likelihood of error, and probably in turn, of adverse outcomes. Within medicine, much of the research has come from anesthesia, which has made major improvements in safety. Examples of successful systems changes in medication delivery include implementation of computerized physician order entry (CPOE), clinical decision support systems (CDSS), unit dosing, barcoding of medications, and implementation of "smart pumps" that can recognize what medication is being delivered. These technologies can track medication use, and more importantly, the frequencies and types of warnings as they alarm.

Overall, the area of safety has a different philosophy and several different tools than classic epidemiology. For improving safety, culture is extremely important, and tools such as root cause analysis and failure mode and effects analysis—which can be used to project what the problems with a process may be before they occur—are highly valuable. When combined with epidemiologic data, such tools may be extremely powerful for improving the safety of care.

Patient safety concepts as applied to pharmacoepidemiology

While pharmacoepidemiology techniques have most often been used to study the risks and benefits of drugs, they can also be used to study medication errors and preventable ADEs (i.e., those due to errors). Approaches to detecting medication errors include manual or automatic screening of claims data, administrative databases, medical records, electronic health records, incident reports mostly by providers in hospitals, patient monitoring, direct observation often by pharmacists, and spontaneous (self-reporting) approaches. All of these approaches have inherent advantages and pitfalls and there is no single approach that is considered the gold standard for detecting medication errors or ADEs. Factors which might influence the identification of medication errors and ADEs include the setting (ambulatory vs. inpatients; routine care vs. research studies), the expected types of medication errors (prescribing vs. administration errors), and the projected costs of detection. In addition, the type of detection method influences which types of medication errors are found (e.g., only those resulting in patient harm) and with which frequency.

Screening of claims data, administrative databases, medical records, and electronic health records is used to evaluate large data sets, but is generally done retrospectively. The quality of the available information, however, varies between different data sources (see Chapters 8 and 9) which restricts opportunities to comprehensively detect medication errors, more of some types than others. Especially in the outpatient setting, claims data can be obtained for very large numbers of individuals. Weaknesses include that it cannot be determined with certainty whether or not the patient actually consumed the medication, and, if not linked to other information sources, clinical detail is often minimal (e.g., information on weight or renal function might be missing), making it hard to answer questions that relate to a patient's clinical condition.

In the inpatient setting, manual chart review is a well-established method to detect ADEs and medication errors. With most relevant patient information at hand, the appropriateness of drug prescribing and administration can be assessed, although documentation may still be incomplete, especially for assessing issues such as appropriateness. The main problems with chart review are that it is time-consuming and expensive. When electronic health records are in place, the manual screening of paper-based information can be replaced by semi-automated approaches. The level of standardization and the extent to which clinical information is stored by using controlled vocabulary determines the feasibility and effectiveness of automated, algorithm-based data analyses of ADEs and medication errors.

When electronic health records include electronic prescribing applications with clinical decision support, data from these applications can readily be used to detect many types of medication errors at the stage of prescribing. However, the specificity of these systems will also depend on the availability of information accessible via the electronic health records.

Spontaneous reporting (self-reported) of medication errors is comparatively easy to be set in place and to maintain, both in inpatient and outpatient settings. However, both ADEs and medication errors are substantially underreported (see also Chapter 7). Indeed, the major barrier for reporting medication errors are staff's perception that reporting might be associated with disciplinary actions, even if the hospital pursues a nonpunitive policy.

Thus, spontaneous reporting is only useful for getting samples of errors and cannot be used to assess the underlying rate of medication errors in a sample. However, patient monitoring using their self-reporting for ADEs has been successful, and can identify more ADEs than chart review.

Direct observation is primarily done during research studies at inpatient sites and offers a comprehensive assessment of medication dispensing and administration errors. While being both cost and personnel intensive, direct observation has been successfully and reliably used to classify complex medication errors, and it is particularly useful at stages that are not sensitive to other detection methods (e.g., drug preparation and drug administration).

Many of the early medication error and ADE studies were performed in the hospital setting. In the inpatient adult setting, patients are vulnerable to medication errors because of the severity of their illness, the complexity of their disease process and medication regimens, and at times because of their age (e.g., the elderly are particularly susceptible). In pediatric drug use, the system-based factors that may contribute to a higher rate of near misses include the need for weight-based dosing and dilution of stock medicines, as well as decreased communication abilities of young children.

Knowledge about errors in the ambulatory setting is increasing (see Case example 22.7), although research lags behind the inpatient setting due to the difficulties of accessing patients once they leave a doctor's office. Some work has already been done about errors at the point of transition from hospitals to ambulatory settings and vice versa. Handoffs, in which the clinical care of a patient is transferred from one health provider or entity to another, are always vulnerable to errors. However, comparisons among studies are challenging because of variations in data quality and methodology.

Clinical problems to be addressed by pharmacoepidemiologic research

Medication errors can occur at any stage of the medication use process, including prescribing, transcribing, dispensing, administering, and monitoring. Of these stages, prescribing errors in the hospital have been documented to cause the most harm, although errors at any stage can do so, and monitoring errors (i.e., errors caused by lack of proper monitoring) are quite prominent outside the hospital. The greater proportion of harmful errors at the drug prescribing stage may be a consequence of the data collection methodology employed in these studies, which were multi-pronged but excluded direct observation, the most sensitive technique for administration error detection.

Important types of errors include dosing, route, frequency, drug-allergy, drug–drug interaction, drug–laboratory (including renal dosing), drug–patient characteristic, and drug administration during pregnancy. Although these errors occur most frequently at the drug ordering stage, they can occur at any stage in the medication use process.

In several studies, *dosing errors* have represented the most frequent category. To determine whether or not a dosing error is present, most often some clinical context is needed, for example the patient's age, gender, weight, level of renal function, prior response to the medication (if it has been used previously), response to other similar medications, clinical condition, and often the indication for the therapy. While many of these data elements can be obtained from review of the medical chart, many are not typically available from claims data alone.

Route of administration problems also represent a common type of error. Many drugs can be given by one or a few routes and not by many others. Some such errors—such as giving benzathine penicillin that contains suspended solids intravenously instead of intramuscularly—would often be fatal, and though they have caused fatalities, are fortunately very rare. Other route errors—such as grinding up a sustained released preparation (which can negate the slow release properties of the drug) to give it via a tube—are much more frequent, and can have serious consequences. Route errors are especially problematic at the administration stage of the medication use process, and administration errors are both difficult to detect and much less often intercepted than prescribing errors. The best approach for detecting administration errors has long been direct observation.

Case Example 22.7: For the use of pharmacoepidemiology to study medication errors

Background

- Most of the data on the frequency of adverse drug events have come from the inpatient setting, and many outpatient studies have relied on chart review or claims data to detect ADEs. Gandhi's 2003 study on the frequency of adverse drug events in a community-living population used a different approach.

Issue

- The goal of the study was to assess the frequency of adverse drug events in an ambulatory primary care population.

Approach

- The frequency of adverse drug events was assessed by calling patients after a visit at which medications were prescribed, to determine whether or not an adverse drug event had occurred, and in addition to review the chart at 3 months.

Results

- Adverse drug events occurred at a rate of 20.9 per 100 patients.
- About 8 times as many adverse drug events were identified by calling patients as by reviewing charts.
- While the severity of the ADEs overall was fairly low, about a third were preventable, and 6% were both serious and preventable.

Strengths

- The key strength of this approach was that, by calling patients, it was possible to identify many adverse drug events that were not noted in the chart.

Limitations

- The key weakness of this approach is that many of the effects patients attributed to their medications may not have been due to the medications at all, but due to other things such as their underlying conditions. The authors attempted to address this by asking the patient's physician in each instance whether they believed the symptoms related to the medication.

Key points

- Calling patients—though expensive and time-consuming—identifies many adverse drug events that are not identified through chart review.
- Almost none of the visits was associated with an ICD-9 code suggesting the presence of an ADE, suggesting that claims data should not be used to estimate the frequency of ADEs of all types in the outpatient setting.
- More work is need to facilitate assessment of whether a specific patient complaint is related to a medication.

Dosing frequency errors can occur either at the prescribing, dispensing, or administration stage. While these errors probably cause less harm cumulatively than dose or route errors, they can be problematic. Some frequency errors at the prescribing or dispensing stage can be detected even with claims or prescription data. Such errors have greater potential for harm when drugs are given with a greater frequency than intended. However, the therapeutic benefit may not be realized when given with too low frequency, and extremely negative effects can occur for some drugs, for example with antiretrovirals, to which resistance develops if they are given at a low frequency.

Allergy errors represent a particularly serious type of error, even though most of the time when a drug is given to a patient with a known allergy, the patient does well. Allergy errors typically cannot be detected with claims data, since allergy information on patients is not available. Thus, these errors have to be detected either through chart review, which is laborious, or more often through electronic medical record data.

Drug–drug interaction exposures represent an interesting and difficult area, both for research and interventions, to decrease errors. While many interactions have been reported, the severity varies substantially from minor to life-threatening. If a conscious decision is made to give patients two medications despite the knowledge that they interact, this cannot be considered an error except in very limited circumstances, for example with meperidine and monoamine oxidase inhibitors. Also, it is legitimate to give many medications together despite clear interactions with important consequences if there are no good alternatives, or if dose alterations are made, or if additional monitoring is carried out (for example, with warfarin and many antibiotics). However, the necessary alterations in dosing or additional monitoring are often omitted, which can have severe consequences. It is possible in large claims data sets to detect situations in which simultaneous exposures appear to have occurred, but not possible to determine if this actually occurred, as a physician may give patients instructions to cease the use of one of the drugs.

Drug–laboratory errors (e.g., monitoring of potassium represent an important category of errors, but can be difficult to detect electronically because of poor interfaces between laboratory and pharmacy information. Such errors are relatively straightforward to identify when large pharmacy and laboratory databases can be linked, although again assessment of clinical outcomes is difficult unless these data are also available.

Renal dosing errors represent a specific subtype of drug–laboratory errors and are especially important; these errors can also be and often are considered dosing errors. In one large inpatient study (Chertow *et al.*, 2001), nearly 40% of inpatients had at least mild renal insufficiency, and there are many medications that require dosing adjustment in the presence of decreased glomerular filtration. In that study, without clinical decision support, patients received the appropriate dose and frequency of medication only 30% of the time.

Many studies of drug–patient characteristic checking have focused on the use of medications in the presence of specific diseases. However, in the future, genomic testing will undoubtedly dominate, as many genes have profound effects on drug metabolism (see Chapter 14). Currently, few large data sets can be linked with genotype information, but this is becoming increasingly frequent in

clinical trials and a number of cohorts are being established as well.

Another important type of error may inadvertently result from *system-based interventions* such as the introduction of information technology. For instance, workflow changes, misunderstanding of functionalities and inappropriate handling of CPOEs and CDSS may induce new risks and therefore the implementation and routine use of information technology should be thoughtfully planned and closely monitored.

Methodological problems to be addressed by pharmacoepidemiologic research

Information bias

In performing drug analyses, the present conventions preclude the determination of total daily dose in several ways. Physicians may prescribe a greater amount of medicine than is required for the time period prescribed. For example, if a patient requires 50 mg of atenolol per day, the doctor may actually write a prescription for 100 mg of atenolol per day and verbally convey instructions to the patient to divide the pills. This is particularly problematic with drugs that must be titrated to the appropriate therapeutic dose (e.g., warfarin). If either physicians or pharmacists were required to document an accurate total daily dose, this would improve the ability to perform research.

Another important methodological issue is measurement of patient adherence to medications (see also Chapter 20). Since prescribing and dispensing data are seldom jointly available, determining patient adherence is extremely difficult. Improving clinician access to data from pharmacy benefit managers might be very useful, as might availability of electronic prescription data to pharmacies.

Many medications are contraindicated in pregnancy. Here, the greatest difficulty for the investigator is assessing whether or not the patient is actually pregnant at the time of the exposure, although this can be assessed retrospectively by identifying the date of birth, assuming a term pregnancy, and then working backward. The outcomes of interest are often not represented in ways that make it easy to perform analyses, although data on medication exposures and on births are readily available and can often be linked.

Another important piece of clinical information for pediatrics is a child's weight. Most pediatric medications are dosed on the basis of weight. Standardized documentation of this information is unavailable, hindering not only analyses of pediatric dosing but also actual dosing by pediatricians.

A final issue is the coding of allergies. It is important for both clinical care and research that allergies are differentiated from sensitivities or intolerances through codes rather than free text. Continued drug use in the presence of drug sensitivity may be perfectly appropriate, whereas the same treatment in the presence of an allergy is likely an error. It is particularly important that severe reactions, such as anaphylaxis, are clearly coded and identifiable in the medical records. New allergies need to be captured in better ways. The eventual aim is to have one universal allergy list in an electronic format for each patient, rather than multiple disparate lists.

Sample size issues

Sample sizes are often small in medication error and ADE studies, primarily due to the high costs of primary data collecting studies. Electronic databases will be an important tool to improve sample sizes in a cost effective manner. Computerized physician order entry systems, electronic health records, test result viewing systems, computerized pharmacy systems, bar-coding systems, pharmacy benefit managers, and claims systems will all be important sources of such data. There will be important regulatory issues that will need to be addressed before actual construction and use of these systems.

Generalizability

Many existing medication error studies have limited generalizability due to setting or methodology. For example, many studies have been performed in tertiary care, academic hospital settings. It is unclear how findings from this setting translate to other settings. Also, methodologies vary widely from study to study, hindering comparisons.

Examples of currently available solutions

Several data sources can be used to assess the frequency of medication errors. These include claims data, claims data linked with other types of clinical information such as laboratory data, electronic medical record information including that from computerized order entry or pharmacy systems, chart review, and direct observation. Spontaneous reporting can also be used, but underreporting is so great that it is only useful for getting samples of errors, and cannot be used to assess the underlying rate of medication errors in a population (see Chapter 7).

Claims data have the great advantage that they can be obtained for very large numbers of individuals (see Chapter 8). However, it cannot be determined with certainty whether or not the patient actually consumed the medication, and clinical detail is often minimal, making it hard to ask questions that relate to a patient's clinical condition. Searches can be performed for specific diagnoses, but the accuracy of coding is limited for many of the diagnoses of interest, for example renal failure and depression, as well as for outcomes such as renal insufficiency.

Linking claims and other types of data—particularly laboratory results—can substantially expand the range of medication errors that may be detected. For example, it may be possible to assess what proportion of patients exposed to a certain medication has a serum creatinine above a specific level at the time of their initial exposure. Nonetheless, the lack of detailed clinical data can still limit the usefulness of these linked datasets.

Chart review can provide valuable additional clinical information, and can be done to supplement claims studies or studies that link claim information with laboratory information. With the chart, it is possible to understand the clinical context, for example the indication for starting a medication, which can sometimes be inferred but rarely determined with certainty with more limited data sources. Chart review is time consuming and expensive, however.

Electronic medical records can provide the clinical detail available with paper-based chart review, but often at much lower cost. It is also possible to search electronic medical records for specific diagnoses, laboratories, and key words suggesting the presence of outcomes. Such records are only used in a minority of outpatient offices today, but they have become the standard in many other countries in primary care, for example the UK, and are increasing globally. It will be possible to use these records to detect both medication errors and ADEs at much lower costs than was previously possible.

The future

The future of pharmacoepidemiologic research will include large databases that allow linking of prescription information with clinical and claims data. These types of databases will facilitate the studies of medication errors and ADEs. They will also be critical for detecting rare ADEs. Sources of data for these databases will include systems of computerized physician order entry, computerized pharmacy, bar-coding, pharmacy benefit managers, and electronic health records. Standardized coding of data, that is, the uniform coding of drug names, as well as doses and concentrations, will be an important advancement to allow easy analysis.

Other important issues that must be addressed are representing prescriptions in ways that allow determination of total daily dose, joint documentation of prescriptions and dispensing data to allow determination of patient adherence, clear documentation of conditions like pregnancy or weights of pediatric patients, and improved coding of allergies.

Key points for the use of pharmacoepidemiology to study medication errors

• Medication errors are very common, compared to adverse drug events, and relatively few result in injury.
• In most studies, about a third of adverse drug events are preventable.
• The epidemiology of medication errors and adverse drug events has been fairly well described for hospitalized adults, but less information is available for specific populations, and for the ambulatory setting.

• It is possible now to detect many medication errors using large claims databases, and as it becomes possible to link these data with more types of clinical data including especially laboratory and diagnosis data, it will be feasible to more accurately assess the frequency of medication errors across populations.
• The increasing use of electronic health records should have a dramatic effect on our ability to do research in this area using pharmacoepidemiologic techniques.

FDA's Sentinel Initiative: enhancing safety surveillance

In 2008, the US Department of Health and Human Services announced the launch of the Food and Drug Administration's (FDA's) Sentinel Initiative to create the national electronic system for medical product safety surveillance mandated by Congress in the FDA Amendments Act of 2007 (FDAAA). This section describes the goals of the Sentinel Initiative and the associated methodological and operational challenges.

Overview

FDA is responsible for protecting and promoting health by ensuring the safety and efficacy of human drugs, biological products, and medical devices as well as other FDA-regulated products. Postmarketing safety surveillance—monitoring the safety of medical products once they reach the market—is a key component in this effort (see Chapter 7). For decades, FDA has relied primarily on spontaneous reporting systems (see Chapter 7). Yet the information FDA receives from these systems is highly variable and there is substantial underreporting. With the growth in data systems and information technology (IT) and the advances in the science of safety, it has become increasingly practicable to create a framework for active surveillance. A critical milestone occurred in 2007, when Congress passed FDAAA, Section 905 of which called for active postmarketing drug safety surveillance.

From the start, the Sentinel Initiative has been envisioned as a collaborative effort that will explore, and then implement, how to develop a national electronic system, the *Sentinel System*, for monitoring FDA-regulated medical product safety. The system leverages existing automated healthcare data, including administrative claims data, electronic health record (EHR) data, and registries, collected for other purposes (i.e., reimbursement, clinical care, and quality evaluations)—see Chapters 8 and 9. Its role is to augment FDA's existing postmarketing safety surveillance systems by giving FDA a tool to *proactively* gather and evaluate information about the postmarketing safety of its regulated medical products.

Despite a number of critical scientific, technical, and policy challenges, which are discussed in more detail here, significant progress has been made since the initiative's launch in 2008. A critical milestone was reached when the Mini-Sentinel pilot program implemented its rapid response capability in 2011. The pilot project is a collaboration of FDA and over 30 collaborating institutions, of which 17 of those are data partners from across the country and encompass the data of over 130 million patients. Mini-Sentinel is already demonstrating rapid analysis of medical product safety questions (see Case example 22.8). FDA scientists are getting responses to their queries in a matter of weeks, as compared to months or even longer using traditional surveillance methods, realizing a key benefit of an active surveillance system.

The Sentinel System: implementing active surveillance

Active surveillance allows assessments in specific populations using comparator groups and can be conducted using a variety of methodological approaches. Active surveillance can be medical product-based, identifying adverse events in patients taking certain products; setting-based, identifying adverse events in certain healthcare settings where patients are likely to present for treatment (e.g., emergency departments); or event-based, identifying adverse events likely to be associated with medical products (e.g., acute liver failure).

The initial approach being tested in Sentinel Initiative pilots (e.g., Mini-Sentinel) combines medical product- and event-based approaches. Active surveillance of postmarketing medical product safety typically involves a series of steps, including *signal generation, signal refinement,* and *signal evaluation*. FDA has defined a *safety signal* as a concern about an excess of adverse events compared to what is expected to be associated with a product's use. For purposes of this discussion, adverse event means any untoward medical occurrence associated with the use of a drug in humans, whether or not considered drug related. *Signal generation* is an approach that uses statistical methods to identify a possible safety signal, often times without prespecifying a particular medical product exposure or adverse outcome. *Signal refinement* is a process by which an identified safety signal is further evaluated to determine whether evidence exists to support a relationship between the exposure and the outcome. Depending on how and when during a product's life cycle a safety signal is identified, a number of approaches for signal refinement (e.g., re-examination of data from the clinical development program or conduct of a pharmacoepidemiologic study) can be pursued. Should the signal refinement assessment provide evidence supporting an association between the product exposure and the adverse outcome, it may be necessary to conduct additional analyses to further evaluate the signal. *Signal evaluation* is conducted to ensure that the medical product adverse outcome relationship is not spurious; this process will also likely provide more information about the safety signal, particularly if source record verification is included.

Information gained from any source, including the Sentinel System, is considered along with all other data about the safety signal coming from a variety of other sources, including the premarketing development program, spontaneous reports, and other postmarketing studies to help FDA staff make a regulatory decision.

Investigations informing foundational aspects of the Sentinel System

The launch of the Sentinel Initiative has raised a number of administrative, organizational, and procedural challenges. From the start, FDA has encouraged the participation of all interested stakeholders, recognizing that success will depend on

---

Case Example 22.8: For FDA's Sentinel Initiative

Background

- Olmesartan (Benicar), an angiotensin II receptor blocker (ARB) is approved for the treatment of hypertension, alone or with other antihypertensive agents. Several Adverse Event Reporting System (AERS) cases reporting celiac disease in association with olmesartan use were identified. Similar cases were not identified with use of other ARBs, indicating a potential signal for risk of celiac disease with olmesartan.

Question

- Is the rate of celiac disease higher in incident users of olmesartan than other drugs in the same class?

Approach

- To improve programming efficiency and facilitate rapid querying of data held by Mini-Sentinel Data partners, the Mini-Sentinel Operations Center has developed modular programs to accomplish common tasks. Each program has several required input parameters and the output contains summary-level counts stratified by various parameters (e.g., age group, sex, year).

- The modular program used evaluates the rate of specified outcomes (defined by ICD-9-CM diagnosis codes) among those with incident use of specified products in the outpatient pharmacy dispensing file (defined by National Drug Codes, NDC), with or without a preexisting condition (defined by ICD-9-CM diagnosis codes).

- To be able to identify incident users, those with a prescription within the previous 365 days were excluded. Analyses were also conducted using a washout period of 91 and 183 days.

- In order to identify incident cases, those with a diagnosis of celiac disease (ICD-9 code 579.0) within the previous 365 days were excluded.

Results

- The rates of celiac disease were similar in the olmesartan and other ARB groups.

- These results provide a level of reassurance that the signal detected in AERs (olmesartan and celiac disease) is not supported with claims data.

Strengths

- Rapid results from Mini-Sentinel provide useful information to contribute to FDA's overall knowledge and evaluation of a potential safety issue.

Limitation

- No source record validation was completed to ensure the predictive value of the algorithm used to identify cases of celiac disease. Therefore, the capture of events may be incomplete or may include irrelevant events.

Key points

- The Mini-Sentinel assessment using a modular program provided useful information to FDA that contributed to its understanding of a potential safety issue.

---

the ability to engage national expertise and secure the commitment of all interested parties. As FDA has worked to develop Sentinel, the guiding principles have included:

- *Integrity*: The management structure and data analysis components of Sentinel must be insulated from undue influence.
- *Privacy protection and data security*: It is a fundamental part of FDA's ongoing responsibilities as FDA fulfills its mission to protect public health, including under Sentinel, to safeguard the privacy and security of directly identifiable data and all information FDA receives.

- *Systems approach*: Effective life-cycle safety surveillance of medical products requires a systems approach, including participation of all stakeholders.
- *Transparency*: Sentinel's governance structure and processes should incorporate a broad range of expertise and experience as well as address both apparent and actual conflicts of interest.

A key finding from initial outreach activities was that a *distributed data system* would be the preferred approach for organizing the active surveillance system. A distributed system allows data to be maintained in the local environment, as opposed to a centralized approach which would consolidate data into one physical location. The benefits of this distributed approach include the maintenance of patient privacy by keeping directly identifiable patient information behind local firewalls in its existing protected environment. And because the data partners are completely familiar with their healthcare systems, the distributed system enables their involvement in running analyses, ensuring an informed approach to interpreting results.

In 2009, FDA took the first steps to establish Sentinel and competed and awarded a contract to Harvard Pilgrim Health Care Institute (HPHC) to pilot a miniature Sentinel System (Mini-Sentinel). As part of the pilot, HPHC is using a distributed data system. A goal of the Mini-Sentinel pilot is to create a laboratory that gives FDA the opportunity to test epidemiologic and statistical methods and learn more about some of the barriers and challenges, both internal and external, to establishing the Sentinel System. Another important goal of the Mini-Sentinel is to pilot the Coordinating Center model that will enable FDA to submit queries to participating data partners who in turn return data, usually in the form of rates or counts.

The Mini-Sentinel Coordinating Center (MSCC) and participating data partners are using a common data model as the basis for their analytic approach. This approach requires data partners to transform their data into a standard format. With all data in a common format, the MSCC writes computer programs for a given query, and each participating data partner runs the query in their dataset. Participating organizations send only summaries of their results to the MSCC for further evaluation and to compile the findings to send to FDA. The use of a common analytic program minimizes the potential for differences in results across data partners. HPHC is ensuring that data use complies with the Health Insurance Portability and Accountability Act (HIPAA, see Chapter 15). As currently envisioned, all analyses of data are to be performed by the data partners in their secure environments with minimal, if any, transfer of directly identifiable data.

Clinical problems to be addressed by pharmacoepidemiologic research

Marketed medical products are required by federal law to be safe for their intended use in the intended population. A *safe* medical product is one that has reasonable risks, given the magnitude of the benefit expected and the alternatives available. Despite the rigorous US drug development and approval process (see Chapters 1 and 6), well-conducted, randomized, controlled clinical trials cannot uncover every medical product-related safety problem, nor are they expected to do so. In most cases, clinical trials aren't large enough, diverse enough, or long enough in duration to provide all the information on a product's performance and safety. Clinical trials are unlikely to detect relatively rare, serious adverse events that would not be expected to occur in a population the size of a premarketing development program, nor would clinical trials identify adverse events with long latency periods or in subpopulations who have not participated in studies. Furthermore, as new medical products enter the market, the potential for interactions with other drugs, biologics, medical devices, and foods increases. Evaluating and updating the evolving safety profile of a medical product, as larger numbers of more diverse patients are exposed during marketing, is a substantive clinical problem. FDA must make sure that patients and providers have the up-to-date information they need to inform the safe use of medical products.

Over the past decade, our understanding of disease origins at the molecular level and our increasing knowledge about the role genes play in how drugs are metabolized are expanding our understanding of how and why medical products cause unintended effects (see Chapter 14). Advances in statistical and epidemiologic methods for active surveillance, combined with advances in medical informatics, are enabling researchers to generate and confirm hypotheses about the existence and causes of safety signals with specific products in defined populations. FDA has begun applying these new techniques to its process for monitoring medical product performance and safety, beginning when a medical product is first being developed on through the application and marketing phases. This life-cycle approach allows safety signals generated at any point during development or marketing to be considered within benefit–risk considerations to inform regulatory decisions and patient care. FDA regards improving the quantification of the benefit–risk analysis to be one of the important facets of the science of safety that urgently requires additional development.

The science of safety also offers new opportunities for addressing a fundamental dilemma: the tradeoff between safety and access. A clear example of this occurs when FDA, after analysis of a safety signal, considers whether or not to withdraw a drug from the market for safety reasons. Although withdrawal eliminates the possibility of further adverse events, it also deprives those patients for whom the drug may be of benefit despite the risks involved. If, using methods being developed today, we can determine that an adverse event is restricted to a small, identifiable segment of the population, the drug, biologic, or device could potentially remain on the market and continue to benefit those who are not subject to the event.

Methodological problems to be addressed by pharmacoepidemiologic research

The complex requirements of the Sentinel System have raised a number of technologic, methodological, and operational challenges. Particularly significant methodological challenges include achieving the goal of real-time or near real-time surveillance; designing an active surveillance assessment that produces actionable information in a reasonable time frame; validating a potential safety signal; managing uncertainties in interpreting summary measures from multiple observational data sources; and developing new methods for signal generation. There are also a number of data-related challenges: developing and implementing harmonized data standards; linking data sources to enhance the duration of observation; and enabling access to outcomes that might not be captured in the local database (e.g., device registries, National Death Index). Operational challenges that must be addressed involve facilitating a national dialogue on issues and establishing relevant policies, developing a governance approach, and ensuring privacy and data security.

Factors affecting the ability to conduct near real-time surveillance

The timing of safety assessment in the postmarketing period will vary by medical product. For some products, the premarketing development database will suggest that certain signals need immediate postmarketing assessment. For other products, assessments will be needed at a later point during product marketing when an unexpected safety signal emerges. The ability to conduct near real-time surveillance using the Sentinel System will be affected by how quickly a medical product is *taken up* into the marketplace as well as how often data sources are *updated* with new exposures and outcomes of interest as they occur.

Validating a safety signal

It is crucial to minimize the opportunity for false positive results. When applying the Maximized Sequential Probability Ratio Test (maxSPRT) that has been developed for real-time monitoring of vaccine-related adverse outcomes (see "Vaccine safety" section in this chapter), investigators often use two types of control groups: matched controls and historical expected counts. Recognizing that the claims data submitted on a weekly basis for monitoring become more complete over time, subsequent confirmatory analyses are sometimes conducted later in the evaluation period to take advantage of more mature data. Another technique that has been applied to assess potential biological plausibility of a safety signal is the use of a temporal scan statistic to test for temporal clustering in the postexposure time period. Additionally, logistic regression analyses, adjusting for relevant covariates, are sometimes conducted to assess potential associations. Validation of coded diagnoses against source records may also be conducted. If a signal persists, investigators may conduct additional analyses or design a full study to test the hypotheses raised by the signal.

Many similar issues will have to be considered as safety signals emerge from active surveillance assessments conducted for drugs, biologics, and devices. Assessments of safety signals for medical products used in sick patients (in contrast to vaccines, which are generally given to healthy individuals) will present additional methodological issues, in particular, confounding by indication.

An additional issue that must be grappled with is the question of whether the same database can be used for both signal generation and signal evaluation. One practice is to split a database so that different data are used for signal generation component and the hypothesis confirmation component. However, other researchers advocate for the use of an independent data source to test hypotheses. Work is ongoing to determine the optimal approach to this complex issue.

Interpreting summary measures from multiple observational data sources

In a distributed system, data partners run assessment on their data and return only summaries to the Coordinating Center. Some methods used to assess safety signals may generate counts that would then be summed by the Coordinating Center, whereas other methods would generate a summary relative incidence estimate at each individual site.

How to interpret varying estimates of the strength of the safety signal from individual sites remains unclear. As noted above, the data being leveraged for surveillance are being collected for other purposes (e.g., insurance reimbursement, clinical care). Because each institution has a unique way in which it uses its formularies and applies diagnostic coding practices, variations in the results of a safety signal assessment may be driven by variations in institutional practices.

Additionally, in considering whether and how such results can be combined, one source of information is the guidelines on meta-analyses of observational studies (see Chapter 19). Meta-analysis of any type of data require consideration of various important issues. Observational studies have additional complexities because observational studies are prone to certain confounding and biases that are not an issue with randomized trials. One of the major concerns, heterogeneity of study design, is addressed by the use of a centralized analytic

approach run on data that have been standardized in a common data model. However, evaluation of other sources of heterogeneity (e.g., patient population, formulary variation, prescribing practices, approach to diagnostic coding) must be assessed. Ultimately, a combined estimate of the strength of the safety signal is informative. However, understanding of heterogeneous results across data partners, if it occurs, may also be informative

Developing new methods for signal generation

Based on strategic and resource considerations, FDA has elected to focus initially on developing signal refinement capabilities. Ultimately, however, the initiative will turn its attention to signal generation.

Statistical methods for signal generation are used in many fields—developing spam filters and identifying credit card misuse are two examples. However, the risk attendant to any signal generation effort with medical product safety is the potentially significant public health effect of a false–positive signal. In addition to the resources, both financial and personnel, required to discern true positive signals from false positive signals, there are consequences that must be considered when determining when to communicate a safety signal identified using signal generation techniques. Patients who learn that their medical therapy is being evaluated for a safety risk may inappropriately discontinue the therapy. The discontinuation may be inappropriate because the safety concern is not substantiated or because even with that particular risk, the potential benefit to the patient justifies the potential risk. Additionally, in this era of increased access to information, we must be mindful of the potential effect on healthcare practitioners related to alert fatigue. FDA would like to minimize the risk of desensitizing healthcare practitioners and the public to alerts of public health importance by not communicating false–positive safety signals.

Over the past decade, those working in pharmacovigilance (e.g., FDA, pharmaceutical companies, academia, vendors, see Chapter 6), have developed data mining methods for signal generation as part of their efforts to analyze spontaneous reports.

More recently, these methods are being applied to health care databases. FDA will be examining research to maximize the collection of actionable information from signal generation methods while minimizing the occurrence of false positives.

Data infrastructure needs to conduct active surveillance

To achieve a modern health information environment, we need to enhance and integrate three key information management domains: (1) *access* to information; (2) *interfaces*, or user-friendly tools, supported by a robust IT architecture, to convert information efficiently into knowledge; and (3) *standards* that are used by all to facilitate information exchange. These three domains interact to influence our efficiency at receiving, managing, and communicating information.

Data structure

Because the Sentinel System is intended to be a distributed system with data held in local environments, FDA evaluated the optimal characteristics of a possible database model for such a system. The conclusions were that a common data model would facilitate the conduct of active surveillance assessments. A common data model standardizes specific data elements used for surveillance, allowing for the development of centralized analytic programs that can be run in participating data partner environments. A common data model has a number of advantages, including, for example, reducing the need for complex metadata and data mapping activities; ensuring that all data partners are using the same terms to describe the same concepts; enabling a centralized analytic approach; and creating common language for use across data sources for assessments. However, this also requires substantial start-up effort and continued resources to perform data updates since near real-time active surveillance requires updating data elements on a regular schedule.

Data Standards

The Sentinel System is predicated on the secondary use of existing automated healthcare data to obtain a better understanding of medical product safety. The lack of a standard format for the storage and exchange of data slows the sharing of information among key stakeholders, making it cumbersome and manually labor intensive. The development and use of terminology standards for important data elements used by the Sentinel System, particularly for electronic health records (EHRs), will greatly facilitate the creation of analytical tools. Standardizing data elements and terminologies is critical to any attempt to achieve a modern electronic approach to monitoring medical product safety.

Database linkages

As part of the foundational work that FDA is doing to inform the Sentinel System, the agency must understand what data are collected, the duration of patient observation, and the completeness of data. This is particularly important given our fragmented healthcare system where Americans receive healthcare from a myriad of organizations. The ability to link individuals across health insurer systems (as they switch insurance carriers) and EHR systems (as they switch providers) enables long-term follow-up and removes a substantial limitation of current observational studies using routinely collected healthcare information. It would also diminish the risk of patients being double counted because they appear in more than one healthcare system or administrative claims database. Beyond linking across healthcare practitioners and systems, there is also the need for the Sentinel System to link to external data sources such as vital statistics databases or registries (e.g., National Center for Health Statistics, birth and death registries, tumor registries) to capture patient data beyond that found in administrative claims databases or EHRs.

Although integration of multiple disparate sources could improve the understanding of each patient as he or she encounters the healthcare system, such integration across systems requires surmounting substantial regulatory, privacy, and technical challenges (see also Chapter 15). In order for the Sentinel System to realize its full potential, it will have to overcome these obstacles related to linking information at the patient level.

Operational challenges

In addition to the methodological challenges noted above, there are numerous operational challenges underlying the development of a system such as the one envisioned. FDA has, with public input, begun creating the foundation for what is hoped to be a valuable national resource to help improve the informed, safe use of medical products.

Governance

Although FDA is taking the lead in the Sentinel Initiative, as already mentioned, collaboration is critical, and expertise and resources need to be shared to the greatest extent possible. FDA has also concluded that its statutory mandates require it to exert substantial control over certain activities. Thus, a portion of Sentinel operations must remain under agency control. This model is also being tested as part of the Mini-Sentinel contract. A major challenge in the years ahead will be to develop a governance framework for the national resource portion that ensures broad participation and reflects a sustainable business model.

Privacy and security

Since the launch of the Sentinel Initiative, FDA has engaged thought leaders in the privacy and security field. One of the first contracts awarded under the initiative involved identifying and analyzing potential privacy issues (see Chapter 15). We have already described above how a distributed system approach maintains patient privacy by maintaining directly identifiable patient information with data partners behind local firewalls.

However, as we have begun to grapple with the realities of conducting active medical product surveillance, we have come to understand that there may be infrequent occurrences when de-identified datasets may not be sufficient. For example, if it becomes necessary to validate a coded outcome against source records, it may be necessary to access protected health information (PHI). In some cases, if claims data are used for an assessment, some elements of PHI (e.g., month, year of an exposure) may need to be transferred from the healthcare environment that delivered the care to the claims environment that is conducting the assessment for validation of findings. There may also be instances when information must be shared between data partners and a Coordinating Center, or among data partners, as noted previously. FDA is actively exploring methods and techniques to ensure that only the minimum amount of PHI leaves its local environment to meet the needs of a specific assessment.

In addition to HIPAA (see Box 22.1), other privacy and security regulations will apply to the Sentinel System. The Sentinel System will have to be protected in accordance with the Federal Information Security Management Act (FISMA), issued in 2002. FDA recognizes that attention must also be paid to computer security with respect to the transmission of queries and result summaries, and FDA will require implementation of policies and procedures to ensure such security at each stage of the process.

Examples of currently available solutions

Today, FDA uses a number of programs and tools to carry out postmarketing surveillance, but efforts focus primarily on its spontaneous adverse events reporting system, a mostly passive system comprising the Adverse Event Reporting System (AERS) (see Chapter 7), the Vaccine Adverse Event Reporting System (VAERS) (see "Vaccine safety" section in this chapter), and the Manufacturer and User Facility Device Experience (MAUDE) Database (see "Epidemiologic studies of implantable medical device" section). As efforts to develop the Sentinel System continue, FDA is increasingly looking to learn from active surveillance programs already in place to help inform the development of the Sentinel System. Programs such as the Vaccine Safety Datalink (VSD) have grappled with data infrastructure, methods, and operational challenges that will face the Sentinel System. FDA is studying these programs closely to benefit from the lessons they have learned along the way and apply those lessons to facilitate the development of the Sentinel System.

Box 22.1 HIPPA de-identification

HIPPA allows for de-identification of a dataset by removing the following identifiers of the individual or of relatives, employers, or household members of the individual.

(A) Names
(B) All geographic subdivisions smaller than a State, including street address, city, county, precinct, zip code, and their equivalent geocodes, except for the initial three digits of a zip code if, according to the current publicly available data from the Bureau of Census
   (1) the geographic units formed by combining all zip codes with the same three initial digits contains more than 20 000 people; and
   (2) the initial three digits of a zip code for all such geographic units containing 20 000 or fewer people is changed to 000
(C) All elements of dates (except year) for dates directly related to the individual, including birth date, admission date, discharge date, date of death; and all ages over 89 and all elements of dates (including year) indicative of such age, except that such ages and elements may be aggregated into a single category of age 90 or older;
(D) Telephone numbers;
(E) Fax numbers;
(F) Electronic mail addresses:
(G) Social security numbers;
(H) Medical record numbers;
(I) Health plan beneficiary numbers;
(J) Account numbers;
(K) Certificate/license numbers;
(L) Vehicle identifiers and serial numbers, including license plate numbers;
(M) Device identifiers and serial numbers;
(N) Web Universal Resource Locators (URLs);
(O) Internet Protocol (IP) address numbers;
(P) Biometric identifiers, including finger and voice prints;
(Q) Full face photographic images and any comparable images; and ® any other unique identifying number, characteristic, or code, except as permitted for re-identification purposes provided certain conditions are met.

In addition to the removal of the above-stated identifiers, the covered entity may not have actual knowledge that the remaining information could be used alone or in combination with any other information to identify an individual who is subject of the information.

   ∗ 45 CFR 164.514(b)(2)

The future

Sentinel is a long-term, complex initiative that, by necessity, is being implemented in stages; the initiative is evolving as capabilities, methods, public awareness, public acceptance, and data standardization increase. Although the initiative is already providing FDA with important new capabilities, it is important to balance eagerness for progress with the very real risks inherent in overreaching current capabilities. The overarching challenge of the Sentinel System will be to ensure that it is sufficiently nimble to meet the changing needs of a nation in which the healthcare system is rapidly evolving. This means that the Sentinel System must be poised for integration into other national efforts aimed at secondary uses of healthcare data. Within

that context, it is important to note that this effort will not optimally serve the public until the nation has learned how to integrate clinical care with clinical research. However, if implemented thoughtfully, the initiative can play a major role in ensuring that the ehealth revolution fulfills its promise of addressing the country's broad public health problems.

Key points for FDA's Sentinel Initiative

• Despite a number of scientific, technical, and policy challenges, the Sentinel Initiative reached a critical milestone in 2011 when the Mini-Sentinel pilot program implemented rapid response capabilities, and the pilot is already demonstrating rapid analysis of medical product safety questions for its participants.

• A governance framework must be established for the Sentinel System that permits a portion of the Sentinel System to rest exclusively under FDA control while allowing FDA to partner on those aspects — research on methods and IT infrastructure — that are most logical and efficient to be shared as a national resource.

• It is critical that we train the next generation of experts in this and related fields.

Comparative effectiveness research

The history of comparative effectiveness research in the US

Efforts to increase the use of scientific evidence to inform clinical decisions have been characterized by labels such as *outcomes research, effectiveness research, evidence-based research, health technology assessment,* and, most recently, *comparative effectiveness research* (CER). To combat the perception that the main agenda behind the push for comparative

---

Case Example 22.9: ZODIAC study by Strom *et al.* (2008)

Background

• A novel antipsychotic drug (ziprasidone) with demonstrated efficacy in treatment of schizophrenia and bi-polar mania was known since its development to cause QT prolongation, which may be a risk factor for serious cardiovascular events.

Question

• Does the known modest QT prolongation effect increase the risk of serious cardiovascular morbidity and mortality?

Approach

• Used a randomized large simple trial to assign patients with schizophrenia enrolled in 18 countries to receive either ziprasidone or olanzapine (a second-generation antipsychotic agent without evidence of QT prolongation effect).

• Other than the random assignment to the two treatment groups, physicians and patients were free to change regimens and dosing based on patients' responses to the assigned medication and free to use any concomitant medications.

• Used broad inclusion criteria to enroll patients.

• Neither physicians nor patients were blinded to the treatment allocation.

Results

• Cardiovascular risk factors including hypertension, hyperlipidemia, diabetes, obesity, and smoking were seen to be highly prevalent in this patient population at baseline.

• Use of antihypertensives or statins were reported by a small proportion of patients, suggesting undertreatment of hypertension and hyperlipidemia.

Strengths

• Real world research with patients receiving routine medical care in naturalistic 'real world' practice.

• Limited data collection during the trial did not burden the physicians and patients.

• Random allocation of patients minimized selected bias or channeling bias.

Limitation

• Detailed patient characteristics at baseline were not collected, relying instead on the randomization to create balanced study groups.

• Outcomes other than the primary study outcome of interest were not systematically recorded.

Key Points

• The comparison here between two drugs used for the same indication, one with a known effect on QT prolongation and one without an effect on QT prolongation, can provide more useful information on the association with cardiovascular disease than a comparison between the study drug and a placebo.

effectiveness research is to drive down the cost of health care, Congress has rebranded CER as *patient-centered outcomes research* (PCOR). The major objective of CER is to provide scientific information to patients and clinicians to assist in health care decisions. In this chapter, we will use the more commonly accepted term at the time of this book's publication, comparative effectiveness research.

Earlier government initiatives for effectiveness research in the US were attempted first by the Congressional Office of Technology Assessment, then by the National Center for HealthCare Technology, then by the Agency for Health Care Policy and Research (renamed later the Agency for Healthcare Research and Quality—AHRQ). The next development was the Medicare Prescription Drug, Improvement, and Modernization Act (MMA) of 2003, authorizing AHRQ to support research in the form of systematic reviews and syntheses of the scientific literature, with focus on "outcomes, comparative clinical effectiveness, and appropriateness of health care items such as pharmaceuticals and health care services, including prescription drugs" and the manner in which they are organized, managed, and delivered. Substantial federal funding was provided as well. Separately, the Department of Veterans Affairs (VA) and the Centers for Medicare and Medicaid Services (CMS) developed CER programs. The private sector (e.g., Blue Cross/Blue Shield Technology Evaluation Center, and others) similarly initiated evidence-based medicine projects, and CER publications have been increasing since at least the early 1980s.

Congress advanced CER by creating the Federal Coordinating Council for Comparative Effectiveness Research to coordinate CER across the Federal government, and by commissioning the Institute of Medicine (IOM) to formulate national priorities for CER to guide the allocation of research funds productively. The reports from the Federal Coordinating Council and the IOM provided a working definition of CER and a list of 100 research priorities. As part of the 2010 Patient Protection and Affordable Care Act, Congress created the Patient Centered Outcomes Research Institute (PCORI) to implement the national agenda for CER funded by public and private sources.

History of comparative effectiveness research outside the US

CER has also been adopted formally by the governments of other countries, primarily in Europe. The National Institute for Health and Clinical Excellence (NICE) in the United Kingdom (UK), created in 1999, represents one model for using CER to inform policy research and practice. To help reduce variation in clinical practice and to standardize the quality of care, the primary mandate for NICE has been to evaluate health technology, surgical and diagnostic procedures, and public health interventions for disease prevention, and to develop evidence-based clinical guidelines for these.

Other European governments have also made considerable efforts to incorporate CER into health policy decisions, using different approaches for organizing these efforts. These countries differ on the degree to which they "produce" CER (i.e., conduct evidence synthesis, systematic reviews, and clinical and economic studies (in the UK, Germany, Sweden) or "use" existing CER, relying principally on evidence submitted by the manufacturers (in Denmark, France, the Netherlands). These countries favor comparative evidence obtained from randomized clinical trials, separate entities for handling the evaluation of drugs and of medical technologies, and linking evaluations ultimately to reimbursement decisions.

Definition of effectiveness

In contrast to an investigation of *drug efficacy* which asks whether a drug *has the ability* to bring about the intended effect (i.e., in an ideal world, with perfect adherence, no interactions with other drugs or other diseases, etc., *could* the drug achieve its intended effects?), an investigation of *drug effectiveness* asks whether, in the real world, a drug *in fact* achieves its desired effect. For example, a drug given in experimental conditions might be able to lower blood pressure, but if it causes such severe sedation that patients refuse to ingest it, it will not be effective. Thus, an efficacious drug may lack effectiveness.

Definitions of comparative effectiveness research

The US Congressional Budget Office report of December 2007 defined comparative effectiveness research as:

> a rigorous evaluation of the impact of different options that are available for treating a given medical condition for a particular set of patients. Such a study may compare similar treatments, such as competing drugs, or it may analyze very different approaches, such as surgery and drug therapy.

In the IOM report of December 2010, CER was defined as:

> The generation and synthesis of evidence that compares the benefits and harms of alternative methods to prevent, diagnose, treat, and monitor a clinical condition or to improve the delivery of care. The purpose of CER is to assist patients, clinicians, purchasers, policy-makers, and the public to make informed decisions that will improve health care at both the individual and population levels.

In the US Federal Coordinating Council report of December 2010, CER was similarly defined as:

> the conduct and synthesis of research comparing the benefits and harms of different interventions and strategies to prevent, diagnose, treat and monitor health conditions in "real world" settings. The purpose of this research is to improve health outcomes by developing and disseminating evidence-based information to patients, clinicians, and other decision-makers, responding to their expressed needs, about which interventions are most effective for which patients under specific circumstances.

By these definitions, CER includes three key elements: (1) evidence synthesis (identifying and summarizing existing data addressing a question), (2) evidence generation (creating new data addressing a question), and (3) evidence dissemination (distributing the available data, with the goal of modifying patient care). Its key elements include the study of effectiveness, rather than efficacy, and that it compares among alternative strategies.

Another key element invoked by the recent US CER initiative is that of inclusiveness of participants in the process. As conceived in the IOM's recommendations for "a robust national CER enterprise," this should involve a continuous process that considers and prioritizes topics for CER research and funding to address current knowledge gaps about diseases and conditions, and a process that continuously includes the participation by caregivers, patients, and consumers to provide input regarding issues of public concern. Slutsky *et al.* (2010) states that priorities for CER research must be based on input from all stakeholders in health care; research and synthesis must apply to a wide range of health care services; and the results must be made accessible to multiple audiences. However, most other countries have excluded the vendors of the technologies being evaluated from the CER process, to avoid commercial bias.

Most CER to date has dealt with the effects of medications, which is one reason why the field is of great interest to pharmacoepidemiologists. However, the full scope of CER is much broader as it seeks to address the continuum of medical interventions and seeks to encompass beneficial and adverse outcomes as well as economic implications, and encourages the use of new data, new analyses of existing data, and systematic reviews of research reports (published or unpublished), and focuses attention not only on knowledge creation but also on strategies for implementation.

Clinical problems to be addressed by pharmacoepidemiologic research

In one sense, CER is narrower than pharmacoepidemiology because it places emphasis on "head-to-head" comparisons of the safety and benefits of treatments and diagnostic strategies, to identify "best-in-class" treatments, in the real world, whereas pharmacoepidemiology often compares users to non-users. Yet, CER extends beyond pharmacoepidemiology because it can include nondrug interventions, comparing not only similar treatments but also different diagnostic tests, care delivery systems, etc.

The goals of CER are therefore: (a) to inform decisions among alternative clinical options, (b) to put new technology into proper perspective versus older technology, (c) to increase use of more effective clinical options and decrease use of less effective treatments, and (d) to identify subgroups of patients more likely to respond to some treatments than others. A consequence of achieving these goals could also be a reduction in health care costs through avoidance of treatments that do not work or are less effective than alternatives.

Current deficiencies in health care highlight the contributions that CER can make to address these. According to a 2007 IOM report, "the rate with which new interventions are introduced into the medical marketplace is currently outpacing the rate at which information is generated on their effectiveness and circumstances of best use," and "less than half of all medical care is based on or supported by adequate evidence about its effectiveness."

The major gaps in the current knowledge base about treatment interventions, according to Slutsky, are lack of information about how a treatment works in actual clinical practice, in contrast with how it works in the contrived settings of clinical trials; lack of information about the comparative effectiveness of treatment options; and lack of information about how variation in patient characteristics affects treatment effectiveness. The disparities in utilization of various treatments, observed among hospitals, providers, and geographic locations, may be attributed partly to these knowledge gaps.

CER investigations will aim to redress these information gaps, while including all relevant stakeholders and decision makers. However, inclusion of all stakeholders and decision makers in the process of priority setting, study design, and implementation of results may be over-simplistic and possibly counterproductive. The involvement of participants from such range of backgrounds, orientations, and value judgments may create a cumbersome process, bogged by conflict, and likely to prolong the discovery process and introduce commercial bias. How these conflicting goals, inclusiveness vs. expediting unbiased results, will be reconciled remains to be resolved.

As also envisioned in the IOM's report, CER will measure benefits and harms that are important to patients and will produce "results at the population and subgroup levels, and clinical prediction rules to identify patients likely to benefit from an intervention." Traditional efficacy studies typically report average effects, disregarding variability in patient responses. However, providers must make decisions about treatment choices for patients whose profiles are not comparable to the average of study participants in the efficacy trials. An important goal for CER is to explore heterogeneity, looking for subgroups of patients who benefit more (or less) from a given intervention. CER should be used to explore patient variability, and with advances in molecular biology, this may become increasingly possible (see Chapter 14).

To increase generalizability, CER should include data from patients and physicians from a wide range of care settings. Traditional clinical trials are typically conducted by investigators affiliated with tertiary care hospitals. The vision for CER is that it will provide opportunities for community hospitals and practices to become involved.

Methodological problems to be addressed by pharmacoepidemiologic research

Issues for evidence synthesis

The synthesis of new and existing information features prominently in definitions of CER. Meta-analysis specifies an approach for performing structured, systematic reviews of published data and for the synthesis of analytic findings by means of formal statistical analysis, to provide an overall measure of effect as a summary of those findings, when appropriate. The advantages of combining results are increased statistical power to detect significant effects of treatments and increased precision of estimates, by virtue of the large number of patients pooled across studies. The advantage of large numbers from studies based on multiple population groups also makes possible the detection of effects in subgroups of patients. Meta-analysis also considers the variations in study design, study settings, and methods of analysis, to explain possible sources of variation among study findings and contradictory conclusions in the literature. To be most useful, meta-analyses should include a broad range of data sources, including unpublished data.

However, the strengths of meta-analyses are mitigated by their own methodological problems. As discussed by Simmonds *et al.* (2005), these include disagreement among experts about which studies to include or exclude from a meta-analysis, which outcome end-points to consider, how to pool studies that differ in design and method—all of which can affect the summary findings of meta-analyses. In addition, limitations in the original studies can influence conclusions from the pooled studies. Also, reviewers of the same studies may reach different conclusions because of varying expertise or because of differences in values. In addition, meta-analysis requires regular updates to keep it relevant for clinical guidelines as new information continuously becomes available. Also, the conclusions from pooled published results tend to be biased because of preferential selectivity to publish studies with statistically significant results and with stronger treatment effects.

Issues for evidence generation

Nonexperimental studies

Most CER studies to date have been conducted using nonexperimental study designs. Indeed, since CER seeks to study the effects of interventions in the real world, nonexperimental approaches can be uniquely useful. Further, since one is comparing the effects of different interventions, rather than comparing an intervention to an unexposed group, one is looking to detect smaller differences, and this in turn will require larger sample sizes. Here, too, nonexperimental study designs can be logistically more feasible.

As noted by the IOM report, CER studies should rely on multiple types of data sources, including primary data sources (medical and pharmacy records, electronic medical records, and *de novo* data generated through clinical trials or observational studies) and secondary data sources (administrative claims and clinical registries). Using linked multiple data sources can provide still more powerful tools, enriching the data and enlarging the samples for study. However, the challenge to linking data from multiple sources is the need for standardized variables to permit identical computerized queries to be submitted and executed across data resources and standardized format for returning responses from different databases. To be able to access the data and to be able to interpret the analytic findings from the data correctly, familiarity with the logical organization and content of disparate databases is required. There are also logistical problems in accessing these data sources, including issues of ownership of data, difficulty in obtaining institutional review board approval, infrastructure, governance, data security, and privacy.

Nonrandomized CER studies of intended effects, however, are more susceptible to confounding by indication than nonrandomized studies of unintended effects. Studies of intended drug effects present a special methodological problem of confounding by the indication for therapy. In these situations, the risk factor under study is the drug being evaluated and the outcome variable under study is the clinical condition that the drug is supposed to change (cure, ameliorate, or prevent). In clinical practice, if one assumes prescribers are rational, one would expect treated patients to differ from untreated patients, as the former have an indication for the treatment. To the extent that the indication is related to the outcome variable as well, the indication can function as a confounding variable.

Confounding by the indication for the treatment is less of a problem when a study is focusing on unintended drug effects, or side effects, whether they are harmful or beneficial. In this situation, the indication for treatment is less likely to be related to the outcome variable under study.

Confounding by the indication for the treatment also may seem less of a problem when doing comparisons among alternative treatments, since both study groups have the indication for treatment. However, this is not to say that nonrandomized studies comparing therapeutic alternatives are necessarily free from confounding by indication. The true indication for a treatment is much more subtle than simply the regulator-approved indication. For example, people prescribed a calcium channel blocker as initial treatment for their hypertension are likely to be different from those prescribed a diuretic, with the former being more likely to have preexisting angina and less likely to have diabetes. Unless choice between the alternatives is effectively random, confounding by indication remains an issue in comparative studies. Indeed, given one is looking to detect differences that are likely to be smaller (compared to studies comparing exposed subjects to unexposed subjects), subtle confounding by indication can be even more problematic.

Considerable effort has been undertaken to develop more effective methods for controlling confounding, e.g., propensity scores, instrumental variables, etc., in studies based on administrative or other observational data. However, it is important to keep in mind that most approaches (including propensity scores) are still dependent on identifying and measuring those variables that are the true predictors of therapeutic choice. Identifying and measuring, and thereby adjusting for, everything important is often not possible. Approaches like instrumental variables are promising alternatives. However, finding valid instruments in pharmacoepidemiology is extremely difficult. Much more work is needed in these areas, to advance the field of CER.

Standards for performing and reporting observational studies were provided by several professional associations.

Experimental studies

For the reasons described above, the use of clinical trial designs will always be of paramount importance for generating new evidence on CER. However, CER will focus on using clinical trial designs that are flexible, adaptive, pragmatic, practical, efficient (all the different terms used to refer to this new design), in contrast to the traditional randomized, blinded, placebo-controlled clinical trials.

Traditional clinical trials are typically inadequate to address comparative effectiveness. The major limitation of traditional randomized clinical trials is their rigid protocols. These include eligibility criteria that exclude patients with comorbid conditions,

pregnant women, or ethnic minorities; specification of only a few study outcomes, and mostly short-term outcomes; and artificial study settings that do not resemble clinical practice in the "real world" and do not resemble patient adherence with recommended therapy regimen in the "real world." Traditional clinical trials are also complex and time-consuming, and thus not feasible for comparing interventions as evidence accumulates over longer periods of time about the natural history of the medical conditions and the treatments studied. In contrast, pragmatic clinical trials include patients with comorbid conditions and from diverse demographic backgrounds, providers from community settings instead of only tertiary settings, comparator treatments that are in use in clinical practice (rather than placebo controls), variations in the treatment as patients respond differently, and outcomes that matter to patients and clinicians rather than investigators and drug companies. These aspects of pragmatic clinical trials represent normal real world conditions.

Pragmatic clinical trials raise their own problems. The liberal inclusion criteria characteristic of this study design assures greater representativeness of the study groups, but this increased heterogeneity can decrease the probability of detecting a given treatment effect as statistically significant. The larger samples used by pragmatic trials make them more expensive than smaller trials. Pragmatic clinical trials emphasize evaluation of long-term outcomes, which requires greater resources because of the need to follow-up study groups over long periods. Loss to follow-up over time and/or nonadherence over time can introduce bias. The lack of blinding in pragmatic trials creates potential for biased observations and a threat to internal validity. Another limitation of this type of trial results from the flexible treatment protocols preferred. Specifically, these trials involve the participation of community providers in their usual practice. Accordingly, they can vary the treatment process to different patients depending on the variable responses to therapy and they can vary the dose and regimen in the same patients over time. This flexibility enables assessment of outcomes of the composite treatment, but precludes assessment of particular components within the treatment process.

Other limitations are inherent in all clinical trials. Some interventions cannot be investigated with clinical trials because of ethical considerations, even though such trials may be preferred scientifically. Further, the strength of a clinical trial is also one of its weaknesses; it can answer only a very focused question, and there are inevitably many others that also need to be answered, to place a treatment in its appropriate context in our therapeutic armamentarium. Finally, given the cost of clinical trials, it is not practical to undertake them for most CER questions. Thus, much of CER will continue to use the techniques of nonexperimental pharmacoepidemiology for the foreseeable future, but their limitations must always be kept in mind in interpreting the emerging results.

Issues for evidence dissemination

Dissemination has several distinct goals. One goal involves identifying priority topics and information available on these topics and developing objective interpretations of this information, as provided by the Cochrane Collaboration reviews, for example. The output from this research becomes the source information for dissemination to clinicians, patients, and policy-makers. Another goal involves knowledge translation, using this information to draft clinical guidelines. The IOM proposed standards for developing trustworthy clinical practice guidelines. A third goal involves knowledge exchange and utilization, achieved by the actual distribution of information to educate clinicians, patients, and policy-makers about current knowledge and best practice. A final goal involves monitoring and assessment of whether the above efforts translate into actual good practice and to identify which means of dissemination have a greater chance to create an impact. Each of these goals presents challenges that will require creative approaches to accomplish successfully.

Examples of currently available solutions

Organizational approaches

AHRQ's EHC program has supported since 1997 Evidence-Based Practice Centers (EPCs), which focus on evidence synthesis. These centers produce comparative effectiveness reviews on medications, devices, and other health care services.

AHRQ's John M. Eisenberg Center for Clinical Decisions and Communications Science translates comparative effectiveness reviews and research reports created by the EHC program into short, easy-to-read guides and tools that can be used by consumers, clinicians, and policy-makers.

AHRQ's EHC program also has supported the DEcIDE (Developing Evidence to Inform Decisions about Effectiveness) Network, a collection of research centers created in 2005. These centers gather new knowledge and information on specific treatments. The DEcIDE Network conducts studies on the outcomes, effectiveness, safety, and usefulness of medical treatments and services.

AHRQ's Centers for Education and Research on Therapeutics (CERTs) is a national initiative to increase awareness of the benefits and harms of new, existing, or combined uses of therapeutics (drugs, medical devices, and biological products) through education and research.

The NIH has also been involved in CER. Historically, NIH has used its CER funding to fund mostly clinical trials, but some nonexperimental studies were funded as well. Given the scale of NIH (budget over $30 billion/year) and its decentralized organization, there is no way to succinctly summarize all of its work in CER, as most of the 27 NIH institutes/centers have been involved. One new locus of CER in NIH is the network of Clinical and Translational Science Awards (CTSAs), which have increasingly been interested in such work. The CTSAs prepared a white paper with recommendations for advancing the CER concepts into practice, in particular promoting the translation of results of clinical and translational research into practice and public policy. NIH also funds multiple different clinical trial research networks, e.g., in HIV/AIDS, asthma, leukemia, drug-induced liver injury, maternal-fetal medicine, and many, many more. As noted above, of the $1.1 billion made available in the Stimulus Act for CER, $400 million was targeted to NIH, supplementing the CER activities it was already doing.

In addition, PCORI is a nonprofit organization charged to fund research projects that provide evidence on how diseases, disorders, and other health conditions can effectively and appropriately be prevented, diagnosed, treated, monitored, and managed. Members of the PCORI Board of Governors have been selected from academia, hospitals, health care industry, and patient organizations, with only two government officials (from NIH and AHRQ) included. The creation of a Methodology Committee of PCORI was also mandated by Congress, to develop standards and methods for the conduct of research, and the translation of research results in a useful and understandable way. PCORI will be funded by the Patient-Centered Outcomes Research Trust Fund, which was allocated $10 million for 2010, $50 million for 2011, and $150 million for 2012. In future years, the Trust Fund will include an annual $2 fee per Medicare beneficiary transferred from the Medicare Trust Fund, and an annual $2 fee per-covered-life assessed on private health plans, adjusted for health expenditure inflation. In total, annual funding for PCORI could be more than $650 million.

Finally, the question of who should be funding CER studies has given rise to a thorny debate, partly motivated by political ideology and partly by business considerations. Some argue that CER should not be funded by government. Since the goal is to compare the benefits and harms of alternative products or medical technologies, it is argued that sponsorship for such studies belongs in the private sector. The counter argument can be made, however, that if the government will not be funding such research, this type of research is not likely to take place, or will not be unbiased. In general, it is often not in the interest of a manufacturer to risk subjecting its product to head-to-head comparison against a competitor's product, with the possibility of losing out in this competition. Further, such comparisons are less likely to be commercially biased if they are funded, designed, and conducted by organizations without an inherent conflict of interest.

Current applications of CER

A survey by Hochman and McCormick of recently published studies of comparative effectiveness found that only one third of studies evaluating medications qualified as comparative effectiveness research and only a minority compared pharmacologic and nonpharmacologic therapies, emphasizing the need for expanding CER. As noted also by the IOM committee, the US "lacks a national infrastructure for learning from the delivery of health care" through research.

The future

Funding

Currently, the predominant source of funding for CER in the US is the federal government, but PCORI is now beginning to provide funding as well. Much of the funding for clinical efficacy research comes from industry sources. In the future, the CER enterprise could be expanded even further if industry were to routinely conduct and sponsor comparative trials with products being proposed for marketing. In this new CER environment, given the results of CER studies will be used by payors and providers, it is possible that companies will also invest resources, allowing them to compete on the utility of their products rather than competing just on their marketing ability.

In view of these prospects for expanded funding of CER, the future of CER seems promising. However, the effectiveness of this program will depend also on building an infrastructure to sustain CER in the long term.

Human capital development

As noted by the Federal Coordinating Council, training will be required of new researchers to apply the specialized methods of CER and to develop CER methods. Specialized skills are needed to perform traditional randomized clinical trials and novel pragmatic trials; to perform formal meta-analyses and nonexperimental studies; to access and link various databases; to translate the findings into practice guidelines and for dissemination. CER's emphasis on community participation and inclusion will require experts from many different fields and backgrounds to find a common language to communicate productively with each other. Thus, it is necessary to develop and support training programs for researchers seeking careers in CER.

Cost containment

A major issue for the future is the use of CER results to control health care costs. Critics of CER fear that the results of CER will inevitably affect reimbursement decisions by public and private payers, being used for rationing health services. However, in fact, health care rationing already occurs, either implicitly or explicitly; therefore it is better if rationing is based on clinical data.

Regardless, the primary goal of CER is to lead to better care, not necessarily cheaper care. The goal of CER is to find out what works better. As the emphasis is on comparative research, CER is not going to dictate that one not intervene in certain settings, but rather how best to intervene in those settings. This could result in abandoning expensive technologies that are no better than less expensive options. However, it also could result in paying for a more expensive technology because the evidence shows it is better.

Ultimately, CER is not by itself going to solve the world's health care spending problem. In some cases, the studies will find that the more expensive treatment is best. However, over time, it should save money by preventing wasteful spending on treatments that are less effective.

Reasonable expectations of CER

Though the research community is energized, expectations must be tempered by several limits to what CER can realistically solve. It is infeasible to expect that CER can address all therapeutic questions; health care is too complex. If it were possible to base the practice of medicine entirely on science, it would take into account not only complex pathophysiology, but also behavioral factors such as values, perceptions, and attitudes about risks, quality of life preferences, cost tradeoffs, etc. However, as the science underlying current medical practice is not sufficiently complete, art comes into practice when subjective judgment is required. Therefore, even in situations where complete evidence-based information is available to guide clinical decisions, providers or patients may still opt for a decision based on personal choices that they value irrespective of the science.

Finally, over-emphasis on scientific evidence can lead to a paralysis when such evidence is unavailable. In the face of uncertainty, variation among reasonable but unproven options should be tolerated and even encouraged, as it will facilitate later evaluation. This is contrary to the vision of a knowledge state that is sufficiently complete to guide all decisions about effective interventions at the individual patient level. We also need to be sure that the desire for scientific evidence does not paralyze medical practice when such evidence is absent. In such circumstances, the resulting variability in practice can provide the data underlying future CER studies.

Key points

- CER seeks to improve patient care through increasing the use of scientific evidence to inform clinical decisions about alternative treatment options.
- Key elements of CER include *evidence synthesis* (identifying and summarizing existing data addressing a question), *evidence generation* (creating new data addressing a question), and *evidence dissemination* (distributing the available data, with the goal of modifying patient care).
- CER aims to focus on scientific comparisons of the gamut of medical options (including drugs, biologics, devices, surgeries, diagnostic tests, traditional medicine, prevention strategies, and health delivery systems), to the relative effectiveness of these medical options in "real world" settings.
- CER advocates the inclusion of the gamut of relevant stakeholders and decision makers in the processes of setting priorities for research, selecting appropriate study designs, and disseminating and implementing the results from comparative effectiveness investigations.
- Through these foci and activities, CER aims to rationalize medical care and potentially reduce health care costs.

Further reading

Studies of drug utilization

Beer C, Hyde Z, Almeida OP, Norman P, Hankey GJ, Yeap BB, Flicker L (2011) Quality use of medicines and health outcomes among a cohort of community dwelling older men: an observational study. *Br J Clin Pharmacol* **71**: 592–9.

Brown TR (ed.) (2006) *Handbook of Institutional Pharmacy Practice*, 4th edn. Bethesda, MD: American Society of Health System Pharmacists.

Dartnell JGA (2001) *Understanding, Influencing and Evaluating Drug Use*. Australia: Therapeutic Guidelines Limited.

Hennessy SM, Bilker WB, Zhou L, Weber AL, Brensinger C, Wang Y, Strom BL (2003) Retrospective drug utilization review, prescribing errors, and clinical outcomes. *JAMA* **290**: 1494–9.

Kauffman DW, Kelly JP, Rosenberg L, Anderson TE, Mitchell AA (2002) Recent patterns of medication use in the ambulatory adult population of the United States: the Slone survey. *JAMA* **287**: 337–44.

Kidder D, Bae J (1999) Evaluation results from prospective drug utilization review: Medicaid demonstrations. *Health Care Financ Rev* **20**: 107–18.

World Health Organization (1993) *How to Investigate Drug Use in Health Facilities: Selected Drug Use Indicators*. WHO/DAP/93.1. Geneva: World Health Organization.

World Health Organization (2009) *Medicines Use in Primary Care in Developing and Transitional Countries: Fact Book Summarizing Results from Studies Reported between 1990 and 2006*. WHO/EMP/MAR/2009.3. Geneva, Switzerland: World Health Organization.

World Health Organization International Working Group for Drug Statistics Methodology, WHO Collaborating Centre for Drug Statistics Methodology, WHO Collaborating Centre for Drug Utilization Research and Clinical Pharmacology (2003) *Introduction to Drug Utilization Research*. Geneva: World Health Organization.

Evaluating and improving physician prescribing

Auerbach AD, Landefield CS, Shojania KG (2007) The tension between needing to improve care and knowing how to do it. *N Engl J Med* **357**: 608–13.

Black AD, Car J, Pagliari C, Ananddan C, Cresswell K, et al. (2011) The impact of eHealth on the quality and safety of healthcare: a systematic overview. *PLoS Med* **8**: 387–97.

Cabana MD, Rand CS, Power NR, Wu AW, Wilson MH, Abboud PC, et al. (1999) Why don't physicians follow clinical practice guidelines? *JAMA* **282**: 1458–65.

Donner A, Birkett N, Buck C (1981) Randomization by cluster—samples size requirements and analysis. *Am J Epidemiology* **114**: 906–14.

Eccles M, McColl E, Steen N, Rousseau N, Grimshaw J, Parkin D, et al. (2002) Effect of computerized evidence based guidelines on management of asthma and angina in adults in primary care: a cluster randomized controlled trial. *BMJ* **325**: 941–8.

Farmer AP, Legare F, Turcot L, Grimshaw J, Harvey E, McGowan JL, Wolf F (2009) Printed educational materials: effect on professional practice and healthcare outcomes. (Cochrane Database of Systematic Reviews). In: *The Cochrane Collaboration*, Issue 2. New York: John Wiley & Sons, Inc.

Fordis M, King JE, Ballantyne CM, Jones PH, Schneider KH, Spann SJ, et al. (2005) Comparison of the instructional efficacy of internet-based CME with live interactive CME workshops: a randomized controlled trial. *JAMA* **294**: 1043–51.

Godin G, Belanger-Gravel A, Eccles M, Grimshaw J (2008) Healthcare professionals' intentions and behaviours: a systematic review of studies based on social cognitive theories. *Implement Sci* **3**: 36–46.

Gonzales R, Steiner JF, Lum A, Barrett PH (1999) Decreasing antibiotic use in ambulatory practice: impact of a multidimensional intervention on the treatment of uncomplicated acute bronchitis in adults. *JAMA* **281**: 1512–19.

Greer AL (1988) The state of the art versus the state of the science: the diffusion of new medical technologies into practice. *Int J Technol Assess Health Care* **4**: 5–26.

Grimshaw JM, Shirran L, Thomas R, Mowatt G, Fraser C, Bero L, et al. (2001) Changing provider behavior: an overview of systematic reviews of interventions. *Med Care* **39** (suppl 2): 2–45.

Kiefe CI, Allison JJ, Williams OD, Person SD, Weaver MT, Weissman NW (2001) Improving quality improvement using achievable benchmarks for physician feedback: a randomized controlled trial. *JAMA* **285**: 2871–9.

Majumdar SR, McAlister FA, Furberg CD (2004) From knowledge to practice in chronic cardiovascular disease–a long and winding road. *J Am Coll Cardiol* **43**: 1738–42.

Rousseau N, McColl E, Newton J, Grimshaw J, Eccles M (2003) Practice based, longitudinal, qualitative interview study of computerized evidence based guidelines in primary care. *BMJ* **326**: 314–22.

Serumaga B, Ross-Degnan R, Avery AJ, Elliot RA, Majumdar SR, Zhang F, Soumerai SB (2011) Has pay-for-performance improved the management and outcomes of hypertension in the United Kingdom? *BMJ* **342**: 322–9.

Soumerai SB, McLaughlin TJ, Gurwitz JH, Guadagnoli E, Hauptman PJ, Borbas C, et al. (1998) Effect of local medical opinion leaders on quality of care for acute myocardial infarction: a randomized controlled trial. *JAMA* **279**: 1358–63.

Spinewine A, Schmader KE, Barber N, Hughes C, Lapane KL, Swine C, Hanlon JT (2007) Appropriate prescribing in the elderly: how well can it be measured and optimized. *Lancet* **370**: 173–84.

Special methodological issues in pharmacoepidemiologic studies of vaccine safety

Baggs J, Gee J, Lewis E, Fowler G, Benson P, Lieu T, Naleway A, Klein NP, Baxter R, Belongia E, Glanz J, Hambidge SJ, Jacobsen SJ, Jackson L, Nordin J, Weintraub E (2011) The Vaccine Safety Datalink: a model for monitoring immunization safety. *Pediatrics* **127**: S45–S53.

Bate A, Evans SJW (2009) Quantitative signal detection using spontaneous ADR reporting. *Pharmacoepidemiology and Drug Safety* **18**: 427–36.

Baylor NW, Midthun K (2008) Regulation and testing of vaccines. In: Plotkin S, Orenstein WA, Offit P, eds, *Vaccines*, 5th edn. Philadelphia, PA: W.B. Saunders, pp. 1611–28.

Centers for Disease Control and Prevention (1999) Intussusception among recipients of rotavirus vaccine–United States, 1998–1999. *MMWR Morb Mortal Wkly Rep* **48**: 577–81.

Evans SJ, Waller PC, Davis S (2001) Use of proportional reporting ratios (PRRs) for signal generation from spontaneous adverse drug reaction reports. *Pharmacoepidemiology and Drug Safety* **10**: 483–6.

Fine PE, Chen RT (2001) Confounding in studies of adverse reactions to vaccines. *Am J Epidemiol* **136**: 121–35.

Glanz JM, McClure DL, Magid DJ, Daley MF, France EK, Salmon DA, et al. (2009) Parental refusal of pertussis vaccination is associated with an increased risk of pertussis infection in children. *Pediatrics* **123**: 1446–51.

Glanz JM, McClure DL, Xu S, Hambridge SJ, Lee M, Kolczak MS, Kleinman K, Mullooly JP, France EK (2005) Four different study designs to evaluate vaccine safety were equally validated with contrasting limitations. *J Clinical Epidemiology* **59**: 808–18.

Greene SK, Kulldorff M, Lewis EM, Li Rong, Yin R, Weintraub ES, Fireman BH, Lieu TA, Nordin JD, Glanz JM, Baxter R, Jacobsen SJ, Broder KR, Lee GM (2010) Near real-time surveillance for influenza vaccine safety: proof-of-concept in the Vaccine Safety Datalink Project. *Am J Epidemiol* **171**: 177–88.

Halsell JS, Riddle JR, Atwood JE, Gardner P, Shope R, Poland GA, et al. (2003) Myopericarditis following smallpox vaccination among vaccinia-naive US military personnel. *JAMA* **289**: 3283–9.

Howson CP, Howe CJ, Fineberg HV, eds (1991) *Adverse Effects of Pertussis and Rubella Vaccines: A Report of the Committee to Review the Adverse Consequences of Pertussis and Rubella Vaccines*. IOM (Institute of Medicine). 1991 Washington, DC: National Academy Press.

Huang WT, Chen WW, Yang HW, Chen WC, Chao YN, Huang YW, et al. (2010) Design of a robust infrastructure to monitor the safety of the pandemic A(H1N1) 2009 vaccination program in Taiwan. *Vaccine* **28**: 7161–6.

Kramarz P, France EK, DeStefano F, Black SB, Shinefield H, Ward JI, et al. (2001) Population-based study of rotavirus vaccination and intussusception. *Pediatr Infect Dis J* **20**: 410–16.

Larson HJ, Cooper LZ, Eskola J, Katz SL, Ratzan S (2011) Addressing the vaccine confidence gap. *Lancet.* **378** (9790): 526–35.

Murch SH, Anthony A, Casson DH, Malik M, Berelowitz M, Dhillon AP, et al. (2004) Retraction of an interpretation. *Lancet* **363**: 750.

Murphy TV, Gargiullo PM, Massoudi MS, Nelson DB, Jumaan AO, Okoro CA, et al. (2001) Intussusception among infants given an oral rotavirus vaccine. *N Engl J Med* **344**: 564–72.

Schonberger LB, Bregman DJ, Sullivan-Bolyai JZ, Keenlyside RA, Ziegler DW, Retailliau HF, et al. (1979) Guillain–Barre syndrome following vaccination in the National Influenza Immunization Program, United States, 1976–1977. *Am J Epidemiol* **110**: 105–23.

Stratton K, Ford A, Rusch E, Clayton EW (eds) (2011) *Adverse Effects of Vaccines: Evidence and Causality*. IOM (Institute of Medicine). Washington, DC: The National Academies Press.

Walker AM (2010) Signal detection for vaccine side effects that have not been specified in advance. *Pharmacoepidemiology and Drug Safety* **19**: 311–17.

Xu S, Zhang L, Nelson J, Zeng C, Mullooly J, McClure D, et al. (2010) Identifying optimal risk windows for self-controlled case series studies of vaccine safety. *Stat Med* **30**: 142–52.

Epidemiologic studies of implantable medical devices

Resnic FS, Gross TP, Marinac-Dabic D, Loyo-Berrios N, Donnelly S, Normand S-LT, Matheny ME (2010) Automated surveillance to detect post procedure safety signals of approved cardiovascular devices. *JAMA* **304** (18): 2019–27.

Sedrakyan A, Marinac-Dabic D, Normand S-LT, Mushlin A, Gross T (2010) A framework for evidence evaluation and methodological issues in implantable device studies. *Medical Care* **48**: S121–S128.

Normand S-LT, Marinac-Dabic D, Sedrakyan A, Kaczmarek R (2010) Rethinking analytical strategies for surveillance of medical devices: the case of hip arthroplasty. *Medical Care* **48**: S58–S67.

Sedrakyan A, Normand S-LT, Dabic S, Jacobs S, Graves S, Marinac-Dabic D (2011) Comparative assessment of implantable hip devices with bearing surfaces: systematic appraisal of evidence. *British Medical Journal* **343**: d7434.

Studies of drug-induced birth defects

Chambers C, Braddock SR, Briggs GG, Einarson A, Johnson YR, Miller RK, *et al.* (2001) Postmarketing surveillance for human teratogenicity: a model approach. *Teratology* **64**: 252–61.

FDA (2012) Guidance for industry: establishing pregnancy exposure registries. Available from http://www.fda.gov/downloads/ScienceResearch/SpecialTopics/WomensHealthResearch/UCM133332.pdf (accessed July 10, 2012).

Heinonen OP, Slone D, Shapiro S (1977) The women, their offspring, and the malformations. In: Kaufman DW, ed. *Birth Defects and Drugs in Pregnancy*. Littleton, MA: Publishing Sciences Group.

Holmes LB (2012) *Common Malformations*. New York: Oxford University Press.

Holmes LB (1983) Teratogen update: Bendectin. *Teratology* **27**: 277–81.

Hook EB, Healy KB (1976) Consequences of a nationwide ban on spray adhesives alleged to be human teratogens and mutagens. *Science* **191**: 566–7.

Kelley KE, Hernández-Díaz S, Chaplin EL, Hauser R, Mitchell AA (2012) Identification of phthalates in medications and dietary supplement formulations in the U.S. and Canada. *Environ Health Perspect* **120**: 379–84.

Lenz W (1962) Thalidomide and congenital abnormalities. *Lancet* **1**: 45.

Louik C, Gardiner P, Kelley K, Mitchell AA (2010) Use of herbal treatments in pregnancy. *Am J Obstet Gynecol* **202**: 439.e1–10.

Mitchell AA (2010) Proton-pump inhibitors and birth defects–some reassurance, but more needed (editorial). *N Engl J Med* **363**: 2161–3.

Mitchell AA (2012) Studies of drug-induced birth defects. In: Strom BL, Kimmel SE, Hennessy S, eds. *Pharmacoepidemiology*. 5th edn. West Sussex, UK: Wiley-Blackwell, pp. 487–504.

Mitchell AA (2003) Systematic identification of drugs that cause birth defects—a new opportunity. *N Engl J Med* **349**: 2556–9.

Mitchell AA, Cottler LB, Shapiro S (1986) Effect of questionnaire design on recall of drug exposure in pregnancy. *Am J Epidemiol* **123**: 670–6.

Mitchell AA, Gilboa SM, Werler MM, Kelley KE, Louik C, Hernández-Díaz S, and the National Birth Defects Prevention Study (2011) Medication use during pregnancy, with particular focus on prescription drugs: 1976–2008. *Am J Obstet Gynecol* **205**: 51.e1–8.

Schatz M, Chambers CD, Jones KL, Louik C, Mitchell AA (2011) The safety of influenza immunizations and treatment during pregnancy: the Vaccines and Medications in Pregnancy Surveillance System. *Am J Obstet Gynecol* **204**: S64–8.

Slone D, Shapiro S. Miettinen OS, Finkle WD, Stolley PD (1979) Drug evaluation after marketing. *Ann Intern Med* **90**: 257–61.

Warkany J (1974) Problems in applying teratologic observations in animals to man. *Pediatrics* **53**: 820.

Werler MM, Mitchell AA, Hernández-Díaz S, Honein MA, and the National Birth Defects Prevention Study (2005) Use of over-the-counter medications during pregnancy. *Am J Obstet Gynecol* **193**: 771–7.

Risk management

Directive 2001/83 EC, Article 1 (28b).

European Medicines Agency and Heads of Medicines Agencies (2012) Guideline on Good Pharmacovigilance Practices, Module V – Risk Management Systems (published July 2012. http://www.ema.europa.eu/docs/en_GB/document_library/Scientific_guideline/2012/06/WC500129134.pdf

Institute of Medicine. Kohn LT, Corrigan JM, Donaldson MS (eds) (2000) *To Err Is Human: Building a Safer Health System*. Institute of Medicine, Washington DC: National Academies Press.

National Coordinating Council for Medication Error Reporting and Prevention website, http://www.nccmerp.org/aboutMedErrors.html.

Ovation Pharmaceuticals, Inc. Advisory Committee Briefing Document. Sabril® (vigabatrin) Tablet and Powder for Oral Solution For Adjunctive Treatment of Refractory Complex Partial Seizures in Adults (NDA 20-427), For Monotherapy Treatment of Infantile Spasms (NDA 22-006). Peripheral and Central Nervous System Advisory Committee January 7–8, 2009. Available at http://www.fda.gov/downloads/AdvisoryCommittees/CommitteesMeetingMaterials/Drugs/PeripheralandCentralNervousSystemDrugsAdvisoryCommittee/UCM153780.pdf

US Food and Drug Administration. Guidance for Industry (2005) *Development and Use of Risk Minimization Action Plans*.

US Department of Health and Human Services. Food and Drug Administration. Guidance. Drug Safety Information–FDA's Communication to the Public. March 2007. Available at http://www.fda.gov/downloads/Drugs/GuidanceComplianceRegulatoryInformation/Guidances/UCM072281.pdf

The use of pharmacoepidemiology to study medication errors

Aronson JK (2009) Medication errors: definitions and classification. *Br J Clin Pharmacol* **67**: 599–604.

Bates DW, Boyle DL, Vander Vliet MB, Schneider J, Leape LL (1995) Relationship between medication errors and adverse drug events. *J Gen Intern Med* **10**: 199–205.

Bates DW, Cullen D, Laird N, Petersen LA, Small S, Servi D, *et al.* (1995) Incidence of adverse drug events and potential adverse drug events: implications for prevention. *JAMA* **274**: 29–34.

Bates DW, Leape LL, Cullen DJ, Laird N, Petersen LA, Teich JM, *et al.* (1998) Effect of computerized physician order entry and a team intervention on prevention of serious medication errors. *JAMA* **280**: 1311–16.

Berwick DM (1989) Continuous improvement as an ideal in health care. *N Engl J Med* **320**: 53–6.

Chertow GM, Lee J, Kuperman GJ, Burdick E, Horsky J, Seger DL, Lee R, Mekala A, Song J, Komaroff AL, Bates DW (2001) Guided medication dosing for inpatients with renal insufficiency. *JAMA* **286**: 2839–44.

Cypress BW (1982) *Drug Utilization in Office Visits to Primary Care Physicians: National Ambulatory Medical Care Survey, 1980*. Department of Health and Human Services publication (PHS) 82–1250. Public Health Service.

Falconnier AD, Haefeli WE, Schoenenberger RA, Surber C, Martin-Facklam M (2001) Drug dosage in patients with renal failure optimized by immediate concurrent feedback. *J Gen Intern Med* **16**: 369–75.

Forster AJ, Murff HJ, Peterson JF, Gandhi TK, Bates DW (2003) The incidence and severity of adverse events affecting patients after discharge from the hospital. *Ann Intern Med* **138**: 161–7.

Gandhi TK, Weingart SN, Borus J, Seger AC, Peterson J, Burdick E, *et al.* (2003) Adverse drug events in ambulatory care. *N Engl J Med* **348**: 1556–64.

Hazlet TK, Lee TA, Hansten PD, Horn JR (2001) Performance of community pharmacy drug interaction software. *J Am Pharm Assoc* **41**: 200–4.

Hennessy S, Bilker WB, Zhou L, Weber AL, Brensinger C, Wang Y, *et al.* (2003) Retrospective drug utilization review, prescribing errors, and clinical outcomes. *JAMA* **290**: 1494–9.

Institute of Medicine. Kohn LT, Corrigan JM, Donaldson MS (eds) (1999) *To Err Is Human: Building a Safer Health System*. Washington, DC: National Academy Press.

Kaushal R, Bates DW, Landrigan C, McKenna KJ, Clapp MD, Federico F, *et al.* (2001) Medication errors and adverse drug events in pediatric inpatients. *JAMA* **285**: 2114–20.

Kopp BJ, Erstad BL, Allen AM, Theodorou AA, Priestley G (2006) Medication errors and adverse drug events in an intensive care unit: direct observation approach for detection. *Crit Care Med* **34**: 415–25.

Koppel R, Metlay JP, Cohen A, Abaluck B, Localio AR, Kimmel SE, *et al.* (2005) Role of computerized physician order entry systems in facilitating medication errors. *JAMA* **293**: 1197–1203.

Krähenbühl-Melcher A, Schlienger R, Lampert M, Haschke M, Drewe J, Kraehenbuehl S (2007) Drug-related problems in hospitals: a review of the recent literature. *Drug Saf* **30**: 379–407.

Kuperman GJ, Gandhi TK, Bates DW (2003) Effective drug-allergy checking: methodological and operational issues. *J Biomed Inform* **36**: 70–9.

Montesi G, Lechi A (2009) Prevention of medication errors: detection and audit. *Br J Clin Pharmacol* **67**: 651–5.

Peterson JF, Bates DW (2001) Preventable medication errors: identifying and eliminating serious drug interactions. *J Am Pharm Assoc* **41**: 159–60.

Potylycki MJ, Kimmel SR, Ritter M, Capuano T, Gross L, Riegel-Gross K, *et al.* (2006) Nonputitive medication error reporting: 3-year findings from one hospital's primum non nocere initiative. *J Nurs Adm* **36**: 370–6.

Schiff GD, Klass D, Peterson J, Shah G, Bates DW (2003) Linking laboratory and pharmacy: opportunities for reducing errors and improving care. *Arch Intern Med* **163**: 893–900.

Seidling HM, Storch CH, Bertsche T, Senger C, Kaltschmidt J, Walter-Sack I, *et al.* (2009) Successful strategy to improve the specificity of electronic statin-drug interaction alerts. *Eur J Clin Pharmacol* **65**: 1149–57.

FDA's Sentinel Initiative

Behrman RE, Benner JS, Brown JS, McClellan M, Woodcock J, Platt R (2011) Developing the Sentinel System — a national resource for evidence development. *New England Journal of Medicine* **364**: 498–499.

FDA's Sentinel website http://www.fda.gov/Safety/FDAs-SentinelInitiative/default.htm?utm_campaign=Google2&utm_source=fdaSearch&utm_medium=website&utm_term=Sentinel%20initiative&utm_content=1

Mini-Sentinel website http://mini-sentinel.org/

Platt R, Carnahan R (2012) The U.S. Food and Drug Administration's Mini-Sentinel Program. *Pharmacoepidem. Drug Safe*, **21**: 1–303. doi: 10.1002/pds.3230.

Public Law 110-85. 110th Congress. US Food and Drug Administration Amendments Act of 2007, September 2007.

Comparative effectiveness research

Benner JS, Morrison MR, Karnes EK, Kocot SL, McClellan M (2010) An evaluation of recent federal spending on comparative effectiveness research: priorities, gaps, and next steps. *Health Aff* (Millwood) **29**: 1768–76.

Chalkidou K, Walley T (2010) Using comparative effectiveness research to inform policy and practice in the UK NHS: Past, present and future. *Pharmacoeconomics* **28**: 799–811.

Congressional Budget Office (2007) Research on the comparative effectiveness of medical treatments Nov 2007. Available at: http://www.cbo.gov/ftpdocs/88xx/doc8891/12-18-ComparativeEffectiveness.pdf (accessed January 2011).

Conway PH, Clancy C (2010) Charting a path from comparative effectiveness funding to improved patient-centered health care. *JAMA* **303**: 985–6.

Federal Coordinating Council for Comparative Effectiveness Research (2009) Report to the President and the Congress. Washington, DC: Department of Health and Human Services, June 2009. Accessed December 14, 2010. Available at http://www.hhs.gov/recovery/programs/cer/cerannualrpt.pdf

Institute of Medicine (2007) Learning what works best: The nation's need for evidence on comparative effectiveness in health care. September 2007. Available at: http://www.iom.edu/~/media/Files/Activity%20Files/Quality/VSRT/ComparativeEffectivenessWhitePaper-ESF.pdf

Institute of Medicine (2008) Knowing what works in health care: A roadmap for the nation. January 2008. Available at: http://www.iom.edu/Reports/2008/Knowing-What-Works-in-Health-Care-A-Roadmap-for-the-Nation.aspx

Institute of Medicine (2009) Initial national priorities for comparative effectiveness research. Washington, DC: National Academies Press, 2009. Accessed December 14, 2010; Available at http://www.iom.edu/Reports/2009/ComparativeEffectivenessResearchPriorities.aspx

Institute of Medicine (2011) *Clinical Practice Guidelines We Can Trust*. Washington, DC: The National Academies Press.

Institute of Medicine (2011) *Finding What Works in Health Care: Standards for Systematic Reviews*. Washington, DC: The National Academies Press.

Kerridge I, Lowe M, Henry H (1998) Ethics and evidence based medicine. *BMJ* **316**: 1151–3.

Luce BR, Drummond M, Jönsson B, Neumann PJ, Schwartz JS, Siebert U (2010) EBM, HTA, and CER: clearing the confusion. *Milbank Q* **88**: 256–76.

Luce BR, Kramer JM, Goodman SN, Connor JT, Tunis S, Whicher D, Schwartz JS (2009) Rethinking randomized clinical trials for comparative effectiveness research: the need for transformational change. *Ann Intern Med* **151**: 206–9.

Manchikanti L, Falco FJ, Boswell MV, Hirsch JA (2010) Facts, fallacies, and politics of comparative effectiveness research: Part I. Basic considerations. *Pain Physician* **13**: E23–54.

National Pharmaceutical Council. A brief history of comparative effectiveness research and evidence-based medicine. Available at: http://www.npcnow.org/Public/Issues/i_cer/cer_toolkit/A_Brief_History_of_Comparative_Effectiveness_Research_And_Evidence-Based_Medicine.aspx (accessed January 14, 2011).

Selker HP, Strom BL, Ford DE, Meltzer DO, Pauker SG, Pincus HA, Rich EC, Tompkins C, Whitlock EP (2010) White paper on CTSA consortium role in facilitating comparative effectiveness research: September 23, 2009 CTSA consortium strategic goal committee on comparative effectiveness research. *Clin Transl Sci* **3**: 29–37.

Slutsky JR, Clancy CM (2010) Patient-centered comparative effectiveness research. *Arch Intern Med* **170**: 403–4.

Strom BL, Faich GA, Reynolds RF, Eng SM, D'Agostino RB, Ruskin JN, Kane JM (2008) The Ziprasidone Observational Study of Cardiac Outcomes (ZODIAC): design and baseline subject characteristics. *J Clin Psychiatry* **69**: 114–21.

Teutsch SM, Berger ML, Weinstein MC (2005) Comparative effectiveness: asking the right questions, choosing the right method. *Health Affairs* **24**: 128–32. Available at: http://content.healthaffairs.org/content/24/1/128.

CHAPTER 23

The Future of Pharmacoepidemiology

Brian L. Strom, Stephen E. Kimmel, and Sean Hennessy
Perelman School of Medicine at the University of Pennsylvania, Philadelphia, PA, USA

"We should all be concerned about the future because we will have to spend the rest of our lives there."
                                        Charles Franklin Kettering, 1949

Speculating about the future is at least risky and possibly foolish. Nevertheless, the future of pharmacoepidemiology seems apparent in many ways, judging from past trends and recent events. Interest in the field by the pharmaceutical industry, government agencies, new trainees, and the public is truly exploding, as is realization of what pharmacoepidemiology can contribute. Indeed, international attention on drug safety remains high, important safety questions involving widely used drugs continue to emerge, and questions concerning the effectiveness of systems of drug approval and drug safety monitoring remain.

As the functions of academia, industry, and government have become increasingly global, so has the field of pharmacoepidemiology. The number of individuals attending the annual International Conference on Pharmacoepidemiology has increased from approximately 50 in the early 1980s to over 1200 in 2012. The International Society for Pharmacoepidemiology (ISPE), established in 1991, has grown to over 1400 members from 54 countries. It has developed a set of guidelines for Good Epidemiologic Practices for Drug, Device, and Vaccine Research in the United States in 1996, and updated these guidelines most recently in 2008. Many national pharmacoepidemiologic societies have been formed as well. The journal *Clinical Pharmacology and Therapeutics*, the major US academic clinical pharmacology journal, actively solicits pharmacoepidemiologic manuscripts, as does the *Journal of Clinical Epidemiology*. The major journal devoted to the field, *Pharmacoepidemiology and Drug Safety*, ISPE's official journal, is indexed on Medline and achieved an impact factor of 2.527 in 2009, similar to that of the *Journal of Clinical Epidemiology* and remarkably high for a niche field.

The number of individuals seeking to enter the field continues to increase, as is their level of training. The number of programs of study in pharmacoepidemiology is increasing in schools of medicine, public health, and pharmacy. While in the 1980s the single summer short course in pharmacoepidemiology at the University of Minnesota was sometimes cancelled because of insufficient interest, later the University of Michigan School of Public Health summer course in pharmacoepidemiology attracted 10% of all students in the entire summer program, and thereafter McGill University, Erasmus University in Rotterdam, and the Johns Hopkins Bloomberg School of Public Health all conduct summer short courses in pharmacoepidemiology. Several other short courses are given as well, including by ISPE itself. Regulatory bodies around the world have expanded their internal pharmacoepidemiologic programs.

The number of pharmaceutical companies with their own pharmacoepidemiologic units has also increased, along with their support for academic units and their funding of external pharmacoepidemiologic studies. Requirements that a drug be shown to be cost-effective have been added to many national health care systems, provincial health care systems, and managed care organizations (see Chapter 9), either to justify reimbursement or even to justify drug availability. Drug utilization review is being widely applied, and many hospitals are becoming mini-pharmacoepidemiologic practice and research laboratories. The US Congress has recognized the importance of pharmacoepidemiology, requiring FDA to build a new data resource, containing at least 100 million lives, for evaluating potential adverse effects of medical products (see "FDA's Sentinel Initiative" in Chapter 22).

Thus, from the perspective of those in the field, the trends in pharmacoepidemiology are remarkably positive, although many important challenges remain. In this chapter, we will briefly give our own view on the future of pharmacoepidemiology from the perspectives of academia, the pharmaceutical industry, regulatory agencies, and then the law.

The view from academia

Scientific developments

Methodological advances

The array of methodological approaches available for performing pharmacoepidemiologic studies will continue to grow. Each of the methodological issues discussed in Part III can be expected to be the subject of further research and development. The future is likely to see ever more advanced ways of performing and analyzing epidemiologic studies across all content areas, as the field of epidemiology continues to expand and develop. Some of these new techniques will, of course, be particularly useful to investigators in pharmacoepidemiology (see Chapter 21). The next few years will likely see expanded use of propensity scores, instrumental variables, sensitivity analysis, and novel methods to analyze time-varying exposures and confounders. In addition, we believe that we will see increasing application of pharmacoepidemiologic insight in the conduct of clinical trials, as well as increased use of the randomized trial design to examine questions traditionally addressed by observational pharmacoepidemiology (see Chapter 16), especially given the controversies resulting from inconsistencies between nonexperimental studies vs. experimental studies, and given the emerging field of comparative effectiveness research (see Chapter 22).

Drug regulators have enthusiastically embraced therapeutic risk management (see Chapter 22). Yet, this field is very much in its infancy, with an enormous amount of work needed to develop new methods to measure, communicate, and manage the risks and benefits associated with medication use. Rigorous studies (i.e., program evaluations) of the effectiveness of risk management programs remain the exception rather than the rule. Development of this area will require considerable effort from pharmacoepidemiologists as well as those from other fields.

We may see developments in the processes used to assess causality from individual case reports (see Chapters 7 and 13). "Data mining" approaches will be used increasingly in spontaneous reporting databases to search for early signals of adverse reactions. Hopefully, we will see studies evaluating the utility of such approaches. The need for newer methods to screen for potential adverse drug effects, such as those using health care claims or medical record data, is also clear (see Chapter 22).

We are likely to see increasing input from pharmacoepidemiologists into policy questions about drug approval. We anticipate that emphasis will shift from studies evaluating whether a given drug is associated with an increased risk of a given event to those that examine patient-and regimen-specific factors that affect risk. Such studies are crucial because, if risk factors for adverse reactions can be better understood before a safety crisis occurs, or early in the course of a crisis, then the clinical use of the drug may be able to be repositioned, avoiding the loss of useful drugs.

With recent developments in molecular biology and bioinformatics, and their application to the study of pharmacogenetics, exciting developments have occurred in the ability of researchers to identify biologic factors that predispose patients to adverse and beneficial drug effects (see Chapter 14). However, few of these discoveries have yet been shown useful in improving patient care, and new studies and methods must be pursued to determine the clinical utility of genetic testing. Pharmacogenetics has evolved from studies of measures of slow drug metabolism as a contributor to adverse reactions to the study of molecular genetic markers. This has been aided by the development of new, noninvasive methods to collect and analyze biosamples, making population-based genetic studies feasible. We believe that clinical measurement of biologic factors will ultimately complement existing approaches to tailoring therapeutic approaches for individual patients. However, it is unlikely that genotype will be the only, or even the major, factor that determines the optimal drug or dose for a given patient. Future years are likely to see much more of this cross-fertilization between pharmacoepidemiology and molecular biology. From a research perspective, we can easily envision pharmacogenetic studies added to the process of evaluating potential adverse reactions. We also anticipate the availability of genotypic information for members of large patient cohorts for whom drug exposures and clinical outcomes are recorded electronically, and even for selected patients from automated databases, such as those described in Chapter 9 of this book.

New content areas of interest

There are a number of new content areas that are likely to be explored and developed more. Studies of drug utilization will continue and will continue to become more innovative (see Chapter 22). Particularly as the health care industry becomes more sensitive to the possibility of overutilization, underutilization, and inappropriate utilization of drugs, and the risks associated with each, one would expect to see an increased frequency of and sophistication in drug utilization review programs, which seek to improve care, potentially incorporating techniques from molecular pharmacoepidemiology (see Chapter 14). This is especially likely to be the case for studies of antibiotic misuse, as society becomes ever more concerned about the development of organisms resistant to currently available drugs.

The US Joint Commission on Accreditation of Healthcare Organizations revolutionized US hospital pharmacoepidemiology through its standards requiring adverse drug reaction surveillance and drug use evaluation program in every hospital. Hospitals are also now experimenting with different methods of organizing their drug delivery systems to improve their use of drugs, e.g., use of computerized clinical decision support and the addition of pharmacists to patient care teams.

Interest in the field of pharmacoeconomics, i.e., the application of the principles of health economics to the study of drug effects, is continuing (see Chapter 17). Society is realizing that the acquisition cost of drugs is often a very minor part of their economic impact, and that their beneficial and harmful effects can be vastly more important. Further, more governments and insurance programs are increasingly requiring economic justification before permitting reimbursement for a drug. As a result, the number of studies exploring this is increasing. As the methods of pharmacoeconomics become increasingly sophisticated, and their applications clear, this could be expected to continue to be a popular field of inquiry.

More non-experimental studies of beneficial drug effects, particularly of drug effectiveness, can be expected, as the field becomes more aware that such studies are possible. This is being encouraged by the rapid increase in the use of propensity scores to adjust for measured covariates, although investigators using this method often place more confidence in that technique than is warranted, some not recognizing that its ability to control for confounding by indication remains dependent on one's ability to *measure* the true determinants of exposure (see Chapter 21). It is also being encouraged by the development of comparative effectiveness research (see Chapter 22). Other approaches to controlling for confounding are similarly likely to become more common as they are further developed (see Chapter 21).

We will also see more use of pharmacoepidemiologic approaches prior to drug approval, e.g., to understand the baseline rate of adverse events that one can expect to see in patients who will eventually be treated with a new drug (see "The View from regulatory agencies" in Chapter 6).

Recent years have seen an explosion in the worldwide use of herbal and other complementary and alternative medications. These are essentially pharmaceuticals sold without conventional standardization, and with no required premarketing testing of safety or efficacy. In a sense, for these products, this is a return to a preregulatory era. Society will continue to turn to pharmacoepidemiologists to help evaluate the use and effects of these products.

Research interest in the entire topic of patient nonadherence with prescribed drug regimens goes back to about 1960, but little fruitful research could be done until about 1990 because methods for ascertaining drug exposure in individual ambulatory patients were grossly unsatisfactory. The methodological impasse was broken by two quite different developments. The initial one was to use very low doses of a very long half-life agent, phenobarbital, as a chemical marker; since a single measurement of phenobarbital in plasma is indicative of aggregate drug intake during the prior two weeks. The other, more recent, advance has been to incorporate time-stamping microcircuitry into pharmaceutical containers, which records the date and time each time that the container is opened. Perhaps as a consequence of its inherent simplicity and economy, electronic monitoring is increasingly emerging as the *de facto* gold standard for compiling dosing histories of ambulatory patients, from which one can evaluate the extent of adherence to the prescribed drug regimen. Future years are likely to see a continuing increase in the use and improvement of this technique and technology (see Chapter 20) in research, and perhaps in clinical practice.

The next few years are also likely to see the increasing ability to target drug therapy to the proper patients. This will involve both increasing use of statistical methods, and increasing use of laboratory techniques from other biological sciences, as described above. Statistical approaches will allow us to use predictive modeling to study, from a population perspective, who is most likely to derive benefit from a drug, and who is at greatest risk of an adverse outcome. Laboratory science will enable us to measure individuals' genotypes, to predict responses to drug therapy (i.e., molecular susceptibility). From the perspective of pre-approval testing, these developments will allow researchers to target specific patient-types for enrollment into their studies, those subjects most likely to succeed with a drug. From a clinical perspective, it will enable health care providers to incorporate biological factors in the individualization of choice of regimens.

The past few years have seen the increased use of surrogate markers, presumed to represent increased risk of rarer serious adverse effects when drugs are used in broader numbers of patients. These range from mild liver function test abnormalities, used as predictors of serious liver toxicity, to electrocardiographic QTc prolongation as a marker of risk of suffering the arrhythmia torsades des pointes, which can lead to death. Indeed, some drugs have been removed from the market, or from development, because of the presence of these surrogate markers. Yet, the utility of these markers as predictors of serious clinical outcomes is poorly studied. The next few years are likely to see the increased use of both very large observational studies and large simple trials after marketing, to study important clinical outcomes (see Chapter 16 and "Comparative effectiveness research" in Chapter 22).

In addition, with the growth of concerns about patient safety (see "The use of pharmacoepidemiology to study medication errors" and "Risk management" in Chapter 22), there has been increasing attention to simultaneous use of pairs of drugs that have been shown in pharmacokinetic studies (see Chapter 4) to cause increased or decreased drug levels. Yet, population studies informing the clinical importance and pharmacologic aspects of drug–drug interactions have only been performed in the past few years. The next few years are likely to see the emergence of more studies to address such questions.

Finally, in the last few years, society has increasingly turned to pharmacoepidemiology for input into major policy decisions. For example, pharmacoepidemiology played a major role in the evaluations by the Institute of Medicine of the US National Academy of Sciences of the Anthrax Vaccine (deciding whether the existing vaccine was safe to use and, thereby, whether the military vaccine program should be restarted) and the Smallpox Vaccine program (deciding the shape of the program intended initially to vaccinate the entire US population). This is likely to occur even more often in the future.

Logistical advances

Logistically, with the increased computerization of data in society in general and within health care in particular, and the increased emphasis on using computerized databases for pharmacoepidemiology (see Part II), some data resources will disappear (e.g., The Rhode Island Drug Use Reporting System and the inpatient databases discussed in prior editions of this book have disappeared, with new ones added, and Group Health of Puget Sound has become less commonly used as a data resource, as much larger health maintenance organization (HMO) databases have emerged), and a number of new computerized databases have emerged as major resources for pharmacoepidemiologic research (e.g., commercial insurance databases (see Chapter 9), medical record databases (see Chapter 9), and the databases from Canada, Holland, and Denmark (see Chapter 9)). The importance of these databases to pharmacoepidemiology is now clear: they enable researchers to address, quickly and relatively inexpensively, questions about drug effects in different settings that require large sample sizes, with excellent quality data on drug exposures. Registries will also become increasingly important for pharmacoepidemiologic research. With the initiation of US Medicare Part D in 2006, which provides prescription drug coverage to US Medicare recipients, the availability of this data resource is potentially "game changing" for hypothesis testing studies, as it is so large relative to other resources; nearly 27 million Medicare beneficiaries were already subscribed to Part D coverage in 2009 (see Chapter 9). It has created an enormous new data resource for pharmacoepidemiology, as well as increased interest from the US government in what pharmacoepidemiology can do. The development of FDA's Sentinel Initiative (see Chapter 22) will, similarly, provide a vast new data resource, eventually intended for hypothesis generating.

Nevertheless, even as the use of databases increases, it is important to keep in mind the importance of studies that collect data *de novo* (see

Chapters 10 and 11). Each approach to pharmacoepidemiology has its advantages and its disadvantages, as described in Part II. No approach is ideal in all circumstances, and often a number of complementary approaches are needed to answer any given research question. To address some of the problems inherent in any database, we must maintain the ability to perform ad hoc studies, as well. Perhaps better, less expensive, and complementary approaches to ad hoc data collection in pharmacoepidemiology will be developed. For example, a potential approach that has not been widely used is the network of regional and national poison control centers. In particular, poison control centers would be expected to be a useful source of information about dose-dependent adverse drug effects. Others will probably be developed as well, leveraging, for example, electronic medical records.

It is likely that new types of research opportunities will emerge. For example, as the US finally implemented a drug benefit as part of Medicare, its health program for the elderly, US government drug expenditures suddenly increased by $49.5 billion in 2007. Outside the US, as well, many different opportunities to form databases are being developed. There is also an increased interest in the importance of pharmacoepidemiology in the developing world. Many developing world countries spend a disproportionate amount of their health care resources on drugs, yet these drugs are often used inappropriately. There have been a number of initiatives in response to this, including the World Health Organization's development of its list of "Essential Drugs."

Funding

For a number of years, academic pharmacoepidemiology suffered from limited research funding opportunities. In the early 1980s, the only available US funding for the field was an extramural funding program from FDA with a total of $1 million/year. Industry interest and support were similarly limited. With the increasing interest in the field, this situation appears to be changing rapidly. FDA is markedly expanding its intramural and extramural pharmacoepidemiologic program, and US National Institutes of Health (NIH) is increasingly funding pharmacoepidemiologic studies as well. Much more industry funding is available, as perceived need for the field within industry grows (see below). This is likely to increase, especially as the FDA expands its own pharmacoepidemiologic program, and more often requires industry to perform postmarketing studies.

There is, of course, a risk associated with academic groups becoming too dependent on industry funding, both in terms of choice of study questions and credibility. Fortunately, in the US, the Agency for Health Care Research and Quality (AHRQ) began to fund pharmacoepidemiologic research as well, as part of an initiative in pharmaceutical outcomes research. In particular, the AHRQ Centers for Education and Research on Therapeutics (CERTs) program provides federal support for ongoing pharmacoepidemiologic activities (see also Chapter 1). While still small relative to industry expenditures on research, it is large relative to the US federal funding previously available for pharmacoepidemiology (see "Comparative effectiveness research" in Chapter 22).

Even the US NIH has begun to fund pharmacoepidemiologic projects more often. NIH is the logical major US source for such support, as it is the major funding source for most basic biomedical research in the US. Its funds are also accessible to investigators outside the US, via the same application procedures. However, NIH's current organizational structure represents an obstacle to pharmacoepidemiologic support. In general, the institutes within NIH are organized by organ system. Earlier in the development of pharmacoepidemiology, the National Institute of General Medical Sciences (NIGMS) provided most of the US government support for our field. It remains, conceptually, perhaps the most appropriate source of such support, since it is the institute that is intended to fund projects that are not specific to an organ system, and it is the institute that funds clinical pharmacologic research. However, over the past few years there has been limited funding from NIGMS for epidemiologic research. A notable exception is the NIGMS-funded Pharmacogenetics Research Network (PGRN), which has increasingly been performing larger scale pharmacogenetic epidemiologic studies. Further, NIGMS now funds one

pharmacoepidemiologic training program, as part of its clinical pharmacologic training. In the meantime, NIH funding continues to be available if one tailors a project to fit an organ system or in some other way fits the priorities of one of the individual institutes.

Finally, but of critical importance, there is increasing concern about patient privacy in many countries. The regulatory framework for human research is actively changing, in the process. As discussed in Chapter 15, this is already beginning to make pharmacoepidemiologic research more difficult, whether it is access to medical records in database studies, or access to a list of possible cases with a disease to enroll in ad hoc case-control studies. This will be an area of great interest and rapid activity over the next few years as electronic health records become much more commonplace, and one in which the field of pharmacoepidemiology will need to remain very active, or risk considerable interference with its activities.

Personnel

With the major increase in interest in the field of pharmacoepidemiology, accompanied by an increased number of funding opportunities, a major remaining problem, aggravated by the other trends, is one of inadequate personnel resources. There is a desperate need for more well-trained people in the field, with employment opportunities available in academia, industry, and government agencies. Some early attempts were made to address this. The Burroughs Wellcome Foundation developed the Burroughs Wellcome Scholar Award in Pharmacoepidemiology, a faculty development award designed to bring new people into the field. This program, now discontinued, did not provide an opportunity for fellowship training of entry-level individuals, but was designed for more experienced investigators. Unfortunately, it is no longer an active program.

Outside of government, training opportunities are limited. In the US, the NIH is the major source of support for scientific training. As noted above, NIGMS, which funds training programs in clinical pharmacology, now supports one program in pharmacoepidemiology. The National Institute of Child Health and Human Development also funds training in pediatric pharmacoepidemiology. However, pharmacoepidemiologic training is still too dependent on nonfederal sources of funds, especially at a time when such funding is becoming harder to obtain. There is a growing number of institutions now capable of carrying out such training, for example universities with faculty members interested in pharmacoepidemiology, including those with clinical research training programs supported by, for example, an NIH Clinical and Translational Science Award (CTSA) and organ system-specific training grants. Young scientists interested in undergoing training in pharmacoepidemiology, however, can only do so if they happen to qualify for support from such programs. No ongoing support is normally available from these programs for training in pharmacoepidemiology *per se*. This has been addressed, primarily through the leadership and generosity of some pharmaceutical companies. Much more is needed, however. Fortunately, with the rapid rise in interest in comparative effectiveness research (see Chapter 22), additional training support is emerging from both NIH and AHRQ.

The view from industry

It appears that the role of pharmacoepidemiology in industry is and will continue to be expanding rapidly. All that was said above about the future of pharmacoepidemiology scientifically, as it relates to academia (see Chapter 6), obviously relates to industry, as well (see Chapter 6). The necessity of pharmacoepidemiology for industry has become apparent to many of those in industry. In addition to being useful for exploring the effects of their drugs, manufacturers are beginning to realize that the field can contribute not only to identifying problems, but also to documenting drug safety and developing and evaluating risk management programs. An increasing number of manufacturers are undertaking pharmacoepidemiologic studies "prophylactically," to have safety data available in advance of when crises may occur. Proper practice would argue for postmarketing studies for all newly marketed drugs used for chronic diseases, and all drugs expected to be either pharmacologically

novel or sales blockbusters, because of the unique risks that these situations present. Pharmacoepidemiology also can be used for measuring beneficial drug effects and even for marketing purposes, in the form of descriptive market research and analyses of the effects of marketing efforts. Perhaps most importantly for the industry's financial bottom line, pharmacoepidemiologic studies can be used to protect the major investment made in developing a new drug against false allegations of adverse effects, protecting good drugs for a public that needs them. Further, even if a drug is found to have a safety problem, the legal liability of the company may be diminished if the company has, from the outset, been forthright in its efforts to learn about that drug's risks. Finally, as noted in Chapter 1, FDA now has new authority to require postmarketing pharmacoepidemiologic studies, so one can expect to see many more required of industry by regulators.

In light of these advantages, most major pharmaceutical firms have formed their own pharmacoepidemiologic units. Of course, this then means that industry confronts and, in fact, aggravates the problem of an insufficient number of well-trained personnel described above. Many pharmaceutical companies increased their investment in external pharmacoepidemiologic data resources, so that they will be available for research when crises arise. This has been declining, however. A risk of the growth in the number of pharmacoepidemiologic studies for industry is the generation of an increased number of false signals about harmful drug effects. This is best addressed by having adequately trained individuals in the field, and by having personnel and data resources available to address these questions quickly, responsibly, and effectively, when they are raised.

The view from regulatory agencies

It appears that the role of pharmacoepidemiology in regulatory agencies is also expanding (see Chapter 6). Again, all of what was said above about the future of pharmacoepidemiology scientifically, as it relates to academia, obviously relates to regulatory agencies, as well. In addition, there have been a large number of major drug crises, many described throughout this book. Many of these crises resulted in the removal of the drugs from the market. The need for and importance of pharmacoepidemiologic studies have become clear. Again, this can be expected to continue in the future. It has even been suggested that postmarketing pharmacoepidemiologic studies might replace some premarketing Phase III studies in selected situations, as was done with zidovudine. As noted, regulatory agencies are being given increased authority to require such studies after marketing. Regulatory bodies are also expanding their pharmacoepidemiologic staffing, and seeking training in pharmacoepidemiology for those already employed by the agencies.

We are also seeing increasing governmental activity and interest in pharmacoepidemiology, outside the traditional realm of regulatory bodies. For example, in the US, pharmacoepidemiology now plays an important role within the AHRQ, the Centers for Disease Control and Prevention, and the NIH, and there has been intermittent debate for 30 years about the wisdom of developing an independent new Center for Drug Surveillance.

As noted above, the use of therapeutic risk management approaches (see Chapter 22) has been aggressively embraced by regulatory bodies around the world. This will continue to change regulation as more experience with it is gained.

Finally, there is an enormous increase in attention to drug safety, most recently driven by drug safety issues identified with COX-2 inhibitors and even traditional nonsteroidal anti-inflammatory drugs, and then by the thiazolidinediones, used for treatment of diabetes. The net result has been major regulatory change, and even new legislation.

The view from the law

Finally, the importance of pharmacoepidemiology to the law has also been increasing. The potential financial risk to drug manufacturers posed by lawsuits related to adverse drug effects is very large. Some financial payments have been enormous, and indeed put large multinational companies at risk. It is clear that the interest in the field and the need for more true experts in the field will, therefore, increase accordingly.

Conclusion

"There are no really 'safe' biologically active drugs. There are only 'safe' physicians."

Harold A. Kaminetzsky, 1963

All drugs have adverse effects. Pharmacoepidemiology will never succeed in preventing them. It can only detect them, hopefully early, and thereby educate health care providers and the public, which will lead to better medication use. Pharmacoepidemiology can also lead to safer use of medications through a better understanding of the factors that alter the risk:benefit balance of medications. The net results of increased activity in pharmacoepidemiology will be better for industry and academia but, most importantly, for the public's health. The next drug disaster cannot be prevented by pharmacoepidemiology. However, pharmacoepidemiology can minimize its adverse public health impact by detecting it early. At the same time, it can improve the use of drugs that have a genuine role, protecting against the loss of useful drugs. The past few decades have demonstrated the utility of this field. They also have pointed out some of its problems. Hopefully, the next few years will see the utility accentuated and the problems ameliorated.

Key points

• The discipline of pharmacoepidemiology has been growing and will likely continue to grow within academia, industry, and government.
• Methodological advances are expected to continue in order to support pharmacoepidemiologic studies as well as newer approaches such as risk management programs and molecular pharmacoepidemiology.
• Content areas such as pharmacoeconomics, medication adherence, risk management, and intermediate surrogate markers will grow as interest and need for these foci increases.

- Both automated databases and *de novo* studies will continue to be important to the field and will serve as important complements to each other.
- Challenges faced by pharmacoepidemiology include limited funding opportunities, regulatory restrictions and privacy concerns surrounding human research, limited training opportunities, and inadequate personnel resources.
- All sectors responsible for the public health, including academia, industry, and government, must address the challenges facing pharmacoepidemiology, and must support its continued development in order to maximize the benefit and minimize the risk inherent in all medications and medical devices.

Further Reading

Andrews EB, Avorn J, Bortnichak EA, Chen R, Dai WS, Dieck GS *et al.* (1996) Guidelines for good epidemiology practices for drug, device, and vaccine research in the United States. *Pharmacoepidemiol Drug Saf* **5**: 333–8.

Bates DW, Leape LL, Cullen DJ, Laird N, Petersen LA, Teich JM, Burdick E, Hickey M, Kleefield S, Shea B, Vander Vliet M, Seger DL (1998) Effect of computerized physician order entry and a team intervention on prevention of serious medication errors. *JAMA* **280**: 1311–16.

Classen DC, Pestotnik SL, Evans RS, Burke JP (1991) Computerized surveillance of adverse drug events in hospital patients. *JAMA* **266**: 2847–51.

Committee on Smallpox Vaccination Program Implementation, Board on Health Promotion and Disease Prevention; Baciu A, Anason AP, Stratton K, Strom B (eds) (2005) *The Smallpox Vaccination Program: Public Health in an Age of Terrorism.* Washington, DC: The National Academies Press.

Food and Drug Administration, eHealth Foundation, and the Brookings Institute (2008) Sentinel Initiative: structure, function and scope. Washington, D.C. December 16, 2008. http://www.fda.gov/oc/initiatives/critical-path/transcript121608.pdf

Howard NJ, Laing RO (1991) Changes in the World Health Organization essential drug list. *Lancet* **338**: 743–5.

Institute of Medicine (2005) *The Smallpox Vaccination Program: Public Health in an Age of Terrorism.* Washington, DC: National Academies Press.

ISPE (2008) Guidelines for good pharmacoepidemiology practices (GPP). *Pharmacoepidemiol Drug Saf* **17**: 200–8.

Joellenbeck LM, Zwanziger LL, Durch JS, Strom BL (eds) (2002) *The Anthrax Vaccine: Is it Safe? Does it Work?* Washington, DC: National Academies Press.

Leeder JS, Riley RJ, Cook VA, Spielberg SP (1992) Human anti-cytochrome P450 antibodies in aromatic anticonvulsant-induced hypersensitivity reactions. *J Pharmacol Exp Ther* **263**:360–7.

Lunde PKM (1984) WHO's programme on essential drugs. Background, implementation, present state and prospectives. *Dan Med Bull* **31** (suppl 1): 23–7.

Pullar T, Feely M (1990) Problems of compliance with drug treatment: new solutions? *Pharm J* **245**: 213–15.

Spielberg SP (1992) Idiosyncratic drug reactions: interaction of development and genetics. *Semin Perinatol* **16**: 58–62.

Strom BL, Carson JL (1990) Use of automated databases for pharmacoepidemiology research. *Epidemiol Rev* **12**: 87–107.

Strom BL, Gibson GA (1993) A systematic integrated approach to improving drug prescribing in an acute care hospital: a potential model for applied hospital pharmacoepidemiology. *Clin Pharmacol Ther* **54**: 126–33.

Strom BL, West SL, Sim E, Carson JL (1989) The epidemiology of the acute flank pain syndrome from suprofen. *Clin Pharmacol Ther* **46**: 693–9.

Urquhart J (1997) The electronic medication event monitor–lessons for pharmacotherapy. *Clin Pharmacokinet* **32**: 345–56.

Woosley RL, Drayer DE, Reidenberg MM, Nies AS, Carr K, Oates JA (1978) Effect of acetylator phenotype on the rate at which procainamide induces antinuclear antibodies and the lupus syndrome. *N Engl J Med* **298**: 1157–9.

Young FE (1988) The role of the FDA in the effort against AIDS. *Public Health Rep* **103**: 242–5.

Yudkin JS (1980) The economics of pharmaceutical supply in Tanzania. *Int J Health Serv* **10**: 455–77.

Yudkin JS (1984) Use and misuse of drugs in the Third World. *Dan Med Bull* **31** (suppl 1): 11–17.

APPENDIX A
Sample Size Tables

Table A1 Sample sizes for cohort studies[a].

Incidence in control group	Relative risk to be detected															
	0.2	0.3	0.5	0.75	1.25	1.5	2.0	2.5	3.0	3.5	4.0	5.0	7.5	10.0	20.0	50.0
0.00001	1 970 717	2 788 497	6 306 290	29 429 320	37 837 603	10 510 431	3 153 120	1 634 946	1 051 034	756 742	583 904	394 133	211 445	142 727	61 134	22 318
0.00005	394 133	557 684	1 261 219	5 885 657	7 567 179	2 101 980	630 585	326 965	210 189	151 334	116 768	78 816	42 280	28 538	12 220	4 458
0.0001	197 060	278 832	630 585	2 942 699	3 783 376	1 050 923	315 268	163 467	105 083	75 657	58 376	39 401	21 135	14 264	6 106	2 225
0.0005	39 401	55 751	126 078	588 332	756 333	210 078	63 015	32 669	20 999	15 117	11 662	7 870	4 219	2 845	1 215	439
0.001	19 694	27 865	63 015	294 037	377 953	104 973	31 483	16 320	10 488	7 549	5 823	3 928	2 104	1 418	603	216
0.005	3 928	5 557	12 564	58 600	75 249	20 888	6 257	3 240	2 080	1 495	1 152	775	412	276	114	37
0.01	1 957	2 769	6 257	29 170	37 411	10 378	3 104	1 605	1 028	738	568	381	201	133	53	15
0.05	381	538	1 212	5 627	7 140	1 969	582	297	188	133	101	65	32	19	4	–
0.10	184	259	582	2 684	3 357	918	266	133	82	57	42	26	10	4	–	–
0.15	118	166	372	1 703	2 095	568	161	79	47	32	23	13	–	–	–	–
0.20	85	120	266	1 212	1 465	393	109	52	30	19	13	6	–	–	–	–
0.25	65	92	203	918	1 086	287	77	35	19	12	7	–	–	–	–	–
0.30	52	73	161	722	834	217	56	24	12	6	–	–	–	–	–	–
0.35	43	60	131	582	654	167	41	16	7	–	–	–	–	–	–	–
0.40	36	50	109	477	519	130	30	11	–	–	–	–	–	–	–	–
0.45	30	42	91	395	414	101	21	6	–	–	–	–	–	–	–	–
0.50	26	36	77	329	329	77	14	–	–	–	–	–	–	–	–	–
0.55	22	31	66	276	261	58	8	–	–	–	–	–	–	–	–	–
0.60	19	27	56	231	203	42	2	–	–	–	–	–	–	–	–	–
0.65	17	23	48	194	155	29	–	–	–	–	–	–	–	–	–	–
0.70	15	20	41	161	113	17	–	–	–	–	–	–	–	–	–	–
0.75	13	17	35	133	77	7	–	–	–	–	–	–	–	–	–	–
0.80	11	15	30	109	46	–	–	–	–	–	–	–	–	–	–	–
0.85	10	13	25	87	18	–	–	–	–	–	–	–	–	–	–	–
0.90	8	11	21	68	–	–	–	–	–	–	–	–	–	–	–	–
0.95	7	9	17	51	–	–	–	–	–	–	–	–	–	–	–	–

[a] $\alpha = 0.05$ (two-tailed), $\beta = 0.10$ (power = 90%), control : exposed ratio = 1:1. The sample size listed is the number of subjects needed in the exposed group. An equivalent number would be included in the control group.

Table A2 Sample size for cohort studies[a].

Incidence in control group	Relative risk to be detected															
	0.2	0.3	0.5	0.75	1.25	1.5	2.0	2.5	3.0	3.5	4.0	5.0	7.5	10.0	20.0	50.0
0.00001	1 529 057	2 153 636	4 825 616	22 279 822	28 149 090	7 764 537	2 302 889	1 183 563	755 529	540 883	415 381	278 329	147 626	99 000	41 938	15 197
0.0001	152 896	215 349	482 527	2 227 804	2 814 625	776 367	230 258	118 337	151 093	108 167	83 068	55 659	29 520	19 795	8 384	3 036
0.0005	30 570	43 057	96 475	445 402	562 673	155 196	46 024	23 651	75 539	54 077	41 528	27 825	14 756	9 895	4 189	1 516
0.001	15 280	21 521	48 218	222 602	281 179	77 550	22 994	11 815	15 095	10 805	8 297	5 558	2 946	1 974	834	300
0.005	3 047	4 292	9 613	44 362	55 984	15 433	4 571	2 346	7 540	5 396	4 143	2 774	1 469	984	414	148
0.01	1 518	2 138	4 787	22 082	27 834	7 668	2 268	1 163	1 496	1 069	820	548	288	192	79	26
0.05	295	415	927	4 258	5 315	1 456	426	216	740	528	404	269	141	93	37	11
0.10	142	200	444	2 030	2 500	680	196	97	136	95	72	47	23	14	3	–
0.15	91	128	283	1 287	1 561	421	119	58	60	41	31	19	8	3	–	–
0.20	66	92	203	916	1 092	291	80	38	35	23	17	9	–	–	–	–
0.25	50	70	155	693	811	214	57	26	22	14	10	4	–	–	–	–
0.30	40	56	123	545	623	162	42	18	14	9	5	–	–	–	–	–
0.35	33	46	100	439	489	125	31	12	9	4	–	–	–	–	–	–
0.40	27	38	82	359	388	97	22	8	5	–	–	–	–	–	–	–
0.45	23	32	69	297	310	76	16	–	–	–	–	–	–	–	–	–
0.50	20	27	58	248	248	58	11	–	–	–	–	–	–	–	–	–
0.55	17	23	49	207	196	44	5	–	–	–	–	–	–	–	–	–
0.60	15	20	42	173	154	32	–	–	–	–	–	–	–	–	–	–
0.65	13	17	36	145	117	22	–	–	–	–	–	–	–	–	–	–
0.70	11	15	31	120	86	13	–	–	–	–	–	–	–	–	–	–
0.75	9	13	26	99	59	–	–	–	–	–	–	–	–	–	–	–
0.80	8	11	22	80	35	–	–	–	–	–	–	–	–	–	–	–
0.85	7	10	18	64	–	–	–	–	–	–	–	–	–	–	–	–
0.90	6	8	15	49	–	–	–	–	–	–	–	–	–	–	–	–
0.95	5	7	12	36	–	–	–	–	–	–	–	–	–	–	–	–

[a] $\alpha = 0.05$ (two-tailed), $\beta = 0.10$ (power = 90%), control : exposed ratio = 2 : 1. The sample size listed is the number of subjects needed in the exposed group. Double this number would be included in the control group.

Table A3 Sample sizes for cohort studies[a].

Incidence in control group	Relative risk to be detected															
	0.2	0.3	0.5	0.75	1.25	1.5	2.0	2.5	3.0	3.5	4.0	5.0	7.5	10.0	20.0	50.0
0.00001	1 369 471	1 930 847	4 322 614	19 888 657	24 913 372	6 843 626	2 014 756	1 029 014	653 418	465 696	356 275	237 254	124 571	83 030	34 793	12 510
0.00005	273 886	386 158	864 495	3 977 589	4 982 452	1 368 657	402 927	205 788	130 673	93 131	71 248	47 445	24 910	16 602	6 955	2 499
0.0001	136 938	193 072	432 230	1 988 706	2 491 087	684 286	201 449	102 885	65 330	46 560	35 619	23 719	12 452	8 299	3 476	1 248
0.0005	27 380	38 603	86 418	397 599	497 995	136 790	40 266	20 563	13 055	9 303	7 117	4 738	2 486	1 656	692	247
0.001	13 685	19 294	43 192	198 711	248 859	68 352	20 118	10 272	6 521	4 646	3 554	2 365	1 240	825	344	122
0.005	2 729	3 847	8 611	39 600	49 549	13 603	4 000	2 040	1 294	921	703	467	244	161	66	21
0.01	1 359	1 916	4 288	19 711	24 636	6 759	1 985	1 011	640	455	347	230	119	78	31	9
0.05	264	372	830	3 800	4 705	1 284	373	188	117	82	62	40	19	12	2	–
0.10	127	179	398	1 811	2 213	600	171	85	52	36	26	16	7	3	–	–
0.15	81	114	254	1 148	1 383	372	104	50	30	20	14	8	–	–	–	–
0.20	58	82	181	817	968	257	71	33	19	12	8	4	–	–	–	–
0.25	45	63	138	618	719	189	50	23	13	7	4	–	–	–	–	–
0.30	36	50	109	485	552	143	37	16	8	4	–	–	–	–	–	–
0.35	29	41	89	391	434	111	27	11	4	–	–	–	–	–	–	–
0.40	24	34	73	319	345	86	20	7	–	–	–	–	–	–	–	–
0.45	20	28	61	264	275	67	14	–	–	–	–	–	–	–	–	–
0.50	17	24	52	220	220	52	9	–	–	–	–	–	–	–	–	–
0.55	15	21	44	184	175	39	–	–	–	–	–	–	–	–	–	–
0.60	13	18	37	154	137	29	–	–	–	–	–	–	–	–	–	–
0.65	11	15	32	128	105	19	–	–	–	–	–	–	–	–	–	–
0.70	10	13	27	106	77	10	–	–	–	–	–	–	–	–	–	–
0.75	8	11	23	87	53	–	–	–	–	–	–	–	–	–	–	–
0.80	7	10	19	71	31	–	–	–	–	–	–	–	–	–	–	–
0.85	6	8	16	56	–	–	–	–	–	–	–	–	–	–	–	–
0.90	5	7	13	43	–	–	–	–	–	–	–	–	–	–	–	–
0.95	4	6	11	31	–	–	–	–	–	–	–	–	–	–	–	–

[a] $\alpha = 0.05$ (two-tailed), $\beta = 0.10$ (power = 90%), control : exposed ratio = 3 : 1. The sample size listed is the number of subjects needed in the exposed group. Triple this number would be included in the control group.

Table A4 Sample sizes for cohort studies[a].

Incidence in control group	Relative risk to be detected															
	0.2	0.3	0.5	0.75	1.25	1.5	2.0	2.5	3.0	3.5	4.0	5.0	7.5	10.0	20.0	50.0
0.00001	1 285 566	1 815 876	4 068 209	18 690 665	23 293 643	6 381 472	1 869 238	950 463	601 217	427 061	325 766	215 895	112 429	74 554	30 945	11 048
0.00005	257 106	363 164	813 616	3 737 999	4 658 521	1 276 231	373 825	190 079	120 234	85 404	65 147	43 174	22 482	14 907	6 186	2 207
0.0001	128 548	181 575	406 791	1 868 916	2 329 131	638 076	186 899	95 031	60 111	42 697	32 569	21 583	11 238	7 451	3 091	1 102
0.0005	25 702	36 304	81 332	373 649	465 619	127 552	37 358	18 993	12 013	8 532	6 507	4 311	2 244	1 487	615	218
0.001	12 846	18 145	40 650	186 741	232 680	63 737	18 665	9 488	6 000	4 261	3 249	2 152	1 119	741	306	107
0.005	2 562	3 618	8 104	37 214	46 329	12 684	3 711	1 884	1 190	844	643	425	220	145	58	19
0.01	1 276	1 802	4 035	18 523	23 035	6 303	1 842	934	589	417	318	209	107	70	27	8
0.05	248	349	781	3 571	4 399	1 198	346	174	108	76	57	36	17	10	2	–
0.10	119	168	374	1 702	2 070	560	159	78	48	33	24	15	6	2	–	–
0.15	76	107	238	1 079	1 294	347	97	47	28	19	13	7	–	–	–	–
0.20	55	77	171	767	905	240	66	31	18	11	8	3	–	–	–	–
0.25	42	59	130	580	672	177	47	21	12	7	4	–	–	–	–	–
0.30	33	47	103	456	517	134	34	15	7	–	–	–	–	–	–	–
0.35	27	38	83	366	406	103	25	10	3	–	–	–	–	–	–	–
0.40	23	32	69	300	323	81	18	6	–	–	–	–	–	–	–	–
0.45	19	27	58	248	258	63	13	–	–	–	–	–	–	–	–	–
0.50	16	23	48	206	206	48	8	–	–	–	–	–	–	–	–	–
0.55	14	19	41	172	164	37	–	–	–	–	–	–	–	–	–	–
0.60	12	16	35	144	128	27	–	–	–	–	–	–	–	–	–	–
0.65	10	14	30	120	98	18	–	–	–	–	–	–	–	–	–	–
0.70	9	12	25	99	72	7	–	–	–	–	–	–	–	–	–	–
0.75	8	10	21	81	50	–	–	–	–	–	–	–	–	–	–	–
0.80	6	9	18	66	29	–	–	–	–	–	–	–	–	–	–	–
0.85	6	8	15	52	–	–	–	–	–	–	–	–	–	–	–	–
0.90	5	6	12	39	–	–	–	–	–	–	–	–	–	–	–	–
0.95	4	5	10	28	–	–	–	–	–	–	–	–	–	–	–	–

[a] $\alpha = 0.05$ (two-tailed), $\beta = 0.10$ (power = 90%), control : exposed ratio = 4 : 1. The sample size listed is the number of subjects needed in the exposed group. Quadruple this number would be included in the control group.

Table A5 Sample sizes for cohort studies[a].

Relative risk to be detected

Incidence in control group	0.2	0.3	0.5	0.75	1.25	1.5	2.0	2.5	3.0	3.5	4.0	5.0	7.5	10.0	20.0	50.0
0.00001	1 472 091	2 082 958	4 710 686	21 983 178	28 264 016	7 851 105	2 355 325	1 221 276	785 104	565 273	436 166	294 411	157 946	106 615	45 666	16 672
0.00005	294 411	416 580	942 108	4 396 481	5 652 548	1 570 142	471 036	244 238	157 008	113 044	87 224	58 875	31 583	21 318	9 129	3 330
0.0001	147 201	208 283	471 036	2 198 144	2 826 115	785 022	235 500	122 108	78 496	56 515	43 606	29 433	15 788	10 656	4 562	1 663
0.0005	29 433	41 645	94 178	439 474	564 968	156 925	47 071	24 404	15 686	11 292	8 712	5 879	3 152	2 126	908	329
0.001	14 711	20 816	47 071	219 641	282 325	78 413	23 518	12 191	7 835	5 639	4 350	2 935	1 572	1 060	451	162
0.005	2 935	4 152	9 385	43 774	56 210	15 604	4 675	2 421	1 554	1 117	861	579	309	207	86	28
0.01	1 463	2 069	4 675	21 790	27 946	7 752	2 319	1 199	769	552	425	285	151	100	40	12
0.05	285	402	906	4 204	5 334	1 471	435	222	141	100	76	49	24	15	3	–
0.10	138	194	435	2 005	2 508	686	200	100	62	43	32	20	8	4	–	–
0.15	89	125	278	1 273	1 566	425	121	59	36	24	17	10	–	–	–	–
0.20	64	90	200	906	1 095	294	82	39	23	15	10	5	–	–	–	–
0.25	49	69	152	686	812	215	58	27	15	9	6	–	–	–	–	–
0.30	40	55	121	540	623	163	42	19	10	–	–	–	–	–	–	–
0.35	33	45	99	435	489	125	31	13	–	–	–	–	–	–	–	–
0.40	27	38	82	357	388	97	23	8	–	–	–	–	–	–	–	–
0.45	23	32	69	295	309	76	16	–	–	–	–	–	–	–	–	–
0.50	20	27	58	247	247	58	11	–	–	–	–	–	–	–	–	–
0.55	17	24	50	207	195	44	–	–	–	–	–	–	–	–	–	–
0.60	15	20	42	173	152	32	–	–	–	–	–	–	–	–	–	–
0.65	13	18	36	145	116	22	–	–	–	–	–	–	–	–	–	–
0.70	11	15	31	121	85	13	–	–	–	–	–	–	–	–	–	–
0.75	10	13	27	100	58	6	–	–	–	–	–	–	–	–	–	–
0.80	9	12	23	82	35	–	–	–	–	–	–	–	–	–	–	–
0.85	8	10	19	66	14	–	–	–	–	–	–	–	–	–	–	–
0.90	7	9	16	51	–	–	–	–	–	–	–	–	–	–	–	–
0.95	6	8	14	38	–	–	–	–	–	–	–	–	–	–	–	–

[a] $\alpha = 0.05$ (two-tailed), $\beta = 0.20$ (power $= 80\%$), control : exposed ratio $= 1:1$. The sample size listed is the number of subjects needed in the exposed group. An equivalent number would be included in the control group.

Table A6 Sample sizes for cohort studies.

Incidence in control group	\multicolumn{16}{c}{Relative risk to be detected}															
	0.2	0.3	0.5	0.75	1.25	1.5	2.0	2.5	3.0	3.5	4.0	5.0	7.5	10.0	20.0	50.0
0.00001	1 190 356	1 663 432	3 680 447	16 792 779	20 878 641	5 726 194	1 683 582	859 799	546 209	389 547	298 242	198 909	104 767	69 986	29 458	10 630
0.00005	238 065	332 677	736 066	3 358 436	4 175 543	1 145 183	336 697	171 948	109 233	77 903	59 643	39 777	20 950	13 994	5 889	2 124
0.0001	119 028	166 332	368 018	1 679 143	2 087 655	572 556	168 336	85 967	54 611	38 947	29 818	19 886	10 473	6 995	2 943	1 061
0.0005	23 799	33 257	73 580	335 708	417 346	114 455	33 648	17 182	10 914	7 783	5 958	3 973	2 091	1 396	586	210
0.001	11 895	16 622	36 775	167 779	208 557	57 193	16 812	8 584	5 452	3 887	2 975	1 983	1 043	696	292	104
0.005	2 372	3 315	7 332	33 436	41 526	11 382	3 343	1 705	1 082	771	589	392	205	136	56	19
0.01	1 182	1 651	3 651	16 643	20 647	5 656	1 659	845	536	381	291	193	100	66	26	8
0.05	230	321	707	3 208	3 944	1 075	312	157	99	69	52	34	17	10	2	–
0.10	111	154	339	1 529	1 856	503	144	71	44	30	23	14	6	3	–	–
0.15	71	99	216	969	1 160	312	88	43	26	17	13	7	–	–	–	–
0.20	51	71	155	689	812	216	60	28	17	11	8	4	–	–	–	–
0.25	39	54	118	522	603	159	43	20	11	7	4	–	–	–	–	–
0.30	31	43	93	410	464	121	32	14	7	4	–	–	–	–	–	–
0.35	26	35	76	330	365	93	23	10	4	–	–	–	–	–	–	–
0.40	21	29	63	270	290	73	17	6	–	–	–	–	–	–	–	–
0.45	18	25	52	223	232	57	13	–	–	–	–	–	–	–	–	–
0.50	15	21	44	186	186	44	9	–	–	–	–	–	–	–	–	–
0.55	13	18	38	155	148	34	5	–	–	–	–	–	–	–	–	–
0.60	11	16	32	130	116	25	–	–	–	–	–	–	–	–	–	–
0.65	10	13	27	108	89	18	–	–	–	–	–	–	–	–	–	–
0.70	9	12	23	90	66	11	–	–	–	–	–	–	–	–	–	–
0.75	8	10	20	74	46	–	–	–	–	–	–	–	–	–	–	–
0.80	7	9	17	60	28	–	–	–	–	–	–	–	–	–	–	–
0.85	6	7	14	47	–	–	–	–	–	–	–	–	–	–	–	–
0.90	5	6	12	36	–	–	–	–	–	–	–	–	–	–	–	–
0.95	4	5	9	26	–	–	–	–	–	–	–	–	–	–	–	–

[a] $\alpha = 0.05$ (two-tailed), $\beta = 0.20$ (power $= 80\%$), control : exposed ratio $= 2 : 1$. The sample size listed is the number of subjects needed in the exposed group. Double this number would be included in the control group.

Table A7 Sample sizes for cohort studies[a].

Incidence in control group	Relative risk to be detected															
	0.2	0.3	0.5	0.75	1.25	1.5	2.0	2.5	3.0	3.5	4.0	5.0	7.5	10.0	20.0	50.0
0.00001	1 088 323	1 516 254	3 330 831	15 057 392	18 412 768	5 014 203	1 455 566	736 622	464 207	328 848	250 342	165 451	85 870	56 861	23 565	8 410
0.00005	217 658	303 242	666 145	3 011 370	3 682 391	1 002 792	291 297	147 315	92 835	65 764	50 064	33 087	17 171	11 370	4 711	1 681
0.0001	108 825	151 615	333 059	1 505 617	1 841 094	501 366	145 638	73 651	46 413	32 879	25 029	16 541	8 584	5 684	2 355	839
0.0005	21 759	30 314	66 590	301 015	368 057	100 225	29 111	14 721	9 276	6 570	5 001	3 305	1 714	1 134	469	166
0.001	10 875	15 151	33 281	150 439	183 927	50 082	14 545	7 354	4 634	3 282	2 498	1 650	855	566	233	82
0.005	2 169	3 021	6 635	29 979	36 623	9 968	2 892	1 461	920	651	495	326	168	111	45	15
0.01	1 080	1 505	3 304	14 922	18 210	4 954	1 436	725	456	322	245	161	83	54	21	6
0.05	210	292	639	2 876	3 480	942	271	135	84	59	44	29	14	8	2	–
0.10	101	140	306	1 370	1 638	441	125	62	38	26	19	12	5	2	–	–
0.15	65	90	195	868	1 025	274	76	37	22	15	11	6	–	–	–	–
0.20	46	64	139	617	718	190	52	25	14	9	6	3	–	–	–	–
0.25	36	49	106	466	534	140	37	17	10	6	4	–	–	–	–	–
0.30	28	39	84	366	411	107	28	12	6	3	–	–	–	–	–	–
0.35	23	32	68	294	323	83	21	9	4	–	–	–	–	–	–	–
0.40	19	26	56	240	257	65	15	6	–	–	–	–	–	–	–	–
0.45	16	22	47	199	206	51	11	–	–	–	–	–	–	–	–	–
0.50	14	19	39	165	165	39	8	–	–	–	–	–	–	–	–	–
0.55	12	16	33	138	132	30	–	–	–	–	–	–	–	–	–	–
0.60	10	14	28	115	104	23	–	–	–	–	–	–	–	–	–	–
0.65	9	12	24	96	80	16	–	–	–	–	–	–	–	–	–	–
0.70	8	10	20	79	60	9	–	–	–	–	–	–	–	–	–	–
0.75	7	9	17	65	42	–	–	–	–	–	–	–	–	–	–	–
0.80	6	7	14	52	26	–	–	–	–	–	–	–	–	–	–	–
0.85	5	6	12	41	–	–	–	–	–	–	–	–	–	–	–	–
0.90	4	5	10	31	–	–	–	–	–	–	–	–	–	–	–	–
0.95	3	4	8	22	–	–	–	–	–	–	–	–	–	–	–	–

[a] $\alpha = 0.05$ (two-tailed), $\beta = 0.20$ (power $= 80\%$), control : exposed ratio $= 3 : 1$. The sample size listed is the number of subjects needed in the exposed group. Triple this number would be included in the control group.

Table A8 Sample sizes for cohort studies[a].

Incidence in control group	Relative risk to be detected															
	0.2	0.3	0.5	0.75	1.25	1.5	2.0	2.5	3.0	3.5	4.0	5.0	7.5	10.0	20.0	50.0
0.00001	1 034 606	1 440 316	3 154 116	14 188 116	17 178 604	4 657 092	1 342 104	674 194	422 454	297 814	225 764	148 182	76 019	49 975	20 438	7 223
0.00005	206 915	288 054	630 802	2 837 520	3 435 570	931 374	268 406	134 830	84 485	59 558	45 149	29 633	15 201	9 993	4 086	1 443
0.0001	103 454	144 022	315 388	1 418 696	1 717 691	465 659	134 194	67 410	42 238	29 776	22 572	14 815	7 599	4 995	2 042	721
0.0005	20 685	28 795	63 057	283 636	343 387	93 087	26 824	13 473	8 442	5 950	4 510	2 960	1 518	997	407	143
0.001	10 338	14 392	31 515	141 754	171 599	46 516	13 402	6 731	4 217	2 972	2 253	1 478	757	497	203	71
0.005	2 061	2 870	6 282	28 248	34 169	9 259	2 665	1 338	837	590	446	292	149	98	39	13
0.01	1 027	1 429	3 128	14 059	16 990	4 601	1 323	663	415	292	221	144	73	48	19	6
0.05	199	277	605	2 709	3 247	876	250	124	77	53	40	26	12	8	2	–
0.10	96	133	289	1 290	1 529	410	115	57	35	24	17	11	5	2	–	–
0.15	61	85	184	817	957	255	71	34	20	14	10	6	–	–	–	–
0.20	44	61	132	581	670	177	48	23	13	9	6	3	–	–	–	–
0.25	34	47	100	439	499	130	35	16	9	5	3	–	–	–	–	–
0.30	27	37	79	344	384	99	26	11	6	–	–	–	–	–	–	–
0.35	22	30	64	277	302	77	19	8	3	–	–	–	–	–	–	–
0.40	18	25	53	226	241	60	14	5	–	–	–	–	–	–	–	–
0.45	15	21	44	186	193	47	10	–	–	–	–	–	–	–	–	–
0.50	13	18	37	155	155	37	7	–	–	–	–	–	–	–	–	–
0.55	11	15	31	129	124	28	–	–	–	–	–	–	–	–	–	–
0.60	9	13	26	108	97	21	–	–	–	–	–	–	–	–	–	–
0.65	8	11	22	89	75	15	–	–	–	–	–	–	–	–	–	–
0.70	7	9	19	74	56	7	–	–	–	–	–	–	–	–	–	–
0.75	6	8	16	60	39	–	–	–	–	–	–	–	–	–	–	–
0.80	5	7	13	48	24	–	–	–	–	–	–	–	–	–	–	–
0.85	4	6	11	38	–	–	–	–	–	–	–	–	–	–	–	–
0.90	4	5	9	28	–	–	–	–	–	–	–	–	–	–	–	–
0.95	3	4	7	20	–	–	–	–	–	–	–	–	–	–	–	–

[a] $\alpha = 0.05$ (two-tailed), $\beta = 0.20$ (power = 80%), control : exposed ratio = 4 : 1. The sample size listed is the number of subjects needed in the exposed group. Quadruple this number would be included in the control group.

Table A9 Sample sizes for case–control studies[a].

Prevalence in control group	Odds ratio to be detected															
	0.2	0.3	0.5	0.75	1.25	1.5	2.0	2.5	3.0	3.5	4.0	5.0	7.5	10.0	20.0	50.0
0.00001	1 970 728	2 788 519	6 306 363	29 429 793	37 838 497	10 510 715	3 153 225	1 635 011	1 051 081	756 780	583 937	394 159	211 464	142 743	61 147	22 330
0.00005	394 143	557 705	1 261 292	5 886 130	7 568 072	2 102 264	630 690	327 029	210 236	151 372	116 801	78 842	42 300	28 555	12 234	4 469
0.0001	197 070	278 853	630 659	2 943 172	3 784 269	1 051 207	315 373	163 532	105 130	75 696	58 409	39 427	21 155	14 281	6 120	2 237
0.0005	39 412	55 772	126 151	588 806	757 227	210 362	63 120	32 734	21 046	15 155	11 695	7 896	4 238	2 862	1 228	451
0.001	19 704	27 887	63 088	294 510	378 847	105 257	31 588	16 384	10 535	7 587	5 856	3 954	2 124	1 435	617	228
0.005	3 939	5 579	12 638	59 074	76 145	21 173	6 363	3 304	2 127	1 533	1 184	801	432	293	128	49
0.01	1 968	2 790	6 331	29 646	38 309	10 663	3 210	1 669	1 076	777	601	407	221	150	67	27
0.05	391	560	1 288	6 111	8 059	2 261	690	363	237	172	135	93	52	37	18	9
0.10	195	281	659	3 181	4 302	1 219	379	202	133	98	77	54	32	23	13	8
0.15	129	189	451	2 215	3 072	879	278	150	100	75	60	43	26	19	11	8
0.20	97	143	348	1 741	2 476	716	230	126	85	64	52	37	23	18	11	8
0.25	77	116	287	1 465	2 137	624	203	113	77	59	48	35	23	18	12	9
0.30	64	98	248	1 289	1 930	569	188	106	73	56	46	34	23	18	13	10
0.35	56	86	222	1 174	1 802	536	180	103	72	56	46	35	24	19	14	11
0.40	49	77	203	1 097	1 727	519	177	102	72	56	47	36	25	20	15	12
0.45	44	70	191	1 048	1 694	513	178	104	74	58	49	38	27	22	17	14
0.50	40	66	182	1 023	1 696	519	182	108	77	61	52	40	29	24	19	16
0.55	38	62	178	1 019	1 732	535	191	114	82	66	56	44	32	27	21	18
0.60	36	61	177	1 035	1 806	562	203	123	89	72	61	49	36	31	25	21
0.65	35	60	180	1 077	1 927	605	222	135	99	80	69	56	42	36	29	25
0.70	34	61	188	1 149	2 110	669	248	153	113	92	79	64	49	43	35	31
0.75	35	64	203	1 268	2 390	764	287	178	133	109	94	77	59	52	43	38
0.80	37	70	230	1 465	2 831	913	348	218	164	135	117	97	75	66	55	49
0.85	43	82	278	1 811	3 591	1 168	451	285	216	179	156	129	101	90	75	68
0.90	54	108	379	2 527	5 143	1 687	659	420	320	266	233	195	154	137	116	105
0.95	93	190	690	4 717	9 851	3 257	1 288	828	635	531	466	391	313	280	238	217

[a] $\alpha = 0.05$ (two-tailed), $\beta = 0.10$ (power = 90%), control : case ratio = 1 : 1. The sample size listed is the number of subjects needed in the case group. An equivalent number would be included in the control group.

Table A10 Sample sizes for case–control studies[a].

Prevalence in control group	Odds ratio to be detected															
	0.2	0.3	0.5	0.75	1.25	1.5	2.0	2.5	3.0	3.5	4.0	5.0	7.5	10.0	20.0	50.0
0.00001	1 529 065	2 153 652	4 825 672	22 280 178	28 149 758	7 764 749	2 302 966	1 183 610	755 564	540 911	415 405	278 348	147 639	99 012	41 948	15 205
0.00005	305 811	430 731	965 148	4 456 162	5 630 233	1 553 041	460 628	236 743	151 128	108 194	83 091	55 678	29 534	19 807	8 393	3 044
0.0001	152 904	215 366	482 583	2 228 160	2 815 293	776 578	230 335	118 385	75 573	54 105	41 552	27 844	14 770	9 906	4 199	1 524
0.0005	30 578	43 073	96 531	445 759	563 340	155 407	46 101	23 698	15 130	10 833	8 321	5 577	2 960	1 986	843	307
0.001	15 288	21 537	48 274	222 959	281 846	77 761	23 072	11 862	7 574	5 424	4 167	2 793	1 483	996	424	155
0.005	3 055	4 308	9 669	44 719	56 653	15 644	4 649	2 393	1 530	1 097	844	567	302	204	88	34
0.01	1 526	2 154	4 843	22 440	28 505	7 880	2 346	1 210	775	556	428	289	155	105	46	19
0.05	303	431	984	4 623	6 001	1 674	506	264	171	124	97	66	37	26	13	7
0.10	150	216	503	2 405	3 207	904	279	148	97	71	56	39	23	17	9	6
0.15	100	145	343	1 673	2 292	653	205	111	74	55	44	31	19	14	8	6
0.20	74	110	265	1 313	1 849	533	170	93	63	47	38	28	17	13	8	6
0.25	59	89	218	1 104	1 597	465	151	84	57	44	35	26	17	13	9	6
0.30	49	75	188	971	1 443	425	140	79	55	42	34	26	17	14	9	7
0.35	42	65	168	883	1 349	401	135	77	54	42	34	26	18	14	10	8
0.40	37	58	154	825	1 294	388	133	77	54	42	35	27	19	15	11	9
0.45	33	53	144	788	1 270	385	133	78	56	44	37	28	20	17	13	10
0.50	31	50	137	768	1 272	389	137	81	58	46	39	31	22	19	14	12
0.55	28	47	133	764	1 301	402	144	86	62	50	42	33	24	21	16	14
0.60	27	45	133	775	1 357	423	154	93	68	55	47	37	28	24	19	16
0.65	26	45	135	805	1 449	456	168	103	76	61	52	42	32	28	22	19
0.70	26	45	140	859	1 588	505	188	116	86	70	61	49	38	33	27	23
0.75	26	47	151	947	1 799	577	218	136	102	84	72	59	46	40	33	29
0.80	28	51	170	1 092	2 133	690	265	166	125	104	90	74	58	51	42	38
0.85	31	60	205	1 349	2 708	884	343	218	165	137	120	100	78	70	58	53
0.90	39	78	279	1 880	3 881	1 278	503	322	246	205	180	150	119	107	90	82
0.95	66	137	506	3 505	7 438	2 472	984	635	489	410	360	303	243	218	186	169

[a] $\alpha = 0.05$ (two-tailed), $\beta = 0.10$ (power = 90%), control : case ratio = 2 : 1. The sample size listed is the number of subjects needed in the case group. Double this number would be included in the control group.

Table A11 Sample size for case–control studies[a].

Prevalence in control group	Odds ratio to be detected															
	0.2	0.3	0.5	0.75	1.25	1.5	2.0	2.5	3.0	3.5	4.0	5.0	7.5	10.0	20.0	50.0
0.00001	1369478	1930861	4322663	19888975	24913964	6843813	2014824	1029056	653448	465720	356295	237271	124583	83040	34800	12517
0.00005	273893	386172	864545	3977907	4983044	1368844	402996	205830	130703	93155	71268	47461	24922	16612	6963	2506
0.0001	136945	193086	432280	1989023	2491679	684473	201517	102927	65360	46584	35640	23735	12464	8309	3483	1254
0.0005	27387	38617	86468	397917	498587	136977	40334	20604	13086	9328	7137	4754	2498	1666	700	253
0.001	13692	19309	43242	199028	249451	68540	20186	10314	6551	4671	3574	2382	1252	836	352	128
0.005	2736	3862	8661	39918	50143	13790	4068	2082	1324	945	724	484	256	171	73	28
0.01	1367	1931	4338	20030	25231	6947	2054	1053	671	480	368	246	131	88	39	16
0.05	271	387	881	4125	5313	1477	444	231	149	108	84	57	32	22	11	6
0.10	134	194	450	2145	2841	799	245	129	85	62	49	34	20	14	8	5
0.15	89	130	307	1491	2031	577	180	97	64	48	38	27	16	12	7	5
0.20	66	98	236	1171	1639	471	150	82	55	41	33	24	15	12	7	5
0.25	53	79	195	984	1417	412	133	74	50	38	31	23	15	12	8	6
0.30	44	67	168	865	1281	376	124	70	48	37	30	23	15	12	8	6
0.35	38	58	150	786	1197	355	119	68	47	37	30	23	16	13	9	7
0.40	33	52	137	734	1149	345	118	68	48	37	31	24	16	14	10	8
0.45	30	47	128	700	1128	342	119	69	49	39	32	25	18	15	11	9
0.50	27	44	122	682	1131	346	122	72	52	41	35	27	19	16	12	10
0.55	25	42	119	679	1156	357	128	76	55	44	38	30	22	18	14	12
0.60	24	40	118	689	1207	377	137	83	60	49	41	33	25	21	17	14
0.65	23	40	119	715	1289	406	150	91	67	55	47	38	28	24	20	17
0.70	23	40	124	762	1414	450	168	104	77	63	54	44	33	29	24	21
0.75	23	42	133	839	1602	515	195	121	91	75	65	53	41	36	29	26
0.80	24	45	150	968	1900	616	236	149	112	93	80	66	52	45	38	34
0.85	27	52	180	1194	2413	789	307	195	148	123	107	89	70	62	52	46
0.90	34	68	245	1664	3459	1142	450	288	220	184	161	134	107	95	80	72
0.95	57	119	444	3100	6632	2208	881	569	438	367	323	271	217	194	165	150

[a] $\alpha = 0.05$ (two-tailed), $\beta = 0.10$ (power = 90%), control : case ratio = 3 : 1. The sample size listed is the number of subjects needed in the case group. Triple this number would be included in the control group.

Table A12 Sample sizes for case–control studies[a].

Prevalence in control group	Odds ratio to be detected															
	0.2	0.3	0.5	0.75	1.25	1.5	2.0	2.5	3.0	3.5	4.0	5.0	7.5	10.0	20.0	50.0
0.00001	1 285 573	1 815 890	4 068 256	18 690 963	23 294 197	6 381 647	1 869 301	950 501	601 245	427 084	325 786	215 910	112 440	74 563	30 952	11 054
0.00005	257 112	363 178	813 662	3 738 297	4 659 075	1 276 406	373 889	190 118	120 262	85 427	65 166	43 189	22 493	14 916	6 193	2 213
0.0001	128 555	181 589	406 838	1 869 214	2 329 685	638 251	186 963	95 070	60 139	42 720	32 588	21 599	11 249	7 461	3 098	1 108
0.0005	25 709	36 318	81 379	373 947	466 173	127 727	37 422	19 032	12 041	8 554	6 526	4 326	2 255	1 496	622	224
0.001	12 853	18 159	40 697	187 039	233 234	63 912	18 729	9 527	6 028	4 284	3 269	2 167	1 130	750	313	113
0.005	2 568	3 632	8 151	37 513	46 884	12 860	3 775	1 923	1 219	867	662	440	231	154	65	25
0.01	1 283	1 816	4 082	18 823	23 592	6 479	1 906	973	618	440	337	224	118	79	34	14
0.05	255	363	829	3 876	4 969	1 378	412	214	137	99	77	52	29	20	10	5
0.10	126	182	423	2 015	2 658	746	228	120	78	57	45	31	18	13	7	4
0.15	83	122	289	1 401	1 901	539	168	90	60	44	35	25	15	11	7	4
0.20	62	92	222	1 099	1 534	440	140	76	51	38	31	22	14	11	7	5
0.25	50	74	183	923	1 326	385	125	69	47	36	29	21	14	11	7	5
0.30	41	63	158	812	1 200	352	116	65	45	34	28	21	14	11	7	6
0.35	35	55	140	738	1 122	333	111	63	44	34	28	21	14	12	8	6
0.40	31	49	128	688	1 077	323	110	63	45	35	29	22	15	13	9	7
0.45	28	44	120	657	1 058	320	111	65	46	36	30	23	17	14	10	8
0.50	25	41	114	640	1 060	324	114	67	48	38	32	25	18	15	11	10
0.55	23	39	111	636	1 084	335	120	72	52	41	35	28	20	17	13	11
0.60	22	38	110	645	1 132	354	128	78	57	46	39	31	23	20	15	13
0.65	21	37	111	669	1 209	381	140	86	63	51	44	35	26	23	18	16
0.70	21	37	116	713	1 326	422	158	97	72	59	51	41	31	27	22	19
0.75	21	39	125	786	1 504	483	183	114	85	70	61	50	38	33	27	24
0.80	22	42	140	905	1 784	579	222	140	105	87	75	62	48	42	35	31
0.85	25	48	168	1 117	2 266	742	289	183	139	115	101	83	65	58	48	43
0.90	31	63	228	1 556	3 248	1 073	423	271	207	173	151	126	100	89	75	67
0.95	52	110	412	2 897	6 229	2 076	829	536	412	345	303	255	203	182	154	139

[a] $\alpha = 0.05$ (two-tailed), $\beta = 0.10$ (power = 90%), control : case ratio = 4 : 1. The sample size listed is the number of subjects needed in the case group. Quadruple this number would be included in the control group.

Table A13 Sample sizes for case–control studies[a].

Prevalence in control group	Odds ratio to be detected															
	0.2	0.3	0.5	0.75	1.25	1.5	2.0	2.5	3.0	3.5	4.0	5.0	7.5	10.0	20.0	50.0
0.00001	1 472 099	2 082 974	4 710 741	21 983 531	28 264 683	7 851 317	2 355 404	1 221 324	785 139	565 302	436 191	294 430	157 960	106 627	45 676	16 681
0.00005	294 418	416 596	942 163	4 396 835	5 653 216	1 570 354	471 115	244 286	157 043	113 073	87 248	58 894	31 598	21 330	9 139	3 339
0.0001	147 208	208 299	471 091	2 198 497	2 826 782	785 234	235 579	122 156	78 531	56 544	43 631	29 452	15 803	10 668	4 572	1 671
0.0005	29 440	41 661	94 233	439 828	565 636	157 137	47 150	24 452	15 721	11 321	8 736	5 899	3 166	2 138	918	337
0.001	14 719	20 831	47 126	219 994	282 992	78 625	23 596	12 239	7 870	5 668	4 375	2 954	1 587	1 072	461	171
0.005	2 943	4 168	9 441	44 128	56 879	15 816	4 753	2 469	1 589	1 146	885	599	323	219	96	37
0.01	1 470	2 085	4 730	22 145	28 617	7 966	2 398	1 248	804	581	449	305	165	113	50	20
0.05	293	419	962	4 566	6 020	1 690	516	272	177	129	101	70	39	28	14	7
0.10	146	211	493	2 377	3 214	911	283	151	100	74	58	41	24	18	10	6
0.15	97	142	337	1 655	2 295	657	208	113	75	56	45	32	20	15	9	6
0.20	73	107	260	1 301	1 850	535	172	95	64	48	39	28	18	14	9	6
0.25	58	87	215	1 095	1 597	466	152	85	58	44	36	27	17	14	9	7
0.30	49	74	186	964	1 442	425	141	80	55	42	35	26	18	14	10	8
0.35	42	65	166	877	1 346	401	135	77	54	42	35	26	18	15	11	9
0.40	37	58	152	820	1 291	388	133	77	54	42	35	27	19	16	12	10
0.45	33	53	143	784	1 266	384	133	78	56	44	37	29	20	17	13	11
0.50	31	50	137	765	1 267	388	137	81	58	46	39	31	22	19	15	12
0.55	29	47	133	761	1 294	400	143	85	62	50	42	33	25	21	16	14
0.60	27	46	133	774	1 350	421	152	92	67	54	46	37	28	24	19	16
0.65	26	45	135	805	1 440	453	166	101	75	61	52	42	32	27	22	19
0.70	26	46	141	859	1 577	500	186	115	85	69	60	49	37	32	26	23
0.75	27	48	152	948	1 785	571	215	134	100	82	71	58	45	39	33	29
0.80	28	53	172	1 095	2 115	682	260	163	123	101	88	73	57	50	42	37
0.85	32	62	208	1 353	2 683	873	337	213	162	134	117	97	76	68	57	51
0.90	41	81	283	1 888	3 842	1 260	493	314	240	200	175	146	116	103	87	79
0.95	70	142	516	3 524	7 359	2 433	962	619	475	397	349	293	234	210	179	162

[a] $\alpha = 0.05$ (two-tailed), $\beta = 0.20$ (power = 80%), control : case ratio = 1 : 1. The sample size listed is the number of subjects needed in the case group. An equivalent number would be included in the control group.

Table A14 Sample sizes for case–control studies[a].

Prevalence in control group	Odds ratio to be detected															
	0.2	0.3	0.5	0.75	1.25	1.5	2.0	2.5	3.0	3.5	4.0	5.0	7.5	10.0	20.0	50.0
0.00001	1 190 363	1 663 444	3 680 489	16 793 046	20 879 138	5 726 351	1 683 639	859 834	546 235	389 568	298 260	198 923	104 777	69 995	29 465	10 635
0.00005	238 071	332 689	736 108	3 358 703	4 176 039	1 145 339	336 754	171 983	109 259	77 923	59 660	39 791	20 960	14 003	5 896	2 129
0.0001	119 034	166 344	368 060	1 679 410	2 088 152	572 713	168 393	86 001	54 637	38 967	29 835	19 899	10 483	7 004	2 950	1 066
0.0005	23 805	33 269	73 622	335 976	417 842	114 612	33 705	17 216	10 939	7 803	5 975	3 986	2 101	1 405	593	216
0.001	11 901	16 635	36 817	168 047	209 054	57 349	16 869	8 618	5 477	3 907	2 993	1 997	1 053	705	298	109
0.005	2 378	3 327	7 374	33 704	42 024	11 540	3 400	1 740	1 107	791	607	406	215	145	63	24
0.01	1 188	1 664	3 693	16 911	21 146	5 814	1 717	880	561	402	308	207	211	75	33	14
0.05	236	333	750	3 482	4 455	1 237	371	193	125	91	70	48	27	19	10	5
0.10	117	167	383	1 810	2 383	669	205	109	71	53	41	29	17	13	7	5
0.15	77	112	261	1 258	1 704	484	152	82	54	41	32	23	14	11	7	5
0.20	58	84	201	987	1 376	396	126	69	47	35	28	21	13	10	7	5
0.25	46	68	166	829	1 190	346	112	62	43	33	27	20	13	10	7	5
0.30	38	57	143	729	1 076	316	105	59	41	32	26	20	13	11	7	6
0.35	33	50	127	662	1 006	299	101	58	40	31	26	20	14	11	8	7
0.40	29	45	116	618	966	290	99	58	41	32	27	21	15	12	9	7
0.45	26	41	108	590	949	288	100	59	42	33	28	22	16	13	10	8
0.50	24	38	103	574	951	292	103	61	44	35	30	24	17	15	11	10
0.55	22	36	100	571	973	301	108	65	47	38	32	26	19	16	13	11
0.60	21	34	99	579	1 016	318	116	70	52	42	36	29	22	19	15	13
0.65	20	34	101	601	1 085	343	127	78	58	47	40	33	25	22	18	16
0.70	20	34	105	640	1 190	380	143	89	66	54	47	38	29	26	21	19
0.75	20	35	112	705	1 350	435	166	104	78	64	56	46	36	32	26	23
0.80	21	38	126	812	1 601	520	201	127	96	80	70	58	45	40	34	30
0.85	23	44	152	1 002	2 034	667	261	167	127	106	93	77	61	55	46	42
0.90	29	58	205	1 395	2 916	965	383	246	189	158	139	117	94	84	71	65
0.95	48	100	371	2 598	5 592	1 868	750	487	376	316	279	236	190	171	147	134

[a] $\alpha = 0.05$ (two-tailed), $\beta = 0.20$ (power = 80%), control:case ratio = 2:1. The sample size listed is the number of subjects needed in the case group. Double this number would be included in the control group.

Table A15 Sample sizes for case–control studies[a].

Prevalence in control group	Odds ratio to be detected															
	0.2	0.3	0.5	0.75	1.25	1.5	2.0	2.5	3.0	3.5	4.0	5.0	7.5	10.0	20.0	50.0
0.00001	1 088 329	1 516 265	3 330 869	15 057 631	18 413 208	5 014 341	1 456 616	736 652	464 229	328 865	250 357	165 463	85 879	56 868	23 570	8 415
0.00005	217 664	303 253	666 182	3 011 608	3 682 831	1 002 930	291 347	147 345	92 856	65 782	50 079	33 098	17 180	11 377	4 717	1 685
0.0001	108 831	151 626	333 096	1 505 856	1 841 534	501 504	145 688	73 681	46 435	32 896	25 044	16 553	8 592	5 691	2 360	844
0.0005	21 764	30 325	66 628	301 253	368 496	100 363	29 161	14 751	9 298	6 588	5 016	3 316	1 723	1 141	474	171
0.001	10 881	15 162	33 319	150 678	184 367	50 220	14 595	7 384	4 655	3 299	2 513	1 662	864	573	239	87
0.005	2 174	3 032	6 672	30 218	37 064	10 107	2 943	1 491	942	668	510	338	177	118	50	19
0.01	1 086	1 516	3 342	15 161	18 652	5 093	1 486	755	478	340	259	173	91	61	27	11
0.05	215	303	678	3 120	3 932	1 085	323	167	107	77	60	41	23	16	8	4
0.10	107	152	345	1 620	2 105	588	179	94	62	45	35	25	15	11	6	4
0.15	70	101	235	1 125	1 507	426	132	71	47	35	28	20	12	9	6	4
0.20	52	76	181	882	1 218	349	111	60	41	31	25	18	11	9	6	4
0.25	42	62	149	741	1 053	305	99	55	37	29	23	17	11	9	6	5
0.30	35	52	128	650	954	280	92	52	36	28	23	17	12	9	7	5
0.35	30	45	114	590	892	265	89	51	36	28	23	18	12	10	7	6
0.40	26	40	104	550	857	257	88	51	36	28	24	18	13	11	8	6
0.45	23	36	97	525	843	256	89	52	37	30	25	19	14	12	9	7
0.50	21	34	92	511	846	259	92	55	39	32	27	21	15	13	10	7
0.55	19	32	89	507	866	268	97	58	42	34	29	23	17	15	12	9
0.60	18	30	88	514	905	283	104	63	46	38	32	26	19	17	13	10
0.65	18	30	89	533	967	306	114	70	52	42	36	30	23	20	16	12
0.70	17	30	92	567	1 061	339	128	80	60	49	42	35	27	23	19	14
0.75	17	31	99	624	1 204	389	149	93	70	58	51	42	32	29	24	17
0.80	18	33	111	718	1 429	466	181	115	87	72	63	52	41	37	31	21
0.85	20	38	132	884	1 817	598	235	151	115	96	84	70	56	50	42	28
0.90	25	50	179	1 230	2 607	867	345	223	172	144	127	107	85	77	65	59
0.95	41	85	323	2 288	5 002	1 678	678	442	342	288	255	215	174	157	134	123

[a]α = 0.05 (two-tailed), β = 0.20 (power = 80%), control : case ratio = 3 : 1. The sample size listed is the number of subjects needed in the case group. Triple this number would be included in the control group.

Table A16 Sample sizes for case–control studies[a].

Prevalence in control group	Odds ratio to be detected															
	0.2	0.3	0.5	0.75	1.25	1.5	2.0	2.5	3.0	3.5	4.0	5.0	7.5	10.0	20.0	50.0
0.00001	1 034 611	1 440 327	3 154 151	14 188 340	17 179 015	4 657 221	1 342 151	674 222	422 474	297 830	225 778	148 193	76 026	49 982	20 443	7 227
0.00005	206 920	288 065	630 838	2 837 745	3 435 981	931 503	268 452	134 858	84 505	59 574	45 162	29 644	15 209	9 999	4 091	1 447
0.0001	103 459	144 032	315 424	1 418 920	1 718 102	465 788	134 240	67 438	42 259	29 792	22 585	14 825	7 607	5 002	2 047	725
0.0005	20 690	28 806	63 092	283 861	343 799	93 216	26 870	13 501	8 462	5 966	4 524	2 970	1 525	1 003	412	147
0.001	10 344	14 403	31 551	141 978	172 011	46 645	13 449	6 759	4 237	2 988	2 266	1 489	765	504	207	75
0.005	2 067	2 880	6 318	28 473	34 581	9 388	2 712	1 366	858	606	460	303	157	104	44	17
0.01	1 032	1 440	3 164	14 285	17 404	4 731	1 370	691	435	308	234	155	81	54	23	10
0.05	205	288	641	2 938	3 670	1 009	298	153	98	70	54	37	20	14	7	4
0.10	101	144	327	1 525	1 966	547	166	87	57	41	32	23	13	10	5	3
0.15	67	96	222	1 059	1 408	397	123	66	43	32	26	18	11	8	5	4
0.20	50	72	171	830	1 138	325	103	56	38	28	23	17	10	8	5	4
0.25	39	58	140	696	985	285	92	51	35	26	21	16	10	8	6	4
0.30	33	49	121	611	892	261	86	48	33	26	21	16	11	9	6	5
0.35	28	42	107	554	836	248	83	47	33	26	21	16	11	9	7	5
0.40	24	38	97	517	803	241	82	48	34	26	22	17	12	10	7	6
0.45	22	34	91	492	790	240	83	49	35	28	23	18	13	11	8	7
0.50	20	32	86	479	793	243	86	51	37	30	25	20	14	12	9	8
0.55	18	30	83	475	812	252	91	55	40	32	27	22	16	14	11	9
0.60	17	28	82	481	849	266	97	59	44	35	30	24	18	16	13	11
0.65	16	28	83	498	908	288	107	66	49	40	34	28	21	18	15	13
0.70	16	28	86	530	997	319	121	75	56	46	40	33	25	22	18	16
0.75	16	29	92	583	1 131	366	140	88	67	55	48	39	31	27	22	20
0.80	17	31	103	670	1 343	439	171	108	82	68	60	50	39	35	29	26
0.85	18	35	123	826	1 708	564	222	143	109	91	80	67	53	47	40	36
0.90	23	45	166	1 148	2 452	817	327	211	163	137	120	101	81	73	62	56
0.95	37	78	298	2 133	4 707	1 583	641	419	325	273	242	205	165	149	127	116

[a] $\alpha = 0.05$ (two-tailed), $\beta = 0.20$ (power $= 80\%$), control : case ratio $= 4 : 1$. The sample size listed is the number of subjects needed in the case group. Quadruple this number would be included in the control group.

Table A17 Tabular values of 95% confidence limit factors for estimates of a Poisson-distributed variable.

Observed number on which estimate is based (n)	Lower limit factor (L)	Upper limit factor (U)	Observed number on which estimate is based (n)	Lower limit factor (L)	Upper limit factor (U)	Observed number on which estimate is based (n)	Lower limit factor (L)	Upper limit factor (U)
1	0.0253	5.57	21	0.619	1.53	120	0.833	1.200
2	0.121	3.61	22	0.627	1.51	140	0.844	1.184
3	0.206	2.92	23	0.634	1.50	160	0.854	1.171
4	0.272	2.56	24	0.641	1.49	180	0.862	1.160
5	0.324	2.33	25	0.647	1.48	200	0.868	1.151
6	0.367	2.18	26	0.653	1.47	250	0.882	1.134
7	0.401	2.06	27	0.659	1.46	300	0.892	1.121
8	0.431	1.97	28	0.665	1.45	350	0.899	1.112
9	0.458	1.90	29	0.670	1.44	400	0.906	1.104
10	0.480	1.84	30	0.675	1.43	450	0.911	1.098
11	0.499	1.79	35	0.697	1.39	500	0.915	1.093
12	0.517	1.75	40	0.714	1.36	600	0.922	1.084
13	0.532	1.71	45	0.729	1.34	700	0.928	1.078
14	0.546	1.68	50	0.742	1.32	800	0.932	1.072
15	0.560	1.65	60	0.770	1.30	900	0.936	1.068
16	0.572	1.62	70	0.785	1.27	1000	0.939	1.064
17	0.583	1.60	80	0.798	1.25			
18	0.593	1.58	90	0.809	1.24			
19	0.602	1.56	100	0.818	1.22			
20	0.611	1.54						

APPENDIX B
Glossary

The *accuracy* of a measurement is the degree to which the measurement approximates the truth.

Ad hoc studies are studies that require primary data collection.

Active surveillance is surveillance carried out via a continuous, defined process in a specific population, using one of several approaches. Active surveillance can be medical product-based, identifying adverse events in patients taking certain products; setting-based, identifying adverse events in certain healthcare settings where patients are likely to present for treatment (e.g., emergency departments); or event-based, identifying adverse events likely to be associated with medical products (e.g., acute liver failure).

Actual knowledge, in a legal sense, is defined as literal awareness of a fact. Actual knowledge can be demonstrated by showing that the manufacturer was cognizant of reasonable information suggesting, for example, a particular risk.

An *adverse drug event, adverse drug experience, adverse event*, or *adverse experience* is an untoward outcome that occurs during or following clinical use of a drug. It does not necessarily have a causal relationship with this treatment. It may or may not be preventable.

An *adverse drug reaction* is an adverse drug event that is judged to be caused by the drug.

Studies of *adverse effects* examine case reports of adverse drug reactions, attempting to judge subjectively whether the adverse events were indeed caused by the antecedent drug exposure.

Agreement is the degree to which different methods or sources of information give the same answers. Agreement between two sources or methods does not imply that either is valid or reliable.

Analyses of secular trends examine trends in disease events over time and/or across different geographic locations, and correlate them with trends in putative exposures, such as rates of drug utilization. The unit of observation is usually a subgroup of a population, rather than individuals. Also called ecological studies.

Analytic studies are studies with control groups, such as case-control studies, cohort studies, and randomized clinical trials.

Anticipated beneficial effects of drugs are desirable effects that are presumed to be caused by the drug. They usually represent the reason for prescribing or ingesting the drug.

Anticipated harmful effects of drugs are unwanted effects that could have been predicted on the basis of existing knowledge.

An *association* is when two events occur together more often than one would expect by chance.

Textbook of Pharmacoepidemiology, Second Edition. Edited by Brian L. Strom, Stephen E. Kimmel, and Sean Hennessy.
© 2013 John Wiley & Sons, Ltd. Published 2013 by John Wiley & Sons, Ltd.

Autocorrelation is where any individual observation is to some extent a function of the previous observation.

Bias is any systematic (rather than random) error in a study.

Biological inference is the process of generalizing from a statement about an association seen in a population to a causal statement about biological relationships.

Case-cohort studies are studies that compare cases with a disease to a sample of subjects randomly selected from the parent cohort.

Case-control studies are studies that compare cases with a disease to controls without the disease, looking for differences in antecedent exposures.

Case-crossover studies are studies that compare cases at the time of disease occurrence to different time periods in the same individuals, looking for differences in antecedent exposures.

Case reports are reports of the experience of individual patients. As used in pharmacoepidemiology, a case report usually describes a patient who was exposed to a drug and experienced a particular outcome, usually an adverse event.

Case series are reports of collections of patients, all of whom have a common exposure, examining what their clinical outcomes were. Alternatively, case series can be reports of patients who have a common disease, examining what their antecedent exposures were. No control group is present.

An exposure *causes* a health event when it truly increases the probability of that event in some individuals. That is, there are at least some individuals who would experience the event given the exposure who would not experience the event absent the exposure.

Changeability is the ability of an instrument to measure a difference in score in patients who have improved or deteriorated.

Channeling bias is a type of selection bias, which occurs when a drug is claimed to be safe and therefore is used in high-risk patients who did not

tolerate other drugs for that indication. It is sometimes used synonymously with *confounding by indication*.

Drug *clearance* is the proportion of the "apparent" volume of distribution that is cleared of drug in a specified time. Its units are volume per time, such as liters per hour. The total body clearance is the sum of clearances by different routes, e.g., renal, hepatic, pulmonary, etc.

Clinical pharmacology is the study of the effects of drugs in humans.

Cohort studies are studies that identify defined populations and follow them forward in time, examining their frequencies (e.g., incidence rate, cumulative incidence) of disease. Cohort studies generally identify and compare exposed patients to unexposed patients or to patients who receive a different exposure.

Confidence interval is a range of values within which the true population value lies, with some probability.

Confidentiality is the right of patients to limit the transfer and disclosure of private information.

A *confounding variable*, or *confounder*, is a variable other than the risk factor and outcome variable under study that is related independently both to the risk factor and to the outcome. A confounder can artificially inflate or reduce the magnitude of association between and exposure and outcome.

Confounding by indication can occur when the underlying diagnosis or other clinical features that affect the use of a certain drug are also related to the outcome under study.

Construct validity refers to the extent to which results from a given instrument are consistent with those from other measures in a manner consistent with theoretical hypotheses.

Constructive knowledge, from a legal perspective, is knowledge that a person did not have, but could have acquired by the exercise of reasonable care.

A *cost* is the consumption of a resource that could otherwise be used for another purpose.

Cost-benefit analysis of medical care compares the cost of a medical intervention to its benefit. Both costs and benefits must be measured in the same monetary units (e.g., dollars).

Cost-effectiveness analysis of medical care compares the cost of a medical intervention to its effectiveness. Costs are expressed in monetary units, while effectiveness is determined independently and may be measured in terms of any clinically meaningful unit. Cost-effectiveness analyses usually examine the additional cost per unit of additional effectiveness.

Cost-identification analysis enumerates the costs involved in medical care, ignoring the outcomes that result from that care.

Criterion validity refers to the ability of an instrument to measure what it is supposed to measure, as judged by agreement with a reference (gold) standard.

Cross-sectional studies examine exposures and outcomes in populations at one point in time; they have no time sense.

The *defined daily dose* (DDD) is the usual daily maintenance dose for a drug for its main indication in adults.

Descriptive studies are studies that do not have control groups, namely case reports, case series, and analyses of secular trends. They are contrasted with analytic studies.

Detection bias is an error in the results of a study due to a systematic difference between the study groups in the procedures used for ascertainment, diagnosis, or verification of disease.

Differential misclassification occurs when the degree of misclassification of one variable (e.g., drug usage) varies according to the level of another variable (e.g., disease status).

The *direct medical costs* of medical care are the costs that are incurred in providing the care.

Direct nonmedical costs are nonmedical care costs incurred because of an illness or the need to seek medical care. They can include the cost of transportation to the hospital or physician's office, the cost of special clothing needed because of the illness,

and the cost of hotel stays and special housing (e.g., modification of the home to accommodate the ill individual).

Discriminative instruments are those that measure differences among people at a single point in time.

Disease registries are registries characterized by inclusion of subjects based on diagnosis of a common disease or condition.

A *drug* is any exogenously administered substance that exerts a physiologic effect.

Drug utilization, as defined by the World Health Organization (WHO), is the "arketing, distribution, prescription and use of drugs in a society, with special emphasis on the resulting medical, social, and economic consequences."

Drug utilization evaluation (DUE) programs are ongoing structured systems designed to improve drug use by intervening when inappropriate drug use is detected. See also drug utilization review programs.

Drug utilization evaluation studies are ad hoc investigations that assess the appropriateness of drug use. They are designed to detect and quantify the frequency of drug use problems.

Drug utilization review programs are ongoing structured systems designed to improve drug use by intervening when inappropriate drug use is detected.

Drug utilization review studies are ad hoc investigations that assess the appropriateness of drug use. They are designed to detect and quantify any drug use problems. See also drug utilization evaluation programs.

Drug utilization studies are descriptive studies that quantify the use of a drug. Their objective is to quantify the present state, the developmental trends, and the time course of drug usage at various levels of the health care system, whether national, regional, local, or institutional.

Ecological studies examine trends in disease events over time or across different geographic locations and correlate them with trends in putative exposures, such as rates of drug utilization. The unit of observation is a subgroup of a population, rather than individuals. See also analyses of secular trends.

Effect modification occurs when the magnitude of effect of a drug in causing an outcome differs according to the levels of a variable other than the drug or the outcome (e.g., sex, age group). Effect modification can be assessed on an additive and/or multiplicative scale. See interaction.

A study of drug *effectiveness* is a study of whether, in the usual clinical setting, a drug in fact achieves the effect intended when prescribing it.

A study of drug *efficacy* is a study of whether, *under ideal conditions*, a drug has the ability to bring about the effect intended when prescribing it.

A study of drug *efficiency* is a study of whether a drug can bring about its desired effect at an acceptable cost.

Epidemiology is the study of the distribution and determinants of diseases or health-related states in populations.

Evaluative instruments are those designed to measure changes within individuals over time.

Experimental studies are studies in which the investigator controls the therapy that is to be received by each participant, generally using that control to randomly allocate participants among the study groups.

Face validity is a judgment about the validity of an instrument, based on an intuitive assessment of the extent to which an instrument meets a number of criteria including applicability, clarity and simplicity, likelihood of bias, comprehensiveness, and whether redundant items have been included.

Fixed costs are costs that are incurred regardless of the volume of activity.

General causation, from a legal perspective, addresses whether a product is capable of causing a particular injury in the population of patients like the plaintiff.

Generic quality-of-life instruments aim to cover the complete spectrum of function, disability, and

distress of the patient, and are applicable to a variety of populations.

Half-life $(T_{1/2})$ is the time taken for the drug concentration to decline by half. Half-life is a function of both the apparent volume of distribution and clearance of the drug.

Hawthorne Effect is when study subjects alter their behavior simply because of their participation in a study, unrelated to the study procedures or intervention.

Health profiles are single instruments that measure multiple different aspects of quality-of-life.

Health-related quality-of-life is a multifactorial concept which, from the patient's perspective, represents the end-result of all the physiological, psychological, and social influences of the disease and the therapeutic process. Health-related quality-of-life may be considered on different levels: overall assessment of well-being; several broad domains–physiological, functional, psychological, social, and economic status; and subcomponents of each domain—for example pain, sleep, activities of daily living, and sexual function within physical and functional domains.

A *human research subject*, as defined in US regulation, is "a living individual, about whom an investigator (whether professional or student) conducting research obtains either: 1) data through intervention or interaction with the individual, or 2) identifiable private information." [Title 45 US Code of Federal Regulations Part 46.102 (f)]

Hypothesis-generating studies are studies that give rise to new questions about drug effects to be explored further in subsequent analytical studies.

Hypothesis-strengthening studies are studies that reinforce, although do not provide definitive evidence for, existing hypotheses.

Hypothesis-testing studies are studies that evaluate in detail hypotheses raised elsewhere.

Incidence/prevalence bias, a type of selection bias, may occur in studies when prevalent cases rather than new cases of a condition are selected for a study. A strong association with prevalence may be related to the duration of the disease rather than to its incidence, because prevalence is proportional to both incidence and duration of the disease.

The *incidence rate* of a disease is a measure of how frequently the disease occurs. Specifically, it is the number of new cases of the disease which develop over a defined time period in a defined population at risk, divided by the number of people in that population at risk.

Indirect costs are costs that do not stem directly from transactions for goods or services, but represent the loss of opportunities to use a valuable resource in alternative ways. They include costs due to morbidity (e.g., time lost from work) and mortality (e.g., premature death leading to removal from the work force).

Information bias is an error in the results of a study due to a systematic difference between the study groups in the accuracy of the measurements being made of their exposure or outcome.

Intangible costs are those of pain, suffering, and grief.

Interaction, see effect modification.

Interrupted time-series designs include multiple observations (often 10 or more) of study populations before and after an intervention.

Knowledge, as used in court cases, can be actual or constructive; see those terms.

Medication errors are any error in the process of prescribing, transcribing, dispensing, administering, or monitoring a drug, regardless of whether an injury occurred or the potential for injury was present.

Meta-analysis is a systematic, structured review of the literature and formal statistical analysis of a collection of analytic results for the purpose of integrating the findings. Meta-analysis is used to identify sources of variation among study findings and, when appropriate, to provide an overall measure of effect as a summary of those findings.

Misclassification bias is the error resulting from classifying study subjects as exposed when they truly are unexposed, or vice versa. Alternatively,

misclassification bias can result from classifying study subjects as diseased when they truly are not diseased, or vice versa.

Molecular pharmacoepidemiology is the study of the manner in which molecular biomarkers alter the clinical effects of medications.

An *N-of-1 RCT* is a randomized controlled trial within an individual patient, using repeated assignments to the experimental or control arms.

Near misses are medication errors that have high potential for causing harm but didn't, either because they were intercepted prior to reaching a patient or because the error reached the patient who fortuitously did not have any observable untoward sequelae.

Nondifferential misclassification occurs when the misclassification of one variable does not vary by the level of another variable. Nondifferential misclassification usually results in bias toward the null.

Non-experimental studies are studies in which the investigator does not control the therapy, but observes and evaluates the results of ongoing medical care. The study designs that are used are those that do not involve random allocation, such as case reports, case series, analyses of secular trends, case-control studies, and cohort studies.

Observational studies (or nonexperimental studies) are studies in which the investigator does not control the therapy, but observes and evaluates the results of ongoing medical care. The study designs that are used are those that do not involve randomization, such as case reports, case series, analyses of secular trends, case-control studies, and cohort studies.

The *odds ratio* is the odds of exposure in the diseased group divided by the odds of exposure in the nondiseased group. When the underlying risk of disease is low (about 10% or lower) it is an unbiased estimator of the relative risk. It is also an unbiased estimator of the rate ratio in a nested or population-based case-control study in which controls are selected at random from the population at risk of disease at the time that the case occurred.

One-group, post-only study design consists of making only one observation on a single group which has already been exposed to a treatment.

An *opportunity cost* is the value of a resource's next best use, a use that is no longer possible once the resource has been used.

A *p-value* is the probability that a difference as large as or larger than the one observed in the study could have occurred purely by chance if no association truly existed.

Pharmacodynamics is the study of the relationship between drug level and drug effect. It involves the study of the response of the target tissues in the body to a given concentration of drug.

Pharmacogenetic epidemiology is the study of the effects of genetic determinants of drug response on outcomes in large numbers of people.

Pharmacoepidemiology is the study of the use of and the effects of drugs and other medical products in large numbers of people. It is also the application of the research methods of clinical epidemiology to the content area of clinical pharmacology, and the primary science underlying the public health practice of drug safety surveillance.

Pharmacogenetics is the study of genetic determinants of responses to drugs. Although it is sometimes used synonymously with pharmacogenomics, it often refers to a candidate-gene approach as opposed to a genome-wide approach.

Pharmacogenomics is the study of genetic determinants of responses to drugs. Although it is sometimes used synonymously with pharmacogenetics, it often refers to a genome-wide approach as opposed to a candidate-gene approach.

A *pharmacokinetic compartment* is a theoretical space into which drug molecules are said to distribute, and is represented by a given linear component of the log-concentration versus time curve. It is not an actual anatomic or physiologic space, but is sometimes thought of as a tissue or group of tissues that have similar blood flow and drug affinity.

Pharmacokinetics is the study of the relationship between the dose administered of a drug and the concentration achieved in the blood, in the serum, or at the site of action. It includes the study of the processes of drug absorption, distribution, metabolism, and excretion.

Pharmacovigilance is the identification and evaluation of drug safety signals. More recently, some have also used the term as synonymous with pharmacoepidemiology. WHO defines *pharmacovigilance* as the science and activities relating to the detection, assessment, understanding and prevention of adverse effects or any other possible drug-related problems [WHO. Safety monitoring of medicinal products. *The importance of pharmacovigilance*. Geneva, World Health Organization, 2002]. Mann defines *pharmacovigilance* as "the study of the safety of marketed drugs under the practical conditions of clinical usage in large communities" [*Pharmacovigilance*. Mann RD, Andrews EB, eds. John Wiley & Sons Ltd, Chichester, 2002].

Pharmacology is the study of the effects of drugs in a living system.

Pharmacotherapeutics is the application of the principles of clinical pharmacology to rational prescribing, the conduct of clinical trials, and the assessment of outcomes during real-life clinical practice.

Pharmionics is the study of how patients use or misuse prescription drugs in ambulatory care.

Population-based databases or studies refers to whether there is an identifiable population (which is not necessarily based in geography), all of whose medical care would be included in that database, regardless of the provider. This allows one to determine incidence rates of diseases, as well as being more certain that one knows of all medical care that any given patient receives.

Postmarketing surveillance is the study of drug use and drug effects after release onto the market. This term is sometimes used synonymously with "pharmacoepidemiology," but the latter can be relevant to premarketing studies, as well. Conversely, the term "postmarketing surveillance" is sometimes felt to apply to only those studies conducted after drug marketing that systematically screen for adverse drug effects. However, this is a more restricted use of the term than that used in this book.

Potency refers to the amount of drug that is required to elicit a given response. A more potent drug requires a smaller milligram quantity to exert the same response as a less potent drug, although it is not necessarily more effective.

Potential adverse drug events are medication errors that have high potential for causing harm but didn't, either because they were intercepted prior to reaching a patient or because the error reached the patient who fortuitously did not have any observable untoward sequelae.

The *power (statistical power)* of a study is the probability of detecting a difference in the study if a difference really exists (either between study groups or between treatment periods).

Precision is the degree of absence of random error. Precise estimates have narrow confidence intervals.

Pre-post with comparison group design includes a single observation both before and after treatment in a nonrandomly selected group exposed to a treatment (e.g., physicians receiving feedback on specific prescribing practices), as well as simultaneous before and after observations of a similar (comparison) group not receiving treatment.

Prescribing errors refer to issues related to underuse, overuse, and misuse of prescribed drugs, all of which contribute to the suboptimal utilization of pharmaceutical therapies.

The *prevalence* of a disease is a measurement of how common the disease is. Specifically, it is the number of existing cases of the disease in a defined population at a given point in time or over a defined time period, divided by the number of people in that population.

Prevalence study bias, a type of selection bias that may occur in studies when prevalent cases rather than new cases of a condition are selected for a study. A strong association with prevalence may be related to the duration of the disease

rather than to its incidence, because prevalence is proportional to both incidence and duration of the disease.

Privacy, in the setting of research, refers to each individual's right to be free from unwanted inspection of, or access to, personal information by unauthorized persons.

Procedure registries are registries characterized by inclusion of subjects based on receipt of specific services, such as procedures, or based on hospitalizations.

Product registries are registries characterized by inclusion of subjects based on use of a specific product (drug or device) or related products in a given therapeutic area.

Propensity scores are an approach to controlling for confounding that uses mathematical modeling to predict exposure based on observed variables, and uses the predicted probability of exposure as the basis for matching or adjustment.

Prospective drug utilization review is designed to detect drug-therapy problems before an individual patient receives the drug.

Prospective studies are studies performed simultaneously with the events under study; namely, patient outcomes have not yet occurred as of the outset of the study.

Protopathic bias is interpreting a factor to be a result of an exposure when it is in fact a determinant of the exposure, and can occur when an early sign of the disease under study led to the prescription of the drug under study.

Publication bias occurs when publication of a study's results is related to the study's findings, such that study results are not published or publication is delayed because of the results.

Qualitative drug utilization studies are studies that assess the *appropriateness* of drug use.

Quality-of-life is the description of aspects (domains) of physical, social, and emotional health that are relevant and important to the patient.

Quantitative drug utilization studies are descriptive studies of *frequency* of drug use.

Random allocation is the assignment of subjects who are enrolled in a study into study groups in a manner determined by chance.

Random error is error due to chance.

Random selection is the selection of subjects into a study from among those eligible in a manner determined by chance.

Randomized clinical trials are studies in which the investigator randomly assigns patients to different therapies, one of which may be a control therapy.

Recall bias is an error in the results of a study due to a systematic difference between the study groups in the accuracy or completeness of their memory of their past exposures or health events.

Referral bias is error in the results of a study that occurs when the reasons for referring a patient for medical care are related to the exposure status, e.g., when the use of the drug contributes to the diagnostic process.

Registries are organized systems that use observational study methods to collect uniform data (clinical and other) to evaluate specified outcomes for a population defined by a particular disease, condition, or exposure, and that serves one or more predetermined scientific, clinical, or policy purposes. Registries can be thought of as both the process for collecting data from which studies are derived, as well as referring to the actual database.

Regression to the mean is the tendency for observations on populations selected on the basis of an abnormality to approach normality on subsequent observations.

The *relative rate* is the ratio of the incidence rate of an outcome in the exposed group to the incidence rate of the outcome in the unexposed group. It is synonymous with the terms *rate ratio* and *incidence rate ratio*.

The *relative risk* is the ratio of the cumulative incidence of an outcome in the exposed group to the cumulative incidence of the outcome in the unexposed group. It is synonymous with the term *cumulative incidence ratio*.

Reliability is the degree to which the results obtained by a measurement procedure can be replicated. The measurement of reliability does not require a gold standard, since it assesses only the concordance between two or more measures.

A *reporting rate* in a spontaneous reporting system is the number of reported cases of an adverse event of interest divided by some measure of the suspect drug's utilization, usually the number of dispensed prescriptions. This is perhaps better referred to as a *rate of reported cases*.

Reproducibility is the ability of an instrument to obtain more or less the same scores upon repeated measurements of patients who have not changed.

Research, as defined in US regulation, is any activity designed to "develop or contribute to generalizable knowledge." [Title 45 US Code of Federal Regulations Part 46.102 (d)]

A *research subject* is "a living individual, about whom an investigator (whether professional or student) conducting research obtains either: 1) data through intervention or interaction with the individual, or 2) identifiable private information"[35] [US Code of Federal Regulations 46.102 (f)].

Responsiveness is an instrument's ability to detect change.

Retrospective drug utilization review compares past drug use against predetermined criteria to identify aberrant prescribing patterns or patient-specific deviations from explicit criteria.

Retrospective studies are studies conducted after the events under study have occurred. Both exposure and outcome have already occurred as of the outset of the study.

Risk is the cumulative probability that something will happen.

A judgment about *safety* is a personal and/or social judgment about the degree to which a given risk is acceptable.

Safety signal is a concern about an excess of adverse events compared to what is expected to be associated with a product's (drug or device) use.

Service registries are registries characterized by inclusion of subjects based on receipt of specific services, such as procedures, or based on hospitalizations.

Sample distortion bias is another name for selection bias.

Scientific inference is the process of generalizing from a statement about a population, which is an association, to a causal statement about scientific theory.

Selection bias is error in a study that is due to systematic differences in characteristics between those who are selected for the study and those who are not.

Sensibility is a judgment about the validity of an instrument, based on an intuitive assessment of the extent to which an instrument meets a number of criteria including applicability, clarity and simplicity, likelihood of bias, comprehensiveness, and whether redundant items have been included.

Sensitivity is the proportion of persons who truly have a characteristic, who are correctly classified by a diagnostic test as having it.

Sensitivity analysis is a set of procedures in which the results of a study are recalculated using alternate values for some of the study's variables, in order to test the sensitivity of the conclusions to altered specifications.

A *serious adverse experience* is any adverse experience occurring at any dose that results in any of the following outcomes: death, a life-threatening adverse experience, inpatient hospitalization or prolongation of existing hospitalization, a persistent or significant disability/incapacity, or congenital anomaly/birth defect.

Signal is a hypothesis that calls for further work to be performed to evaluate that hypothesis.

Signal detection is the process of looking for or identifying signals from any source.

Signal generation, sometimes referred to as data mining, is an approach that uses statistical methods to identify a safety signal. No particular medical product exposure or adverse outcome is prespecified.

Signal refinement is a process by which an identified safety signal is further evaluated to determine whether evidence exists to support a relationship between the exposure and the outcome.

Specific causation, from a legal perspective, addresses whether the product in question actually caused an alleged injury in the individual plaintiff.

Specific quality-of-life instruments are focused on disease or treatment issues specifically relevant to the question at hand.

Specificity is the proportion of persons who truly do **not** have a characteristic, who are correctly classified by a diagnostic test as not having it.

Spontaneous reporting systems are maintained by regulatory bodies throughout the world and collect unsolicited clinical observations that originate outside of a formal study.

Statistical inference is the process of generalizing from a sample of study subjects to the entire population from which those subjects are theoretically drawn.

Statistical interaction, see effect modification.

A *statistically significant difference* is a difference between two study groups that is unlikely to have occurred purely by chance.

Steady state, within pharmacokinetics, is the situation when the amount of drug being administered equals the amount of drug being eliminated from the body.

Systematic error is any error in study results other than that due to random variation.

The *therapeutic ratio* is the ratio of the drug concentration that produces toxicity to the concentration that produces the desired therapeutic effect.

Therapeutics is the application of the principles of clinical pharmacology to rational prescribing, the conduct of clinical trials, and the assessment of outcomes during real-life clinical practice.

Type A adverse reactions are those that are the result of an exaggerated but otherwise predictable pharmacological effect of the drug. They tend to be common and dose-related.

Type B adverse reactions are those that are aberrant effects of the drug. They tend to be uncommon, not dose-related, and unpredictable.

A *type I statistical error* is concluding there is an association when in fact one does not exist, i.e., erroneously rejecting the null hypothesis.

A *type II statistical error* is concluding there is no association when in fact one does exist, i.e., erroneously accepting the null hypothesis.

Unanticipated beneficial effects of drugs are desirable effects that could not have been predicted on the basis of existing knowledge.

Unanticipated harmful effects of drugs are unwanted effects that could not have been predicted on the basis of existing knowledge.

Uncontrolled studies refer to studies without a comparison group.

An *unexpected adverse experience* means any adverse experience that is not listed in the current labeling for the product. This includes an event that may be symptomatically and pathophysiologically related to an event listed in the labeling, but differs from the event because of greater severity or specificity.

Utility measures of quality-of-life are measured holistically as a single number along a continuum, e.g., from death (0.0) to full health (1.0). The key element of a utility instrument is that it is preference-based.

Validity is the degree to which an assessment (e.g., questionnaire or other instrument) measures what it purports to measure.

Variable costs are costs that increase with increasing volume of activity.

Apparent *volume of distribution* (V_D) is the apparent volume that a drug is distributed in after complete absorption. It is usually calculated from the theoretical plasma concentration at a time when all of the drug was assumed to be present in the body and uniformly distributed. This is calculated from back extrapolation to time zero of the plasma concentration time curve after intravenous administration.

Voluntariness is the concept in research ethics, that investigators must tell subjects that participation in the research study is voluntary, and that subjects have the right to discontinue participation at any time.

Index

Textbook of Pharmacoepidemiology, Second Edition. Edited by Brian L. Strom, Stephen E. Kimmel, and Sean Hennessy.
© 2013 John Wiley & Sons, Ltd. Published 2013 by John Wiley & Sons, Ltd.